T0195330

Treatment of Infertility with Chinese Medicine

Content Strategist: Claire Wilson
Content Development Specialist: Veronika Watkins
Project Manager: Sruthi Viswam
Designer/Design Direction: Christian Bilbow
Illustration Manager: Jennifer Rose
Illustrator: Richard Tibbits

Treatment of Infertility with Chinese Medicine

Second edition

Written by

Jane Lyttleton

BSc (Hons) (NZ) MPhil (UK) Dip TCM (Aus) Cert Acup (China) Cert Herbal Med (China)

Practitioner of Traditional Chinese Medicine, Sydney, Australia;
Director Acupuncture IVF Support clinics, Guest Lecturer, University of Westminster, UK; University of
Western Sydney, Australia

Forewords by:

Steven Clavey

BA (Colorado) DipAdv Acupuncture (Nanjing)

Specialist in Traditional Gynecology (Zhejiang College of TCM); Private Practitioner, Melbourne, Australia

Gavin Sacks

MA(Cantab) BMBCh (Ox) PhD (Ox)MRCOG FRANZCOG CCSST (UK)

Fertility specialist and obstetrician

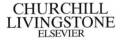
CHURCHILL
LIVINGSTONE
ELSEVIER

Edinburgh   London   New York   Oxford   Philadelphia   St Louis   Sydney   Toronto   2013

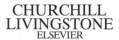

First edition 2004
Second edition 2013

ISBN 978-0-7020-3176-2

British Library Cataloguing in Publication Data

A catalogue record for this book is available from the British Library

Library of Congress Cataloging in Publication Data

A catalog record for this book is available from the Library of Congress

Notices

Knowledge and best practice in this field are constantly changing. As new research and experience broaden our understanding, changes in research methods, professional practices, or medical treatment may become necessary.

Practitioners and researchers must always rely on their own experience and knowledge in evaluating and using any information, methods, compounds, or experiments described herein. In using such information or methods they should be mindful of their own safety and the safety of others, including parties for whom they have a professional responsibility.

With respect to any drug or pharmaceutical products identified, readers are advised to check the most current information provided (i) on procedures featured or (ii) by the manufacturer of each product to be administered, to verify the recommended dose or formula, the method and duration of administration, and contraindications. It is the responsibility of practitioners, relying on their own experience and knowledge of their patients, to make diagnoses, to determine dosages and the best treatment for each individual patient, and to take all appropriate safety precautions.

To the fullest extent of the law, neither the Publisher nor the authors, contributors, or editors, assume any liability for any injury and/or damage to persons or property as a matter of products liability, negligence or otherwise, or from any use or operation of any methods, products, instructions, or ideas contained in the material herein.

your source for books, journals and multimedia in the health sciences

www.elsevierhealth.com

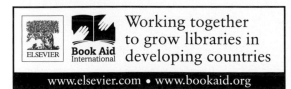

Working together to grow libraries in developing countries

www.elsevier.com • www.bookaid.org

The publisher's policy is to use paper manufactured from sustainable forests

Printed in India
Last digit is the print number: 13

Contents

CONTENTS

CONTENTS

Foreword to the 2nd edition

It is an honor to be asked to write a foreword for the second edition of this wonderful book – a book which, from a science perspective, peels away some of the layers of mystery surrounding Traditional Chinese Medicine (TCM). It is a book which brings TCM into the modern world of reproductive medicine. In some ways, I am a strange choice of author. I am not a practitioner of Traditional Chinese Medicine (TCM). In fact, I am an IVF specialist with a science background, and I do not advocate TCM for everyone. However, I am also a clinician who is, above all, interested in the art of healing. And over the last few years I have been lucky enough to get to know Jane Lyttleton and many of her patients, and they have demonstrated the powerful potential of synergy between TCM and modern Western medicine. A recent survey in my Sydney IVF clinic showed that over 60% of patients used complementary therapies, most of them TCM. It was interesting that very few (of those who used it, and also those who did not) had an opinion or cared whether or not TCM was proven to be effective or not. This illustrates the problem Western medicine has with TCM. Large numbers of patients seem to be very keen on trying it, with relatively little concern about actual effectiveness.

In my IVF clinic, it is not uncommon for patients to ask – before they have even completed their tests or new treatment protocol – 'What else can I do?' My offering of the latest and most sophisticated fertility treatments imaginable does not seem to cut the mustard. My promise of the best success rates that can possibly be achieved; my discussion of new scientific papers and mechanisms of new drugs; my very presence in an upmarket, gleaming and famous clinic, does not give enough confidence. Something else is needed. What?

The thing that modern patients miss, is for them to be taken seriously as an individual. This is not difficult to appreciate, but very difficult to address adequately. The success of Western diagnostic and therapeutic regimes is clear to all, and few patients would fully turn their back on that approach. But in reality, none of us like the idea of 'playing the odds' with our health. In other words, if a specialist tells a patient that she would have a 30% chance of success with an IVF cycle, rather than accepting the odds, she (as most of us) would immediately start to think of ways of 'getting into that 30% group.' Some would regard this as irrational. After all, if we truly knew how to get our patients into that 30% group, we would do whatever is necessary to do it. But the point is that IVF, infertility treatment and medicine in general, simply cannot guarantee outcomes. Our impotence is the reason we discuss statistics.

This is the time to be frank – TCM does not guarantee outcomes either. But rather than focusing simply on the 'outcome' or 'endpoint', TCM showcases the 'journey'. It puts the patient center stage, so that whatever the outcome, the patient can see that she has done the best for herself. She has tried to address the mystery of illness and pain from a personal perspective, and so feels empowered. This is often the opposite of feelings in conventional Western medicine, when failure of treatment (and sometimes even success) leaves a feeling of being put on a conveyor belt, squeezed into a difficult place and spat out the other side – the feeling of being 'just another statistic.'

TCM has the longest tradition of all complementary therapies. It has a unique diagnostic system that is still inexplicable to Western science. It regards every condition in every patient as a particular set of circumstances that cannot be generalized. It is in some ways, the antithesis of statistics. Its success in the management of infertility is therefore difficult to assess. But let us consider what we mean by success. While the bottom line of achieving a live birth is clearly fundamental, there are other markers which seem to matter a lot to our patients, such as: (1) hands on support and confidence boosting; (2) the reassurance that whole body function is being considered; (3) alternative diagnostic pathways that leave open the possibility that individualized success rate can be improved. Even hard-nosed scientists would surely not begrudge any of these potential gains, especially if the end result is to get their patients to keep on trying. Those who keep trying will be more likely to succeed. This is the cynical scientific view of TCM.

Advocates of TCM make far greater claims of course, such as its ability to improve egg and sperm quality, endometrial receptivity, IVF success rates and even livebirth rates. These claims have huge implications, and need to be explored in an open and rational manner. This process has so far stumbled on the wide gap that still exists between the vested interests of Western medicine and complementary practitioners. Some randomized trials with acupuncture have been done (remarkable efforts in themselves) and some have demonstrated benefit – the increased success rate following acupuncture on the day of IVF embryo transfer is perhaps the best known. But we will all gain so much more through greater integration, respect and willingness to explore the unknown. This applies to both the scientific community and the TCM community. The enormous achievement of this book is the way in which science and TCM are used together to explain the various aspects of female infertility. The problems are therefore accessible to both sides of the chasm, and should encourage each side to learn more about the other.

There is little to gain in advocates of TCM or Western medicine sticking firmly to their side of the divide. That simply creates suspicion and conflict, and confusion for our patients. As a scientist, I would like to see more TCM trials, and if trials are difficult, then at least more audits and reporting of TCM outcomes. We need all practitioners to rationally assess their interventions, and not to be afraid to change them as indicated. This book is an immense achievement because not only does it give an excellent account of TCM, but it does it in the context of Western anatomy and physiology, it describes cases and anecdotal reports, and also the clinical trials that have been done. It is an essential reference for any modern fertility clinic.

Gavin Sacks, 2012

Foreword to the 1st edition

The practice of Chinese medicine is maturing in the West. In the quarter century since it began to be known outside of the communities of overseas Chinese, we have watched it move into mainstream Western culture, seen the establishment of high-level education in Chinese medical studies at a number of universities around the world, and welcomed an increasing recognition of both its limitations and its benefits.

This book marks the beginning of a new phase: the publication of the fruits of the long-term personal experience in a clinic, by non-Chinese physicians specialising in one of the various departments of Chinese medicine. Gynaecology is certainly an appropriate beginning, for both its relevance and effectiveness, but we should soon be seeing books recounting the personalised techniques, tools and theories developed over decades of use in Western settings by workers in other departments of Chinese medicine, such as dermatology, paediatrics, orthopaedics and ophthalmology.

This, of course, is only a new thing for us in the West. The tradition within China extends back well over 700 years, following the establishment of distinct specialties in separate departments of Chinese medicine by the imperial court of the Song dynasty. Since that time, texts from the brushes of a multitude of specialists with 30–50 years of experience in a given department have done much to inform, improve and even revolutionise the practice of their time and people.

The key to the popularity of Chinese medicine is its effectiveness, its ability to restore the normal functioning of the human body. This very effectiveness, however, is the fruit of the practicality and flexibility of its theoretical approach, which, in turn, is based squarely on a human being's experience of her- or himself. Physical sensations, emotions, the observation of the various substances that flow out of the body; all of these are the tools with which a Chinese physician works to observe patterns in human functioning. In gynaecology, for example, a woman's observation of the colour and texture of her menstrual blood are important clues to internal functioning. My own teacher told me: 'A good Chinese gynaecologist can tell the internal condition of a woman from her menstrual characteristics alone'. In this case, not only are colour and texture involved, but the timing and duration of the cycle as well.

While there is no denying the value of Western surgical techniques or pharmaceutical measures in gynaecological treatment, particularly in emergency situations or severe conditions, there are many gynaecological disorders for which these techniques are less subtle than might be desired. For disorders such as these, which can be greatly debilitating despite their 'nonlife-threatening' status in the eyes of modern medicine, traditional Chinese gynaecology has many benefits for women. Infertility is one such area.

Here in Australia, after quiet grass-roots work for two decades by practitioners such as Jane Lyttleton, Western gynaecologists have realised that the strengths of Western medicine are just those areas in which Chinese medicine is weak, while the weaknesses of Western medicine are also precisely those areas where Chinese medicine has the most to offer. In other words, the two disciplines complement each other exceedingly well, with very little overlap. Those patients over whom a Western gynaecologist is most likely to despair are often considered quite straightforward by Chinese medicine practitioners; similarly, a Chinese gynaecologist will encourage surgical treatment when it is indicated for an individual patient.

In this ground-breaking book, Jane's approach is to marry the best of both Chinese and Western medicine. She documents in detail the complementary process for the treatment of infertility, drawing upon her 20 years' experience in the use of Chinese medicine to help women conceive. She demonstrates both her in-depth working knowledge of Chinese and Western medicine in this area, and her great compassion for women going through this trial of the spirit.

Included are details of techniques derived from her work with the great Xia Gui-Cheng, the famous contemporary Nanjing gynaecologist, and many equally valuable approaches formed through the many years she has worked with her own patients in Sydney. The description of how the basal body temperature chart is used as a precise indication of yin and yang fluctuations in various function complexes in the body is fascinating and immediately applicable in clinic. While the focus of the book is infertility, a variety of other gynaecological disorders that interfere with fertility are dealt with, including polycystic ovaries, endometriosis, and difficulties with ovulation.

Male infertility is notoriously difficult for Western medicine to treat: IVF is generally recommended. By contrast, for the great majority of patients, male infertility due to a variety of causes is considered relatively easy to treat in Chinese medicine (azoospermia being a notable exception). Jane devotes an entire chapter to the various diagnostic and therapeutic techniques required for restoring, or at least improving, the fertility of the male.

To conclude as we began: the maturing of Chinese medicine in the West can be gauged by its fruits, and this book is a rich harvest of focussed experience notable for its clarity and applicability. Like a good fruit, may it spread its seeds far and wide, to the benefit of women – and – men everywhere!

Steven Clavey
Melbourne, 2004

About the Author

Jane Lyttleton, who comes from a family of scientists and doctors, struck out on a radical limb when she abandoned her career in science in the late 1970s, to study Chinese medicine. This study was a challenge for a mind trained to think in black and white terms using logical linear reasoning – a far cry from the circular reasoning in shades of gray of Chinese medicine. However, internships in Traditional Chinese Medicine (TCM) hospitals in Nanjing, Hangzhou, and Guangzhou at different times over the next 12 years, steeped her in the reality of a living thriving medical system – in its own way, internally cohesive and rational. She has attempted to bring the best of this medicine to a clinical practice in the West, addressing the healthcare needs of Western women. Some 30 years on, she sits comfortably with the logic of both Chinese medicine and Western science and feels both can contribute greatly to positive therapeutic outcomes for the patient.

The medical climate of Sydney, Australia, combined with the demands of well-informed patients, has allowed a useful degree of inter-professional exchange, wherein Jane has been able to share expertise and patient care with GPs and specialists in the area of gynecology and infertility.

She practises acupuncture and herbal medicine in a group practice in central Sydney and runs Support Clinics in a number of locations for patients preparing for and doing IVF. She lives in a beachside suburb with her husband, visited occasionally by her two daughters when they swing by the country.

Acknowledgments

The advent of this book is owed entirely to my teachers, beginning in 1978 here in Australia with Chris Madden – who died far too young, leaving a long trail of saddened but well-trained doctors – and continuing to present day China, with Dr Xia Gui Cheng, the director (now retired) of the Gynecology Department in a large TCM hospital in Nanjing. Much of this book is based on his knowledge and clinical experience, which he generously imparted in his own clinic and also in my clinic in Sydney, where he tackled the uniquely Western attitudes and foibles of some of my most difficult patients. The inimitable Tao Jing Ren, interpreter extraordinaire and friend, made Dr Xia's expertise entirely accessible.

Grateful thanks to my TCM colleagues and friends Sue Cochrone, Will Maclean, and Felicity Moir, who spent painstaking hours editing and correcting different chapters and also to Shona Barker, Miriam Camara, Kerry Carmody, Steve Clavey, and Cathy Davitt who contributed much valued opinions. Siddhi Saraswati, Kerry Kennedy, and Denise Hare contributed helpful lay-person's perspectives. Margaret Bruce and Norbert Ivanyi did some of the illustrations. Professor Shan is the wise old doctor wielding the file in the introduction.

I also want to thank the inspiring team of practitioners who make up the Support Clinics, including Delia McCarthy, Sage Andreason, Machelle Boothroyd, Marienne Cox, Kaitlin Edin, Maggie Godin, Bert Loyeung, Louise Jeffrey, Melinda MacDonald, Rochelle Wagstaff, Cherie Lawrence, Jaclyn Macpherson (and also those who came before and who will come in the future). This dedicated group has now seen several thousands of IVF patients through their journeys and has responded to the clinical challenges, the joy and the heartbreak, with skill and compassion. They truly embody what makes Chinese medicine a vocation and not a job.

Finally, thanks to my family:

- To my mother who overcame her own infertility and look what she got!
- To my sisters (the aunties) – Anna who held the fort single-handedly at times so it wouldn't all fall down, and Sally and Andrea who are always there when needed.
- To my husband David, who found the time to do the final edit in the 2nd edition, whose truly saintly support never wavered, and without whom I wouldn't have reached even first base.
- To Lara, my own Chinese medicine miracle baby and my constant inspiration, and to Charlie, another treasured miracle who came to our family by her own route.

Introduction

The first edition of this text was written more than 10 years ago – a long time in a rapidly developing field like reproductive medicine, where advances sit at the cutting edge of medical technology – but a very short time in Chinese medicine. I am grateful that in this complex and ever changing world, the goalposts don't keep shifting in Chinese medicine! However, the context in which we apply it does keep changing. And this is especially the case in reproductive medicine. Hence, some chapters of the first edition warranted significant updating.

While this text aims to cover all the different aspects of infertility treatment, including essential background theory and professional, philosophical and ethical considerations, it also aims to be a useful clinical reference book. To facilitate this, the new edition features an easy to find symbol ( ) located on the top of those pages that contain the treatment protocols and guidelines you might want to access quickly when you are in the clinic with your patient.

The basic premise of treating functional infertility with TCM remains unchanged. As I outline in Chapter 2, it requires a deep understanding of menstrual and reproductive physiology. And then, as outlined in Chapter 4, it requires a thorough familiarity with the ways we can affect these processes with Chinese medicine. This doesn't change. However, our medical understanding of some gynecological disorders, which we discuss in Chapter 5, such as polycystic ovarian syndrome and endometriosis, has developed a little and this further informs our TCM analysis and treatment of these conditions.

Polycystic Ovarian Syndrome (PCOS) is now a much more commonly diagnosed cause of infertility than it was 10 or more years ago. This condition is an extremely challenging one on many fronts, since it adversely affects not only the reproductive system but also several other physiological systems. We are a long way from completely unravelling the PCOS puzzle but here, we examine the many ways it can present in the clinic, what we currently know about the condition and what causes it, and how we as doctors of Chinese medicine can approach its treatment holistically.

Endometriosis is another common cause of infertility and while surgical techniques for managing this disease are improving all the time, medical treatments are not. TCM steps into this breach effectively for many women and we shall discuss in some expanded detail, different approaches to treatment according to circumstance.

Treatment of male infertility has largely been made redundant by the advent of IVF techniques, whereby healthy active sperm are no longer necessary for fertilization of an egg. This alarms some urologists and andrologists, and some TCM doctors. Fortunately, there has been some very convincing research demonstrating that acupuncture can produce significant improvements in sperm health. We look at these and other updates in Chapter 7.

Chapter 8, which examines miscarriage, its causes and prevention, now includes more discussion of immune infertility and the role that acupuncture and Chinese medicine may play. At this stage of our medical knowledge, autoimmune disease presents more questions than answers but Chinese medicine, because it influences multiple body systems simultaneously holds enormous potential in this area.

The treatment of IVF patients with Chinese medicine has become much more commonplace in the last 10 years, and it is timely for us to closely examine this phenomenon. We need to be clear about what it means to apply a traditional medicine 'on top of' an induced iatrogenic state, and the ethics and philosophical questions it poses. Recognizing that this is uncharted territory (or 'coalface' medicine), Chapters 9, 10 and 11 take the time to examine the values, context, and therapeutic techniques inherent in the different approaches of IVF and TCM and out of this understanding, suggest some guidelines for clinical protocols.

There is much focus now on aspects of our environment and lifestyle and how that impacts our reproductive health and capacity. I have tried to include all current information in Chapter 12, although by the time this book is in print there will no doubt be more!

TCM treatment of functional infertility is not a simple topic and adding ART techniques to what is already complex can present a considerable clinical challenge. I have attempted to come up with strategies that are manageable for both the practitioner and the patient, and I look forward to more developments in this area as more and more doctors of Chinese Medicine explore treatment strategies that will help the IVF patient.

Jane Lyttleton
2012

SECTION

The Fundamentals

1

A tale of two clinics – the treatment of infertility with Chinese medicine or Western medicine

An infertility clinic in China is worlds away from an infertility clinic in the West in just about every way but one: the desperation to have a child where nature has failed to provide. This human response is the same everywhere. The biological imperative to reproduce has no cultural boundaries.

The treatment offered by an infertility clinic in a traditional Chinese medicine (TCM) hospital of the early twenty-first century is basic and minimally-invasive: herbs are prescribed; acupuncture or Qi Gong exercises may be recommended; lifestyle or dietary changes are advised if necessary; pathology tests may be ordered for analysis of blood or semen; surgery may in some cases be recommended. The patient drinks a decoction of herbs twice every day (probably for several months), returns to the clinic weekly, fortnightly or monthly to see if the prescription needs changing and is encouraged to lead a healthy life.

CASE HISTORY – THE WONGS

One couple I remember distinctly is the Wongs, who visited Dr Chong one day when I was sitting in on her morning clinic. Dr Chong, a gynecologist specializing in infertility, works in a large municipal hospital in south China. She sees dozens of patients each morning in her tiny room, furnished with just a table, two benches and one light bulb. The waiting patients huddle around the door and often listen in on consultations. There is little privacy here, even though patients are discussing details of their menstrual cycle and sex life.

The Wongs were country folk who seemed extremely nervous about their visit to the big city hospital. They had been married for 4 years but had not had a child. When asked about her menstrual cycle, Mrs Wong told us it was irregular and long. I noticed that she was slightly plump and somewhat more hairy than the average Chinese woman, and I wondered if she had polycystic ovary syndrome. But Dr Chong was busy asking her about her diet, digestion and general health. After feeling the pulses at her wrist and looking at her tongue, the doctor prescribed a formula of herbal medicines, which were to be taken over the next 2 weeks. The herbs, she explained, would encourage Mrs Wong's periods to come more often. Mr Wong was sent for a semen analysis.

The next time the Wongs came to the clinic, they seemed more relaxed and greeted us with a bag of delicious strawberries from their small farm – no doubt one of the main reasons I remember this couple in particular. Dr Chong had the not too welcome news for Mr Wong that his sperm count was low and that the sperm motility was poor. Dr Chong asked him some more questions, discovering that he suffered chronic lower back pain and had a low libido. She wrote out a script for herbs for him as well.

Mrs Wong reported that the herbs she had been taking had provoked the production of more clear vaginal discharge for several days. Dr Chong looked pleased.

The couple came in from their farm to visit the clinic once a month after that. Apart from these visits and drinking a cup of herbs twice a day, their infertility treatment intruded little on their lives. They both said they felt more energetic and healthy while taking the herbs, and Mr Wong's libido improved. But after 4 months, they were becoming frustrated that they had still not conceived and the pressure from their parents, anxious to meet their one permitted grandchild, was increasing. Dr Chong pointed out that their progress had in fact been very good. Mrs Wong's menstrual cycle was much shorter (closer to 4 and a half weeks now compared to the 6 or 7 weeks at the outset). This, plus an improved sex life, meant greatly increased chances of conceiving.

I was no longer in China when Mrs Wong's pregnancy was announced – but I heard the news on the grapevine. After 6 months of daily treatment, the Wongs had achieved their goal and 9 months later they were the thrilled parents of baby Chen. Two sets of grandparents could relax!

The approach of the assisted reproduction technology (ART) or in vitro fertilization (IVF) clinic in the West, on the other hand, is more sophisticated and the procedures are quite involved. The specialist will prescribe drugs and perhaps perform surgery. He or she will rely on the expertise of nursing staff to administer injections and take blood samples, radiologists to perform ultrasounds, embryologists to monitor fertilization of the egg by the sperm and embryo development in the laboratory. The patient's visits to the clinic are timed around the cycle and are quite frequent during the 4–6 week program, during which time they will receive medication, be monitored for their response and have procedures such as intrauterine insemination, egg collection or embryo transfer carried out.

CASE HISTORY – THE SMITHS

I met Madeline Smith briefly when she sought help for coping with the stress she was experiencing during her IVF attempts. Her story is one that we typically hear in the West. At age 39, she and her 40-year-old husband Frank, after trying unsuccessfully for a year to conceive, had decided they had better get some help. They were worried they may have left it a bit late. A specialist at a state-of-the-art IVF clinic diagnosed Madeline with polycystic ovary syndrome after seeing an ultrasound of her ovaries and blood test results. Because of her infrequent ovulations and her age, he suggested they embark on an IVF program without delay. Madeline, a health and fitness enthusiast, was reluctant but in her eagerness to have a baby, she decided she would do whatever it took. She injected the drugs in her belly every day, visited the clinic for ultrasounds and blood tests regularly, complained about the headaches and abdominal discomfort and cried more than usual (this is the point at which she came to my clinic for acupuncture to help relieve the side-effects).

But when it came time to 'harvest' her eggs she was sedated and the doctor, wielding a needle attached to a pump removed a bumper crop of seven from her ovaries. The embryologist then introduced the sperm (freshly donated by a rather nervous Frank in a back room) into the Petri dish, the eggs all fertilized and four of them developed into embryos. Two were transferred back to Madeline's uterus and two were frozen for the future.

After an interminable wait, Madeline had blood taken for a pregnancy test! Then, after what seemed another endless wait, came the phone call: 'I'm sorry your test is negative.' After such a huge emotional and physical investment, this news was profoundly disappointing.

It took a while for Madeline and Frank to recover from the experience, but in a couple of months they were back at the IVF clinic. They opted for a so-called natural (no drugs) cycle for the transfer of their frozen embryos. Although she was not taking drugs, Madeline still had to attend the clinic for frequent blood tests and ultrasounds. Being more familiar with the process and not having to deal with any drug side-effects she coped much better. Even the failure of one of her frozen embryos to thaw properly at the time of transfer did not dampen her optimism too much – optimism that was well placed because this last embryo was the one that made it. Her pregnancy was not uneventful and baby Rory was born early and tiny, but he survived and Madeline and Frank were the proudest parents on the ward.

From the perspective of the patient, the experience of infertility treatment with TCM or with IVF is altogether different; so is the philosophy of the medicine underpinning these treatments.

The China of today still has its soul deeply rooted in the traditions and beliefs of an era 2000 years ago – a reality that is evident not only in the philosophy and mores of its society but also in its medicine. The medical system that was developed at that time became the inspiration for many other medical systems in Asia. Traditional Chinese medicine is practised not just in China and other parts of Asia but also in the West, often as a complementary approach to the prevailing orthodox medical system.

Modern medicine as we know it has a relatively short history. Medical science has contributed hugely to our knowledge about the structure, function and diseases of the body and medical scientists have developed extraordinary technological systems used in diagnosis, surgery and the manipulation of body functions; nowhere more so than in ART. You might call these advances brilliant or terrifying, depending on your perspective. And TCM, you might call primitive or subtly sophisticated, again depending on your perspective.

The two medical systems have quite different strengths and weaknesses and when called on to address the same maladies, do so using different approaches. The two case histories above illustrate how TCM and Western medicine deal with infertility in startlingly different ways.

An old Chinese professor friend of mine once compared the two systems figuratively in the following scenario:

> Imagine our patient is a round table, which in its diseased state, has grown sharp corners. It now looks like a square table – oh dear!
>
> The table goes to see the specialist in corners.
>
> 'No problem at all, my dear table. We'll have you round again in no time at all.' Well, right he was, more or less. The operation was performed the very next day. The surgeon, wielding a saw, quickly removed the table's corners. The procedure was quite painful but over and done with rapidly and efficiently. Unfortunately, he cut a little too close on the fourth corner and the table lost part of one of its legs. The top, however, while not entirely round and smooth, no longer had sharp corners.
>
> But imagine if the table had come to see the old Chinese professor himself.
>
> 'Tut tut, how did this corner business come about?' he would have enquired and then carefully and thoroughly felt the wood of the table's corners, top and legs.
>
> 'Yes,' he might say quietly after some time, 'I can help you to be a round table again.' Then he would pull out a small file, apply it to one corner and begin to file. He would file and file. And even though it might be tedious and require a lot of patience on the part of both the table and the doctor, and it might take up to 1 year before the table would be truly its old round self again, eventually it would be beautifully smooth and strong and perfectly round again.

The side-effects of Western medicine – the rough contours and the damaged legs – are sometimes a high price to pay for immediately effective treatment. But this promise of a fast and effective result is what makes us choose this type of treatment so often, despite the risks.

Of course, if having 'corners' is a life-threatening situation, then fast and effective is exactly what we want. But where corners are not so critical, but are more of a threat to the quality of our life, then the slower and more subtle approach has its advantages.

Professor Robert Jansen, one of the world's leading experts in the treatment of infertility, describes the strengths and pitfalls of Western medicine, thus, in his excellent book *Getting Pregnant*.[1] (*additions* in parentheses are mine):

> The slighter the variation from normal, the more trouble (*Western*) medicine has in correcting it. Returning a circumstance that's a departure from normal back to towards normal is most likely to be successful when the departure from normal is major (*such as pronounced corners on a round table*). Because any medical or surgical

intervention risks introducing disturbances attributable to the intervention (*like damage to legs*), the less the departure from normal the less likely the intervention will improve the situation and not make it worse.

And what Professor Jansen says is obviously true; we all know that Western medicine can perform what seem to be miracles, especially in the kinds of dire circumstances that leave us praying for such miracles. But in less critical situations, for example those that produce undesirable but not severe or life-threatening symptoms, then there is every likelihood that drugs and surgery will produce side-effects rather than miracles.

What needs to be added to Professor Jansen's assessment of medical treatment is that in cases where the variation from normal is not so great, the slower and more 'holistic' forms of medicine often excel. If the table in our Chinese professor's scenario had not developed such marked corners but just some irregularities in its contour, then the treatment with the file could have been effective and rapid. Or if the table had come for treatment as soon as the corners had started to form, the filing would have achieved satisfactory results in a short time.

Professor Jansen, going on to talk more specifically about fertility treatments, explains further (again, *additions* in parentheses are mine):

> We can show in theory and in practice that the worse a diagnosed cause of infertility is, the better the chance of getting pregnant naturally will end up being after (*Western medical*) treatment – provided that the treatment corrects the problem properly and provided that the treatment does not, through side actions, interfere with any other aspects of reproduction.

Most of our *(Western medical)* treatments can have side-effects and these side-effects are more likely to tip the balance unfavorably when the condition being treated is relatively trivial. This principle is particularly prominent in reproductive medicine and surgery.

So, in infertility as in other specialities, it may be fair to say that using a Western treatment approach such as surgery and drugs, offers reasonable expectation of good results if the cause for infertility is rather severe, e.g., when there is blockage of the fallopian tubes, failure to ovulate or seriously inadequate sperm. In terms of our table analogy, these are very substantial corners made of hardwood that only a saw could have an effect on. Using a file in such cases might take a lifetime to make enough of a difference and, in the case of infertility, we do not have a lifetime to wait. Analyzing the genetic make-up of embryos where there is a family history of an inheritable disorder is another situation requiring the sort of treatment that only the ART clinic can provide.

However, more and more it seems that the saw is being used to fix very small corners or those made of soft wood. Our impatience and/or lack of knowledge of the subtle approaches of holistic medical traditions means that clinics specializing in ART are popping up in every city in the developed world (and some of the developing world) and doing very good business. But many of the infertile couples who receive treatment at these clinics could just as easily increase their chances of conception using the approaches offered by other less-invasive and risky medical systems.

The following chapters explain in detail how the medical system known as Traditional Chinese Medicine approaches the treatment of infertility; then, we revisit the IVF clinic and examine how both medical systems can work with each other to best benefit patients attempting to have a family.

REFERENCES

1. Jansen RPS. *Getting pregnant*. Sydney: Allen and Unwin; 2003, 5.

The menstrual cycle

2

Chapter Contents

BECOMING A SPECIALIST IN FEMALE INFERTILITY

There is an oft quoted saying in Chinese medical texts, 'the treatment of women is ten times more complicated than that of men' (Fig. 2.1). By the time we have examined all the different parts of the menstrual cycle you may feel this is an understatement!

To be a specialist in any field, we have to know our chosen material intimately. In this chapter, I set out what we need to know about the pathways, the fluids, the cells, the tissues, the chemical messages and the changes that happen in every menstrual cycle. We will examine in detail all the complex events that happen in a woman's body when the glands in the brain communicate with the reproductive glands and induce a myriad of different effects in different tissues – an incredible orchestration of events, which require correct timing and constant feedback. The result is a woman's body full of fertile potential (Fig. 2.2).

The theories of both traditional Chinese medicine (TCM) and the Western medical model contribute to our understanding of the physiological processes of the menstrual cycle. When a TCM practitioner is treating a woman for infertility it is very helpful to have a good grasp of the hormonal and anatomical reality of the reproductive processes. At the same time he or she needs to have a deep understanding of the same processes in terms of the Qi and Blood, Yin and Yang.

In this chapter, I consider the roles of the Yin and the Yang, the Qi and the Blood, the Chong and the Ren vessels, the Jing and the Shen, and more. And I also consider estrogen and progesterone, the pituitary and hypothalamus glands, the follicle in the ovary containing the egg, the fallopian tubes and the endometrium lining the uterus.

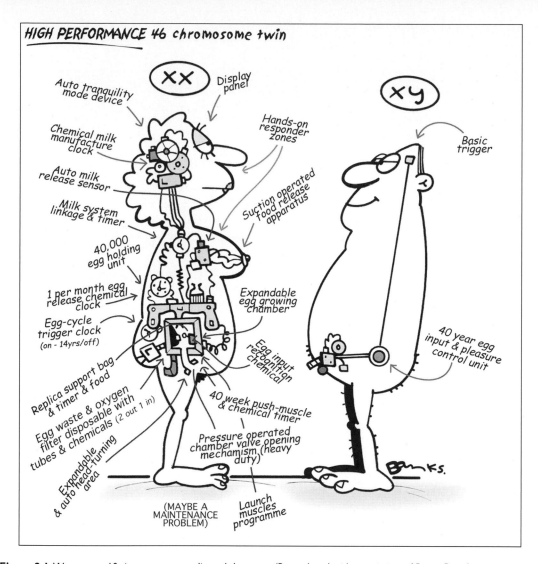

Figure 2.1 Women are 10 times more complicated than men. (Reproduced with permission of Bruce Petty.)

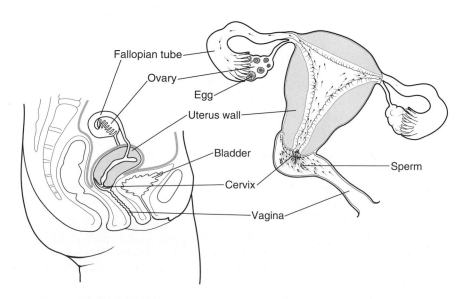

Figure 2.2 Anatomy of the female reproductive tract.

THE CHINESE AND WESTERN MEDICINE APPROACH

Chinese medicine describes processes inside and outside the body in energetic terms: i.e., the tendency to change or develop in a certain direction. Western medicine describes physiologic processes of the body in terms of the biochemical changes that occur and how they influence the actions of organs – this action is also described in terms of the resultant biochemical changes.

Historically, of course, Chinese medicine was practised with very little understanding of the biochemistry of internal physiological processes. All treatments were determined by subtle diagnostic techniques based on careful and detailed observation of external signs. This ability to make a diagnosis based on expert observation of symptoms and signs is one of the very great strengths of TCM (another being the mildness of its treatments and consequent lack of side-effects).

The knowledge we now have available, thanks to recent scientific research in reproductive medicine, adds to this strength. Skilled TCM doctors will still apply their well-tested theoretical framework and treatments but will add another level of sophistication to their clinical approach by using their knowledge of internal reproductive physiology. They will be able to communicate with patients and their gynecologists in a language they understand. Such bridge building, in the end, benefits everyone.

Although it is not appropriate to make exact equivalences between traditional Chinese medicine concepts and modern scientific medical descriptions (representing two profoundly different paradigms) we *can* make parallels – identical processes viewed from different perspectives. These will be summarized once we are familiar with all the terms (see Table 2.2).

The following sections provide a brief explanation of terms used to describe organ systems, channels and substances relevant in TCM gynecology. For further explanation of such TCM concepts, the reader is referred to TCM texts on internal medicine.[1]

THE ORGANS

The Kidney, the Heart and the Uterus

TCM describes all the aspects of female reproduction – the organs, the glands and their secretions, and the psyche – in terms of Kidney function, Heart function and the Uterus. TCM texts say, 'the Uterus, the Heart and Kidney form the core of reproductive activity.'

In broad terms, what the doctors in China 2000 years ago were referring to when they described the Kidney Jing is what modern Western medical science refers to as the gametes or eggs and sperm themselves. Kidney Yin and Yang include the influence of the hormones which regulate the different parts of the cycle.

The Heart encompasses the mind and the activity of the hypothalamus and pituitary, which controls the whole cycle.

The Uterus describes the arena where all of this happens. When we use the term 'Uterus' in a Chinese medicine context, it is a translation of the term *Bao Gong*, which includes all the reproductive organs: uterus, ovaries, fallopian tubes and cervix.

The pathways or channels, called the *Bao Mai* (Uterus vessel) and *Bao Luo* (Uterus channel), provide the means of communication between the Heart, Uterus and Kidneys (Fig. 2.3).

It is interesting to note that old Chinese medicine texts describe the Heart as the master controller (the Emperor) of the other organs. In the same way, Western medicine often refers to the hypothalamus and the pituitary as the master controllers of other glands in the body.

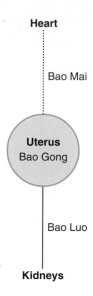

Figure 2.3 The Heart-Uterus-Kidney axis.

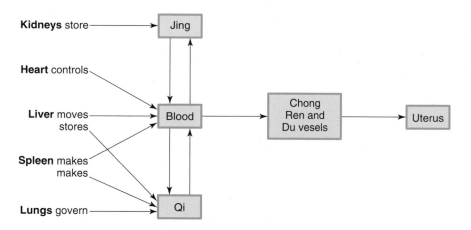

Figure 2.4 Relationship between the Yin organs, Vital substances, Channels, and Uterus.

The other organs

While the kidneys and the heart control the processes necessary for female fertility, they are not the only organs or systems necessary for the effective functioning of the menstrual cycle. Figure 2.4 shows the relationship between all the body's Yin organs and the Uterus.

It is said in TCM that the Kidneys 'dominate reproduction' and are the store of reproductive essence, or Jing, which is discussed below. The Kidney Jing plays a key role in female physiology at all its stages – puberty, pregnancy and menopause. Aspects of Kidney also influence libido and sexual function. The Heart houses the mind or spirit – 'Shen' in TCM terms – and, as such, exerts a subtle but powerful influence over many aspects of the menstrual cycle. The Spleen and Liver also contribute in a less direct way to aspects of reproduction and fertility. The Spleen produces the Blood and the Liver stores and moves it; therefore both can have an effect on the nourishment of the Uterus. The Spleen also controls circulation of Blood in its vessels. The Liver is responsible for smooth movement of Qi and therefore plays a critical role during events surrounding ovulation and menstruation, both of which involve movement and change. The Lungs are less directly involved, but also influence Qi. More detailed explanations of Yin organ function can be found in TCM texts on internal medicine.[1]

THE SUBSTANCES

Jing

Jing is translated as 'reproductive essence'. In Western medical terms, Kidney Jing encompasses the function of the ovaries and some aspects of pituitary function. Plentiful Jing increases fertility and contributes to longevity. It has been observed that women who are successful in having babies in their 40s (i.e. have strong Kidney Jing) often live longer than average.

Kidney Jing is said to be inherited from our parents and stored in the Kidneys. The quality of our Jing determines our genetic predisposition and also reflects how we developed in the womb (this latter, of course, is influenced by our mother's health during the pregnancy). Parents with strong and vital Jing will, barring any unexpected traumas in the womb, pass on strong Jing to their offspring. Less than ideal Jing may be inherited if the parents are older than 40, of poor constitution or if the mother has had many pregnancies close together.

Jing is not only an important first determinant of our basic constitution, but it is also directly related to our ability to produce children of our own. If a girl is born with very deficient Jing, then it is likely that the ovaries or uterus may not develop properly and there will be complete sterility. Puberty, if it comes at all, will be very late, as will development of secondary sexual signs. In women, Jing deficiency (Table 2.1) manifests as primary amenorrhea, resistant ovary syndrome or sporadic and intermittent cycles (oligomenorrhea) or premature menopause (see Ch. 5). Or there may be less severe levels of Jing deficiency, which may manifest as delayed puberty, or very intermittent ovulation or the production of poor quality eggs which do not easily fertilize and make strong embryos. In men, we may see very low sperm counts or even no sperm (see Ch. 7). All degrees of Kidney Jing deficiency spell problems with fertility.

TCM texts say that Kidney Jing is the source of *Tian Gui*. Tian Gui, which translates as 'heavenly water,' is an aspect of Jing which ripens as a young girl reaches puberty. The ripening of the Tian Gui heralds the filling of the Chong vessel with Blood and the Ren vessel with Qi and the periods begin. The quality of the Tian Gui (and hence the Kidney Jing) is important in all the menstrual cycles that follow, and in conception and pregnancy.

According to TCM theory, strong Jing is the basis of healthy Shen or spirit. Human worth can be evaluated in many ways, not just by physical strength and ability to reproduce. Such human attributes as altruism, artistic endeavor and scientific genius make great (non-biological) contributions to human society. Many of these attributes stem from aspects of our spirit or the Shen. Inheritance of good Jing is necessary, therefore, not only for a healthy

Table 2.1   Jing deficiency in women

Severe Jing deficiency	Moderate Jing deficiency	Mild Jing deficiency
No puberty, late puberty	Delayed puberty	Normal puberty and
Primary amenorrhea	Oligomenorrhea	menstrual cycle
Small uterus and ovaries	Premature menopause	Poor or no response to
Underdeveloped secondary	Resistant ovary syndrome	fertility drugs
sexual characteristics	Poor or no response to fertility drugs	Relative infertility
Weak constitution	Possibly poor constitution or small	
Sterility	stature	
No response to fertility drugs	Relative infertility	

physical constitution and the ability to reproduce but also for the development of other human attributes which contribute to humanity in ways other than continuing its genetic lines.

What causes decline in Kidney Jing?

Kidney Jing gets used up with the hundreds of menstrual cycles a woman experiences. Life itself also exhausts our stores of Jing, sometimes more rapidly than others, depending on the nature of the lifestyle and life circumstance.

The mother's Jing (and Blood and Yin) is consumed somewhat during the pregnancy by the rapidly forming fetus and Chinese families were traditionally advised to space out their children (ideally by 5 years) so that the mother's Jing could be replenished before the next baby consumed it again.

The decline of Kidney Jing as we age, is the reason fertility declines in women after more than two decades of producing eggs. It is also the reason that more miscarriages occur and that more babies with genetic disorders like Down syndrome are born to older women. Of course, women in their 20s and 30s can also have miscarriages, or babies with genetic disorders. However, in this case, it is less likely to be Kidney Jing quality which is responsible but other factors, such as sperm quality or external mutagens. By the middle 40s, the Kidney Jing has declined to such a degree that pregnancy is rare. We have all heard stories about miraculous pregnancies to 'mature' women, from Sarah in biblical times, to cover stories in glossy magazines. These stories gain legend status simply because they are extraordinary – and rare.

In my 20 years in the clinic, I have come across just two women who have had babies after 45 (and who have not received donor eggs). In both cases, there had been a long period of amenorrhea, where eggs that might have been spent were conserved.

Kidney Jing can be consumed more rapidly by some types of lifestyle or circumstance than others (see Ch. 12). Epigenetic effects of assisted reproduction technology may also be of concern as far as Jing is concerned (see Chs 9–11).

How is Kidney Jing deficiency treated?

To address inadequacy or decline of Tian Gui, the TCM doctor will treat the Kidney Jing. This is usually done with herbs and sometimes with animal products. As the deficiency is deep, treatment needs to be strong, persistent and lengthy.

When someone is born with very poor Jing and experiences primary amenorrhea, resistant ovary syndrome or sporadic and intermittent cycles, drastic measures are sometimes required to increase the chances of reproducing. It is here that assisted reproduction technology (ART) has produced some startling results. For example, in women who do not ovulate but do have ovaries, drugs can be used to induce ripening of the dormant eggs. If Kidney Jing is not too severe, then sufficient eggs will ripen to be collected for in vitro fertilization (IVF).

In some men with no or very few sperm, testicle biopsies can be taken and immature sperm cells cultured. These can then be used for in vitro fertilization by injecting them directly into the egg (see Ch. 9).

From a TCM perspective, the implications of such techniques can be worrying. If a man or woman has such low Jing energy that they are unable to produce gametes, then it is better from a biological and community point of view that they do not reproduce. This is because, theoretically, the low Jing will be passed onto their offspring born with the aid of ART because the natural brakes to such a possibility have been circumnavigated. One extreme example of this (and a strange paradox), is a congenital form of male infertility (carried on the Y chromosome), which can be passed onto male offspring if certain ART techniques are employed to enable the sperm to fertilize the egg. Thus, a form of Jing deficiency is perpetuated from one generation to the next.

Babies born to parents with congenital gonadal dysfunction or with unexplained infertility with the aid of ART seem to be, in the current broad view, as healthy as other babies. However, research reveals that babies born as a result of these procedures are more at risk of major birth defects[2] and will tend to have lower birth weights.[3] This may reflect the original cause of the infertility as much as the effects of the procedures (for more discussion of these effects, please see Ch. 10).

The majority of IVF children have not yet reached reproductive age, so the quality of some aspects of their Jing is as yet untested in the early twenty-first century.

Yin

Yin is the term used in TCM to describe the cooling, nourishing and moistening, the substantive and internal aspect of body function, and structure. We might say that Yin represents the elixir of youth, which is consumed throughout life, more rapidly by some lifestyles than others.

In the context of the menstrual cycle, Kidney Yin relates to the hormonal triggers which stimulate follicles to develop, as well as to the factors which support the follicle's growth and maturation. The concept of Kidney Yin embraces aspects of pituitary function as well as ovary structure and function. The lining of the uterus and its secretions also reflect the quality of Yin. The function of the glands in the cervix gives us a particularly useful indication of Yin function, as they produce one of the most easily observed of its manifestations, the fertile mucus.

People who have insufficient Yin energy tend to be more dry or hot internally. Often this translates into quantifiable signs like scanty production of vaginal and cervical mucus, or in men, scanty ejaculate. Women who are Yin deficient may have thinner uterine linings which are not secreting adequate nourishment to maintain a pregnancy. TCM texts call this a 'hot dry Uterus'. These women often have scanty periods.

Clinical observations in fertility clinics in China have made a clear connection between ovarian function and Kidney Yin quality. If the Yin energy is inadequate, the follicle in the ovary grows poorly and ovulation may be late (i.e., long cycles) or early if Yin deficiency has given rise to Heat (short cycles) or may happen on a very sporadic basis (intermittent and irregular cycles). A certain threshold quality and quantity of Yin is required before the egg is responsive to hormonal stimulation and can grow to the stage where it is ready to be released and fertilized.

In personality, Yin-deficient people are more restless or anxious; they can be alert and bright-eyed and quick. Often, they are thin and wiry and their skin ages more quickly than others.

What causes Kidney Yin deficiency?

Kidney Yin deficiency may be caused by a constitutional tendency or the Yin may have been damaged by overwork. This is not at all an unusual scenario for women today, particularly those working long hours in stressful conditions. Paid work, for many women, is done before and after the unpaid work of running a household. Add to such conditions poor diet or rushed eating, polluted environment, inadequate sleep and exercise and you have the typical Yin-consuming lifestyle of so many of the women we see in our clinics. Trying to become strong and healthy, let alone pregnant, in such conditions is a challenge.

Kidney Yin may also be damaged by drug abuse and by excess sexual activity or many pregnancies (even if these are terminated). Loss of large quantities of blood (such as prolonged or very heavy periods) or body fluids can damage Yin. Long-term disease in any organ system will eventually damage Kidney Yin.

Yin declines with age, especially from the late 30s. Age-related Yin deficiency is one of the most common reasons for inability to fall pregnant that we see in our clinics in the West.

How is Kidney Yin deficiency treated?

In the clinic, large doses of herbs are prescribed to a Yin-deficient woman to increase the Kidney and Liver Yin so that the ovaries are nourished sufficiently to produce healthy eggs. Such an approach is emphasized in the weeks of the menstrual cycle leading up to ovulation; this treatment also encourages the retention of blood in the uterine lining along with its secretory function. Equally important in the treatment of the Yin is appropriate lifestyle changes. There is usually so little space in our lives these days for stillness and calling a halt to relentless busyness. Even when we say we are resting, we are watching television or movies, and our mind and body, while they may be more relaxed, have not stopped to the point where deep and nourishing rest can replenish reserves. A regular routine and enough sleep are two key first steps in reducing stress and relieving the mind. The capacity to still the mind is an important aim for the Yin-deficient person who is restless and nervous.

A particular challenge of our times, and one which is rarely heeded, is the need to become strong and healthy *before* conceiving. The rush to fit everything in at the last minute often means that pregnancy is embarked upon with little thought to the constitution of the sought-after child. Pregnancy at any cost is often the prevalent attitude of a society used to getting what it wants and now. A TCM doctor will advise a woman who is very Yin-deficient to make adjustments to her lifestyle and build her Yin before attempting to conceive. There is important ground to be laid. This is sometimes a difficult idea for a Western woman to swallow, particularly if she is in her late 30s and the biological clock is ticking loudly.

Fertility drugs and ART programs will often be tried by women in this category (usually in their late 30s or early 40s). However, when the Yin is very low, using strong ovarian-stimulating drugs is a bit like whipping an exhausted horse which has nothing left to give. Seldom are viable eggs produced.

Yang

Yang energy is the counterpart to Yin. Compared with Yin's still, cool, moist, and nourishing nature, it is dynamic, active, and warming. The effect of Yang begins to be felt in the menstrual cycle at ovulation. Dispersing obstructions and aiding unfettered movement are important Yang functions at this time. At the moment of ovulation, there is much dynamic activity – the egg is launched out of its follicle and the fimbrial fingers embrace and guide the egg into the fallopian tube.

The journey of the egg down the tube is also a dynamic one, with both the egg and the tube needing to be able to move smoothly and flexibly. It is the action of Yang which ensures that mucus obstructions in the tube are dissolved to allow free passage to the uterus.

The moment of fertilization also relies on sufficient Yang. Yang is the motivating force for all transformations in the body. The moment a sperm's head finally breaks through the egg's coating, and its DNA fuses with that of the egg, is the greatest transformation of them all – the beginning of a potential human life.

Kidney Yang performs a very important function after ovulation, when a fertilized egg reaches the uterus and implants and develops. The Chinese have for thousands of years ascribed the inability of some women to fall pregnant as 'a Cold womb'. In other words, not enough Kidney Yang energy. Nowadays we know that the Cold womb is one supplied with insufficient progesterone, which means that implantation and early development of the embryo will not be supported. When there is insufficient progesterone produced, the body is demonstrably colder – about 0.4°C colder than when the progesterone levels are high.

What causes Kidney Yang deficiency?

Lack of Kidney Yang may be a constitutional trait or it may result from damage, most commonly by an invasion of external Cold. This initially obstructs the flow of Qi and, eventually, if it is not expelled, affects the body's Yang. Our Western lifestyle provides many opportunities for this so-called Cold invasion, most notably our predilection for icy foods and drinks and the habit many women have of swimming during menstruation. Cold as an external pathogen can enter the body easily via:

- the Stomach (cold foods like ice cream)

- the Uterus (swimming or getting very chilled during the period when the Chong vessel is open)

- the channels on the legs (scanty leg coverings during the period).

The Chinese, and in fact many Asian cultures, strongly advise against behavior which can chill the body during the period. Being chronically exposed to cold, such as living or working in a cold damp environment, can also damage the Yang.

Kidney Yin and Yang depend upon one another and depletion of Kidney Yin will eventually deplete Kidney Yang. This is a commonly seen phenomenon in the infertility clinic, especially in women after their mid-30s. Similarly, when there is prolonged stagnation of Liver or Heart Qi (i.e., emotional disturbances) the Yang of the Kidney can suffer too. The nature of Yang is to move and be active, but in an environment of emotional constraint it cannot move and becomes damaged.

Kidney Yang is consumed by miscarriages, abortions and overtaxing the body physically. Inadequate sleep, specifically going to bed too late, can also be a contributing factor to Kidney Yang deficiency. Certain diseases (e.g. thyroid disease) can compromise the function of Kidney Yang, and prolonged disease of any organ will finally affect the Kidneys, damaging Yin or Yang or both.

How is Kidney Yang deficiency treated?

Herbs, acupuncture and moxa are applied in the treatment of Kidney Yang deficiency. Such treatment has particular relevance in the post-ovulation phase of the menstrual cycle. Women with Kidney Yang deficiency are sometimes prescribed progesterone by specialists in this post-ovulation phase but it is generally recognized that such treatment has limited usefulness. However, herbs which boost Kidney Yang can increase progesterone production and fertility in such women. Treatments to replenish Kidney Yang will never be successful if the patient does not get enough sleep, in the same way that treatments for Kidney Yin will never succeed if the mind is not able to be quietened.

Blood

The Blood, or *Xue*, as it is called in Chinese, embraces the Western notion of blood (the red fluid in our arteries and veins) but goes further to include aspects of tissue nutrition. The Heart is said to govern the Blood (via the circulatory system) and, with the Spleen, plays a role in the production of Blood and therefore contributes to nourishment of the endometrium and thereby the embryo. The Spleen's role is to manufacture Blood from the nutrients it can extract from food. Someone who is Blood deficient will not only be pale but may also be weak and malnourished.

Blood plays an important role in fertility by nourishing the endometrium (the uterine lining), making it a moist, juicy and nutritious place for an embryo to settle in. Shortly before ovulation, peaks of estrogen (released by the developing egg) prime the lining of the uterus – this means the endometrial tissue is provoked by this hormone into proliferating and growing in size, actually producing more blood vessels and laying down more tissue. Without adequate Blood, this process may be retarded or, in fact, stymied completely. Thus, TCM recognizes that it is not only lack of Yin which can lengthen the first half of the cycle and hold up ovulation but also Blood deficiency.

Blood is stored by the Liver, especially when the body is at rest. Some of this store must be passed onto the Uterus before preparation for pregnancy or menstruation can occur. So if the Liver Blood is deficient, then menstruation may be scanty or there may be infrequent or no periods.

The body loses some of its blood stores during the period and so must quickly make good the loss if the newly forming endometrium is to be adequately supplied. In China, it is very common for women across the entire social and professional spectrum to take Blood tonic foods and herbs after periods to ensure this. The Spleen's function in digestion and manufacture of Blood is therefore important at this time.

What causes Blood deficiency?

Inadequate protein in the diet is a frequent cause of Blood deficiency, and it often falls to the TCM doctor to persuade a pale and wan vegetarian patient to try and consume more protein. If a woman experiences very heavy periods over a significant length of time, then she will easily become Blood deficient. Past illness and a constitutional tendency to anemia will also be contributors to Blood deficiency.

How is Blood deficiency treated?

Blood deficiency responds rapidly and well to treatment with Blood tonic herbs and a diet with adequate protein and iron. Of course, causes of heavy menstrual bleeding must be addressed too if the problem is not to reoccur. In the clinic, an emphasis on building Blood occurs in the weeks immediately after the period.

Shen

Shen translates as 'spirit' and encompasses both higher spiritual levels as well as some more mundane aspects of the brain and nervous system. The Shen is related to (and controlled by) the Heart. According to TCM theory, the Heart and the Shen play an integral role (with the Kidneys) in controlling fertility.

A healthy Shen and Heart will create mental stability and contentment. Ovulation relies on the Heart housing the mind (or Shen). When the Heart and the Shen are stable, then the cues for the different stages of the menstrual cycle can proceed smoothly.

What causes Shen instability?

In fertility clinics both in China and the West, the role of the mind is recognized not only in psychological well-being but also in many of the physiological processes leading to successful conception. Emotional stress can play havoc with the menstrual cycle. It can affect the function of the hypothalamus (master control gland in the brain), causing pituitary gland dysfunction, and ovulation may be delayed or completely switched off.

One of the prime requirements for fertility is a balance between Kidney Yin and Kidney Yang. The TCM classics say, 'to maintain balance between Kidney Yin and Kidney Yang, healthy Heart Qi is indispensable.' This refers to the fact that if Kidney Yin does not transform into Kidney Yang at midcycle because of obstructed Heart Qi (i.e. a disturbed Shen), then ovulation will not occur. The Heart and Shen are also involved in ovulation in that they help to catalyze the formation of Tian Gui from Kidney Jing, wherein Kidney energy promotes the development of sperm and eggs.

How is Shen instability treated?

Treatment of the Shen is treatment of the mind. The first step is to regulate sleep patterns, using sedative herbs if necessary. Removal of mental stressors is important too, and, where this cannot be achieved, mind-calming techniques such as yoga, tai chi and meditation become especially important. While treatment of the Shen can be applied at any time, it has particular relevance in the days leading up to ovulation.

Qi

The name the Chinese have given to the energy which circulates in the meridians or channels is *Qi*. It facilitates communication between organ systems and between interior and exterior parts of the body. In the menstrual cycle we are particularly concerned with the movement of Qi in facilitating the movement of the egg from the ovary through the fallopian tube to the uterus at ovulation time. It is also important for the expulsion of menstrual blood from the body.

In clinical terms, it is the Liver Qi, and its unimpeded movement, that becomes a focus of our attention at two pivotal moments in the menstrual cycle – ovulation and menstruation.

What causes Liver Qi stagnation?

Liver Qi is easily impeded by emotional stress. The Liver channel runs through left and right sides of the pelvic cavity, through the ovaries. Obstruction of Qi in these channels can affect the release of the egg from the ovaries and the flexible movement of the fallopian tubes. It is a tenet of Chinese medicine that the Qi leads the Blood and if the Qi of the Liver is obstructed, then the Qi cannot lead the Blood smoothly. Dysmenorrhea results, or the period may flow in a stop-start sort of way. Because movement of Liver Qi is also important in preparing the body for menstruation, Liver Qi stagnation will cause premenstrual symptoms.

How is Liver Qi stagnation treated?

Acupuncture and techniques to relieve stress (such as meditation, yoga, tai chi or exercise) are the treatments of choice to regulate Liver Qi stagnation. Because of the importance of unobstructed Qi flow at the time of ovulation, clinic visits for acupuncture will often be scheduled for this time.

It is also important to pay attention to the Liver Qi towards the end of the menstrual cycle, when Qi stagnation can lead to distressing symptoms such as breast soreness and cramping in the abdomen.

THE CHANNELS

There are 12 main meridians or channels traversing the body, each one related to an organ system. It is on these channels that an acupuncturist finds the many hundreds of points used to treat myriad different disorders. The pathways and points of these channels are described in acupuncture texts.[4]

In addition, TCM texts describe a number of 'extra' channels, some of which play a key role in the functioning of the menstrual cycle and are described here.

The Chong and the Ren vessels

The Chong and the Ren vessels are of primary importance in controlling the menstrual cycle and play an important role in conception and pregnancy. The Chong vessel is sometimes translated as the Penetrating vessel and the Ren vessel as the Conception or Directing vessel. The Chong vessel is known as the 'Sea of Blood' and sometimes as the 'Sea of all 12 Channels'. The Ren vessel is known as the 'Sea of all Yin'.

Both vessels arise from the area between the Kidneys and pass through the uterus to the perineum, exerting strong influence on the abdomen and the organs therein (Figs 2.5, 2.6). Although they also exist in men, their involvement in male reproductive function is not so critical.

The Bao vessel and the Bao channel

The Heart, Kidneys and Uterus are linked by the Bao vessel and the Bao channel (see Fig. 2.3). Traditional Chinese texts describe a channel which runs from the Heart to the Uterus (the Bao vessel or Bao Mai) and from the Kidneys to the Uterus (the Bao channel or Bao Luo). It is via these channels that the Heart Qi and the Kidney Qi exert their influence on the reproductive organs. This influence is described as 'opening' and 'closing' the Uterus. The Uterus is said to open at ovulation time (and thus allows sperm entry) and also at period time (to allow discharge of menses).

After menstruation and after ovulation, the Uterus must close again, as it must after conception (to store the fetus). Such uterine activity relies on the influence of the Heart and the Kidney via the Bao vessel and Bao channel. The closing of the Uterus, especially, relies on the Kidney. When the Kidneys are weak and fail in this function,

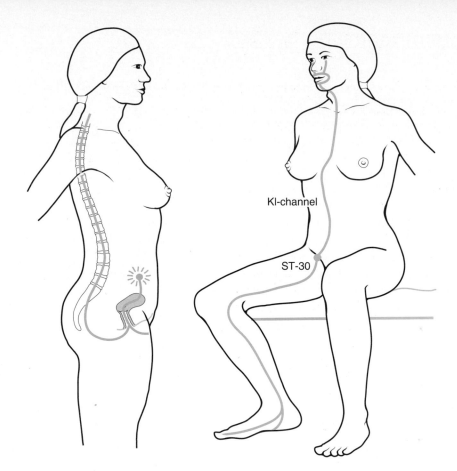

KI-channel

ST-30

Figure 2.5 Pathway of the Chong channel.

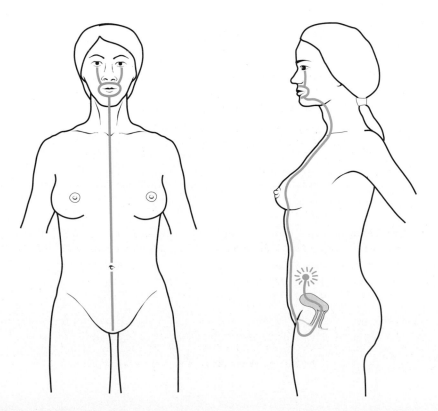

Figure 2.6 Pathway of the Ren channel.

miscarriages occur or there may be spotting during the menstrual cycle. Miscarriages or bleeding due to Kidney weakness can be the result of insufficient hormone support.

On the other hand, the opening of the Uterus relies especially on the Heart. For example, because the Heart plays a crucial role in triggering ovulation, if the Heart Qi is stagnant or obstructed and cannot carry out its function of opening the Uterus, there will be no ovulation. Or, in other words, if the right triggers do not come from the hypothalamus to the pituitary and then to the ovary, the levels of estrogen necessary to provoke the glands in the cervix into making fertile mucus will not be reached. The Uterus will not open to allow entry to the sperm. If there has been no ovulation, then there will be no opening of the Uterus for menstruation either.

Heart Fire (which might occur if the Heart Qi is severely obstructed) may force the opening of the Uterus at inappropriate times or in an undiscriminating way. This may be seen, e.g., if a miscarriage or unregulated bleeding occurs after a woman receives a shock or is under great stress.

The activity of the three extra channels: the Chong, Ren and Bao vessels, is emphasized at different times of the menstrual cycle. The period flow effectively empties the Chong vessel, the Sea of Blood, and it is one of the prime requirements of the post-menstrual phase to make good this Blood loss.

The Bao vessel and Bao channel are active at ovulation time, bringing Jing and Tian Gui from the Kidneys, and Blood from the Heart to the Uterus. The Ren vessel plays a more active role after ovulation, whether in conception and pregnancy or in providing the motive force for menstruation.

The Du and the Dai vessels

The Du vessel and the Dai vessel are two other extra channels that figure in gynecology theory and practice. Points along their pathways are useful in certain situations but their application in the treatment of functional infertility is not central. We shall however revisit them when discussing disorders such as polycystic ovarian syndrome in Chapter 5.

HOW IT ALL BEGINS

In girls who have not yet reached puberty, the ovaries are constantly developing follicles (since follicle-stimulating hormone (FSH) is produced by the pituitary gland even before puberty) which then die; i.e., we could say this demonstrates reproductive potential or a good basis of Kidney energy. However, normal puberty brings with it much greater quantities of pituitary hormones, especially luteinizing hormone (LH), which heralds the beginning of the menstrual cycle. In TCM, we describe this event as the arrival of the 'Tian Gui' and the initiation of the activity of the Chong and Ren vessels. Despite the fact there are sufficient hormones to mature follicles, ovulation seldom occurs in the early months and up to 2 years after puberty. The full expression of Kidney function, especially Kidney Yang, develops more slowly and it takes up to 5 years after the first menstrual period before the luteal phase of the menstrual cycle is fully functional.[5]

THE MENSTRUAL CYCLE

Key events

Modern physiologists describe the menstrual cycle in terms of the hormones made by the ovaries (estrogen and progesterone) and the pituitary gland (FSH and LH) and their actions on the follicles, the tubes and the endometrium or lining of the uterus. The events, starting from the beginning of a cycle, the first day of a menstrual period, can be summarized as shown in Box 2.1.

Box 2.1   Menstrual cycle events

Day 1–5

Levels of the major female hormones estrogen and progesterone are very low at the start of the cycle. This causes:

- the period flow to start (i.e. the uterine lining is no longer maintained)
- the pituitary to start making hormones (FSH and LH) to stimulate the growth of new follicles in the ovary.

Day 7

One of the follicles outstrips the others in growth and starts to produce copious estrogen.

Day 7–12

The high levels of estrogen stimulate:

- the uterine lining to proliferate
- the glands in the cervix to produce fertile mucus.

Day 12 and 13

The continuing high levels of estrogen act on the pituitary, inducing it to produce LH. The surge of LH stimulates the production of lytic enzymes and prostaglandins in the dominant follicle.

Day 14

The egg is released when the enzymes create a break in the follicle wall and the prostaglandins stimulate its expulsion.

Day 15–25

The corpus luteum forms from the empty follicle and produces progesterone (and estrogen) to:

- stimulate the endometrium to secrete nutrients
- inhibit the pituitary from producing any more of the hormones (FSH,LH) which ripen more follicles.

Day 25–28

The corpus luteum dies and the levels of progesterone and estrogen drop, causing:

- the start of period flow as the endometrium disintegrates
- the pituitary to once again start production of FSH and LH to ripen up the next lot of follicles.

We can summarize the various hormone interactions and feedback loops (Fig. 2.7) and chart the ups and downs of the various hormones during the menstrual cycle (Fig. 2.8).

Just as Western physiology describes the menstrual cycle in terms of hormones which influence the ovaries and the uterus, TCM describes it in terms of the effect of Qi and Blood and Yin and Yang on the Uterus. In the broadest terms, the period cycle is seen as just one of many physical manifestations or reflections of the ebb and flow of Yin and Yang energy, like so many aspects of our body functions and lives.

In Chinese medicine, the cycle depends on and reflects the mutual dependence of Yin and Yang: i.e., Yin depends upon the function of Yang and Yang depends upon Yin as its material base. One cannot exist without the other and they complement each other in their functions or roles. As one expands to full expression, the other is consumed, but at its nadir, or point of extinction, gives rise to the other – a dance so elegantly portrayed in the classic Yin/Yang diagram (Fig. 2.9).

This dance creates, in the energetic terms of TCM, the basis of the menstrual cycle: the Yin growing for 14 days, then giving way to the Yang, which depends upon and consumes Yin as it then grows to its maximum after 14 days; then the rise of Yin can begin again. For a woman to be fertile, the Yin and Yang must constantly maintain this balance.

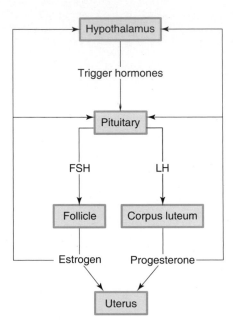

Figure 2.7 Hormone controls in the menstrual cycle.

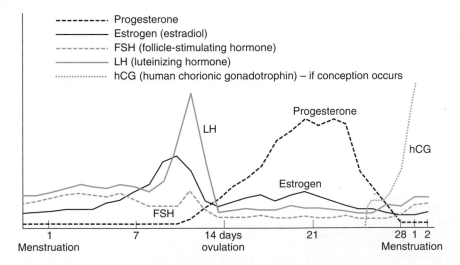

Figure 2.8 Hormone levels during the menstrual cycle.

The length of the cycle

The 28-day cycle (which, by long-held convention, I am using for diagrams and descriptions in this chapter) has been the yardstick for the 'typical' cycle length, habituated as we are to a weekly rhythm. Actually a more correct 'typical' cycle length is 29.5 days – the length of the lunar month. For many women, however, the information that a normal cycle should be 28 or 29 days is meaningless, simply because their cycle is, and always has been, different from the norm. Many women have 24 or 36 day cycles and for them, this represents no problem. In fact, most medical texts usually describe anything from 25 to 35 days as normal. However, from the point of view of Chinese

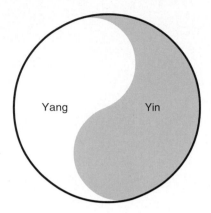

Figure 2.9 Yin and Yang.

medicine, the closer the cycle is to 28 or 29 days the better; this is something the TCM doctor addresses before anything else and is called 'regulating the cycle.'

Phases of the TCM menstrual cycle

When it comes to studying the menstrual cycle, TCM gynecologists break it up into four phases (Fig. 2.10).

The period, post-period and ovulation phases all fall into the follicular phase but have quite precise and unique treatment requirements. When we are considering fertility, the pre-period phase is included in the post-ovulation phase and has no separate treatment principle.

Let us now look at each phase in the menstrual cycle in detail and examine exactly what is required for each phase to be carried out effectively and what evolves from this. The way we apply such knowledge to the treatment of infertility is described in detail in Chapter 4 but as I emphasize there, it is understanding and encouraging the normal movements of Yin and Yang and Qi and Blood during the menstrual cycle that is the foundation of all successful treatment for female infertility.

THE YIN PART OF THE CYCLE

Follicular phase (proliferative or estrogenic phase)

The follicular phase begins on the first day (Day 1) of the period. It is called the follicular phase because it is this part of the cycle in which one or more follicles (and the eggs inside them) in the ovary will grow large enough for ovulation to occur. It is also called the proliferative phase because the lining of the uterus (the endometrium) grows from almost nothing after the period to a thick and receptive padding ready to receive a newly fertilized egg. And from the point of view of hormones, it is the part of the cycle where more estrogen than progesterone is produced (Fig. 2.11).

Shedding of the endometrium

While the follicles in the ovary start their new cycle right from Day 1, in the clinic, we are actually more concerned with what Day 1 means for the endometrium. Treatment applied at this time needs to consider the mechanics of the removal of the uterine lining separately before attention is paid to the follicles in the ovary or the proliferation of the endometrium.

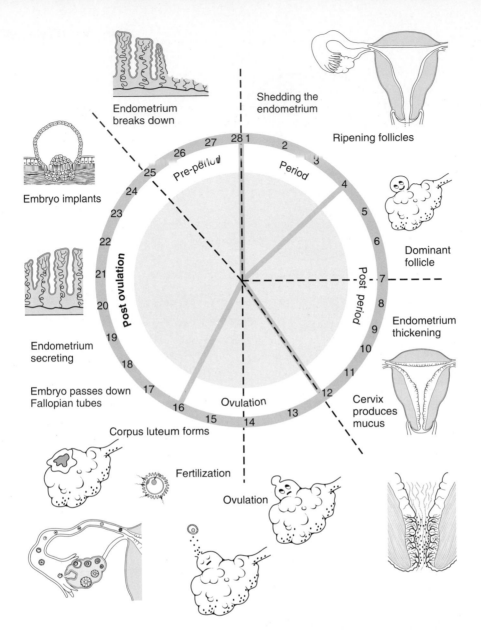

Figure 2.10 Phases of the menstrual cycle.

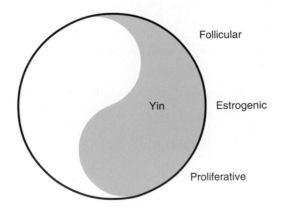

Figure 2.11 The Yin phase.

The first day of the cycle is usually defined as the first day there is menstrual bleeding. Some fertility clinics define Day 1 as the first day a woman wakes up in the morning with bleeding; however, women usually experience the first day there is significant blood loss as Day 1 of the period, whether the bleeding starts at 6 a.m. or 2 p.m. If the period begins in the evening or during the night, however, the next day is called Day 1 of the cycle. Research from the University of Sydney showed that a large majority (>70%) of menstrual cycles do in fact start during the night or within the first 4 h of waking, so in most cases, there is very little room for confusion. The only time when it becomes an issue is when a particular drug protocol requires very precise timing.

Day 1 represents a pivotal and dramatic day, not only from the point of view of the uterine lining, which suddenly begins to disintegrate, but also from the point of view of the Yin and Yang cycle. It is this point on the Yin-Yang cycle that the previous cycle reaches its conclusion, as Yang reaches its zenith, and Yin is born. On this day, one cycle concludes with the discarding of the unused lining and another begins with the signals sent to the ovary to start ripening more eggs.

On Day 1, the Chong vessel (the Sea of Blood) begins to empty. The Qi of the Ren vessel drives the flow of blood downwards through the cervix. The onset of menstrual bleeding reflects the breaking down of the lining in the uterus when the levels of estrogen and progesterone fall. How this actually happens is an extraordinary and intricate dance performed by the spiralling blood vessels of the endometrium. In the 4–24 h preceding menstruation, these coiled blood vessels tighten up and constrict blood flow, effectively starving the endometrium of blood. Consequently, the tissues in the upper portion of the endometrium die. Then these tightly coiled blood vessels relax and expand again, causing the upper layer to become detached from the basal layer (leaving most of the stroma and embedded immune cells intact) and blood to leak from the weakened capillary walls. Tissue, cells, fluid, blood, and blood vessels are shed, resulting in several days of menstrual flow.

The degree of shedding of the endometrium varies from woman to woman. There is no clearly described medical reason why this should be so; however, TCM places great importance in variance of quantity and quality of blood flow during the period and believes it reflects quite accurately key factors in a woman's constitution. If the period flow is problematic in any way, then a clear understanding of this tendency allows for accurate diagnosis and treatment.

The main menstrual flow tends to happen in the first 24 h of the period. The average blood loss per period is 30 or 40 ml but if more than 60 ml are lost each period, there may be a risk of anemia. However, there is more to menstrual flow than just blood. About 50% of the liquid is tissue fluid and serous oozing. The clots that some women experience during a period are not true blood clots but aggregations of glycoproteins and mucin. The clots form when enzymes from the cervix act on the blood proteins to make glycoprotein meshes. Sometimes, small pieces of tissue are seen in the menstrual flow.

The nature of the menstrual flow and symptoms accompanying it are all significant in pinpointing any glitches in the Qi and Blood movement. Any obstructions to the menstrual flow can have implications for infertility. For example, the presence of tissue or clots alerts the TCM doctor to the fact that the flow of the Qi and the Blood is not smooth (known as Qi and Blood stagnation) and may signal a problem in the uterine lining.

In TCM terms, we describe the stretching of the endometrial blood vessels, the breaking down and shedding of the endometrial tissue, the remodeling of what's left and the discharge of menstrual flow as 'movement of the Qi and Blood.' Treatment applied at this time must encourage movement and unobstructed flow to encourage discharge of menstrual flow.

Over the next 2–3 days of the period, the Chong vessel empties and then the building of Yin and Blood begins again until the Chong vessel is completely refilled. After the first few days of the period, clinical focus moves from enabling and encouraging the breakdown of the endometrium and the discharge of the menstrual flow, to building the Yin and the Blood. This is done with herbs and by regulating Chong vessel activity with acupuncture. Diet at this time is especially focussed on nourishing Blood.

Some evolutionary biologists have questioned the role of menstruation in the human.

Menstrual shedding of a uterine lining that has been prepared to receive an embryo (decidualized) occurs in very few species – only humans, monkeys and some bats – and compared with our primate relatives, menstrual blood flow in humans is very heavy. The human placenta implants much more deeply than that of any other species too and this may be related.

Human reproduction has evolved in ways that limit the likelihood of pregnancy while maximizing the frequency of menstruation. Women have a limited and variable fertile window, obscure ovulation signs, a very high incidence of preimplantation embryo loss and low monthly pregnancy rates and on *top* of this many women experience uncomfortable or heavy periods.

From an evolutionary point of view, the purpose of such frequent and often inconvenient menstrual periods is not obvious but some researchers think that this repeated menstrual priming and preconditioning of the uterine lining and its vasculature during non-conception cycles could be important for ensuring successful implantation and placentation in the latter stages of a menstrual cycle in which a conception has occurred.[6]

This concept underpins the importance we as Chinese medicine doctors attach to substantial and smooth movement of Blood during the menstrual phase.

All Chinese medicine *Fu Ke* texts emphasize the regularity and the quality of this menstrual shedding, something that most western gynecologists pay scant regard. What should be recognized is that healthy menstrual periods play an important role in fertility. The above mentioned researchers feel that the period has evolved to protect the uterine tissues from inflammation – oxidative stress inflammatory cells and proinflammatory cytokines and dead cells are found in the menstrual flow.[7]

Extrapolating to TCM concepts, we might say that a good menstrual flow clears Heat and prevents Blood stasis. The tissue remodeling that happens during the period is crucial in providing the correct environment for implantation and deep placentation later in the cycle and this is why we afford it proper clinical attention.

The endometrium in the proliferative phase

During this phase of the menstrual cycle, the uterine lining grows and thickens. The different stages can be described (Fig. 2.12) as:

- shedding during menstruation

- post-menstrual endometrium

- late proliferative endometrium.

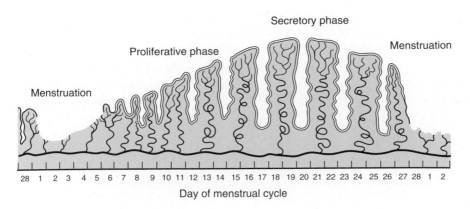

Figure 2.12 The endometrium is shed and then proliferates.

The protocol for prescribing herbs and applying acupuncture at different times of the proliferative phase takes into account these different stages of endometrial development.

Although menstrual bleeding may continue for several days, endometrial regeneration generally begins within 2 days after the onset of menstruation. Initially, the mechanism of this repair process is the same as for normal tissue healing, but by Day 3, estrogen and progesterone receptors form in the glandular epithelium and hormones control it. In other words, rebuilding the endometrium is a specifically Chong/Ren-driven initiative.

By Day 5 the remodeling of the endometrium is complete. At Day 5 or 6, when the period is usually finished, the endometrium is 1–2 mm thick. As estrogen levels rise, more tissue develops, especially in the surface layer.

During the early to mid-proliferative phase, the glands are initially tubular and straight but become more twisted as estrogen levels increase. From about Day 7 or 8 of the cycle, the numbers of ciliated and microvillous cells in the endometrium increase. By the time the proliferation phase is completed and ovulation is imminent a healthy endometrium is at least 8 mm thick.

The proliferation of the endometrium, increasing in thickness and density of blood vessels and glandular cells, reflects the filling of the Chong vessel. To encourage this rebuilding of the uterine lining we use mainly Blood tonics, often with the addition of small amounts of Blood- and Qi-regulating herbs to encourage circulation through all the new blood vessels and tissue being formed. At the same time, acupuncture points on the Chong vessel are often used.

According to our Yin-Yang cycle diagram, the growth of Yin begins right from Day 1 of the cycle. We have referred to the growth of the follicle following stimulation by the pituitary hormones as the Yin aspect of ovarian activity. The new follicles start growing from Day 1 of the cycle or even from the moment that the progesterone and estrogen fall at the end of the previous cycle. However, in the clinic, we usually delay the application of Yin tonics until the menstrual discharge is complete or nearly complete.

The first couple of days of the cycle are characterized by having very little of the two main hormones in circulation. There are some exceptions to the rule of delaying the tonification aspect of treatment in this part of the cycle, e.g., in women who are very Yin deficient, Yin tonics may be used throughout the cycle, even when the endometrium is being discharged.

The ovary in the follicular phase

When we are talking about the events in the ovary, the first half of the cycle is referred to as the follicular phase (Box 2.2).

As the Yin and the Blood grow, so do a number of follicles in response to stimulation from the pituitary hormone FSH. This process is called follicular recruitment. Anti-Mullerian hormone (AMH) produced by the granulosa cells of the ovary inhibits excessive follicular recruitment by FSH and is a useful marker for assessing ovarian reserve.

Box 2.2   **Stages of follicle development**

1. Early follicular phase – follicular recruitment. Between 2 and 50 (depending on the age of the ovary) follicles are chosen for the race to win a trip to the uterus.
2. Mid-follicular phase – dominant follicle selection. A winner (the largest follicle) is selected out of a close bunch of contenders; occasionally two or three follicles tie for first position.
3. Late follicular phase – hormone surge leading to ovulation. The chosen follicle releases its egg into the waiting arms of the fallopian tube.

At the beginning of a cycle, the follicles are less than 4 mm in diameter. Even before a follicle can join the starting line at the outset of a new menstrual cycle, certain growth factors are needed. These factors are necessary to get the follicles to a point where the pituitary hormone FSH takes over their stimulation. In TCM, we might relate these factors to the Kidney Jing, i.e., they represent the *potential* for gamete development. Then FSH (or the growth of Yin) will strongly stimulate the follicle, so that it grows over a period of 2 weeks to 50 times its original size (Fig. 2.13).

The use of Yin tonic herbs appears to help this growth and development process. The quality of Yin, as we have said before, has a bearing on both the quality of the egg itself and the growth of the follicle around it. While the application of Yin tonics is seen quite clearly in the clinic to enhance follicular development, there is little it can do to change the DNA of the egg itself. Since a woman's eggs are formed when she is still an embryo in the womb of her mother and never manufactured again thereafter, the DNA die is well and truly cast. In other words, the DNA in the chromosomes and the mitochondria (the small organelles which are responsible for energy production) of the egg cell are as old as the woman herself and may well be showing the irreversible signs of aging.

In the clinic this can lead to some frustration for older women (over 40 years) trying to conceive. After taking Chinese herbs, these women see many symptoms and signs, which indicate improved fertility, such as regular periods with plentiful fresh red blood, copious fertile mucus, textbook basal body temperature (BBT) charts, improved libido and lubrication, etc. All of this indicates that their Yin and Blood are flourishing and their hormone levels are good but their eggs are still 40-plus years old and are either not easy to fertilize or not good at making viable fetuses.

We know that ovaries and their eggs show the effects of aging much more rapidly than do other parts of the female reproductive system. The uterus and its lining remain quite functional and responsive to hormone stimulation well after the ovaries have retired, as has been demonstrated by successful pregnancies in older post-menopausal women using IVF technology and eggs donated by younger women.

While Kidney Yin declines rapidly with age, especially after 40, some aspects of Kidney Yang endure with vigor, such as the functioning of the endometrium. However, the functioning of the corpus luteum gland (another aspect of Kidney Yang) is affected by age.

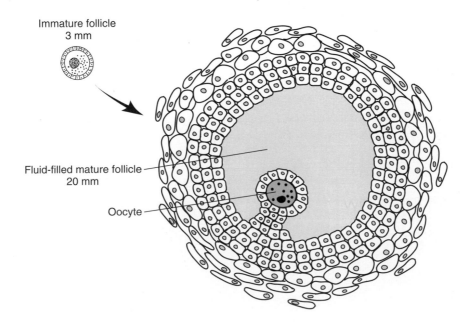

Immature follicle
3 mm

Fluid-filled mature follicle
20 mm

Oocyte

Figure 2.13 Development of the follicle.

In the mid-follicular phase, one follicle becomes dominant (probably due to it having more FSH receptors and a better blood supply). This dominant follicle is the first one to produce estrogen, a certain concentration of which causes the pituitary to produce less FSH, ensuring the demise (atresia) of all other follicles except itself. In cases of multiple ovulations there are two or more follicles exhibiting dominance.

By Day 9, the number of blood vessels in the dominant follicle is twice that of other follicles. It is this growth of extra blood vessels (both here and to a greater extent in the endometrium) which dictates the use of Blood-building and Blood-regulating medicinals around this time. The length of time from selection of the dominant follicle to ovulation is variable. In a 'typical' 28-day cycle, it will take around 5 days, i.e. from about Day 10 to Day 14 (Fig. 2.14).

When concentrations of estrogen secreted by the dominant follicle reach a certain level and are then maintained for about 48 h, a surge of FSH and LH from the pituitary is initiated. This midcycle LH surge triggers events leading to ovulation sometime within the next 36–40 h and increases the ability of the ripe follicle to manufacture progesterone. The LH surge and the beginnings of progesterone production coincide with the approach of the Yang part of the cycle.

Sometimes there is no follicular recruitment at all in this first phase of the menstrual cycle, i.e., there is no response by the follicles in the ovary to FSH or, due to hypothalamus or pituitary gland dysfunction, not enough FSH is produced. These cases are often diagnosed in TCM as Jing deficiency or sometimes as Yin or Blood deficiency and will require special treatment (see Chs 4 and 5). These women experience no periods (amenorrhea) or long erratic cycles (oligomenorrhea).

RELEASING AN EGG LATE – LONG FOLLICULAR PHASE

In women who are Blood or Yin deficient, however, it may take longer for the follicle to get sufficient sustenance to reach maturity. Ovulation will be delayed and menstrual cycles will typically be long. From the TCM doctor's perspective, these patients have diminished fertility due to their Yin or Blood deficiency. In Western physiological terms, we would attribute such slow development of the chosen follicle to sluggish estrogen production, or reduced sensitivity to stimulation by FSH, or perhaps inhibited FSH production by the pituitary.

In some instances, it appears that the egg may mature normally, but ovulation may still be delayed. In this case, the egg is over-ripe by the time it is released and should it be fertilized, there is an increased risk of chromosomal abnormality and miscarriage.[8] Such a delay in ovulation tends to occur as a discrete one-off incident rather than a repeated pattern and may come about for a variety of reasons, such as illness or emotional disturbances, which upset the balance and timing of the hormonal control of ovulation. TCM describes this situation as stagnation of the Heart or Liver Qi, which in some cases then compromises the Kidney Yang and predisposes to miscarriage.

RELEASING AN EGG EARLY – SHORT FOLLICULAR PHASE

In some women, ovulation may have occurred earlier than Day 14. If an unusually short cycle occurred out of the blue, the ovulating follicle reached its required size quickly because it had a head start. That is, it had started

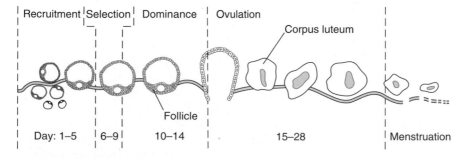

Figure 2.14 The dominant follicle is selected.

growth in the previous cycle but did not become the dominant follicle which ovulated that month. It also escaped the usual atresia.

If early cycles happen on a very regular basis (e.g. the cycle is always around 21 days), we need to consider other mechanisms for early ovulation. Where it is early ovulation that shortens the cycle, there are several possibilities. The pituitary may habitually produce an excess of FSH and the follicles are therefore recruited and matured too rapidly. This sometimes happens in women approaching menopause, although it is not restricted to that group.

Alternatively, some women might have follicles genetically programmed to make more FSH receptors than usual, so they will grow rapidly with less stimulation than usual. Sometimes ovulation is early because an egg is released before it is mature enough – if it is fertilized the fetus often has extra chromosomes and little chance of survival. This may occur more often in situations where there is hormonal imbalance, e.g. polycystic ovary syndrome[9] (see Ch. 5).

In TCM terms early ovulation usually reflects Heat, most often Heat arising as a result of insufficient Yin.

Short menstrual cycles can also be attributed to a shortened luteal phase – this will be covered later when we discuss the luteal phase.

The fallopian tubes in the follicular phase

The tubes themselves are very fine pliable muscles lined with mucus secretions. It is this moisture in the tubes which expresses the Yin aspect of their function and is the aspect which benefits from the use of Yin tonic herbs at this stage of the cycle.

Midcycle phase (ovulation)

The ovary at midcycle

Eventually, the follicle reaches its optimum size – up to 2 cm across (see Fig. 2.13) and the endometrium is thick and blood-laden. In TCM, we would say the Yin is at the peak of its cycle, the Chong vessel is full of Blood and the Yang is just starting to exert its influence.

In the days leading up to ovulation, the growing follicle secretes more and more estrogen – or we may say the Yin grows and grows. In the immediate lead up to ovulation (36 h), and just before Yang arises, the pituitary sends signals (in the form of LH) to the follicle, preparing it to release the egg and stimulating it to produce more progesterone. A small protrusion on the follicle secretes mucus and softens. At the same time, the follicle swells, which weakens the follicle wall, especially at the location of the damp protrusion, and the egg inside is loosened. During the next few hours the follicle ruptures at this weakened site and the egg, which is surrounded with a sticky cloud of 5 million nurse cells, collectively called the cumulus mass, is released into the waiting grasp of the fallopian tube's fingers, the fimbriae (Fig. 2.15).

These events reflect the arrival of the Yang part of the Yin-Yang cycle and it is at this point we start to see Yang tonic herbs appearing in prescriptions. The release of the egg is usually accompanied by a little bleeding from the ovary into the abdomen and this is one of the reasons it is advisable to add Blood-regulating herbs to herbal formulas at ovulation. In TCM, any blood not in its normal place (i.e. in a blood vessel) has the potential to become 'stagnant'.

In TCM theory, the Heart controls the collaterals of the uterus, especially the Bao vessel or Bao Mai. If the Heart Qi is obstructed due to emotional stress, the function of the Uterus will be affected and the processes of ovulation will be derailed. It is the action of the Heart via the Bao Mai that keeps the Uterus 'open' at this time of the month, i.e., the egg can be released and the sperm can be granted passage into the uterus. The Heart is also said to control the Kidney Yin and Kidney Yang. If the switch from Kidney Yin to Kidney Yang at this midcycle point of the menstrual cycle is not orchestrated correctly by the Heart (perhaps as a result of emotional disturbance) ovulation does not occur.

The cervix at midcycle

The cervix responds to increased estrogen levels by opening, and the glands in the endocervix (the canal leading through the cervix to the uterine cavity) respond by producing fertile mucus (Fig. 2.16).

The purpose of the fertile mucus is to aid the survival of sperm and their movement from the vagina through the cervix. In ideal conditions (plenty of estrogen and flourishing Yin), a cascade of mucus pours from the cervical

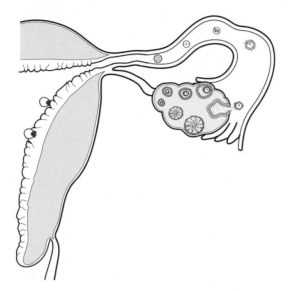

Figure 2.15 The egg is released from the ovary and travels down the tube to the uterus.

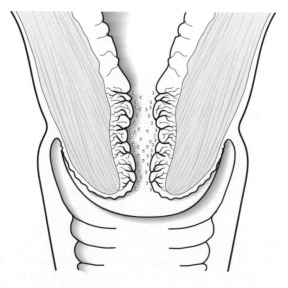

Figure 2.16 Glands in the cervix produce fertile mucus.

glands to the vagina. The chemical and physical nature of this mucus is such that all its mucoprotein strands line up, creating unimpeded passageways along which the sperm can pass.

The alignment of the mucin strands makes the mucus very elastic and it is this quality that is easily checked subjectively by women who are charting their cycles to determine fertile and non-fertile times (see Ch. 3). The secretions also provide a more hospitable pH than the acidic vagina does for the sperm and they contain nutrients which help to activate the sperm and make them swim vigorously.

The arrival of fertile mucus signifies the fertile time of the month. The mucus may be evident for a few hours or several days. For a woman trying to fall pregnant, it is more useful to produce plentiful fertile mucus over several days. This increases the chances of sex occurring at a time when the sperm can survive the acidity of the vagina and can be actively aided in breaching the cervix and traversing the uterus. It is the nature of Yin and Blood herbal tonics to increase the quantity and quality of fertile mucus (presumably via increased estrogen levels) and indeed this is often one of the first changes noticed by women who start taking such herbs.

The estrogen peak, which occurs before ovulation, drops sharply and the cervix responds equally quickly. The cervical secretions dry up over night (so rapidly that they may have disappeared by the very day that the egg is actually released) to be replaced by a thick, dry or pasty discharge. This rapid switch from wet to dry presents a dramatic demonstration of the switch from Yin (moistening) to Yang (warming). Just as sudden is the relocation of the cervix from high in the vagina to a low position. The os (opening) of the cervix closes at the same time. In TCM terms this change of position of the uterus is a reflection of the shift of predominance of activity of the Chong vessel to the Ren vessel.

The fallopian tube at midcycle

It is not only the follicle and the egg that have very active roles to play in the ovulation event – the fallopian tube does not just stand by passively or stiffly. The fingers (fimbriae) of the fallopian tube move to catch the sticky mass and steer it into the head (ampulla) of the tube. And the journey in the tube is not just a blind roll downwards to the uterus. The ciliated and mucusy lining of the tube must carefully usher the egg along its interior, initially to about the half-way point (the isthmus) where the tube becomes much narrower and the mucus is thicker. It is at this junction that the egg is held up to await a passing sperm.

The slowly rising levels of progesterone (Kidney yang) have another important role to play in this fallopian tube arena. The sperm that have made it thus far rely on the action of this progesterone to activate a calcium ion channel in the tail which not only helps the sperm to find the egg but also to penetrate its hard outer coating.[10] The rising Kidney yang of the female cycle feeds and boosts the Kidney yang activity of the sperm.

The zygote or pre-embryo (as the egg will be called after there has been a successful encounter with a sperm) will wait here for 2 or 3 days until the isthmus muscles relax and the secretions are thin enough to allow the zygote's journey to continue to the uterus. The secretions in the tube provide crucial nourishment for the egg and the zygote (Fig. 2.17).

The estrogen produced by the developing follicle is what stimulates the production of this mucus in the fallopian tube in an attempt to protect the fallopian walls from the burrowing instincts of the new embryo and the advent of an ectopic pregnancy. When progesterone starts to be produced by the corpus luteum, this mucus becomes thinner, allowing free and unobstructed passage to the uterus but increasing the risk of the embryo being able to implant in the wall of the tube if for some reason the journey to the uterus is held up (see also Ch. 8).

This is why TCM treatments applied at this stage encourage the removal of obstruction and unfettered, rapid movement. Providing there is a good solid basis of Yin (i.e., the mucus secretions are adequate to hold the egg at the isthmus), there is little risk of the egg traveling too rapidly down the tube, even with enthusiastic acupuncture treatment.

In TCM terms, the release of the egg and its smooth passage down the fallopian tube is said to require free and unobstructed movement of Qi. Therefore at midcycle, Qi-regulating herbs are used, as are acupuncture points which help the Qi to move freely in the abdomen and especially around and through the tubes. Herbs may also be employed at midcycle to help dissolve thick mucusy secretions which have been built up in the follicular phase

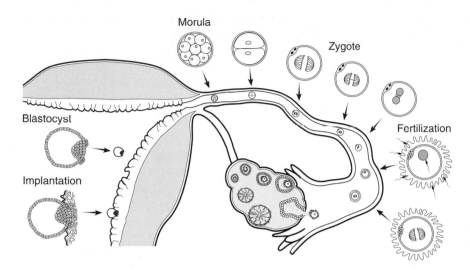

Figure 2.17 The embryo divides as it passes down the tube.

but now need to be dispelled for free passage from the isthmus of the tube to the uterus. If there is a problem like scarring or kinking, or adhesions in or around the tubes which hinder their free movement or obstruct their internal passage, then Blood-regulating herbs, which have more effect on substantial blockages, will be added (see Ch. 6).

The Yang tonics applied from about the time the LH starts to be released also aid in flexibility of the tube and movement of the egg. In particular, they might be supposed to help the muscles in the isthmus relax and its secretions to be dispelled.

As ovulation approaches, we first bear in mind the readiness of the egg to be launched and fertilized, i.e., the quality and quantity of the Yin and the Jing is emphasized. If the Yin or the Jing is deficient and the egg is therefore not optimum quality, there is little in the way of effective treatment to be applied at this stage of the cycle when it is about to be released. Preparatory work for future cycles and future eggs can begin, however, at any point. Blood status is important as ovulation draws near, because the lining of the uterus must be ready to receive the fertilized egg, i.e., the Chong vessel must be full of Blood.

At the culmination of Yin, not only is the egg completely ripe and ready for ovulation but also there is plentiful mucus secretion from the cervix, in the fallopian tube and on the section of the follicle wall, which softens enough to allow the escape of the egg. All these secretions reflect the moistening action of Yin, and can be promoted by the use of Yin tonic herbs.

As the LH surge heralds the imminent release of the egg, the Yang aspect of the cycle is encouraged with the introduction of herbs with Yang activity. These help to moderate somewhat the sticky and potentially obstructive nature of the mucus secretions (called Damp in TCM if they are excessive or lingering), which occur when Yin is at its peak.

THE YANG PART OF THE CYCLE

Luteal phase (progestogenic or secretory phase)

Unlike the rather fickle and changeable nature of the follicular phase, the luteal phase – that period of time between ovulation and the beginning of menstruation – is the most constant and predictable part of the cycle in terms of its length and other measurable parameters. It is in this phase that progesterone is produced by the ovary and nutrients are secreted by the uterine lining (Fig. 2.18).

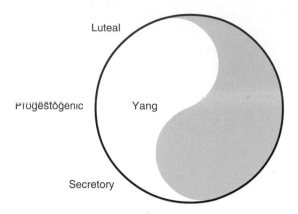

Figure 2.18 The Yang phase.

The ovary in the luteal phase

The empty follicle collapses and forms a gland called the corpus luteum (which is Latin for 'yellow body') inside the ovarian wall. The LH keeps stimulating it to produce progesterone, the most important hormone of this part of the cycle.

Progesterone has three important actions:

- It causes the endometrium to start secreting nutrients in case there is a conception

- It switches off the hormones which would otherwise keep ripening up more eggs

- It provokes changes in the main fertility signs by which women are monitoring their cycle – namely, BBT rises, cervical secretions become thick and pasty and the cervix moves lower in the vagina.

The progesterone produced by the corpus luteum has several actions on the body which are useful if we are monitoring hormonal activities in an attempt to pinpoint ovulation. It acts on the temperature-regulating centers in the hypothalamus in the brain.

Doctors of Chinese medicine first described the importance of a warm womb hundreds of years ago; however, physiologists are not sure why it is beneficial for the embryo or fetus to be in a slightly warmer environment. Chinese medicine describes a 'Cold' uterus as a common cause of infertility. Although this concept of increased 'warmth' in the luteal phase has been borne out by the observations that the body temperature is slightly raised after ovulation, Heat as a physiological parameter in TCM is a broader concept than just temperature. In TCM, the warmth of the uterus refers to its metabolic activity, actively manufacturing and secreting nutrients, and maintaining a highly nurturing home for a fetus.

The corpus luteum, which is responsible for maintaining the endometrium, continues to grow under the initial influence of the LH surge, but peaks in size at around 1.5 cm, about a week after ovulation. Without LH to sustain it, the corpus luteum begins to degenerate and by about Day 26 of a 28-day cycle, its secretory function finishes and the endometrium starts to break down. The life span of the corpus luteum in a normal menstrual cycle usually stays constant for any given woman, varying maybe just 1 or 2 days at the outside.

The corpus luteum seems to be well insulated from the vicissitudes of life's ups and downs in its cosy nook inside the ovarian wall (well away from the brain and all its mental activity) and rarely wavers in its job of producing adequate levels of progesterone for enough time to ensure the implantation and survival of an embryo. The exception to this rule (there always is one, and it is here that the doctor steps in) is the 'inadequate luteal phase' or 'luteal phase defect,' a diagnosis which refers to a short luteal phase because the corpus luteum suffers an early demise. Of course, this means there may not be enough time for an embryo to implant successfully and can be a cause of infertility. Such a failure of Kidney Yang function is easily remedied by TCM treatment.

If a conception occurs and implantation of the embryo is successful, the hormone it produces (human chorionic gonadotrophin, hCG) tells the corpus luteum to remain active for a couple more months until the placenta itself is ready to take over.

The endometrium in the secretory phase

After ovulation, and in response to the hormones produced by the corpus luteum, there is a change in the activity of the endometrium. There is no more proliferation of glandular cells and the lining stops growing thicker. The arterioles continue to grow but because the endometrium does not get any thicker they become more and more compressed and twisted into spiral shapes.

The sequence of changes as the endometrium becomes more secretory are very precise. Four days after ovulation, at about the time the embryo is due to arrive in the uterus, the secretions are enough to fill the cells and appear in the glands. By 10 days after ovulation, the cells of the endometrial tissue are so plumped up with fluid they appear like one smooth surface.

This differentiation process is further characterized by a massive influx of specialized immune cells, especially uterine natural killer (uNK) cells, which are a rich source of growth and angiogenic factors essential for vascular remodeling. The process of decidualization allows simultaneous protection of the embryo against environmental or immunological insults and ensures hemostasis and tissue integrity during deep trophoblast invasion. These functions are highly dependent on good progesterone levels.

The stage of development of the endometrium must match the development of the embryo if implantation is to be effective. It can be viewed as a gatekeeper, allowing embryos to attach only under the right conditions. The so-called Window of Implantation (WOI) occupies a 4–5-day interval in the cycle, at the time when progesterone reaches peak serum concentrations. In a 28-day cycle, this window begins around Day 19 or 20.

If the endometrium has gone past the appropriate stage when the embryo arrives to take up residence, implantation will fail and the embryo will not survive. If the endometrium is lagging a little, or the passage of the pre-embryo down the fallopian tube is too rapid, successful implantation cannot be expected.

Sometimes, even if the timing is right and the embryo is as far as we know 'perfect', the endometrium will not be permissive. Certainly if it is not thick enough this is the case, but even in cases where the thickness is adequate, if an ultrasound shows a homogeneous or 'whited out' look (rather than a trilaminar appearance) it will not be hospitable for the new embryo. A uterine lining, which is not permissive to implantation may have developed in a disorderly way. This is another reason why we place so much emphasis on treatment during the menstrual and postmenstrual phase when the endometrium is being rebuilt.

Obstructions like polyps, fibroids or scarring may interfere with the way in which the endometrium grows. If such impediments to implantation are large or numerous, they will usually be dealt with before attempts at pregnancy.

During the luteal or Yang phase, the main emphasis of prescriptions is on herbs with Yang or warming attributes. One of the observed actions of these Yang herbs is to maintain the progesterone levels at a satisfactory level and thus the uterine lining is kept in a thick, juicy and receptive state in readiness for the possible arrival of the embryo.

Implantation

The most crucial aspect of this part of the cycle, if a conception has occurred, is implantation of the embryo within this cushion-like lining of the uterus. The embryo (in the form of a blastocyst) arrives in the uterus 4–6 days after ovulation and surveys the terrain for a suitable burrowing spot, probably targeting special attachment sites on the epithelial surface. In most successful cases, implantation is completed 8–10 days after ovulation and the majority of implantations that occur more than 11 days after ovulation will not last. On the other hand, a large majority of embryos which implant 9 days after ovulation will develop into healthy fetuses and the pregnancy will be secure.[11] Scientists doing this sort of research think that there is communication between the blastocyst and the prospective mother (via messenger proteins) about where and when to implant. Immune regulating factors are important in creating the right environment and although the mechanism is not understood it appears that an inflammatory reaction in the endometrial cells promotes implantation.[12]

Embryos with strong and abundant Kidney Jing are those most likely to implant and develop quickly (Fig. 2.19).

The process of implantation is aided by the uterus, which presses its front and back walls together, like a closed fist, holding the embryo firmly in place, until it is safely tucked into its endometrial bed. To achieve this snug pressure, all the fluid must be removed from the uterine cavity first. Physiologically, this is achieved very efficiently by the endometrial cells, which 'drink' the endometrial fluid (secretions) – the electron microscopists who take pictures of these gulps call them pinocytosis. If this function is inadequately performed, as may be the case in Kidney and

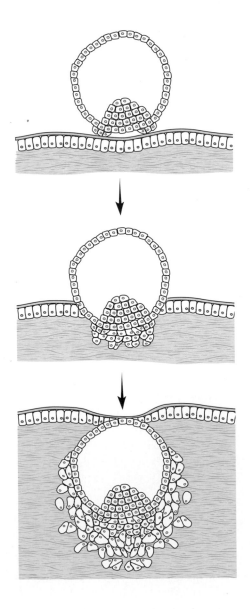

Figure 2.19 The blastocyst implants in the uterine wall.

Spleen Yang-deficient individuals, wherein fluids are not dealt with properly, then the surface of the endometrium may be too slippery or Damp for the fetus to get a foothold.

BACK TO THE DRAWING BOARD

When there is no conception, or if implantation fails, the endometrium will disintegrate and the period will arrive. We are back at Day 1 of another cycle and once again regulating the Blood and Qi will be our primary aim.

PARALLELS BETWEEN TCM AND WESTERN PARAMETERS

Having said at the outset of the chapter that making equivalences between descriptions of physiologic activity in the Western and Chinese medical framework is difficult because of the very different paradigms they are based upon, we *can* make some associations between terms that we are now familiar with applied to the menstrual cycle (Table 2.2).

Many of the actions or manifestations of Yin are what modern Western clinicians call the action of estrogen (Table 2.3). And perhaps we could go a little further and say the action of the pituitary hormones (FSH and LH) represent an aspect of Jing. Likewise, the Yang characteristics of the second part of the cycle are largely attributable to the action of progesterone.

Table 2.2   Summary of parallels between traditional Chinese medicine (TCM) and Western medicine terms

Western physiology	TCM
The gametes	Jing
The influence of the sex hormones	Kidney Yin and Yang
The influence of the hypothalamus and the pituitary	Heart
Ovaries, tubes, endometrium and cervix	Uterus

Table 2.3   Action of estrogen and progesterone in traditional Chinese medicine (TCM) terms

Western physiology	TCM
Estrogen promotes the growth of the follicle and egg (by its positive feedback on the pituitary)	Yin supports action of Jing
Estrogen stimulates the cervical glands to produce fertile mucus	Yin creates Fluids
Estrogen stimulates the cells of the fallopian tubes to produce nutrients and mucus along their linings	Yin creates Fluids
Progesterone lifts the body temperature	Yang warms the Uterus
Progesterone thins out the mucus secretions in the fallopian tube, thereby allowing the embryo passage	Yang transforms Fluids, clears Damp
Progesterone halts the production of fertile mucus from the cervix	Yang dries Fluids

REFERENCES

1. Macioca G. *The foundation of Chinese medicine*. Edinburgh: Churchill Livingstone; 1989.

2. Hansen M, Kurinczuk JJ, Bower C, et al. The risk of major birth defects after intracytoplasmic sperm injection and in vitro fertilization. *N Engl J Med* 2002;**346**(10):725–30.

3. Laura A, Schieve PD, Meikle MD, et al. Low and very low birth weight in infants conceived with use of assisted reproductive technology. *N Engl J Med* 2002;**346**(10):731–7.

4. Deadman P, Al-Khafaji M, Baker K. *A manual of acupuncture*. Hove: Journal of Chinese Medicine Publications Ltd; 1998.

5. Apter D. Development of the hypothalamic-pituitary-ovarian axis. *Ann NY Acad Sci* 1997;**816**:9–21.

6. Brosens JJ, Parker MG, McIndoe A, et al. A role for menstruation in preconditioning the uterus for successful pregnancy. *Am J Obstet Gynecol* 2009;**200**(6):e1–6:615.

7. Brosens JJ, Gellersen B. Death or survival – progesterone-dependent cell fate decisions in the human endometrial stroma. *J Mol Endocrinol* 2006;**36**(3):389–98.

8. Ford JH. *It takes two*. Adelaide: Environmental and Genetic Solutions; 1997, 178.

9. Ford JH. *It takes two*. Adelaide: Environmental and Genetic Solutions; 1997, 182.

10. Lishko PV, Botchkina IL, Kirichok Y. Progesterone activates the principal Ca2+ channel of human sperm. *Nature* 2011;**471**(7338):387–91.

11. Wilcox AJ, Baird D, Weinberg CR. Implantation of the conceptus and loss of pregnancy. *N Engl J Med* 1999;**340**(23):1796–9.

12. Gnainsky Y, Granot I, Paulomi B, et al. Local injury of the endometrium induces an inflammatory response that promotes successful implantation. *Fertil Steril* 2010;**94**(6):2030–6.

Charting the menstrual cycle

3

Chapter Contents

INTRODUCTION

For most women, there are only about 30 days in a year when there is a reasonable chance of conceiving. For a successful pregnancy to eventuate, a whole chain of events need to come together precisely in the woman's body, in her partner's body and in their relationship on one of those days. Being able to accurately identify these relatively rare opportunities raises the odds of success considerably. Watching external clues of the body provides us with a method to do exactly that.

THE BBT CHART

The basal body temperature (BBT) chart records the temperature of the body on waking. It is called basal because it is measured at a time when the body is deeply rested and the body's metabolism and temperature is at its baseline. A woman's basal body temperature rises after she has ovulated and begins to produce progesterone. In a typical menstrual cycle, a BBT chart looks something like that shown in Figure 3.1.

One of the very great strengths of Chinese medicine is discerning what is going on inside the body from watching or feeling what is going on on the outside of the body. Thus, the color and nature of the complexion tells us things about the functioning of the internal organs, as does the glint or lack thereof in the eyes, or the color and nature of the urine or the stools or the menstrual flow, or the strength of the artery at the wrist and inside the ankle, or the look of the tongue, and so on. The Chinese have observed so many minute details and over thousands of years correlated them with disease patterns or tendencies to manifest particular disease patterns but it was only in recent years that doctors in China incorporated into their battery of diagnostic skills two more external signs – namely,

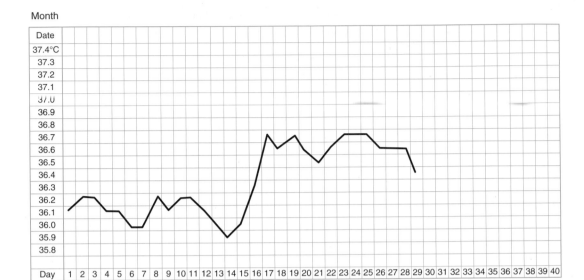

Figure 3.1 Typical basal body temperature (BBT) chart of 29-day cycle.

the change of basal body temperature observed during the menstrual cycle and the production of mucus by the cervix just before ovulation.

TCM gynecologists in China, having to rely on external observations more than pathology tests and investigative surgery, observed BBT patterns with a zeal and focus of attention that would not occur to a Western-trained gynecologist. Thus, the BBT chart has become a tool that reveals to TCM specialists so much more information than it does to a Western specialist. For most specialists in the West, reliance on laboratory results far supersedes reliance on information gathered by the patient and the doctor purely by careful observation. Thus, the BBT chart as a useful diagnostic tool is given little heed by most specialists in the West past indicating an ovulation or not.

Family planning and natural birth control advocates pay the BBT chart greater attention than do gynecologists but their aim is only to discover if, and more particularly when, an ovulation has occurred. The TCM specialist, as we shall discover, uses the BBT chart to discover much more than this.

Basal body temperature charts require no sophisticated equipment and are surprisingly sensitive to many factors related not only to the menstrual cycle but also to lifestyle and events.

Hot on the heels of the discovery of the changes of resting temperature during the menstrual cycle was the 'discovery' of the changes in vaginal secretions according to menstrual phase. Maybe this is one rare instance where Western physicians have noted and used for medical analysis a common external sign before doctors in China have. To be sure the Chinese have observed and said plenty over the last 2000 years about different sorts of vaginal discharges but to my knowledge they did not correlate changes in discharge with the menstrual cycle.

No matter who described the phenomenon first, TCM doctors have wasted little time in incorporating such useful observations into their diagnostic repertoire and have related quantity and quality of fertile mucus secretions to standard TCM diagnostic patterns.[1]

THE HOW'S AND WHY'S OF BBT MEASUREMENTS AND OTHER OBSERVATIONS

Recording the lowest body temperature each morning, and watching the secretions of the cervix and noting the changes in position in the cervix and then charting these observations will, over time, build an individual profile which is as informative as it is interesting. In addition, changes in breast symptoms, abdomen symptoms, bleeding patterns and general symptoms paint a picture that provides an accurate insight into the inner workings of those hormonal tides which ebb and flow each month.

HISTORY OF THE BBT CHART

The first people who started to examine menstrual charting were interested in improving the effectiveness of the rhythm method of contraception recommended by the Catholic religion. The rhythm method assumed that women ovulate on Day 14, or at least some time round the middle of the cycle. It had a woefully low success rate, simply because all women have different rhythms and any individual woman's rhythms can change from one cycle to the next, depending on what is happening in her life. Similarly, couples trying to fall pregnant who believed that intercourse had to occur on Day 14 sometimes had a long wait, especially if the woman had a long cycle and ovulated, say, on Day 18 each month.

Researchers in this field then made the serendipitous discovery that the basal body temperature rose after ovulation, which added a welcome objective verification of ovulation. A method called natural family planning was developed based on this knowledge and women who measured their basal temperature were assured that they could feel quite confident that they were infertile after the basal temperature had risen. The rise in temperature reflects the action on the temperature-regulating centers of the brain by progesterone, a hormone which is produced after ovulation. The action of progesterone in lifting basal body temperature is clearly important enough to be conserved through many thousands of years of natural selection, since this hormone and its thermal activity appears in all our mammalian predecessors.

More advances came when researchers in Australia, the two Dr Billings, examined the relationship of hormonal production, cervical secretions and ovulation.[2] They were able to establish that there was a reliably reproducible cyclic pattern in the cervical discharges (in response to estrogen and progesterone production) and that the most dramatic and easily observed changes occurred before and after ovulation. The work of two professors working at Melbourne and Monash Universities also confirmed that women's own awareness of their cervical mucus could indicate ovulation more accurately than measurements of hormones by blood tests.[3]

Now the contraceptive method, approved by the Catholic Church, could be developed to a sophisticated enough degree that it actually worked. In fact the sympto-thermal method, as it rather clumsily came to be called, boasts a success rate as a contraceptive method of 98%. This compares very favorably with the rate for the condom of 97% and the oral contraceptive pill of 99.5%.[4] Teaching programs sprung up all over the Western world and the method is variously called FAM (fertility awareness method), NFP (natural family planning) or the Billings method. The method not only gave women a wonderful insight into the workings of their own bodies but also liberated them from the need to use chemicals and devices if they did not want to fall pregnant.

Of course the very useful corollary of this method which was developed as a contraceptive aid was that it also could work the other way – it could help women conceive. Knowing when you're fertile and need to avoid intercourse became knowing when you're fertile and need to have intercourse. Not only do the chances of falling pregnant rise dramatically when intercourse is timed appropriately but the pregnancies which result from the precise timing of conception are generally more secure and the incidence of miscarriage is lower.[5]

The more that was learned about the qualities of the fertile mucus, the more was learned about how some aspects of fertility can be enhanced or hindered. For example, observation of the behavior of sperm in the fertile mucus can uncover some impediments to conception. Sometimes the mucus is too acid, or too alkaline, or may contain antibodies. There are various ways these can be overcome. It may be as simple as douching with dilute vinegar, for an alkaline vagina, or sodium bicarbonate for a too acid one. Antibodies in the fertile mucus is a little more difficult to treat and is discussed later.

Let us now revisit the cyclical changes of the cervix, ovaries and uterus. In this section, we wish to focus on the external cues produced by internal physiologic changes and what they tell us about fertility. These close observations are very useful in pinpointing subtle nuances which the TCM practitioner (or other infertility specialist) will use in their diagnosis.

To start, all that is needed is a thermometer, a chart (see, e.g., Fig. 3.2) and a good night's sleep (or at least 3–4 unbroken hours). For those women having regular menstrual cycles, charting starts at the beginning of a cycle, i.e., the first day of bleeding. For women not having periods or having them very sporadically, charting can start immediately but may be followed by a lengthy wait for a pattern to emerge.

Some women find charting their temperature makes them feel too obsessed by and focused on the whole business of getting pregnant; or, on the other hand, if they are not ovulating, too demoralized. To the former, it may be good advice to try charting for just three cycles so a pattern can be established. That pattern may be helpful in pinpointing a reason for a delay in falling pregnant, as we shall see below. Then taking the BBT each day can be dropped if it is truly causing distress. However, in most cases, I find that the woman becomes as curious as I am about her chart and starts to see it as a friendly tool rather than something reminding her of infertility. The journey together becomes an exciting one, as we start to see the effects of treatment on the shape of the chart and on her symptoms and signs.

For those women feeling demoralized by a chart showing no temperature changes, i.e., no ovulation, we will usually drop that method for a few months and concentrate on observing changes in fertile mucus secretions from the cervix. Hopefully, these will happen in response to treatment. As soon as an increase in discharge is noticed, then recording the basal temperature is again encouraged, so that the putative ovulation can be registered by a rise in basal body temperature.

Let us now go through the technique step by step.

The thermometer

In the case of recording and comparing changes in the resting or basal temperature of the body a reliable thermometer is needed – the change is a subtle fluctuation and not one which can be discerned subjectively, as can fever. A mercury or digital thermometer can be used. Digital thermometers are a little easier to read, especially in those groggy first few minutes of the day just after waking, but they are more expensive than the mercury type, and they can be slightly less accurate (although this is not usually a problem for our purposes). It is possible to buy a mercury thermometer designed to measure only the basal body temperature (called a basal body temperature thermometer). In this case the scale covers a narrower range than usual and the gradations are more spread out and easier to read than on a regular thermometer. However, most women use the regular thermometer normally kept in the bathroom cupboard for measuring fevers. Now, however, the thermometer will be kept on the bedside table.

On waking in the morning, after at the very least 3 h uninterrupted sleep, the thermometer is placed in the mouth and left for 3–5 min. BBT can also be measured by placing the thermometer in the vagina or rectum. Because these routes are slightly less convenient, they are less often used. However, if we are finding that the temperature readings are very erratic and it is hard to determine a pattern, then I sometimes recommend the vaginal route, which can give a more stable pattern.

The thermometer is removed, the temperature reading taken and its value noted on the chart under the correct day and date. For a mercury thermometer, it can be placed carefully on the bedside table and the reading taken some time later in the morning or even when going to bed the next evening. This is because most mercury thermometers will remain stable at the temperature they have reached until the mercury is given

Month

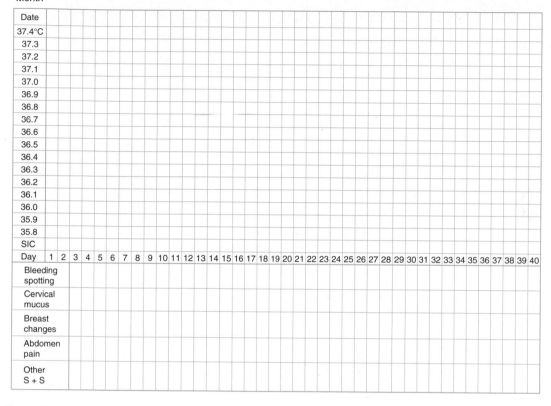

Figure 3.2 BBT chart (blank). S + S = signs and symptoms; SIC = sexual intercourse.

a firm shake down with a sharp flick of the wrist. After reading and recording the temperature, the mercury in the thermometer should be returned to its base level and the thermometer wiped clean ready for the next morning's use.

It is important that the temperature is read at roughly the same time each morning, because later waking raises the basal body temperature. Thus, a very erratic-looking chart may reflect nothing more than a rather erratic sleep and waking pattern. Some studies have shown that the basal temperature rises 0.09°C for each hour of delayed rising in the morning.[6] Thus, BBT charts can be adjusted for different waking times by moving the recorded temperature one square up or down for each hour of waking earlier or later than usual.

The urinary ovulation predictor kit

These kits can be used to test for the rise in luteinizing hormone (LH) prior to ovulation, i.e., at the later stages of the follicular phase. LH produced by the pituitary as the dominant follicle ripens usually does not last very long in circulation and so these kits test for a form of LH that has an extended life span due to transformation in the urine. It is recommended that the urine is tested during the day (not first thing in the morning) after avoiding liquids for about 2 h (so that the urine is not too dilute). A positive reading will show two colored lines with the test line being equal to or darker than the control line. This indicates the LH levels have risen and that an egg will probably be released within 12–48 h. Using the predictor kit in conjunction with the BBT is a useful strategy, especially if the fertile mucus signs are not pronounced. It gives a reliable guide to the most fertile days of the cycle and the best days to be having sex.

The chart

Many different variations of the BBT chart have been developed over the years, initially by those using BBT as a contraceptive tool. Basically, all charts record the basal body temperature and compare the values over the entire menstrual cycle. As other kinds of fertility signals were described (e.g., cervical fluid and position) by the Billings', then provision was made for these to be recorded alongside the temperature readings. Room for other items of personal interest, such as dates of sexual intercourse, or late nights or the occurrence of relevant symptoms has also been added.

Each day the temperature is recorded on the chart, along with other observations related to fluctuations in the hormones (Fig. 3.2), e.g., changes in breast and nipple tenderness or swelling may be noticed or changes in abdomen bloating or discomfort, in sleep patterns, in moods, in food cravings and, most importantly, changes in vaginal lubrication and discharge (this latter can also include spotting of blood).

Fertile mucus

The changes in vaginal discharge which flag changes in fertility are determined both by subjective feelings of moisture at the vulva and by more objective observation of the discharge collected on underclothes, toilet tissue or fingers.

The estrogen peak, which stimulates the production of fertile mucus, usually starts on average 6 days before ovulation. Four different types of mucus are produced by specialized glands in the cervix in response to this estrogen (Fig. 3.3).[7] The cervical discharge produced at infertile times (i.e., at all times except ovulation) is associated with a dry feeling at the vulva. It is called G-type mucus and is thick, pasty and impenetrable. It is produced in crypts of the cervix at the end of the cervical os nearest the vagina (Fig. 3.4). As estrogen levels begin to rise, the cervix produces, from crypts a little higher in the cervix, the more liquid L-type of mucus. This causes the vaginal sensation to be more sticky or wet. As ovulation approaches, crypts still higher in the cervical os produce mucus which is more stretchy and slippery. It is this S-type mucus that is sometimes referred to as the egg-white-like mucus. The sensation at the vulva now is distinctly wet and strings of S mucus, sometimes mixed with clumps of L mucus, may be noticed. The phenomenon which gives this mucus its elasticity is called spinnbarkeit, or 'spinn' for short.

Finally, as ovulation is imminent, the mucus loses its stretch as the cervix produces its P mucus from the very top of the cervical canal. P mucus is so named for its rich potassium content. While this final secretion is less thick and stretchy, it is extremely lubricative and produces a slippery sensation in the vulva. The last day that P mucus is produced is the most fertile day of the whole cycle, i.e., the day before the egg is released or the day it is released.

Fertile mucus forms graphic ferning patterns when it is dried on a smooth surface such as a glass microscope slide. The three different types of fertile mucus crystallize in three distinct patterns: the L mucus makes intricate and many branched ferns; the S mucus makes delicate pine needles lined up close and parallel; and the P mucus makes hexagons (Fig. 3.5).

The function of the branched L mucus is to catch and filter out some of the abnormal or poor-quality sperm before they reach even the uterus. The S mucus, on the other hand, provides a rapid sperm transit system, as it creates clear pathways for them to swim upwards to the uterus. Because it is composed of mucin strands lined up longitudinally it has the unusual quality of being particularly stretchy and adhesive to itself. For example if you tried to pour fertile mucus from one cup to another you would have to cut the flow with scissors if you wanted to stop it halfway.

The P mucus appears to have some quality which gives sperms a final boost or activation as they climb through the cervix to the uterus.

A summary of fertile mucus characteristics is given in Table 3.1.

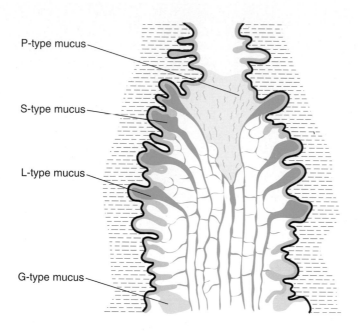

P-type mucus

S-type mucus

L-type mucus

G-type mucus

Figure 3.3 Glands inside the cervix produce different types of mucus.

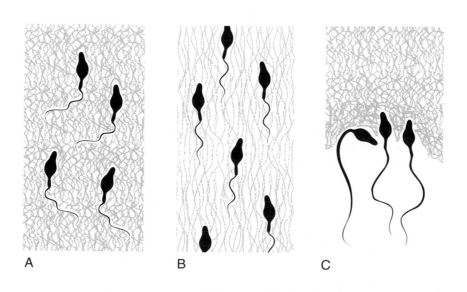

A   B   C

Figure 3.4 Three types of fertile mucus: (A) L-type mucus, (B) S-type mucus, and (C) G-type mucus.

43

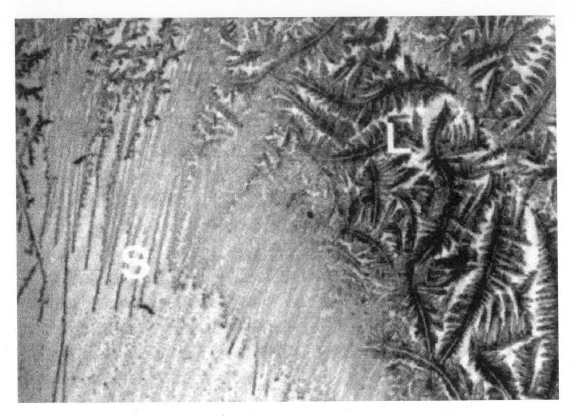

Figure 3.5 Fertile mucus makes (L) fern- or (S) needle-shaped crystals when dried on a slide.

Table 3.1   Summary of fertile mucus characteristics

	Characteristics	Function
G type	Thick, pasty and impenetrable	Blocks entrance to uterus
L type	Sticky or wet. When dried, makes intricate branched ferns	Catches and filters out some of the abnormal or poor-quality sperm before they reach the uterus
S type	Stretchy and slippery like egg white. When dried, makes delicate pine needle shapes	Creates or facilitates pathways for sperm entry to the uterus
P type	Lubricating. When dried, makes hexagons	Activates sperm as they pass through the cervix to the uterus

One easy way to evaluate quality and quantity of cervical secretions is to collect a little from the vaginal entrance (if it is plentiful enough) or gently from the cervical surface itself (if it is less plentiful) with clean fingers and see how much elasticity there is as the fingers are drawn apart (Fig. 3.6). Some women prefer to use toilet tissue to collect the fluid or rely on sensations of moisture alone. Some teachers of the Billings' method stress learning to interpret the subjective sensations of dryness or lubrication at the vulva without further investigations using the fingers (presumably to avoid introducing infection to the vagina or for cultural reasons when this method is taught in developing countries).

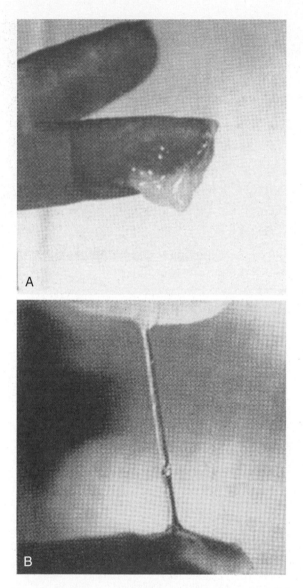

Figure 3.6 Examination of stretchy fertile mucus. (A) G-type mucus – no spinn. (B) S-type mucus – spinn.

The importance of recognizing the changes in the fertile mucus lies in the fact that it precedes ovulation and therefore alerts a woman to her most fertile days. The last day of any fertile mucus, whether seen as a secretion from the vagina or felt as a moist sensation, is often referred to as the 'peak day'. This refers to the day of peak fertility, the day before or the day the egg is released. Nature's design for conception is not random at all but has designed very exact timing. Producing the fertile mucus to facilitate the sperm's journey up the cervix in the days *before* ovulation is aimed at getting these sperm inside the female reproductive tract well before the egg is released (Fig. 3.7). This is because this largest single cell in the body is one of the shortest lived, being fertilizable for only 6–12 h. Some of the millions of lively little sperm cells, on the other hand, have been known to survive for 5 days in the female reproductive tract, although they are most able to fertilize the egg in the first 48 h after delivery to the vagina. So, ideally, there will be a bunch of some hundreds of eager sperm that have survived the hazardous journey as far as the fallopian tubes, lying in wait for the egg as she is launched. Some studies

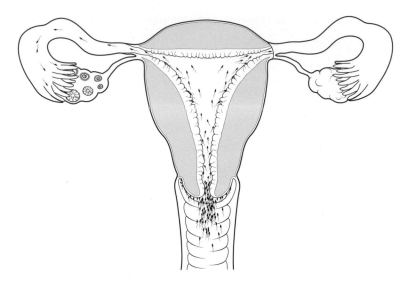

Figure 3.7 Sperm travel from the vagina through the cervix to the uterus and fallopian tubes.

have indicated that the day for sexual intercourse which then leads to the highest conception rate is, in fact, 2 days before ovulation.

The post-coital test

The post-coital test or PCT (also known as Sims–Huhner test) is an interesting test for examining the interaction of cervical mucus with the sperm. Sadly, this simple test is seldom performed in these days of the sophisticated ART clinic although a few facilities still offer it. The PCT looks at the sperm activity in the cervical mucus after sex. Because it must be carried out when there is fertile mucus present, i.e., close to the time of ovulation – the female partner is usually 'tracked' for several days with blood or urine tests to determine her hormonal status. She therefore has accurate warning of approaching ovulation. Fertile mucus leading up to ovulation can be removed on a swab and assessed for a number of criteria such as pH. On the day of ovulation or just before ovulation, the couple are requested to have sexual intercourse and then the woman attends the clinic some hours later for some of the fluid in the cervical canal to be removed and examined. A negative test shows no progressively motile sperm and a positive test shows more than five motile sperm per high power microscope field. Where the test is negative, the female partner sometimes receives the unfortunate label 'hostile' cervix or 'hostile' mucus. What this usually means is that there are antibodies in the mucus which disable or immobilize the sperm.

This test gives us a good idea about fertile mucus quality and sperm performance, and whether there are antibodies to the sperm. However, the useful information we receive from this cheap and non-invasive test does not necessarily influence what ART specialists can offer and so is often dispensed with by such specialists these days. For example, one prominent IVF specialist says,

> Many couples will quite correctly opt for assisted conception whether the PCT is positive or negative. The complexities of timing the PCT, the indirectness of the limited information it provides and probability of recourse to treatment such as IVF irrespective of its result mean that many doctors dispense with it.[8]

In fact, timing the PCT is simple compared to the complexities of tracking with frequent blood tests and ultrasounds the artificially engineered menstrual cycles for IVF procedures. The information it gives us about the quality of the fertile mucus and the behavior of the sperm in it is as direct as any laboratory procedure so far designed in infertility investigations and while the information it provides is of course limited to events at the level of the cervix it is nevertheless useful when the couple are not ready to launch straight into the expensive and demanding technologic route. The relatively non-invasive PCT can provide information which is useful when pursuing other types of treatment. For example, a TCM practitioner can use to good advantage the results of a PCT – it tells us information about the Yin status of the female partner and how the Yin and the Yang of the two partners interact, nourish or facilitate each other. And, theoretically, the more we can refine our diagnosis and hone in exactly on the subtle nuances of this Yin–Yang dance, the more chance we have of exerting an effective influence on the couples' fertility.

The oral contraceptive pill and fertile mucus

Some doctors have observed, and some pill manufacturers have published warnings about, a certain type of fertility impairment after stopping the combined oral contraceptive pill, even after the return of regular periods[9]: this condition occurs only in some women and seems to be independent of the number of years the pill has been taken. It appears that the mucus produced by the cervix in these women having difficulty getting pregnant after being on the pill is largely the G type, even though ovulation may be occurring. Thus, sperm cannot gain entry to the cervix.[10] There is no medical treatment for this condition, which can last for up to 30 months in unfortunate women; however, applying the protocols outlined in Chapter 4 will address many different disorders of fertile mucus, including post-pill disturbances.

Other drugs and fertile mucus

- Antibiotics can provoke an overgrowth of vaginal candida or thrush in sensitive women. If this is severe, it will mask any evidence of fertile mucus. The thrush must be treated with antifungal agents (pharmaceutical or herbal) before the fertile mucus signs become clearly evident again.

- NSAIDs (non-steroidal anti-inflammatory drugs), used as analgesics, lower the prostaglandin levels and, as such, can influence the menstrual cycle and cause fertile mucus to become more scanty in some users.

- Antidepressants – including the selective serotonin reuptake inhibitors (SSRIs) – can also change the cervical mucus pattern, usually reducing the number of days of production of fertile mucus.

- Antihistamines can dry fertile mucus, since they dry most of the mucous membranes in the body.

- Clomifene, a fertility drug which stimulates pituitary activity, acts as an antiestrogen, inhibiting the function of the mucus-producing glands in the cervix.

Chinese medicine and fertile mucus

The TCM doctor is very interested in cervical mucus. The quantity and quality will tell us a lot about some important aspects of female fertility. Specifically, it reflects some aspects of the Yin energy. As we have seen before in Chapter 2, the Yin energy is an important prerequisite for not only ripening a mature, attractive and fertile egg but also for establishing a good ground for implantation – a thick and nourishing uterine lining. Fertile mucus is just one of a number of external cues we can use in assessing the Yin status.

If the fertile mucus is inadequate in quantity or quality, there are Chinese herbal treatments which can be used to address this. Earlier in this chapter, we described the different types of mucus produced by the different glands in the cervix. In Chapter 4, when we look more precisely at how Chinese herbs can influence the steps in the development of the egg and the preparation of the female body, you will see that the Blood and Yin tonics are important in the production of good-quality L mucus (and vaginal lubrication in general) but that small quantities of Yang tonics influence the production of the S mucus and finally, as Yang tonics are taken over a few more days, the P mucus.

Treatment which emphasizes quantity and quality of fertile mucus carries special importance if sperm numbers or motility are low. An environment which maximizes survival of sperm and encourages entry to the uterus may be all the advantage lightly handicapped sperm need.

Position of the cervix

Some women find it useful to observe changes in the cervix itself as ovulation is approached. As the hormones signal the approach of ovulation, the shape, position and texture of the cervix changes. The ligaments that support the uterus respond to the peak of estrogen, which occurs just before ovulation by tightening: this has the effect of pulling the uterus further up in the body, and thus the cervix is positioned higher in the vagina. As the cervix moves higher in the vagina, it is a little more difficult to reach and some women find they need to squat to find its surface (Fig. 3.8). The texture of the surface of the cervix is softer at ovulation.

As the cervical glands release their fluid, the os of the cervix opens. This is clearly apparent to any woman who wishes to palpate the surface of her cervix. This can be checked conveniently at the same time as checking the fertile mucus, probably during the evening shower.

After ovulation, the position of the cervix is once again low in the vagina and quite easily palpated with a finger without resorting to contortionist antics.

PUTTING IT ALL TOGETHER

The advantage of combining the BBT measurements with the observations of the cervix and its secretions is that they provide complementary information and can corroborate each other. Only the fertile mucus and LH predictor kits can indicate that ovulation is about to happen, but only the temperature shift observed in the BBT can show that ovulation has happened.

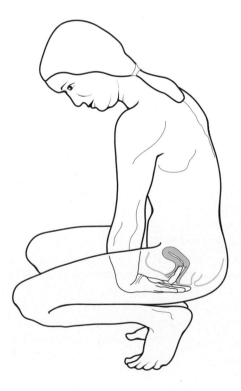

Figure 3.8 Finding the cervix.

Once all these factors have been observed and charted throughout one menstrual cycle, what can we deduce? See, e.g., the chart shown in Figure 3.9. The numbers on this chart indicate:

1. *Follicular phase* – the first half of the cycle before ovulation should record relatively lower temperatures.

2. *Luteal phase* – after ovulation the temperatures should remain at a relatively higher level for 12–14 days.

3. *Ovulation* – the day before the temperatures become elevated is the most likely day of ovulation.

4. *The thermal shift* – the temperature rise should be 0.3°C or 0.4°C.

5. *Sexual intercourse* – frequency of sexual intercourse can be recorded in this column.

6. *Bleeding* – period flow and spotting can be recorded quantitatively with + signs.

7. *Cervical mucus* – changes such as the progression from dry to wet to slippery mucus are recorded. Different women may choose different symbols to record their observations (see below).

8. *Breast changes* – nipple tenderness and breast swelling or soreness can be recorded in this column.

9. *Abdomen discomfort* – ovulation or period pain can be recorded quantitatively with + signs in this column.

10. *Other signs and symptoms* – emotional changes, headaches, lower back pain or insomnia, etc., which may or may not be related to the menstrual cycle can be recorded in this column. A night of insomnia, drinking a lot of alcohol or fever can all push the BBT up. Individual symbols may be chosen. Any other events such as illness, travel or stress which might affect the cycle can also be recorded here.

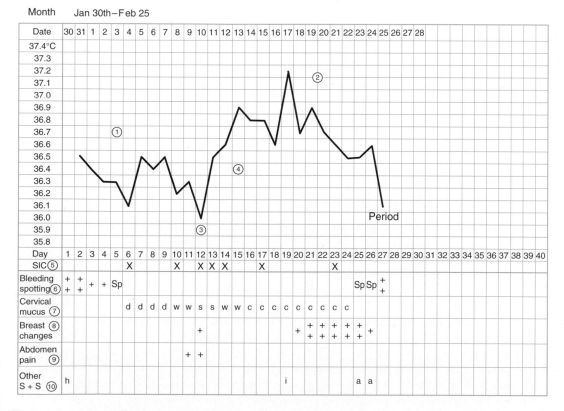

Figure 3.9 Example of BBT chart completed by patient. S + S = signs and symptoms; SIC = sexual intercourse.

In this particular chart (see Fig. 3.9):

1. The follicular phase average temperature was 36.3–36.4°C.

2. The luteal phase average temperature was 36.8°C; the elevated temperatures were maintained for 14 days, which indicates an adequate luteal phase and good progesterone levels.

3. Ovulation occurred on Day 12 or 13.

4. A thermal shift of 0.4°C between the average temperatures occurred.

5. Sexual intercourse occurred on Days 6, 10, 12, 13, 14, 17 and 23.

6. The period lasted 4 days with spotting on the day after the period and 2 days before the next period.

7. Cervical mucus was not evident after the period, i.e., the sensation was dry (d) until Day 10 and 11 when the vaginal sensation became wet (w) then slippery or stretchy (s) on Days 12 and 13. After ovulation the discharge was creamy or crumbly (c).

8. Breast swelling or soreness was experienced on the 6 days leading up to the period.

9. Some abdomen pain was experienced on the first day of the period and at ovulation.

10. A headache (h) occurred on the first day of the period and a night of insomnia (i) the night of Day 18, which pushed the temperature up on Day 19. Premenstrual anger was experienced (a).

BBT CHARTS AND PATTERN DIAGNOSIS

Pattern variations

The following methods of analyzing BBT charts were first described by doctors working in fertility clinics in China[1] in the 1990s.

To begin with, we examine in some detail the sorts of patterns which might occur in the first 2 weeks of a menstrual cycle, i.e., before ovulation.

The follicular or low phase

Day 1 of the menstrual period is the first day of the follicular phase. From the day (or the day before) the menstrual period starts, the BBT should drop to its base level. This level can vary from woman to woman and to a lesser extent from cycle to cycle. Its average range is 36.2–36.5°C.

When the follicular phase is too low

The follicular phase of the cycle is naturally the lower phase of the biphasic graph; however, in some cases, the temperature readings are consistently extremely low (Fig. 3.10). If they are below the bottom level of the chart, i.e., below 36.0°C, this is an indication of a very low metabolic rate and low thyroid activity may be suspected. Accompanying symptoms which may be reported could be lethargy, weight gain and sensitivity to cold. Low thyroid activity is thought to affect fertility. In the most severe cases hypothyroidism can contribute to ovarian failure (this usually involves an autoimmune condition). Chinese medicine will describe this person as generally Yang deficient (or specifically Spleen and Kidney Yang deficient) and will apply treatment throughout the whole

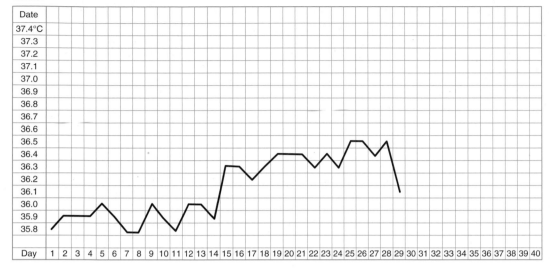

Figure 3.10 Follicular phase is too low.

menstrual cycle to address this fundamental deficiency, i.e., to stimulate metabolism and warm the patient with the use of moxibustion and by using herbs that are heating in nature.

Later, when we examine the luteal phase, we will see a particular and specific type of Yang deficiency that affects the temperature of only the second phase of the cycle and possibly the progesterone levels produced after ovulation. This specific type of Kidney Yang deficiency may not involve general body symptoms and requires a special protocol of timed treatment which will be outlined in the next section.

When the follicular phase is too long

The length of the menstrual cycle is usually determined by the length of the follicular phase, i.e., the length of the follicular phase is variable, reflecting as it does the length of time it takes for the follicle in the ovary to grow to a certain size (around 2 cm) and then release a mature egg. In women with a 28-day cycle the follicular phase will typically be 14 days, but in women with a 35-day cycle this phase will last around 21 days and in women with a 24-day cycle it will be around 10 days. All are thought to be quite acceptable variations from the norm, although TCM treatment will attempt to steer the follicular phase towards 14 days.

Once ovulation has occurred, the luteal phase tends to be a standard 12–14 days, unless there is a defect in the function of the corpus luteum. This situation is described later in the subsection 'Short luteal phase.'

According to TCM if ovulation is delayed (Fig. 3.11), then one of the prerequisite substances or conditions is absent or insufficient or the process of ovulation is obstructed (known as Qi stagnation) or the Shen or Heart is disordered (see Chs 2 and 4).

As described previously, the 'nutrients' required for an egg to develop to the point where it is ripe enough to be released and fertilized are the Kidney Jing, Kidney Yin and the Blood. If the Kidney Jing is insufficient, then ovulation will often be late or missed altogether in severe cases. Fertility can be severely compromised in these cases and even if conception is achieved the fetus may not be viable. The medicinals which strengthen Kidney Jing and Yin and nourish the Blood will be prescribed, often for a lengthy time.

During these cycles with extended follicular phases the woman may notice the fertile type of cervical mucus for longer than usual, or none at all.

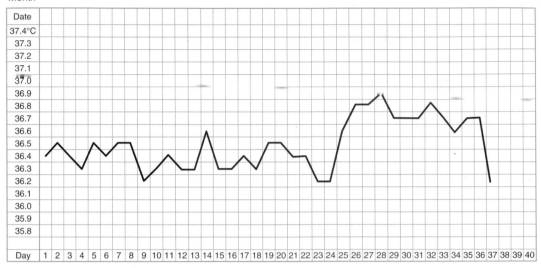

Figure 3.11 Follicular phase is too long.

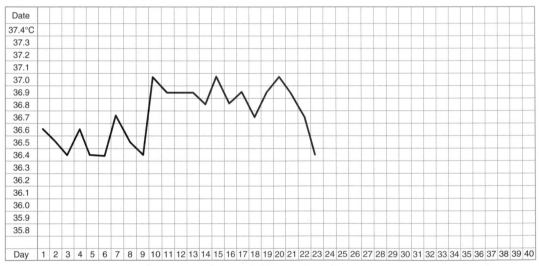

Figure 3.12 Follicular phase is too short.

When the follicular phase is too short

If the follicular phase is consistently short, say only 9 or 10 days (Fig. 3.12), then the TCM practitioner will use treatments to attempt to lengthen it. Often it will be necessary to clear Heat so that ovulations are not provoked prematurely.

The reason for this is that the egg and the follicle must not only grow to a certain size but must also reach a certain level of maturity, which takes time and energy and nourishment. The body loses blood and energy reserves during the period and these must be replaced in the days immediately following. At the same time, Yin and Blood reserves are required to nourish the rapidly developing follicle with its egg. If the egg is released only a few days after the end of the period, chances are it will not be as fully developed as possible. (Sometimes there is an egg already half-ripened from the previous cycle which is ready to leave the rank rather rapidly, but this tends to produce an

Month

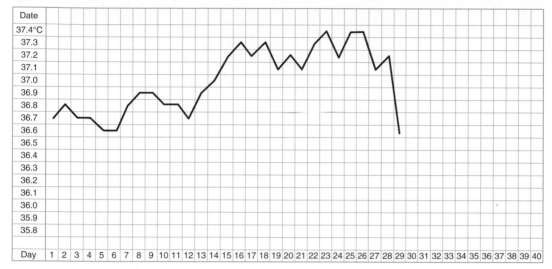

Figure 3.13 Follicular phase is too high.

unusually short cycle rather than a consistently short cycle.) Both herbs and acupuncture can be used to lengthen the follicular phase: to achieve this, treatment needs to begin before the end of the period, preferably around Day 3, so that the functions of the Chong and the Ren vessel can be reprogrammed.

When the follicular phase is too high

Some women have consistently high BBT readings, even in the pre-ovulatory phase (Fig. 3.13). This may reflect a high metabolic rate and possibly hyperactivity of the thyroid gland. The condition may be accompanied by a fast heart beat, feelings of agitation, insomnia or weight loss. In TCM, we generally attribute such a pattern to a phenomenon known as internal Heat. This condition predisposes to production of cervical mucus that is scanty or too acid or which contains antisperm antibodies. In addition, the endometrial lining may be too thin or dry. Therefore, measures must be taken to clear such Heat. This usually means using herbs which 'clear Heat' and reinforce Yin.

At the beginning of the follicular phase, i.e., the beginning of the new cycle, Day 1 of the period, if the temperature has not already dropped (ideally it should drop the day the period begins or the day before) or drops some time during the period or even after the period (i.e., Day 3–7) then some internal imbalance may be suspected (Fig. 3.14).

In TCM terms, this particular phenomenon is described as a failure of Yang transforming to Yin (see Ch. 2) but in clinical practice it can alert us to the possibility of an underlying condition such as endometriosis. The way TCM sees it, it reflects an incomplete discharge of all the endometrial blood, such as happens when endometrial implants outside the uterus bleed into the pelvic cavity or into a cyst. The TCM practitioner will attempt to correct this pattern by applying treatment from Day 1 of the period to facilitate complete discharge of blood and the switch from Yang to Yin. Underlying causes will then be addressed at other times of the cycle.

When the follicular phase is unstable

The values of BBT recorded in the follicular phase should be reasonably steady: not the same each day of course, but not varying (Fig. 3.15) by more than about 0.2 or 0.3°C (0.5°F). Fever, lack of sleep or alcohol consumption will cause unusually high readings.

If there are unexplained peaks and troughs in the chart from day-to-day, we describe these in Chinese medical terms as expressions of Liver- and Heart-Fire. What this means is that at some level the Shen is uneasy and

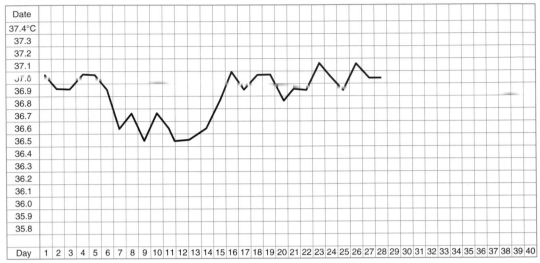

Figure 3.14 Follicular phase starts too high.

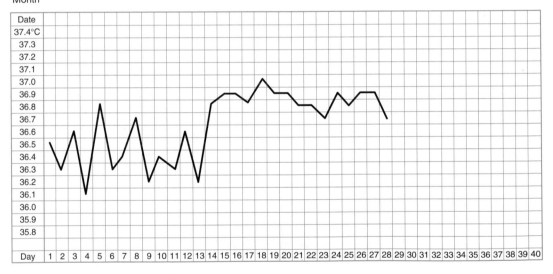

Figure 3.15 Follicular phase is unstable.

treatment which clears Heat and reinforces Yin will be applied at this time to calm the mind. The patient will be encouraged to reduce stress and lead a more regulated life, incorporating relaxation techniques.

A summary of follicular phase patterns is given in Table 3.2.

Ovulation

As the follicle keeps growing (in response to stimulation by FSH from the pituitary), it will produce large quantities of estrogen. In some women, this has the effect of making the BBT drop a little (see Fig. 3.9, Day 12).

Table 3.2   Summary of follicular phase patterns

BBT Pattern	Diagnosis	Treatment
Low follicular phase	Generalized Yang deficiency	Warm Yang throughout cycle
Long follicular phase	Deficiency of Kidney Jing, Yin or Blood	Nourish Blood, reinforce Kidney Jing and Yin after the period
Short follicular phase	Heat, usually Yin-deficient Heat	Clear Heat and nourish Yin from early in cycle
High follicular phase	Heat, usually Yin-deficient Heat	Clear Heat and nourish Yin from early in cycle
High follicular phase initially	Obstruction of transformation of Yang to Yin	Promote Kidney Yang to Yin transformation, regulate period
Unstable follicular phase	Liver- or Heart-Fire	Clear Liver- or Heart-Fire, calm the mind

Some women notice this on their BBT charts and others do not. Because this peak of estrogen only lasts about 12 h its effect may not be detected on an early morning temperature reading if it happened for example between 10 a.m. and 10 p.m. In most women it has the effect of stimulating the cervical glands to produce fertile mucus. Women who are using a urine LH detection kit should notice that it becomes positive around this time.

It is the effect of the next hormone produced by the ovary, progesterone, which brings about a marked change in the BBT. In most women, as soon as progesterone is produced, the BBT rises quite markedly, i.e., 0.4–0.5°C (up to 1°F). We are not sure why basal temperature rises but, whatever the reason is, it is important, because progesterone and its action of warming the body (by acting on the temperature-regulating centers in the hypothalamus) is found throughout the evolution of mammals. Levels of progesterone remain high throughout pregnancy, so it is clearly considered an advantage to the embryo and the developing baby to be in a slightly warmer than usual environment.

The effect of progesterone can also be seen in measurable differences in metabolic rates during sleep – they are lowest at the end of the low phase (follicular phase) and highest at the end of the high phase (luteal phase).[11,12]

Thus, charting tells us at this point, when the waking temperature is registering higher on our chart, that ovulation has occurred.

Once 2 or 3 days of elevated temperatures have been recorded, then attempts at conceiving can be abandoned for another month. The egg survives for a very short time (about 12 h) after it is released and once the body has registered the circulating progesterone by raising its BBT significantly, then the egg has usually been and gone. You can see why charting temperature on its own is not a very useful tool for choosing when to try to conceive. However, several months of BBT graphs convey a good understanding of the hormonal comings and goings of the body and, when combined with observations of other signs, provides an extremely accurate record of the most fertile days.

As soon as progesterone starts to circulate, the cervical mucus dries up rapidly and the entrance to the cervix is blocked with an impenetrable (to sperm) 'Keep Out' sign. This secretion is thick and crumbly and white. The vaginal sensations will tend to be dry.

The drying up of the cervical fluid marks the end of the Yin phase and the rise in temperature indicates the successful switch from Yin to Yang.

The luteal or high phase

The temperature readings taken in this part of the cycle are a little more steady than in the follicular or low part of the cycle. This is because hormone production by the corpus luteum (tucked away inside the ovary) is less affected by external and emotional upheavals than are the hypothalamus and the pituitary (in the brain), which are more vulnerable to the influence of the external world and the emotions. Ideally, BBT values should waver no more than 0.1°C (0.2°F). In general, once the temperature has lifted by 0.3–0.5°C (1°F), it should maintain this level for at least 11 or 12 days, and preferably 13 or 14 days. If a menstrual cycle is shorter than 28 days, it usually means that ovulation has occurred early. However, it sometimes means that the luteal phase is inadequate. The temperature drop which occurs towards the end of a cycle signals the disappearance from the system of progesterone, i.e., the corpus luteum has disintegrated and is no longer producing this hormone. The longest the corpus luteum can be expected to survive in the absence of a pregnancy is 16 days, but 12–14 days is more typical. With the drop in the progesterone, the lining of the uterus loses its glue, so to speak, and will start to disintegrate and the period begins. If a conception has occurred and the embryo has successfully negotiated the trip down through the tubes and is also successful in embedding in the endometrium, the corpus luteum will be given a signal to continue producing progesterone until such time as the developing embryo can produce its own (about 8 weeks later).

The luteal phase is sometimes called the 'inadequate luteal phase' in gynecology texts if the corpus luteum does not keep the production of progesterone up for long enough to allow the newly arrived embryo to implant and develop in the endometrium.

When the second part of the cycle is not ideal, i.e., the temperature climbs too slowly or drops too soon or wavers up and down or doesn't reach a higher enough temperature, it is said in Chinese medicine that the Yang of the Kidney is insufficient. One of the functions of Yang is to warm the body, and any deficiency in heat or metabolism will be ascribed by TCM to Yang deficiency.

Let us now look at the different sorts of patterns which may occur in the luteal phase and how TCM analyzes them.

When the luteal phase is too short

TCM evaluates any degree of Kidney Yang deficiency from the length of the luteal phase (i.e., how far short of 14 days is the period of time between ovulation and the first day of the period). In ideal situations it is a minimum of 12 days, preferably 14 days. If the rise in temperature only lasts for 3 days (Fig. 3.16), then one cannot even be sure that ovulation has occurred.

In such a case, the menstrual cycle may be barely 2½ weeks long. Blood tests may be necessary to determine if ovulation is occurring and, if it is not, the TCM practitioner will treat this case in the same way she would amenorrhoea (see Ch. 5). Kidney Jing, Yin or Yang tonic herbs will be prescribed to improve the quality of ovulation or the use of fertility drugs may be advised.

If the luteal phase is 5 or 6 days (cycle may be about 3 weeks long), then ovulation probably has occurred (Fig. 3.17) but large doses of Kidney tonic herbs will be used at different times of the cycle to improve the corpus luteum function and in some cases simultaneous use of drugs may be recommended.

A luteal phase that typically lasts 8–10 days (Fig. 3.18) reflects a milder Kidney weakness but one which nevertheless can compromise fertility because progesterone support will not be sufficient to ensure implantation.

Clomifene (Clomid), a well-known fertility drug, is often given for problems with ovulation, including inadequate luteal phases. In general the drug works very effectively in lengthening and raising the temperature in the luteal phase.

When the luteal phase is too low

After ovulation and the production of progesterone the temperature should ideally rise 0.4–0.5°C (1°F). The absolute values of temperature readings in the two phases is not as significant as the difference between them.

Month

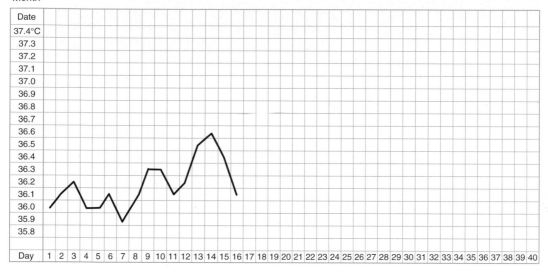

Figure 3.16 Luteal phase is very short.

Month

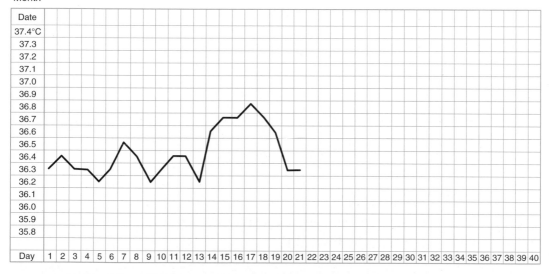

Figure 3.17 Luteal phase is too short.

A rise of 0.3°C is thought to be just adequate and a rise of 0.1 or 0.2°C is called a low luteal phase (Fig. 3.19) and represents a failure of Kidney Yang to properly fulfill its function. In this case, the Kidney Yang is weak right from the beginning of the luteal phase, whereas in the previous pattern it warmed the body to some degree but could not sustain it for long enough. In the case of a low luteal phase, we need to do more than strengthen the Kidney Yang function; we need to strongly build the very foundation of Kidney Yang – namely, Kidney Yin. It is only when Kidney Yin provides a strong base that Kidney Yang can grow out of it. And in some cases (depending on the clinical symptoms) it is the Qi or Blood which needs building before Kidney Yang can develop in the post-ovulatory phase.

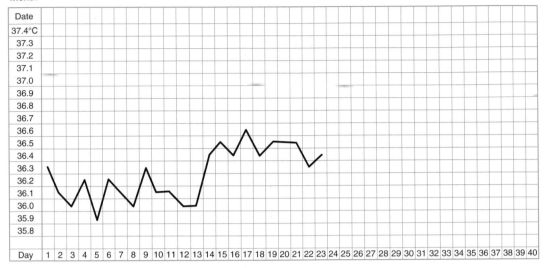

Figure 3.18 Luteal phase is slightly short.

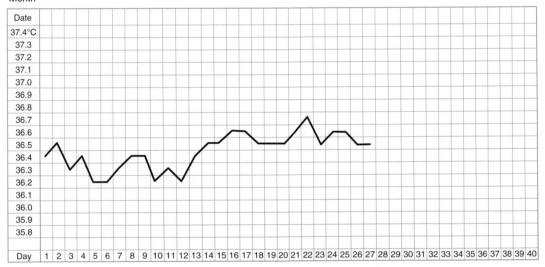

Figure 3.19 Low luteal phase.

When the luteal phase is unstable

In the **sawtooth pattern** (Fig. 3.20) the BBT rises adequately at ovulation but it will drop and rise again over the course of the luteal phase. This pattern represents instability of the Heart and Liver Qi concurrent with Kidney Yang deficiency. The basis of such instability is nearly always emotional and often manifests in the follicular phase as well as the luteal phase especially where there is Kidney Yin deficiency. If luteal phase temperatures are higher then expected, or there are a number of high peaks, Liver Fire must be suspected.

Month

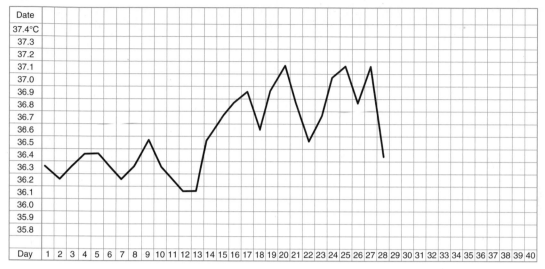

Figure 3.20 Unstable luteal phase – sawtooth pattern.

Month

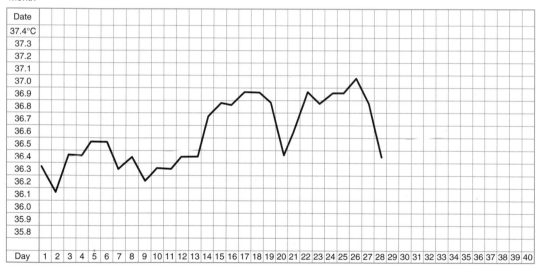

Figure 3.21 Unstable luteal phase – saddle pattern.

Treatment of this pattern may require concomitant relaxation techniques and attention to stress reduction. The best way to stabilize the sawtooth luteal phase is to promote Kidney Yang by nourishing Blood. This involves the use of Blood tonics in combination with Kidney Yang tonics and has the result of calming the Liver and the Heart.

In the **saddle pattern**, the instability in this BBT is shown in a sudden and predictable plunge in the temperature about 1 week after ovulation (Fig. 3.21). There is a second smaller surge of estrogen during the luteal phase, which may in some women cause a drop in BBT for a day. The cervical glands may also respond to this estrogen, and more secretions may be noticed on this day.

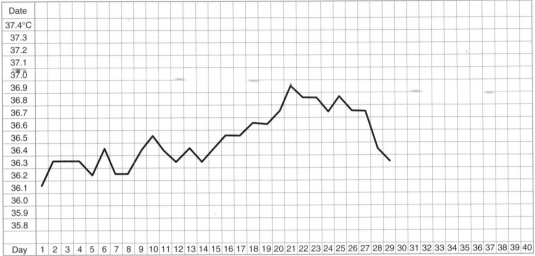

Figure 3.22 Luteal phase with slow rise.

Surges of estrogen or drops in progesterone at this stage of the cycle indicate both lack of firm Kidney Yang and instability in the Heart and Liver. Generally, this is not a serious impediment to fertility because the Kidney Yang is not very deficient, as evidenced by the recovery of a good temperature level that is maintained until the end of the luteal phase (or into early pregnancy). However, because the disruption occurs at such a sensitive time in the cycle, just at the point where implantation is occurring, the TCM practitioner will attempt to change this pattern by boosting Kidney Yang and stabilizing the Heart and the Liver Qi.

When the luteal phase rises too slowly

The luteal phase temperature reached in this pattern (Fig. 3.22) is eventually high enough for us to be convinced that progesterone and Kidney Yang levels are adequate; however, it takes several days (>3) for the temperature to rise after ovulation rather than the usual 1 or 2 days.

Some women observe the changes in the cervix and fertile mucus indicating ovulation well in advance (by some days) of the temperature rise. However, when the temperature rise does come it is quite clear that ovulation has indeed occurred. It is thought that these women may be slow to react to the circulating progesterone, their bodies taking a few days before the BBT is raised.

TCM classifies this pattern as a deficiency of Kidney Yang combined with Spleen Qi and Yang deficiency. In some cases there may be underlying Yin deficiency also or Liver Qi stagnation.

When the luteal phase declines too early

In this pattern (Fig. 3.23), the luteal phase lasts the usual 13 or 14 days until the start of the period but the temperature declines rapidly from its peak shortly after ovulation. It is normal to find that the temperature drops a day before the period starts, but it should not drop before that.

In TCM, this pattern indicates a form of Kidney Yang deficiency combined with Spleen Qi deficiency. Even though the period does not come early, the fact that the temperature has dropped indicates the decline of the Kidney Yang. The lack of Spleen Qi integrity is sometimes the cause of blood not being held securely in the

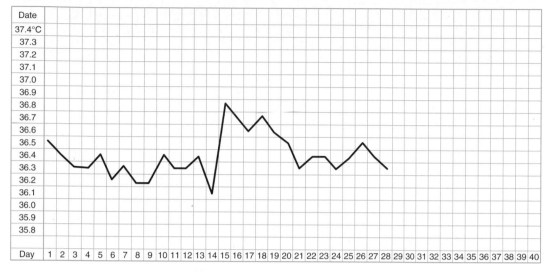

Figure 3.23 Luteal phase with early decline.

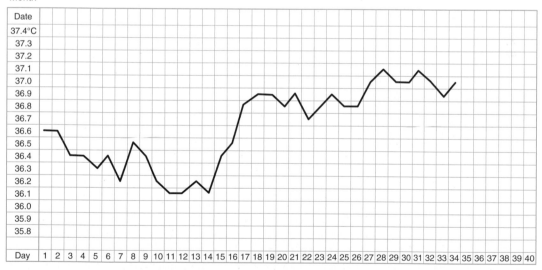

Figure 3.24 Long luteal phase – pregnancy.

endometrial blood vessels and so we may see some premenstrual spotting in this pattern. Of course an early decline of progesterone levels is another way of describing the phenomenon of premenstrual spotting.

When the luteal phase is higher than usual or lasts longer than usual

This pattern represents no irregularities or malfunction; in fact, it indicates pregnancy (Fig. 3.24). There are a couple of other signs which may indicate pregnancy. As mentioned earlier, the egg is fertilized in the fallopian tube and then begins a slow journey down the tube as an embryo, which gradually divides into more and more

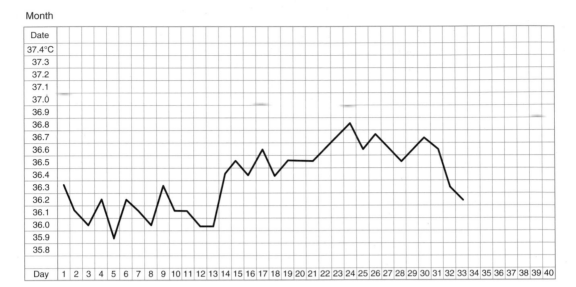

Figure 3.25 Long luteal phase – miscarriage.

cells. It reaches the uterus several days later and implants in the endometrium. When this happens there may be some slight spotting as the endometrium is disturbed. At this point too, the BBT may reach a higher value than recorded before, as more progesterone is produced in response to the implantation. Once 10 high temperatures have been recorded, a sensitive urine test will register the pregnancy hormone, human chorionic gonadotrophin (hCG), produced by the embryo.

Sometimes this pattern is confusing because a period still comes but the temperature does not drop. It is not so very unusual for periods to keep occurring at the expected monthly interval as many as 3 months into the pregnancy. Most often, the bleeding will be scantier than a normal period but occasionally this is not the case. Charting the basal temperature then is really the only way (other than to have frequent blood tests or ultrasounds) to confirm the ongoing existence of the pregnancy.

Some women may pick up a disturbing trend when they begin charting and that is that they are conceiving sometimes but suffering early stage miscarriages (Fig. 3.25).

In these cases, the temperature will stay elevated more than 16 or 17 days but fall not much later, so that it appears to just be a long cycle. If this pattern is repeated, then steps will be taken to prevent it in the future.

In some rare cases, the temperature will stay elevated because a corpus luteum cyst develops. This has the effect of maintaining the corpus luteum and its progesterone output past its usual lifetime; hence the period doesn't come. A pregnancy test will be disappointingly negative but the corpus luteal cyst can be expected to resolve on its own. BBT patterns in the luteal phase are summarized in Table 3.3.

MORE ON DISCHARGES

Some vaginal discharges do not originate in the cervix and some that do originate in the cervix are not the fertile type. For some women there is a marked increase in the thick and rather dry or pasty discharge of the post-ovulatory phase in response to high progesterone levels (which can encourage growth of vaginal yeast organisms). It is not uncommon for women to notice an increase in thin or slippery discharge just before the period. This may just reflect the drop in progesterone as the corpus luteum stops functioning and does not indicate a fertile time. Or this thin discharge may be the beginning of fluid loss from the endometrial lining of the uterus.

Table 3.3   BBT patterns in the luteal phase

BBT pattern	Diagnosis	Treatment
Short luteal phase	Kidney Yang deficiency arising from Yin deficiency	Strongly supplement Kidney Yin in follicular phase to create Yang in luteal phase
Slightly short luteal phase	Kidney Yang deficiency	Boost Kidney Yang in luteal phase
Low luteal phase	Kidney Yang deficiency	Nourish Kidney Yin and Blood, boost Kidney Yang in luteal phase
Unstable luteal phase – sawtooth	Liver/Heart Qi unstable, Kidney Yang deficiency	Regulate Liver/Heart Qi, calm Liver Fire, boost Kidney Yang by nourishing Blood
Unstable luteal phase – saddle	Kidney Yang deficiency, Liver/Heart Qi unstable	Reinforce Kidney Yang, regulate Liver/Heart Qi
Slow-rise luteal phase	Kidney Yang deficiency, Spleen Qi deficiency	Reinforce Kidney Yin after period, invigorate Spleen Qi from early midcycle and boost Kidney Yang in the luteal phase
Early-decline luteal phase	Kidney Yang deficiency, Spleen Qi deficiency	Invigorate Spleen Qi and boost Kidney Yang in luteal phase
Long luteal phase	Pregnancy	Support Kidney Yang if necessary

Other women sometimes report seeing a moist or creamy discharge in the middle of the luteal phase. This may reflect a small surge of estrogen, which can occur at this stage, stimulating the cervical glands. This discharge does not indicate a second fertile period for that cycle.

Yet other women will notice some constant form of discharge all the way through the cycle right from the end of the period. This may be just a natural physiologic discharge which, if it is not associated with any infection or inflammation, is said to be quite normal for that woman. Although this is quite correct from a Western medical point of view, from the TCM point of view any excess discharge of fluid or mucus from the body is thought to reflect a disorder in the fluid metabolism. Often people with excess mucousy discharges (from various orifices) are said to be 'Damp' and it is the job of the TCM practitioner to help to correct this imbalance.

Clearly, determining fertile (and non-fertile) days in women with chronic discharge is not quite as simple as it is for women who have dry days before and after ovulation. A woman prone to Damp must closely observe any changes in the constant discharge, particularly toward wetter or more stretchy type of mucus, in order to ascertain the fertile period. Once again, the peak day of fertility will be the last day that this different sort of mucus is observed before the return of the usual discharge. If treatment clears the Damp successfully, observation of fertile mucus becomes easier.

Sometimes a vaginal discharge can mean an infection. It will usually have a different or offensive smell, may be colored (yellow or green) and may cause inflammation of the vagina or vulva. It is important that such infections are treated promptly (usually with antibiotics or antifungals, although herbs can also be very effective) and that intercourse is avoided until the infection or soreness is resolved. This is to prevent cross-infection and also to avoid discomfort or trauma to the inflamed tissue. Another sort of pathologic discharge may arise from inflammation of the cervix. This may be a watery sort of discharge and will not be offensive like an infection but may still be irritant. Although there is no drug treatment for such a discharge, TCM can treat it effectively with herbal decoctions and douches. For treatments of vaginal discharges, the reader is referred to TCM gynecology texts.[13]

1. Cheng XG. Use of the basal body temperature in pattern discrimination for patients with infertility and amenorrhoea. *Shanghai J TCM* 1992;**10**:18–9.

2. Billings EL, Billings JJ, Brown JB, et al. Symptoms and hormonal changes accompanying ovulation. *Lancet* 1972;**1**:282–4.

3. Billings EL, Westmore A. *The Billings method*. Melbourne. Anne O'Donavon; 1998, 203.

4. Hatcher RA, Trussell J, Stewart F, et al. *Contraceptive technology*. 16th edn New York: Irvington; 1994.

5. Gray RH, Simpson JL, Kambic RT, et al. Timing of conception and the risk of spontaneous abortion among pregnancies occurring during the use of natural family planning. *Am J Obstet Gynecol* 1995;**172**:1567–72.

6. Royston JP, Abrams RM, Higgins MP, et al. The adjustment of basal body temperature measurements to allow for time of waking. *Br J Obstet Gynaecol* 1980;**87**(12):1123–7.

7. Odeblad E, Hoglund A. The dynamic mosaic model of the human ovulatory cervical mucus. *Proc Nordic Fertil Soc* 1978;January.

8. Jansen RPS. *Getting pregnant*. Sydney: Allen and Unwin; 2003, 62.

9. Schering Pty Ltd. *Notes distributed with Triquilar and other combined oral contraceptives*. Tempe: Wood St; 2012.

10. Billings EL, Westmore A. *The Billings method*. Melbourne: Anne O'Donavon; 1998, 174.

11. Meijer GA, Westerterp KR, Saris WH, et al. Sleeping metabolic rate in relation to body composition and the menstrual cycle. *Am J Clin Nutr* 1992;**55**(3):637–40.

12. Bisdee JT, James WP, Shaw MA. Changes in energy expenditure during the menstrual cycle. *Br J Nutr* 1989;**61**(2):187–99.

13. Macioca G. *Obstetrics and gynecology in Chinese medicine*. London: Churchill Livingstone; 1998.

SECTION 2

In The Clinic

Diagnosis and Treatment of Female Infertility

4

Chapter Contents

Part 1 – Making a Diagnosis

INTRODUCTION

Before any TCM treatment is applied, the doctor must be sure of the diagnosis. By gathering together the relevant details of the case history, and looking at the tongue and taking the pulse, the pieces of the puzzle will usually form a picture which roughly approximates one or more of the patterns outlined in this chapter.

We seldom find a clear-cut textbook case in our clinics. Most women we see in infertility clinics in the West have already run the gauntlet of investigations and treatments – some of them quite invasive – and the diagnostic picture may have been complicated by these. Nevertheless, with time and experience, the TCM doctor learns to sniff out what is relevant and ignore what is not, until a diagnosis and a plan of action can be made, as illustrated in the case histories throughout this book.

THE TWO KEY ELEMENTS: OVULATION AND MENSTRUATION

Traditionally, the menstrual cycle, and any disturbances of it, were described in Chinese medicine texts only in terms of the period – the arrival (late, early or on time) or the non-arrival of the period – this being the most clearly observable external sign. Thus, observations of the timing and nature of the menstrual flow were the most important signs upon which a diagnosis could be made. Historically, treatments for infertility also gave great emphasis to the period, i.e., treatments were applied during or just before the menstrual flow.

We can now incorporate more modern ideas based on discoveries about female physiology made by Western doctors and scientists, and base our TCM diagnosis on more than just the menstrual flow. We can follow the menstrual cycle not just by the appearance of the period but also by other key events: most importantly the time that the egg is released from the ovary, i.e., ovulation. When we are concerned with fertility this is the key event of the menstrual cycle.

We have at our disposal in the wealthy Western countries extraordinary diagnostic tools which allow us not only to pinpoint the ovulatory event itself but also all the steps leading up to it. For example, a vaginal ultrasound can track the progress of a follicle from the very first signs of stimulation by the follicle-stimulating hormone (FSH) right up to its full size at maturity when the egg will be released. The ultrasound also reveals the readiness (i.e., thickness and structure) of the lining of the uterus to receive a fertilized egg. Blood tests can track ovulation by measuring:

• FSH, which stimulates follicle growth

• estrogen levels, which increase as the follicle grows

• luteinizing hormone (LH), which heralds the imminent release of the egg

• the progesterone produced by the corpus luteum after the egg has been released.

IVF clinics make full and productive use of all these diagnostic tools on a frequent and regular basis, which is one of the reasons these infertility programmes can be so expensive.

However, we do not need to rely on expensive and invasive tests to monitor the internal events of the menstrual cycle. Although not so quantitative in their measurements, careful observation of certain external signs can give us useful qualitative information (Box 4.1).

Box 4.1 Tracking ovulation

Cervical Mucus Observations

Stretchy mucus released from glands in the cervix tells us a follicle in the ovary is growing and producing estrogen and will soon be ready to be released. Cessation of stretchy mucus tells us the follicle has been released – appearance next of a drier white floccular discharge tells us that the corpus luteum has formed and that it is producing progesterone; the cervix will now be closed.

Urine Tests

Readily available urine tests (ovulation predictor kits) measuring the levels of the pituitary hormone LH, which cues the egg for release, give us even more precise information. These kits, available over the counter at pharmacies, can predict ovulation some 36h ahead.

BBT Charts

Basal body temperature (BBT) charts are described in Chapter 3 and indicate if or when ovulation occurred and how well the corpus luteum is functioning.

It makes good sense to start making our TCM diagnosis, and designing treatments, using these physiological signposts as well as subjective descriptions of symptoms. Questions about the period, the middle of the cycle and about sensations in the ovaries, breasts or genitals will offer valuable information. If our patient is recording her BBT, then we can discern even more information about her condition and the diagnosis of her infertility. The shape of the chart, as we saw in Chapter 3, will tell us about the Kidney Yin and Yang and the Qi of the Heart and Liver.

The Period

The period gives us unique insights into the workings of the reproductive system. The questions we ask are:

- When – regularity and length of cycle (early, late, on time)?

- How long – short or protracted period?

- How much – heavy, medium or scanty flow?

- Looks like – bright red, dark red, purplish, mucusy, clotty?

- Feels like – abdomen pain, backache, dull or sharp pain?

From such information we can already discern aspects of diagnosis related to Blood stagnation, or Qi deficiency or internal Heat or Cold and so on.

Midcycle

Symptoms and signs at midcycle are much more subtle and some women will notice very little until they are requested to watch closely for certain changes. What we want to know about primarily is the quality and quantity of the mucus produced by the glands in the cervix in response to the estrogen coming from the ripening follicles.

We ask the following questions about the fertile mucus and ovulation:

- When – Day 14, earlier, later?

- How long – fertile mucus evident for several days or just a few hours?

- How much – copious or scanty and difficult to detect?

- Looks like – clear stretchy, thick cloudy?

- Feels like – abdomen, genital or breast symptoms?

All of this gives us information about the quality of the Yin and the movement of the Qi and when and how well it is developing in this phase of the cycle.

Pain in the Ovary

Some women feel pain or an ache on one or other side of the abdomen when the ovary on that side is enlarged with several ripening follicles. The pain is usually felt before the egg is released and from that point of view, is a useful indicator of the most fertile time for sexual intercourse. It is a cruel irony that for some women this pain is so strong that the idea of sex is anathema.

Box 4.2   Main categories of infertility

1. Kidney deficiency
2. Heart and Liver Qi stagnation
3. Blood stagnation
4. Phlegm-Damp accumulation

Breast Tenderness

Less commonly, the breasts and nipples react to the peak of estrogen produced by the ripening follicle and they can become swollen and sore. This tells us that there is probably a good amount of estrogen circulating. TCM theory, however, tells us that pain, even when associated with a normal physiological process, is an indicator of Qi being obstructed. In this case, the Liver Qi is not circulating well and the pain represents some stagnation of the Qi in the breasts.

Genital Discomfort

The increased levels of hormones at ovulation can also cause swelling or bearing-down sensations in the vulva region in some women – this may indicate Spleen Qi weakness which, like Liver Qi stagnation, is easily corrected.

TCM CATEGORIES OF FEMALE INFERTILITY

At an infertility clinic in the West, we may describe female infertility using such labels as fallopian tube blockage, polycystic ovaries, inadequate luteal phase, oligomenorrhea or irregular, infrequent ovulation, resistant ovary syndrome, endometriosis and so on. Although these disease labels do not usually translate directly into specific TCM categories of infertility, the symptom pictures they manifest are easily analyzed and categorized to fit a TCM diagnostic pattern.

The section on female infertility in traditional TCM gynecology texts is usually found in the last chapter as one of 'eight miscellaneous diseases.' These texts usually describe four main categories of infertility (and sometimes numerous subcategories), which are given in Box 4.2.

What one sees when prescriptions are handed out to patients in the infertility clinic of the TCM teaching hospital which we visited in Chapter 1, or any other infertility clinic in China, is that nearly all the prescriptions treat the Kidneys. This is not because the last three of the four patterns described in Box 4.2 do not occur in practice but because they usually occur in combination with, or even as a result of, a Kidney weakness. If there is functional infertility, then by definition the Kidney Yin and Yang are depleted or not functioning correctly.

The categories of functional female infertility could be rewritten (Box 4.3):

1. Problems related to ovulation – Kidney Yin deficiency or Heart Qi stagnation (either of these two patterns can be complicated by Liver Qi stagnation, Phlegm-Damp or Blood stagnation)

2. Problems of embryo implantation – Kidney Yang deficiency (possibly complicated with Liver Qi stagnation, Phlegm-Damp or Blood stagnation).

We know there is no (or rare) ovulation if:

• there are no periods

• there are very irregular periods

Box 4.3   TCM diagnoses of functional infertility according to menstrual cycle phase

Problems Related to Ovulation or the First Part of the Menstrual Cycle
- Most commonly related to Kidney Yin deficiency
- Next most common cause is Heart Qi stagnation
- Either can be complicated by Liver Qi stagnation or Phlegm-Damp or Blood stagnation

Problems of Embryo Implantation or the Second Part of the Menstrual Cycle
- Most commonly related to Kidney Yang deficiency
- May also be complicated by Liver Qi stagnation, Phlegm-Damp or Blood stagnation
- Kidney Yang deficiency often accompanied by signs of Spleen weakness

(Refer to Ch. 6 for infertility related to mechanical obstructions)

- the BBT chart shows no biphasic pattern

- blood tests show low estrogen/progesterone levels or high FSH levels.

We know there is 'poor' ovulation if:

- the BBT chart shows a small rise in temperature

- the temperature rise is very short-lived

- blood tests taken in the middle of the luteal phase show low levels of progesterone

- there is spotting in the luteal phase.

We suspect problems with implantation if:

- there is poor ovulation

- there are fibroids or other physical barriers to implantation

- the uterine lining is inadequate on ultrasound and periods are scanty or dark or clotty

- we have eliminated everything else and pregnancy is still not occurring.

The following are general clinical pictures. It is important to remember when making a diagnosis that not all women who suffer from a particular deficiency or stagnation will show all (or even some) of the described symptoms and signs. Every case will manifest a different constellation, depending on where the deficiency or stagnation exerts its influence most.

Kidney Deficiency

The most common cause of functional infertility, Kidney deficiency, often underlies or coexists with other causes. Women with weak Kidney energy will often present with some or all of the following:

- Poor stamina, low reserves of energy

- Lower back weakness or pain

- Some difficulty with urination, e.g., daytime frequency or frequent nocturia or slight incontinence

- Shadows under their eyes.

• Signs and Symptoms

Kidney Jing deficiency will be the diagnosis if there are, in addition to any of the above symptoms, the following:

- obvious developmental disorders in the reproductive organs, or

- little development of secondary sexual signs such as breast development, or

- under-functioning ovaries, even if the ovaries appear normal. Puberty may be late and ovulation may be erratic; sometimes the only sign is an inability of the ovaries to respond to fertility drugs.

• BBT Chart and Fertile Mucus

BBT charts are usually not recorded because the cycle is erratic or absent. However, where charts are completed, there will usually be no pattern or an indistinct biphasic response. Fertile mucus is rarely seen.

• Pulse

The pulse will usually be weak and thready.

• Tongue

The tongue is usually pale.

• Blood Tests

AMH (anti-Mullerian hormone) which is produced by the primary and preantral follicles in the ovary, will be low indicating a low reserve of follicles available for recruitment. In the case that ovaries are not functioning well, estrogen levels (in the follicular phase) and progesterone levels (in the luteal phase) will also be low. FSH may be elevated.

• Signs and Symptoms

This is an increasingly common diagnosis of infertility. Kidney Yin deficiency occurs especially in older women and usually arises out of depletion of resources – working (and playing) too hard without allowing the time and deep rest needed for replenishing body and soul.

A woman who is Yin deficient may complain of some or several of the following symptoms:

- restlessness or anxiety

- difficulty getting good-quality sleep

- flushing easily

- frequently needing to drink fluid.

Often, but not always, she is thin or wiry and may tend to have dry skin or hair due to a lack of the cooling and moistening influence of Yin in the body – this leads to a relative excess of Yang, expressed as Heat or dryness. Yin deficiency often leads to Blood deficiency and the period flow may become scanty. On the other hand, Heat affecting the Blood may cause heavy bright-red periods.

• BBT Chart and Fertile Mucus

The follicular phase of the Yin deficient woman's chart is often unsteady and may be longer than the usual 13 or 14 days if ovulation is delayed. However, if Yin-deficient Heat provokes the release of an immature egg the follicular phase will be shortened.

The average temperature in the low phase may, in some cases, hover around 36.7°C (98°F) instead of the more usual 36.5°C (97.7°F) or lower. When Yin is deficient, it can also contribute to a poorly sustained temperature rise in the luteal phase.

There may be little discernible vaginal lubrication or fertile mucus. Any fertile mucus produced may have a tendency to be too acid in these women.

• Pulse

When the Yin is weak, the pulse will usually be weak, especially on the deep levels. Or the pulse may give the impression of floating superficially under the skin. If there is any Yin-deficient Heat the pulse will also be rapid.

• Tongue

Yin-deficient tongues tend to be dry and small, and are often red with little coat.

• Blood Tests

FSH levels are often elevated in this category and where Kidney yin is very depleted, AMH levels will be low indicating low numbers of follicles available for recruitment.

Kidney Yang Deficiency

• Signs and Symptoms

Kidney Yang deficiency may reflect a constitutional tendency or occurs:

- after an injury to the body by Cold

- if the body is overstrained or

- out of long-term Yin deficiency or Qi deficiency or Heart or Liver Qi stagnation.

When the Kidney Yang is deficient, fluids are not metabolized efficiently and edema may result. Generally, body metabolism slows and it is easier to put on weight and harder to shift it.

Kidney Yang-deficient patients often show signs of:

- Puffiness or overweight

- Lethargy

- Low libido and general motivation

- Lower backache, sometimes accompanied by pain in the knees and legs, which feels worse in the cold weather.

Often, there is diarrhoea and lower back pain just before or at the beginning of the period. Dysmenorrhea can occur if the Yang is insufficient to 'drive' the blood flow. Clots in the menstrual flow, which are composed of tissue rather than blood, are thought by some Chinese doctors to indicate Kidney Yang deficiency also.

• BBT Chart

BBT readings of Kidney Yang-deficient women can be quite low (36.0°C or 96.8°F or less); sometimes the temperature readings are off the bottom of the chart.

The temperature rise at ovulation is not often delayed in cases of Kidney Yang deficiency unless it is combined with Kidney Yin deficiency or Heart Yang deficiency or it is complicated with Damp-Phlegm or Blood Stagnation.

Kidney Yang deficiency often leads to inadequate luteal phase – the BBT readings in the second phase are not as high as they should be, or the temperature does not stay raised for long enough.

Readings on the urine LH detector kit may be inconclusive if the LH surge is inadequate.

• Pulse

The pulse may be slow and deep.

• Tongue

The tongue is usually pale and swollen.

• Blood Tests

Progesterone measured in the luteal phase may be low.

Kidney Yin and Yang Deficiency

• Signs and Symptoms

Often both Kidney Yin and Yang are deficient. In this case there will not be many obvious clinical symptoms of one or the other – in other words, the imbalances tend to cancel each other out so that there is no relative excess of either. Or sometimes there will be a confusing mix of Kidney Yin-deficient symptoms, e.g., hot soles of feet at night – along with Kidney Yang-deficient symptoms such as lethargy with a pale swollen tongue.

The diagnosis will most often be one of Kidney Yin and Yang deficiency when a woman presents with infertility if she:

- is in her late 30s or older

- has few, if any, clear symptoms of Kidney deficiency other than infertility

- has no other known reason for failing to fall pregnant (e.g., blocked tubes or low sperm count).

• BBT Chart and Fertile Mucus

A weakness of Kidney Yang that results from inadequate Kidney Yin typically produces a BBT chart with a reluctant start to the luteal phase, i.e., a very slow climb to the higher temperature level or a very small rise, i.e., only 0.2°C, or a rise which is short-lived. In these women, there is usually little fertile mucus.

• Pulse

The pulse will usually be thready and may show characteristics of Yin or Yang deficiency.

• Tongue

The tongue may be pale and swollen or red and dry.

• Blood Tests

Measures of ovarian activity may all be low in this case – AMH, Estrogen and progesterone. The LH surge may not show clearly on the urine detector kit.

Heart and Liver Qi Stagnation

Heart Qi Stagnation

• Signs and Symptoms

The Heart is a very important organ when it comes to ovulating regularly and on time. TCM describes the importance of communication between Heart and Uterus via the Bao vessel. In Western physiological terms, this refers to the signals the ovary receives from the brain which determine the growth and release of eggs.

If a woman has a history of irregular ovulation, or has stopped ovulating altogether (anovulation), and there are reasons to think there may be an emotional cause then Heart Qi stagnation must be considered a likely diagnosis. Most cases of chronic anovulation (amenorrhoea) from emotional causes and stagnation are due to Heart Qi stagnation.

The TCM doctor will also suspect a Heart disorder if there are emotional factors which have precipitated the amenorrhoea. These factors may be recent, such as a sudden shock or upset, or more chronic, such as ongoing extreme anxiety or agitation. They may also hark back to years before, e.g., during puberty, when severe emotional distress can profoundly affect the incipient functioning of the Chong and the Ren vessels as they begin their reproductive roles.

As with diagnoses of the Kidney dysfunction leading to infertility, diagnoses of Heart Qi stagnation leading to infertility may have few of the typical symptoms, particularly if the Shen-disturbing events which obstructed the Bao vessel occurred a long time ago. However, a very skilled TCM diagnostician will in such cases be able to pick up a Shen disturbance in the eyes and the pulse.

With disturbances of the Heart and Shen, we may expect to see other symptoms such as:

- palpitations

- anxiety

- insomnia.

When Heart Qi stagnation is prolonged or severe, then Heart-Fire develops. There will be more severe signs of Shen disturbance, including:

- hysteria or

- extreme neurosis.

• BBT Chart

Shen disturbance usually shows clearly on the BBT chart in the follicular phase as peaks and troughs or a generally very unsteady graph.

Heart-Fire can take the peaks to levels as high or higher than the luteal phase levels.

• Pulse

The pulse may have a choppy or tight feeling at the left distal position or may be very thready at this position.

• Tongue

The tongue may have a red tip.

• Blood Tests

These might show that the pituitary gland is under- or over-producing FSH or LH and estrogen levels may be low. In a woman in her mid- to late-40s (with Kidney Yin or Jing deficiency) this scenario indicates impending menopause, but in a younger woman it indicates a disorder somewhere along the hypothalamus-pituitary-ovary axis.

Liver Qi Stagnation

• Signs and Symptoms

The Liver, like the Heart, is influenced by the emotions; therefore, Heart Qi and Liver Qi stagnation can occur together. However, Liver Qi stagnation manifests in slightly different ways and can cause symptoms at different times in the menstrual cycle.

Disorder of the Liver Qi is a very common cause of gynecologic conditions generally. Stress easily obstructs the smooth flow of Liver Qi and, since the Liver channel traverses the pelvis, and particularly the reproductive organs, this can throw a spanner in the menstrual cycle works.

The unimpeded flow of Liver Qi is necessary for several of the processes of the normal menstrual cycle. For example, those parts of the cycle which require movement – such as the expulsion of the egg, the trapping of it by the fallopian tubes and the passage of it down to the uterus – all require unobstructed Liver Qi in the pelvic area. When the Liver Qi is unobstructed, the changes in hormone levels are negotiated more smoothly and rapidly and symptoms do not develop. When the Chinese made these observations and developed these theories thousands of years ago they did not know of course that the liver, as we know it in Western physiological terms, is responsible for helping regulate hormone levels. It is in the liver that they are broken down effectively, if there are plentiful enzymes and cofactors.

Emotional stress at the time of ovulation can prevent the release of the egg. We also know that stress can affect the levels of hormones released by the pituitary, which are necessary for the growth and release of an egg. Usually this means an obvious disruption of the menstrual cycle, i.e., the period won't come.

It is also possible for stress to reduce the hormone output to a level where there is just enough LH produced to luteinize the follicle so that it will start behaving as if ovulation has occurred (i.e., produce progesterone and a period will therefore follow) but in fact it hasn't. This situation, known as luteinized unruptured follicle (LUF), may lead to a short (inadequate) luteal phase and is found more often in women with irregular cycles or endometriosis.

Stress at the time of ovulation can also cause the fine muscles of the fallopian tubes to tense and contract such that the egg/zygote is not able to find free passage to the uterus. Similarly, tension in the uterus, cervix and tubes does not help the journey of the sperm in their quest.

The effect of stress on the Liver Qi is more commonly noticed by women towards the end of the cycle, when it manifests as premenstrual syndrome.

The effects of obstructed Liver Qi are prominent before the period, because at this point change needs to be negotiated smoothly – if the Liver Qi is not moving freely, such changes bring with them annoying or distressing symptoms. In some women, it is the inability to adjust quickly enough to the rapid change in hormones that occurs after ovulation – these are the unfortunate women who notice premenstrual symptoms for nearly 2 weeks of every cycle. More often, Liver Qi gets stuck at the point when the body is registering whether a conception has occurred or not and is making the necessary adjustments in the hormones. Specifically, the progesterone starts to fall if there is no conception. The response of the body may be irritability, breast soreness, bloating or headaches in the week before the period.

Although emotional stress is the most common cause of Liver Qi stagnation, it can also be caused by prolonged drug use (prescription or recreational), including the oral contraceptive pill (see Ch. 5).

When Liver Qi stagnation is prolonged or severe, then Liver-Fire develops. This brings with it more intense irritability to the point of uncontrollable anger. There may also be headaches with bloodshot eyes. Liver-Fire often feeds Heart-Fire (according to the Five-Element cycle) bringing with it more severe emotional imbalances.

• BBT Chart

Liver Qi stagnation on its own will not significantly affect the shape of the chart itself, except by lengthening it if ovulation is delayed. However, premenstrual Liver-Fire can lift the luteal phase basal temperatures. Caution is needed in such cases because it can obscure a Kidney Yang deficiency, which would normally be associated with low luteal phase temperatures. Liver-Fire in the earlier parts of the cycle can cause some instability or temperature peaks.

• Pulse

Pulses tend to be wiry when there is Liver Qi stagnation, especially on the left side in the central position.

• Tongue

The tongue only registers the stagnation if it develops into Fire or Blood stagnation, when it becomes red or purple, respectively.

• Blood Tests

These will be normal except in the case that ovulation is disrupted in which case luteal phase progesterone levels will be low.

Blood Stagnation

• Signs and Symptoms

Blood stagnation often develops as the long-term consequence of other disorders (e.g., Cold, Damp-Heat or Kidney deficiency) and is a complex syndrome in any discipline, no less gynecology. So the clinical picture can reflect aspects of several pathologies and may be complicated. Less often, Blood stagnation can be the direct consequence of trauma, e.g., surgery or an accident.

From a TCM point of view, the menstrual cycle will be adversely affected by Blood stagnation in that the Chong vessel (the Sea of Blood) will not be filled smoothly, and will not empty properly. The function of the Heart, which controls Blood circulation, will also be compromised.

Problems with the Chong vessel will be reflected in problems with the endometrium. For example, the way the lining forms and the way it breaks down may be faulty – there will be clots and tissue in the menstrual flow and its discharge may be incomplete, followed by spotting. Or there may be discharge from endometrial implants in the pelvic cavity if the woman has endometriosis. Problems of the Heart will be associated with the pituitary gland, which may send erratic or erroneous signals to the ovary or none at all.

Blood stagnation usually causes pain felt at a confined localized site. Menstrual flow is clotty and unsmooth. The stagnation will often be associated with substantial masses or growths. In clinical terms this category of infertility usually describes an obstruction somewhere in the reproductive tract or in the glands which control it. Endometriosis, uterine fibroids or polyps, fallopian tube blockages, ovarian cysts and tumors and pituitary tumors all fall into this category.

• BBT Chart

BBT charts do not directly register the presence of Blood stagnation. However, if the Chong vessel does not empty completely during the period (as is often the case in endometriosis where blood from endometrial implants remains in the pelvic cavity), then the temperature may not fall to its low level immediately the new cycle starts. Instead it may take several days to gradually fall to the appropriate level of the follicular phase.

• Pulse

The pulse may have a choppy quality or feel tight if there is pain. Often it is easier to detect any associated pathology, such as Kidney deficiency or Phlegm-Damp, than it is to directly detect the Blood stagnation on the pulse.

• Tongue

The tongue may have a purplish hue or show some purple areas.

• Blood Tests

These will usually be normal if the ovaries are still functioning regularly. If the menstrual cycle is disrupted by an ovarian cyst estrogen/progesterone levels may be abnormal and if there is a pituitary tumour prolactin levels may be elevated.

Phlegm-Damp Accumulation

• Signs and Symptoms

Like Blood stagnation, Phlegm-Damp accumulation describes a complex phenomenon (unique to TCM) which includes congealing of fluids at certain sites or in certain systems such that their function is disrupted. When we are considering causes of infertility, such disruption may be found in the pituitary, the ovaries, the uterus or the fallopian tubes causing pituitary tumors, ovarian cysts, endometrial congestion or blocked or edematous tubes.

In normal situations the mucus in the tubes is just sufficient to firstly coat the walls and make them slippery, to stop the embryo sticking and burrowing into them and, at the isthmus where the mucus is thicker, to delay the passage of the fertilized egg for a couple of days during its first few cell divisions. However, in pathological scenarios, the Damp might completely obstruct the tube and not allow passage of the egg to the isthmus or the zygote (if there has been a conception) to the uterus. It may also coat and stick together the fimbriae at the end of the tubes, or even the ovary itself, preventing the egg from being released or being caught by the tube. There is some evidence that this occurs in cases of endometriosis (discussed further in Ch. 5). Polycystic ovary syndrome (PCOS) often falls into this category, as do some tube pathologies such as hydrosalpinx.

Phlegm-Damp most often develops secondarily to other pathologies, such as deficient Kidney Yang, Liver Qi stagnation or Blood stagnation. For this reason it will usually manifest clinically as a mixture of symptoms that reflect the various pathologies.

In some cases, however, Phlegm-Damp accumulation is simply the result of overeating rich, sweet food. Little by little the body's digestive system is damaged by such a diet and will tend to break down food and fluids less and less well, until fatty or mucus deposits (called Phlegm-Damp) begin to disrupt organs and their function. Thus, Phlegm-Damp is often associated with obesity, or at least a tendency to put on weight.

The menstrual periods will often be scanty and thick or mucusy, and may come at irregularly spaced long intervals.

• BBT Chart and Fertile Mucus

BBT charts reflect the effects (e.g., delayed ovulation) or origins (e.g., Kidney Yang deficiency) of Phlegm-Damp. They may appear to have little of the usual biphasic pattern or, if there is a temperature shift at ovulation it will be a small one.

Although Damp conditions often cause an increase in mucous membrane discharges, including vaginal discharges, there is usually very little of the stretchy fertile mucus seen around ovulation time because the cervical glands become obstructed by Phlegm-Damp.

• Pulse

The pulse in a Phlegm-Damp condition is typically slippery and full; however, if the accumulation of Phlegm-Damp is isolated in a discrete location (e.g., one fallopian tube) then it may not register on the pulse. If Kidney Yang deficiency or Liver Qi stagnation are contributing causes of the Phlegm-Damp, their characteristics may be felt on the pulse instead.

• Tongue

The tongue will often be coated with a thick or greasy coat, although if the Damp is isolated to discrete sites in the reproductive tract it may not show on the tongue.

• Blood Tests

These are usually normal unless cysts in the ovary cause abnormal estrogen/progesterone levels or a pituitary tumour causes high prolactin levels. In the case of PCOS, AMH readings are often elevated (reflecting the large number of primary and pre antral follicles in the ovaries).

Part 2 – Traditional Chinese Medicine Treatments for Functional Infertility

SAME DISEASE, DIFFERENT TREATMENTS

In Chinese medicine there is a saying:

> Tong bing yi zhi,
>
> Yi bing tong zhi

which means:

> Different diseases, one treatment
>
> Same disease, different treatments

For example, in the clinic we may see four women all with polycystic ovary disease. But these women's clinical presentation may reflect four different types of TCM diagnosis and therefore four different treatment plans. Three women, on the other hand, who suffer variously from amenorrhoea, menstrual headaches or dysmenorrhea may all receive the same basic TCM diagnosis and be treated using small variations of the same guiding herbal prescription. The treatment of many and diverse women arriving at the fertility clinic likewise will proceed according to their TCM diagnosis and despite the common label 'infertility' they will all receive different individualized treatments. Modern innovations to TCM treatments come from the information we receive about particular events in the menstrual cycle using blood tests, ultrasounds, BBT measurements or cervical mucus examination.

Wide fluctuations in Qi and Blood and Yin and Yang occur during the menstrual cycle, resulting in different imbalances manifesting at different times. Two of the most obvious examples, often seen in the clinic, are Blood deficiency after the period and Liver Qi stagnation before the period. We now know that Kidney Yin deficiency affects, in particular, the processes of the first phase of the cycle, and Kidney Yang deficiency affects, in particular, the processes of the second phase of the cycle. So, naturally, our diagnosis and the emphasis of treatment changes at different times of the cycle – this is why the treatment of women is considered so much more complex than that of men.

In Chinese medicine texts, the Kidney is said to 'dominate reproduction' – the Kidney Yin and Yang must be adequate and balanced for the correct functioning of all aspects of the female (and male) reproductive organs. Consequently, the treatment of Kidney Yin and Yang underpins all Chinese medicine prescriptions for infertility. The exception to this rule is infertility caused by simple obstruction in the reproductive tract with no impairment of gland function. A young woman with blocked fallopian tubes (possibly a result of a non-symptomatic chlamydia infection years earlier) will often fall pregnant very easily once the obstruction is removed (surgically) or circumnavigated (by IVF procedures).

When it comes to treating infertility, or any other gynecologic disorder, no matter what our diagnosis, it is important to always keep the treatments congruent with the phase and stage of the menstrual cycle during which it is being administered. This means following closely the relative activities of the Chong and the Ren vessels and the relative balance of Kidney Yin and Yang.

PRESCRIBING TREATMENT

In this chapter, I present a few guiding formulas and acupuncture treatments which can be applied at different times of the menstrual cycle and which can be modified to make them uniquely fitting for the individual patient. The herbal formulas presented here – all of them used by doctors working in infertility clinics in China today – are age-old century-tested medicines applied according to diagnoses arrived at using the traditional Bian Zheng (or pattern recognition) methods of TCM in combination with modern diagnostic methods.

Sometimes, Western drug therapy is appropriate alongside herbal or acupuncture treatment. This will be mentioned briefly here and in the following chapter, which looks at Western disease categories of infertility. The combination of IVF and other assisted reproduction technology (ART) with Chinese medicine is covered in Chapters 10 and 11. Lifestyle and dietary changes are often crucial too (see Ch. 12). Any practitioner can follow the simple approach outlined in this chapter. Simple prescribing, however, does not mean simplistic. Many very skillful and experienced doctors use simple classical formulas – the skill comes in the timing of their administration and the adjustments that are made to account for individual nuances in the presenting pattern. With experience, specialists in infertility refine their prescriptions elegantly and subtly.

The most useful way to approach prescribing, for practitioners new to this area, is to choose an appropriate guiding formula and then customize it to fit the patient. For example, because we are treating the reproductive system the classical formula Liu Wei Di Huang Wan, which supplements Kidney Yin, will turn up time and time again, but will be modified to suit different patients and the stage of the menstrual cycle.

The treatments presented here are only one set of possible guidelines – historically, there were many approaches taken by infertility doctors, who each developed their own favorite protocols. The following treatments are based on those developed by Professor Xia Gui Cheng from the Jiangsu Province Hospital in Nanjing.[1] They represent one of the more rational and consistent approaches to the treatment of infertility in women, comprising sound, well-tested and proven strategies based on both Chinese medicine and Western medicine knowledge.

Chinese herbs are not always very convenient (or palatable) for Western women, and for those women who have difficulty taking them in decoction there are good alternatives. Responding to a demand by Western consumers for 'convenient' medicines, and increasingly by Chinese patients themselves, factories in China are now producing quality controlled 'instant' preparations of individual herbs which appear to retain a high degree of potency. These granulated herbs can be mixed up into prescriptions which are then dissolved in boiling water to make a ready-to-drink tea, reducing preparation time significantly. And for patients who really cannot tolerate the taste, the granules can be put in capsules.

TIMING OF TREATMENTS

The application of the following treatment schedule is not as complicated as it might at first seem. In an ideal situation, we might try to arrange treatment of the patient to start at the beginning of the period or just after it. Of course, treatment can begin on whichever day the patient first comes to the clinic but we should be aiming at treatment through 3–6 full cycles (if the woman has monthly menstrual cycles and does not fall pregnant during this time), starting from the day the period begins.

Once treatment has been given to help discharge the menstrual flow, then the treatment to prepare for ovulation begins (3 or 4 days into the cycle). In many ways this is the most crucial time of the entire cycle. The basis for ovulation and even the implantation of an embryo is established from these early days. It is helpful to try and arrange clinic visits during this phase so that the practitioner can check the status of Yin and Blood by examining the pulse and the tongue, and the general demeanor and well-being of the patient, and prescribe the appropriate formula.

Changes in vaginal secretions as the cycle proceeds will indicate when the formula should be modified. If a woman has a regular cycle and easily discerned variations in vaginal secretions, appropriately labeled formulas can be given at the time of the post-period clinic visit to be taken in a sequence until ovulation or her next clinic visit.

The next important time for a clinic appointment is at the time of ovulation itself. Different herbs related to ovulation will be prescribed and dispensed at this time and acupuncture given to facilitate movement in the fallopian tubes and to calm the mind.

Post-ovulation prescriptions need to be taken a couple of days after the temperature has risen on the BBT chart and, unless symptoms change, this formula will be the one which is taken until the period comes or there is a positive pregnancy test. If more acupuncture is to be administered, it is most effective (and least risky) during the first week after ovulation.

For patients who do not have a regular cycle and who cannot easily determine the time of ovulation, the schedule of best-timed treatments is not quite so easy to predict or plan. Fertility treatment should start from the beginning of a period and weekly visits scheduled with the flexibility to move these forward if signs of ovulation (particularly cervical mucus) present themselves. Where there is no cycle at all, treatment for amenorrhoea will proceed as described in the next chapter.

PRESCRIPTIONS

You will recall from Chapter 2 that the menstrual cycle is divided into four different phases (Fig. 4.1). Each of these phases has its own treatment characteristics.

PROBLEMS IN THE FOLLICULAR PHASE OR AT OVULATION

Menstrual Phase – Discharging the Lining of the Uterus

Factors operating even at this early part of the cycle can already have a significant influence on events later in the cycle when an embryo might try to implant. So, our first concern in the clinic is to encourage the complete discharge of the menstrual blood so that a new endometrium can grow evenly on a smooth base. Although the Kidney Yin (Fig. 4.2) starts to grow as soon as a new cycle begins, we do not pay it attention immediately.

Clinicians working in ART centers have noticed that fertility is slightly increased in cycles after surgery in which the lining of the uterus is scraped out, a procedure known as dilatation and curettage (D&C). The state and environment of the newly formed endometrium appears to provide more favorable implantation sites for an embryo. In effect the acupuncture points used and the herbs prescribed during the period attempt a 'herbal or acupuncture D&C' – a good basis from which to start the next part of the treatment, which is the building of the Blood in the Chong vessel. Even if there is no evidence of stagnation (i.e., there is no pain or clotting), there may still be therapeutic benefit to be gained by encouraging a thorough 'flushing' of the uterine cavity before a new lining grows.

As we mentioned in Chapter 2, human females tend to have much heavier periods and have placentas that need much deeper invasion into the uterine lining than do other species. It is the priming and preconditioning of the uterine lining that happens during the menstrual phase to prepare for implantation and placental development that is what we wish to influence with out treatment during Phase 1.

Herbal Formula — The following well-known formula (Tao Hong Si Wu Tang) can be given in a patent pill form to encourage complete discharge of menses. However, if there are clinical signs of Blood stagnation, a decocted or granulated herbal preparation would be preferable to pills because they would have a more powerful action.

Tao Hong Si Wu Tang (Persica Carthamus Four Substances decoction)

Dang Gui	9 g	Radix Angelicae Sinensis
Shu Di	12 g	Radix Rehmanniae Glutinosae Conquitae
Chuan Xiong	6 g	Radix Ligustici Wallichii
Bai Shao	12 g	Radix Paeoniae Lactiflorae
Tao Ren	6 g	Semen Persicae
Hong Hua	3 g	Flos Carthami Tinctorii

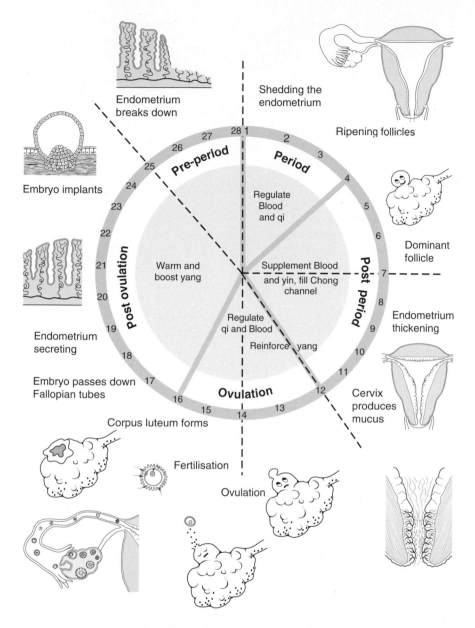

Figure 4.1 Treatment principles in the 4 Phases of the menstrual cycle.

The first four herbs in this prescription constitute Si Wu Tang, which nourishes and invigorates Blood. The addition of Tao Ren and Hong Hua aids in eliminating Blood stasis.

In the case of Qi deficiency, such that Qi does not lead the Blood add:

Dang Shen	9 g	*Radix Codonopsis Pilulosae*
Bai Zhu	9 g	*Rhizoma Atractylodis Macrocephalae*

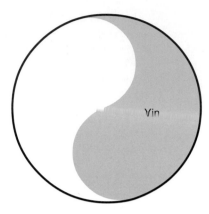

Figure 4.2 The Yin phase.

or add the patent formula:

Si Jun Zi Wan (Four Gentleman Combination).

In the case of Blood stagnation add:

Wu Ling Zhi	9 g	*Excrementum Trogopterori*
Pu Huang	9 g	*Pollen Typhae*
Shan Zha	12 g	*Fructus Crataegi*
Yan Hu Suo	9 g	*Rhizoma Corydalis Yanhusuo*

Acupuncture Points — Choose points from the following (and see Table 4.1):

SP-10	Xuehai
SP-6	Sanyinjiao
SP-8	Diji
CO-4	Hegu
ST-28	Shuidao
KI-14	Siman
Ren-6	Qihai
Tituo	
BL-25	Dachangshu
BL-30	Baihuangshu
BL-32	Ciliao or any of the other sacral points
PC-5	Jianshi

CASE HISTORY – MELINDA

Melinda (32) conceived and gave birth to her son with no difficulty. It was after the birth that difficulties began. Retained placental products gave her a nasty infection and a lot of pain. She spent several days in hospital on intravenous antibiotics. Since her periods had returned (3 months after the birth) they had been painful and clotty and dark, and worse, she had been unable to conceive again in the following 5 years. She described her periods as Hellish! The flow was very heavy and dark and contained large clots, the size of small eggs. Her abdomen pain was acute, sharp and debilitating for more than

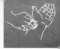

24h and her lower back ached. Before her period, she felt irritable and tired. She saw no distinct signs of ovulation but her breasts became swollen and sore from midcycle until her period came. Her cycle was regular at 28–30 days and her BBT charts (Fig. 4.3) of the last 6 months showed an unstable follicular phase but otherwise were good. Her general health was good, although she rated her stress levels as high and her sleep was restless. Her pulses were rapid and wiry and her tongue looked mauve.

The diagnosis of Melinda's infertility was stagnation of Blood affecting the endometrium. She had not had an ultrasound but it would not have surprised me to find that there were fibroids or polyps or endometriosis developing in such an environment. She exhibited quite a degree of Liver Qi stagnation also. The first aim of treatment was to strongly remove the Blood stagnation and to this end, I asked her to suspend attempts to fall pregnant for a couple of cycles.

From midcycle and during her next period she took herbs to regulate Liver Qi and resolve Blood stagnation.

Chai Hu	12g	Radix Bupleuri
Dang Gui	9g	Radix Angelicae Sinensis
Bai Shao	15g	Radix Paeoniae Lactiflorae
Chuan Xiong	6g	Radix Ligustici Wallichii
Tao Ren	6g	Semen Persicae
Hong Hua	3g	Flos Carthami Tinctorii
Wu Ling Zhi	9g	Excrementum Trogopterori
Pu Huang	9g	Pollen Typhae
Yan Hu Suo	9g	Rhizoma Corydalis Yanhusuo
Xu Duan	9g	Radix Dipsaci
He Huan Pi	9g	Cortex Albizziae Julibrissin
Suan Zao Ren	15g	Semen Ziziphi Spinosae

Acupuncture before the period: LIV-8, LIV-3, LIV-14, SP-6, ST-29, PC-6, PC-7, Yin Tang

Acupuncture during the period: SP-10, SP-6, SP-8, CO-4, ST-29, PC-5

She took Liu Wei Di Huang Wan and Tian Wang Bu Xin Dan in pill form from the end of the period until she ovulated.

Acupuncture between period and ovulation: KI-3, KI-13, SP-6, HT-7, PC-6, Yin Tang

After 2 cycles following this regime, her period flow was much less heavy, had no clots and was quite a lot less painful although not pain free. Her premenstrual symptoms, especially the breast soreness, had improved markedly. She still saw no signs of fertile mucus at midcycle so during the 3rd month she took Gui Shao Di Huang Tang in decocted form after her period. This month her BBT chart showed a stable follicular phase (Fig. 4.4).

It was in this cycle that she conceived. Her second son was born without drama during or after the birth.

Post-Menstrual Phase – Building Kidney Yin and the Blood

In terms of building fertile potential, the post-menstrual, or follicular phase, is the most crucial phase of the cycle. Much careful thought must be given to making treatments as effective as possible at this time. Not only is this the time that the egg matures to its fullest potential for fertilization but it is also the time during which the lining of the uterus prepares from the ground up.

The way the endometrium constructs itself during this crucial post-menstrual phase has bearing on the success of implantation of an embryo and can also determine the nature of the next period flow (in terms of quantity and discomfort). Ideally, the endometrium should be around 10mm thick by the time it has been completely reconstructed at midcycle. Both acupuncture and herbs can influence this orderly growth.

Table 4.1   Acupuncture points used in treatment of infertility: menstrual phase

Treatment goal	Acupuncture point
To open the uterus and encourage strong downward movement and a smooth and thorough discharge of the menstrual flow	CO-4 with SP-6
To moderate this action and hold the Qi	Ren-6
To treat all aspects of the Blood, both its movement and its supplementation and control the extent of the bleeding if there is Heat	SP-10
To remove obstructions to Blood flow	SP-8 (Xi-cleft point of Spleen channel)
To move Blood	KI-14 (the most important point on the Chong channel for moving Blood)
To regulate the Qi in the uterus and moderate the descending action of SP-6	Tituo
To regulate Qi in the lower Jiao	BL-25 and BL-30
To regulate Qi specifically in the Uterus	BL-32
To regulate Qi, particularly if there is pain in the back and sacrum	Baliao
To make Blood flow smoothly, relieve pain and calm the mind	PC-5

Month   February–March

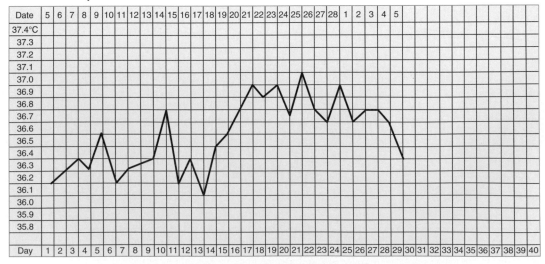

Figure 4.3 Case history – Melinda. This chart shows an unstable follicular phase.

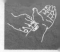

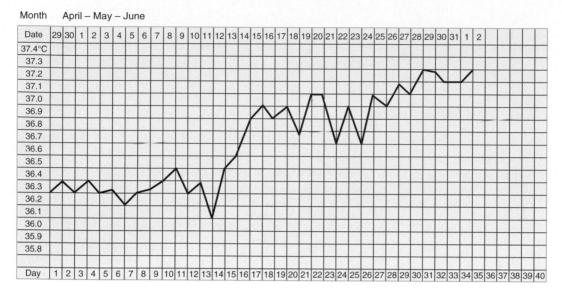

Figure 4.4 Case history – Melinda. She is pregnant in the 3rd month of treatment.

• When do we Start to Reinforce the Yin?

We usually begin building Kidney Yin when the period finishes or is finishing. Typically, this is around Day 4 of the period (Day 1 being the 1st day of menstrual flow). If the bleeding is very scanty or short, it might be appropriate to start the Yin building treatment on Day 3. It is important to allow the endometrium time to completely discharge its unneeded fluids, blood and tissue before using tonics to start stimulating its growth again. On the other hand, if a woman has very long periods that continue well past Day 4 (e.g., for 10 days), starting Yin tonic treatment on Day 4 is recommended regardless. In such cases, giving herbs during the period to encourage it to discharge more efficiently over a shorter period of time is the appropriate course of action.

• How do we know Yin Levels are Increasing?

When the bleeding stops, there is usually very little vaginal discharge, i.e., the Yin levels are still very low. Ideally, the vagina should be quite moist in the week after the period and the thicker stretchy fertile mucus should appear for several days prior to ovulation. Research done at the University of Umea in Sweden[2] has shown us that there are three or four different types of fertile mucus produced by the cervix (see Ch. 3). The first is called the L type and is the type which gradually develops when Yin and Blood tonics are being taken during the first half of the cycle.

Assessing this vaginal discharge (i.e., asking the woman to observe very closely and record any changes) is one of the most useful ways of determining Kidney Yin levels (Table 4.2). The levels of discharge can, to some degree, decide the timing and the doses of the Yin tonic herbs the doctor prescribes.

Herbal Formula — In most fertility clinics, the base formula chosen is the famous Liu Wei Di Huang Tang, a treatment which was formulated hundreds of years ago and has been used ever since to build the Yin. Because we are going to use it just after the period and want to build the Blood as well as the Yin, it is usual to add the Blood tonics Dang Gui and Bai Shao. This makes the formula known as Gui Shao Di Huang Tang:

Gui Shao Di Huang Tang (Angelica Peonia Rehmannia decoction)

Shu Di	12 g	*Radix Rehmanniae Glutinosae Conquitae*
Shan Yao	9 g	*Radix Dioscorea Oppositae*

Shan Zhu Yu	9 g	*Fructus Corni Officinalis*
Fu Ling	6 g	*Sclerotium Poriae Cocos*
Mu Dan Pi	6 g	*Cortex Moutan Radicis*
Ze Xie	6 g	*Rhizoma Alismatis*
Dang Gui	9 g	*Radix Angelicae Sinensis*
Bai Shao	9 g	*Radix Paeoniae Lactiflorae*

Shu Di and Shan Zhu Yu enrich the Yin of the Kidney and Liver and Shan Yao enriches the Yin of the Spleen. To counteract the rich and cloying natures of the tonics (especially Shu Di), Ze Xie and Fu Ling are added. To clear Kidney-and Liver-Fire, Mu Dan Pi is added. The two extra Blood tonics added to this formula balance each other's action: Dang Gui is warm and moist and moves the Blood gently; Bai Shao, on the other hand, while still nourishing the Blood, is cooling and sour and contracting.

If the period flow is still substantial on Day 4 the following herbs, which encourage the flow to finish by regulating the Blood, can be added to the guiding formula for a couple of days:

Chi Shao	9 g	*Radix Paeoniae Rubra*
Yi Mu Cao	9 g	*Herba Leonuri Heterophyll*
Shan Zha (Sheng)	9 g	*Fructus Crataegi*

Some Yin and Blood tonics are hard to digest and, if that proves to be the case, then these formulas should be expanded to contain herbs to help Spleen function, e.g., Shu Di is often better digested if a few grams of Sha Ren are included. Alternatively, a patent medicine like Xiang Sha Lui Jun Zi Wan, which helps digestion by invigorating and regulating the Spleen and Stomach Qi, can be taken at the same time.

Preparing for Ovulation

Typically, the herbs are taken in decoction or granules once or twice a day until there starts to be evidence that the Yin is well established, i.e., until the vaginal discharge starts to become a little more marked. For some women it is difficult to make accurate or objective assessments of cervical mucus; however, with instruction and encouragement, it usually gets easier. And certainly, once the herbs have taken effect, fertile mucus becomes more copious and therefore easier to detect.

Table 4.2   Mucus secretions of the cervix and levels of Yin

	No Yin deficiency	Moderate Yin deficiency	Severe Yin deficiency
1st week follicular phase	After bleeding stops, increasing moisture until middle of the cycle	Some small amount of vaginal discharge	Vaginal dryness. Very little detectable discharge at all
2nd week follicular phase	Approaching ovulation, discharge becomes more copious and stretchy and is apparent for several days	Close to ovulation, small amounts of stretchy discharge appear for 1–2 days	No production of stretchy mucus. No ovulation in more severe cases

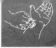

As Yin levels grow, Yang is consumed, i.e., the continuing growth of Yin depends on Yang. Therefore, as we approach the middle part of this phase of the cycle (around Day 8 or 9 say if ovulation is expected on Day 14) we need to start thinking about adding small amounts (5–6 g) of some mild Yang tonics to the guiding formula.

Herbal Formula — Choose two of the following:

Tu Si Zi	6 g	*Semen Cuscatae*
Rou Cong Rong	6 g	*Herba Cistanches*
Xu Duan	6 g	*Radix Dipsaci*

This enhances the formation of stretchy cervical mucus, or S mucus, which, as we saw in Chapter 3, can provide very positive benefit to the sperm attempting to pass up the cervix.

Now as we approach midcycle, Yin is reaching its maximum. The Yin tonics in the base formula can be increased in dose:

Shu Di	15 g	*Radix Rehmanniae Glutinosae Conquitae*
Shan Zhu Yu	12 g	*Fructus Corni Officinalis*

More and stronger Yang tonics can be added now to aid the final and fullest stage of Yin growth (and the birth of Yang), which leads to plentiful fertile mucus, both S and the final P form, the release of LH and ovulation.

On Day 11 or 12 therefore, we add one or two of:

Suo Yang	6 g	*Herba Cynomorii Songarici*
Zi Shi Ying	9 g	*Fluoritum*
Yin Yang Huo	9 g	*Herba Epimedii*
Ba Ji Tian	9 g	*Radix Morindae Officinalis*

While the addition of Yang herbs to formulas prescribed when the egg inside the follicle is reaching maturity is based on an understanding of the cycle of Yin and Yang, researchers have found that these Yang herbs have a particular quality of enhancing energy (ATP) production in the mitochondria. This is precisely what is required in the developing egg cell as it is the mitochondria from the egg that will be responsible for providing the energy to drive the many cell divisions of the embryo in its first few days. Table 4.3 summarizes qualities of different yang herbs that might be used in fertility formulas and includes relative ATP production rates observed in laboratory studies on mice fed with different yang herbs.[3]

Acupuncture Points — There are many points that can be used in the first part of the menstrual cycle. There is documented evidence[3] of increased blood supply to the uterus after acupuncture. Choose points from the following (and see Table 4.4):

Ren-4	Guanyuan
Ren-7	Yinjiao
KI-3	Taixi
KI-5	Shuiquan
KI-8	Jiaoxin
ST-30	Qichong
KI-13	Qixue
ST-27	Daju
BL-23	Shenshu

KI-4	Dazhong
KI-6	Zhaohai
SP-4	Gongsun
SP-6	Sanyinjiao
SP-10	Xuehai
ST-36	Zusanli
LIV-3	Taichong
BL-32	Ciliao or any of the other Baliao

Throughout the post-menstrual phase, continue to use a selection of these points, especially those which reinforce both Kidney Yin and Yang and those which regulate the Chong and Ren vessels.

Table 4.3 Summary of qualities of different Yang herbs

Acts on	Tu Si Zi	Rou Cong Rong	Suo Yang	Bu Gu Zhi	Zi Shi Ying	Du Zhong	Yin Yang Huo	Lu Jiao Shuang	Xu Duan	Xian Mao	BaJi Tian
Jing	X	X	×	×				X			
Blood			×					X	×		
Shen					X						
Yin	X					×	×				
Yang	X	X	X	X	×	X	X	×	X	X	X
Miscarriage	X					X			X		
ATP % increase	222	191	230	175		157	130		120	149	142

Table 4.4 Acupuncture points[a] used in the treatment of infertility – post-menstrual phase

Treatment goal	Acupuncture point
To balance both the Ren and Chong vessels at the outset of the cycle	Choose from: Ren-7, KI-5, KI-8, KI-13
To influence Chong vessel activity	SP-4, ST-30
To encourage Blood production	ST-36, LIV-3 and SP-10
To emphasize development of Kidney Yin	Choose from: KI-3, KI-5, KI-6, SP-6, BL-23, Ren-4
To influence Kidney Jing	ST-27
To regulate Qi in the reproductive organs and supplement the Kidneys	Baliao

[a]Use even method needling.

CASE HISTORY – RANI

Rani (30) was a healthy young university lecturer who was feeling frustrated in the extreme by her infertility. In the 4 years she had been trying to fall pregnant she had had every test possible; the laparoscopy showed a perfectly healthy abdomen, the hysterosalpingogram showed normal uterus and tubes, the blood tests done at different times showed that her hormone levels were all normal, her husband's sperm were plentiful and swam well and the post-coital test was positive.

Rani did three stimulated cycles with IVF, during which she produced a good number of eggs which fertilized well. She also completed three frozen embryo cycles and twice did artificial insemination cycles. Nothing worked: it was truly a case of unexplained infertility. Usually in cases like this it isn't too hard for the TCM doctor to find a reason for the infertility even if it is a subtle one. However, in Rani's case there were few clues to go on. Her cycle was regular, she experienced no premenstrual symptoms, her periods were largely trouble-free, except for a little cramping on Day 1. At ovulation she perceived no signs but a urine ovulation detector kit told her she ovulated regularly on Day 13 or 14. She had not kept any BBT charts. Her general health was excellent and the only stress she experienced was that related to her infertility.

When there are so few symptoms or signs the TCM doctor has to rely on the pulses and tongue and subtle or obscure clues. Rani's pulses were wiry on the Heart and Liver positions and thready on the Kidney position. Her tongue was pale. Rani informed me that when her periods started at 14 she lost a lot of head hair, nearly going bald. Gradually, it regrew but it was still thin. At puberty the Chong vessel fills with Blood; this event deprived the head hair of its nourishment, indicating that Rani's Blood reserves were very low. In addition, poor-quality head hair is a sign of Kidney deficiency. That, with the lack of discernible discharge at midcycle and her pulse and tongue picture, indicated to me that the diagnosis of Rani's infertility was most probably Kidney Yin and Blood deficiency. Because she had no marked symptoms, we simply followed the treatment protocol outlined above without any modifications.

After her period, she took Gui Shao Di Huang Tang. On Day 9 she added:

Rou Cong Rong	6g	Herba Cistanches
Tu Si Zi	6g	Semen Cuscatae

and further on Day 12:

Suo Yang	6g	Herba Cynomorii Songarici
BaJiTian	9g	Radix Morindae Officinalis
Hong Hua	3g	Flos Carthami Tinctorii
Dan Shen	9g	Radix Salviae Miltiorrhizae
Chuan Xiong	6g	Radix Ligustici Wallichii

On Day 16, after the urine testing kit had indicated ovulation, she took a post-ovulation formula, Yu Lin Zhu:

Dang Shen	12g	Radix Codonopsis Pilulosae
Bai Zhu	9g	Rhizoma Atractylodis Macrocephalae
Fu Ling	9g	Sclerotium Poriae Cocos
Dang Gui	9g	Radix Angelicae Sinensis
Bai Shao	9g	Radix Paeoniae Lactiflorae
Chuan Xiong	6g	Radix Ligustici Wallichii
Shu Di	9g	Radix Rehmanniae Glutinosae Conquitae
Tu Si Zi	9g	Semen Cuscatae
Du Zhong	9g	Cortex Eucommiae Ulmoidis
Lu Jiao Pian	9g	Cornu Cervi Parvum
Zhi Gan Cao	6g	Radix Glycyrrhizae Uralensis

During her period, she took Tao Hong Si Wu Wan.

She followed this treatment regimen with minor variations for 3 months, at the end of which time she was pregnant. Rani's was simply a case of reinforcing Kidney Yin and building Blood sufficiently to increase her fertility in a way that drug regimens could not. Her pregnancy was a healthy one and the birth uncomplicated, but after a couple of weeks of breast-feeding (another drain on Chong vessel Blood) she developed marked alopecia – two large bald patches on her head.

Modifications and Variations

If there are any other imbalances present: Heart or Liver stagnation, Blood stagnation or obstruction by Phlegm-Damp, we need to consider additions or subtractions to the basic formula. We also need to consider the relative balance of the Kidney Yin and Yang for each individual.

Kidney Deficiency

KIDNEY YIN DEFICIENCY

The follicular phase, which is concerned with follicle and endometrium development, is the time when prescribed treatment includes building Yin whether there is a gross Yin deficiency or not. Here we discuss modifications to be made if the Yin deficiency is marked. It has long been recognized that Kidney Yin disorders are more difficult to treat successfully than Kidney Yang disorders, especially in women over 35.

Herbal Formula — If there is a functional ovulatory disorder we can assume a pathological deficiency of Kidney Yin. In some cases this will be accompanied by the systemic Yin-deficient signs and symptoms already discussed. In these cases we may need to add more Yin tonics to our base formula.

Add to the base formula (Gui Shao Di Huang Tang):

Nu Zhen Zi	12g	Fructus Ligustri Lucidi
Han Lian Cao	9g	Herba Ecliptae Prostratae
Mai Dong	9g	Tuber Ophiopogonis

Or increase the dose of the emperor herbs of our base formula from the beginning, e.g.:

| Shu Di | 15g | Radix Rehmanniae Glutinosae Conquitae |
| Shan Zhu Yu | 12g | Fructus Corni Officinalis |

and add to these:

| Sheng Di | 15g | Radix Rehmanniae Glutinosae |

To aid digestion of these herbs add:

| Sha Ren | 6g | Fructus seu Semen Amomi |

Acupuncture Points — To directly nourish the Yin, herbs are more effective than acupuncture, but acupuncture is a useful adjunct, particularly where there is Yin deficiency Heat or the Chong and Ren vessel function is not well controlled due to the Kidney weakness. For some very restless or busy Yin-deficient women the half-hour rest on the acupuncture table may be the only time they stop in the day.

Choose points from those in Table 4.4 which emphasize treating the Kidney Yin. For example:

| KI-6 | Zhaohai |
| KI-3 | Taixi |

with reinforcing technique. And where there is Yin deficiency Heat add:

| KI-2 | Rangu |

with mild regulating technique.

Women with ovulatory disturbances (i.e., long irregular cycles) are often given a fertility drug called clomifene (Clomid or Serophene). In a Yin-deficient woman this is unfortunate – while clomifene is very effective in stimulating ovulation, it can be at the cost of the Yin. For example, the lack of fertile mucus and the thinness of the endometrium often seen in Yin-deficient women, can be exacerbated by this drug due to its anti-estrogen action (see Ch. 5). In the more unfortunate of these cases menstrual cycles may cease altogether. Ovulations induced by clomifene in Yin-deficient women rarely produce eggs which are of sufficient quality to produce viable embryos. TCM practitioners are always very wary of recommending the use of this drug for women who are distinctly Yin deficient.

Yin is usually depleted over a long period of time and, likewise, it takes some time to recover it. Yin-deficient women trying to fall pregnant may be looking at 6–12 months of building their Kidney Yin again with tonic herbs and a sensibly paced life.

The TCM practitioner also needs to encourage the woman to get enough good-quality sleep, a regular routine which factors in time for meals and exercise and ideally some down time for the mind. This could include meditation or mind-quietening activities such as yoga, tai chi, walking alone, swimming, etc.

CASE HISTORY – PHOEBE

Phoebe (35) had used no contraception for the 4 years of her marriage but had not succeeded in falling pregnant. A laparoscopy revealed no clues. She had kept BBT charts for a year and these showed a short luteal phase and erratic follicular and luteal phases (Fig. 4.5).

Her cycle was 25 days; premenstrually she experienced swollen breasts, insomnia, fatigue, irritability and abdomen pain. She experienced severe period pain with a heavy, clotty, dark flow and lower back pain. The symptoms were worse with movement and better for rest and massage. She saw no fertile mucus at midcycle. She was a thin, dry, anxious, stressed woman who experienced palpitations.

The cause of infertility in Phoebe's case is Kidney Yin deficiency, leading to Kidney Yang deficiency. The short luteal phase seen on her BBT chart and the lower back pain indicate Kidney Yang deficiency. Her constitution, demeanor and lack of fertile mucus reveal the Kidney Yin deficiency. This is complicated by Heart- and Liver-Fire, evidenced by premenstrual symptoms, a tendency to anxiety and the erratic nature of the follicular phase on her BBT chart. Blood stagnation is evident in the painful and clotty period. The treatment principle was:

- reinforce Kidney Yin and Yang

- regulate Liver and Heart Qi

- regulate Blood.

The post-menstrual formula aimed to strongly reinforce Kidney Yin. To do this successfully, the Shen needed to be pacified.

Suan Zao Ren	15 g	Semen Ziziphi Spinosae
Bai Zi Ren	9 g	Semen Biotae Orientalis
Dang Gui	9 g	Radix Angelicae Sinensis
Long Yan Rou	9 g	Arillus Euphoriae Longanae
Fu Shen	6 g	Sclerotium Poriae Cocos Pararadicis
ShuDi	12 g	Radix Rehmanniae Glutinosae Conquitae
Sheng Di	12 g	Radix Rehmanniae Glutinosae
Shan Zhu Yu	9 g	Fructus Corni Officinalis
Shan Yao	9 g	Dioscorea Oppositae

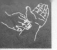

Ze Xie	6g	Rhizoma Alismatis
Mu Dan Pi	6g	Cortex Moutan Radicis
Dan Shen	9g	Radix Salviae Miltiorrhizae

At ovulation, she took herbs to regulate Qi and Blood and to begin building Kidney Yang. At the same time, Kidney Yin tonic herbs were continued, as were Blood tonics.

Xu Duan	6g	Radix Dipsaci
Tu Si Zi	6g	Semen Cuscatae
Wu Ling Zhi	6g	Excrementum Trogopterori
Hong Hua	3g	Flos Carthami Tinctorii
Di Long	6g	Lumbricus
Ji Nei Jin	3g	Endothelium Corneum Gigeraiae Galli
Mai Ya	6g	Fructus Hordei
Dang Gui	9g	Radix Angelicae Sinensis
Bai Shao	6g	Radix Paeoniae Lactiflorae
Shu Di	6g	Radix Rehmanniae Glutinosae Conquitae
Nu Zhen Zi	9g	Fructus Ligustri Lucidi

After ovulation, she took herbs to boost Kidney Yang, maintain Kidney Yin and address Liver Qi stagnation.

Xu Duan	9g	Radix Dipsaci
Tu Si Zi	12g	Semen Cuscatae
Rou Cong Rong	9g	Herba Cistanches
Xiang Fu	9g	Rhizoma Cyperi Rotundi
Mu Xiang	6g	Radix Saussureae seu Vladimiriae
Nu Zhen Zi	9g	Fructus Ligustri Lucidi
He Huan Pi	6g	Cortex Albizziae Julibrissin
Suan Zao Ren	9g	Semen Ziziphi Spinosae
Gou Teng	12g	Ramulus Uncariae Cum Uncis
Chai Hu	6g	Radix Bupleuri
Bai Shao	6g	Radix Paeoniae Lactiflorae

During the period, she took pills, 'Tong Jing Wan,' which contain herbs to resolve Blood stagnation.

The period pain and flow showed immediate improvement — less heavy, less painful. Over the months the improvement continued. Fertile mucus became apparent in the 2nd month of taking herbs. Anxiety and palpitations persisted over some months and it may have been this continued Shen disturbance which held back the recovery of the Kidney Yin. She continued to take variations of the above prescriptions for the following 10 months. Gradually her BBT chart improved (Fig. 4.6).

It took nearly a year for Phoebe's Kidney Yin to develop to the point where she could produce a good-quality egg and then maintain the Kidney Yang and luteal function during implantation and early embryo development. However the long-awaited pregnancy was a dream one, so was her baby girl.

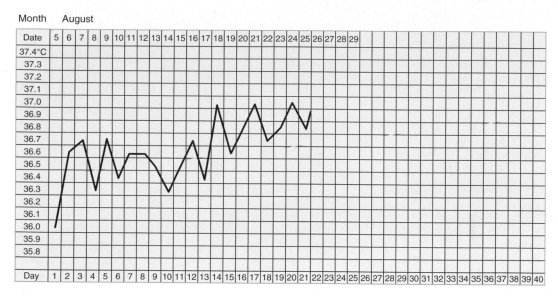

Figure 4.5 Case history – Phoebe. Phoebe's chart shows evidence of marked Heart- and Liver-Fire in the erratic temperature readings of both follicular and luteal phases.

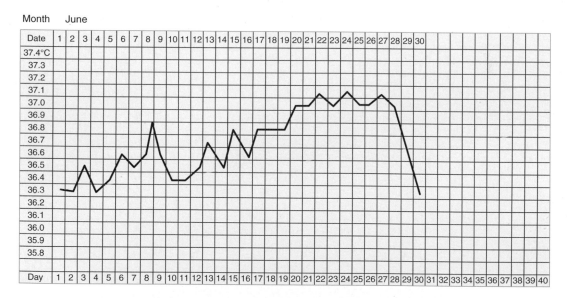

Figure 4.6 Case history – Phoebe. This chart shows a much improved luteal phase due to replenished Kidney Yin and reduced Heart- and Liver-Fire. The following month Phoebe became pregnant.

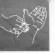

CASE HISTORY – ROBIN

Robin (40 years) had been trying to fall pregnant for 4 years and was getting worried now that she was about to turn 40. Both she and her husband were in the medical profession and they had already arranged all the relevant investigations and organized the prescription for clomifene.

A laparoscopy revealed nothing untoward but blood tests revealed low progesterone levels in the luteal phase. Her BBT charts (Fig. 4.7) indicated this also, i.e., the luteal phase was short and recorded basal temperatures were not much higher than those in the follicular phase.

This improved a lot when she took the clomifene but the side-effects (agitation, palpitations and flushing) were severe enough for her to discontinue it after 2 cycles.

Robin's cycle was usually short: namely, 21–25 days. Ovulation was accompanied by some abdomen pain and she seldom saw any fertile mucus. Premenstrually, she was emotionally volatile and irritable. Her periods were accompanied by dragging pain in the abdomen and the blood tended to be dark, mucusy and sometimes clotty. Other chronic symptoms included frequent urinary tract infections (UTI), which were often provoked by sexual activity.

At first consultation, this woman spoke quickly, had a fidgety demeanor and a marked malar flush. Her pulse was short and tight, slippery and fast (due to the current UTI) and her tongue had a red tip with a dry cracked center.

Her inability to become pregnant stemmed from several factors. Her luteal phase was inadequate, so that even if she conceived the embryo would likely not implant and develop. The appearance of her BBTs with their low luteal phase readings, her low progesterone reading in the luteal phase, her short cycle and the dragging nature of her period pain indicated Kidney Yang deficiency. However, underlying this is the deficiency of Kidney Yin. This Yin deficiency, which is the true basis of her infertility, was apparent in the lack of fertile mucus, her restlessness, her malar flush and her red dry tongue. It is her Yin deficiency that made clomifene such an inappropriate drug, provoking as it did signs of Yin-deficient Heat.

Robin's periods flowed sluggishly in the beginning (creating pain). Yin deficiency and fluid deficiency probably contributed to the thick mucusy flow, as could Damp. There was likely some Damp in the Lower Jiao, as evidenced by the frequent UTIs. Qi stagnation is also apparent in the premenstrual picture and the ovulation and period pain. In summary her diagnosis was:

Kidney Yin deficiency leading to Kidney Yang deficiency complicated by Liver Qi stagnation and Phlegm-Damp accumulation. The main thrust of treatment must be to strongly build Kidney Yin in the follicular phase so that Kidney Yang does not collapse in the luteal phase.

The treatment principle was:

- reinforce Kidney Yin to build Kidney Yang

- clear Phlegm-Damp

- regulate Liver Qi

- regulate Blood during menstruation.

Treatment during the period – herbs to resolve Blood and Qi stagnation, and Damp-Heat (for the active UTI):

Dang Gui	9 g	Radix Angelicae Sinensis
Dan Shen	9 g	Radix Salviae Miltiorrhizae
Yan Hu Suo	9 g	Rhizoma Corydalis Yanhusuo
Wu Ling Zhi	9 g	Excrementum Trogopterori
Mu Dan Pi	9 g	Cortex Moutan Radicis
Huang Bai	9 g	Cortex Phellodendri

Shan Zhi Zi	6g	Fructus Gardeniae Jasminoidis
Che Qian Zi	9g	Semen Plantaginis
Xiang Fu	9g	Rhizoma Cyperi Rotundi
Wu Yao	6g	Radix Linderae Strychnifoliae
Chen Pi	3g	Pericarpium Citri Reticulate

Following the period – herbs to build Yin and Blood (and clear Damp-Heat):

Shu Di	12g	Radix Rehmanniae Glutinosae Conquitae
Sheng Di	15g	Radix Rehmanniae Glutinosae
Bai Shao	9g	Radix Paeoniae Lactiflorae
Dang Gui	9g	Radix Angelicae Sinensis
Shan Yao	9g	Dioscorea Oppositae
Shan Zhu Yu	9g	Fructus Corni Officinalis
Nu Zhen Zi	12g	Fructus Ligustri Lucidi
Mu Dan Pi	9g	Cortex Moutan Radicis
Huang Bai	9g	Cortex Phellodendri
Shan Zhi Zi	3g	Fructus Gardeniae Jasminoidis
Fu Ling	9g	Sclerotium Poriae Cocos
Suan Zao Ren	15g	Semen Ziziphi Spinosae
Ze Xie	9g	Rhizoma Alismatis

As ovulation approached, Robin needed more Qi moving herbs as well as small amounts of Yang tonic herbs to begin the transition from Yin to Yang. In addition, herbs were added to prevent recurrence of the UTIs provoked by sex at midcycle.

Added to the above formula were:

Che Qian Zi	9g	Semen Plantaginis
Mu Xiang	9g	Radix Saussureae seu Vladimiriae
Wu Yao	6g	Radix Linderae Strychnifoliae
Tu Si Zi	9g	Semen Cuscatae
Xu Duan	6g	Radix Dipsaci
Huang Lian	1.5g	Rhizoma Coptidis
Huang Bai	3g	Cortex Phellodendri

and Sheng Di, Shan Zhi Zi and Suan Zao Ren were removed.

After ovulation Robin took the usual herbs for supporting the Kidney Yang. Kidney Yin was nourished and herbs were added to prevent the emotional volatility experienced premenstrually.

Tu Si Zi	9g	Semen Cuscatae
Xu Duan	9g	Radix Dipsaci
Yin Yang Huo	6g	Herba Epimedii
Fu Pen Zi	9g	Fructus Rubi Chingii
Nu Zhen Zi	12g	Fructus Ligustri Lucidi
Sang Ji Sheng	9g	Ramulus Sangjisheng
Gou Qi Zi	12g	Fructus Lycii Chinensis
Yi Yi Ren	15g	Semen Coicis Lachryma-jobi
He Huan Pi	9g	Cortex Albizziae Julibrissin
Gou Teng	12g	Ramulus Uncariae Cum Uncis
Suan Zao Ren	15g	Semen Ziziphi Spinosae
Bai Zi Ren	9g	Semen Biotae Orientalis

Cycle 1 brought an immediate improvement in the amount of fertile mucus (2 days of obvious stretchy mucus). This is not an uncommon response and is an encouraging sign that the Yin can indeed be recovered. However, it usually takes longer than 1 cycle to affect enough of a change to increase fertility. In fact, Robin's BBT chart this cycle showed a very unconvincing and short luteal phase not so different from the one shown in Figure 4.7, i.e., the Kidney Yang was still insufficient.

The next cycle she followed the same regimen with adjustments for incidental symptoms. This time her cycle lengthened considerably to 28 days and the temperature shift at ovulation was clearer, although the final range was still quite low (Fig. 4.8).

Her period this time was much improved, with a smooth flow of blood that was no longer mucusy or thick.

Cycle 3 was complicated by an upper respiratory infection followed by a UTI for which antibiotics were prescribed. There was an early ovulation and early period on Day 21. After this set back, we decided to double the dose of herbs, i.e., she boiled one packet of herbs twice each day. This seemed to do the trick – her BBT remained elevated and a pregnancy test on Day 30 was positive (Fig. 4.9).

Her pregnancy was reasonably uneventful and she delivered a healthy baby at term.

Robin's Kidney Yin was of course drained somewhat by the pregnancy and breast-feeding. Now several years after the birth she is showing the signs of menopause at 45 years.

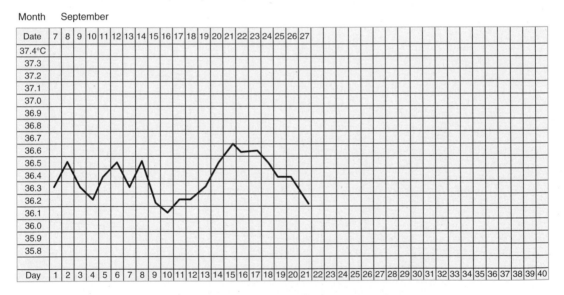

Figure 4.7 Case history – Robin. Robin's chart shows a low and short luteal phase.

KIDNEY YANG DEFICIENCY

Herbal Formula — At the beginning of the cycle most of our treatment emphasis is on building Kidney Yin. However, if a woman is seriously Yang deficient this must be addressed at the same time we are nourishing Kidney Yin. Many women develop weak Spleen Qi and Kidney Yang functions as they age – this is why we often see a mixture of Kidney Yin and Kidney Yang-deficiency symptoms simultaneously in women in their late 30s and onwards. Remember though that the emphasis on building Kidney Yang still belongs mainly to the second half of the cycle and that is when strongest Yang tonic treatment can be applied. If there is a general Yang-deficient constitution, mild Kidney Yang tonics can be added to the base formula (Gui Shao Di Huang Tang) from Day 3 or 4, for example:

| Tu Si Zi | 9 g | *Semen Cuscatae* |
| Rou Cong Rong | 6 g | *Herba Cistanches* |

Month   November – December

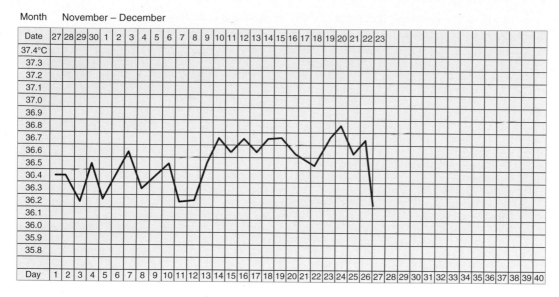

Figure 4.8 Case history – Robin. After 2 cycles of treatment, this chart showed that the luteal phase had improved.

Month   December – January

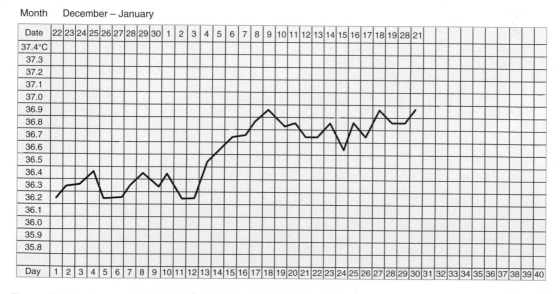

Figure 4.9 Case history – Robin. This chart indicated that she had conceived.

Stronger Kidney Yang tonics will be added only when the Yin base is established, i.e., the vaginal discharge is getting thicker and more stretchy.

If Rou Cong Rong causes diarrhea in someone with Spleen weakness it should be replaced with an alternative Yang tonic.

97

The use of fertility drugs, such as clomifene, is generally not contraindicated in cases of Yang deficiency unless the Yin is also quite deficient. In fact, ovulations induced by clomifene are generally followed by rather good luteal phases, indicating that this drug may indeed be beneficial to Kidney Yang.

Acupuncture Points — Points chosen from the list in Table 4.3 will emphasize those which reinforce both Kidney Yin and Yang, for example:

Ren-4	Guanyuan
KI-3	Taixi

And those which specifically boost Kidney Yang should be added:

BL-23	Shenshu
Ren-3	Zhongji
BL-32	Ciliao and the other Baliao

Reinforcing technique and moxa are applicable for all points.

KIDNEY JING DEFICIENCY

Herbal Formula — The formula Gui Shao Di Huang Tang is very useful for supplementing Yin and Blood (i.e., stimulating the follicle and priming the endometrium) but the Jing (the eggs themselves) may also need attention. If ovulation is very uncertain or erratic, and particularly if that has been the case since puberty, the addition of herbs to nourish Jing is essential. Traditionally, this is done with the addition of animal products such as Gui Ban and Bie Jia. These substances are extracted from the soft part of the tortoise plastron. Since turtles and tortoises all over the world are now considered to be endangered species, the use of Gui Ban and Bie Jia should be restricted unless they come from a farmed source with a CITES certificate. Some practitioners and patients prefer to use the alternative Mu Li, which is made from ground oyster shell. Other substances, which can be added to our base formula when Jing is very low are:

Zi He Che*	1.5–3 g (in powder or pill form)	*Placenta Hominis*
Lu Jiao Jiao	9 g	*Cornu Cervi Parvum*
He Shou Wu	9 g	*Radix Polygoni Multiflori*

Fertility drugs which act directly on the ovary (FSH preparations such as Puregon or Gonal-F) are often employed in these cases. These drugs are very potent stimulators of the ovary and, in most cases, if there are any follicles at all, an ovulation will be induced. However, the quality of the egg is not always good when the Jing is deficient.

Although Chinese herbs are much slower acting than fertility drugs, the ovulations they do eventually promote have a much better chance of being followed by a successful pregnancy.

Because Kidney Jing deficiency represents a deep level of deficiency, treatment will often need to continue for months or years. These cases can be difficult to treat successfully, especially if the reproductive organs are underdeveloped. Nevertheless, I have seen doctors in the fertility clinics in China commence treatment of seemingly very difficult cases of Kidney Jing deficiency to see if there was any response which would encourage further treatment – often there was.

*Zi He Che is used in Chinese infertility clinics but is restricted in many other countries. Many practitioners prefer not to use human or animal substances in which case this and Lu Jiao Jiao can be replaced with plant substitutes such as Huang Jing (Rhizoma Polygonati).

CASE HISTORY – SAMANTHA

Samantha (29) was a small and frail-looking woman who wanted to become pregnant. She had never used contraception and had been actively pursuing pregnancy for 3 years. However, she ovulated very infrequently and, since reaching puberty at the late age of 17, she had experienced several stretches of amenorrhoea. Investigations revealed an underdeveloped uterus. Her periods when they came were scanty and accompanied by lower back pain.

Samantha had many symptoms indicating Kidney deficiency. She needed to urinate four or five times a night and she suffered stress incontinence and lower back pain. Additionally, she had chronic asthma. She was underweight, pale and felt the cold. She was frequently unwell.

The diagnosis of her infertility was Kidney Jing deficiency. She was recommended to take herbs to strongly nourish and build Kidney Jing, Kidney Yin and Yang, and Qi and Blood for 1 year.

Dang Gui	9g	Radix Angelicae Sinensis
Bai Shao	9g	Radix Paeoniae Lactiflorae
Shan Yao	9g	Radix Dioscorea Oppositae
Shu Di	9g	Radix Rehmanniae Glutinosae Conquitae
Sha Ren	6g	Fructus seu Semen Amomi
Shan Zhu Yu	9g	Fructus Corni Officinalis
Mu Dan Pi	9g	Cortex Moutan Radicis
Fu Ling	9g	Sclerotium Poriae Cocos
Chai Hu	6g	Radix Bupleuri
Tai Zi Shen	15g	Radix Pseudostellariae Heteropyllae
Xu Duan	9g	Radix Dipsaci
Tu Si Zi	9g	Semen Cuscatae
Chen Pi	3g	Pericarpium Citri Reticulate
Gui Ban*	15g	Plastrum Testudines
Bie Jia*	15g	Carapax Amydae Sinensis

Quite soon after commencing the herbs, Samantha felt more substantial and not overwhelmingly tired any more. At times she noticed more ovulation-type mucus and her periods came more often, although they did not become monthly and her BBT pattern was often erratic.

She took this and variations of this formula for only 5 months before she became pregnant. This was unexpected and I feared for the pregnancy because her Kidney function was still not strong. She gave birth to a small (2kg) but healthy baby boy at 37 weeks. Nikky is now 6 years old, small for his age but and as energetic and healthy a young boy as any parent would wish.

*Gui Ban and Bie Jia are endangered species although farmed and CITES certified sources are available. Dr Xia prescribed these substances when he saw this patient in my clinic in Sydney.

Acupuncture Points — Some of the points listed for use in the follicular phase in Table 4.4 have an effect on the Jing, for example:

BL-23   Shenshu
Ren-4   Guanyuan
ST-27   Daju

and other points such as:

KI-12   Dahe

can be added but generally herbs have a greater impact on Jing deficiency than acupuncture.

Heart and Liver Qi Stagnation

Building and maintaining the Yin stores for the follicular phase requires a quiet mind. If the Heart Qi is disordered and the Shen is disturbed, it is very difficult to maintain such inner quiet and development of Yin is jeopardized. Women with such Shen disturbance would benefit greatly from a technique like meditation but often that is an impossible request — it is hard enough for them to sit still, let alone quiet the mind. Often it is best to encourage active pursuits which occupy the body and by their repetitive nature gradually quieten the mind, e.g., walking, jogging or swimming. Then, if appropriate, more internal exercises can be introduced like yoga or Tai Qi and then, eventually, may be meditation.

Herbal Formula — To stabilize the Shen and regulate Heart Qi add to the post-menstrual phase guiding formula (Gui Shao Di Huang Tang):

He Huan Pi	12g	*Cortex Albizziae Julibrissin*
Bai Zi Ren	9g	*Semen Biotae Orientalis*
Mu Li	15g	*Concha Ostreae*

or give at the same time the formula Gan Mai Da Zao Tang, which soothes the Heart with sweet flavors.

If there is Heart-Fire add:

Huang Lian	3g	*Rhizoma Coptidis*
Zhi Zi	6g	*Fructus Gardeniae Jasminoidis*
Lian Zi Xin	1.5–3g	*Plumula Nelumbinis Nuciferae*

Liver Qi stagnation tends to cause more problems later in the cycle, but if there is general tension or high stress or pain with ovulation then herbs to regulate Liver Qi can usefully be added in the post-menstrual phase:

He Huan Pi	9g	*Cortex Albizziae Julibrissin*
Suan Zao Ren	12g	*Semen Ziziphi Spinosae*
Chuan Lian Zi	6g	*Fructus Meliae Toosendan*
Qing Pi	6g	*Pericarpium Citri Reticulatae Viridae*

If there is Liver-Fire add:

Mu Dan Pi	9g	*Cortex Moutan Radicis*
Chi Shao	12g	*Radix Paeoniae Rubra*

Acupuncture Points — To the points chosen from Table 4.4, i.e., those which foster Yin and Blood and regulate the Chong and Ren vessels, add points to pacify Liver- and Heart-Fire such as:

LIV-2	Xingjian
HE-5	Tongli
HE-7	Shenmen
PC-6	Neiguan
PC-7	Daling

These points can be needled with mild reducing technique if the patient is not too anxious.

Ovulation disturbances related to stress and emotional states tend not to be very long term and are generally not treated with fertility drugs by specialists (although occasionally an ardent GP will prescribe clomifene). Acupuncture treatment is generally very helpful in calming the mind to allow development of Yin in the post-menstrual phase.

Blood Stagnation

Symptoms of Blood stagnation manifest during the menstrual period and this is the best time to treat them. However, if we think the endometrium has not been smoothly discharged, herbs to regulate blood stagnation can also be added to the formulas we start using early in the follicular phase. Evidence of Blood stagnation could be continued spotting of dark blood after the period should have finished or a BBT chart on which the temperature does not drop with the arrival of the period.

Herbal Formula — In this case we should add to Gui Shao Di Huang Tang the herbs mentioned earlier that provoke more complete discharge of the endometrium:

Yi Mu Cao	15 g	*Herba Leonuri Heterophylli*
Chi Shao	9 g	*Radix Paeoniae Rubra*
Shan Zha	15 g	*Fructus Crataegi*

If there is a known history of substantial Blood stagnation (e.g., endometrioma or ovarian cysts), then more herbs to regulate Blood can be added:

Tao Ren	9 g	*Semen Persicae*
Hong Hua	6 g	*Flos Carthami Tinctorii*
Wu Ling Zhi	9 g	*Excrementum Trogopterori*

If a woman has been diagnosed with antisperm antibodies in the cervical mucus, sperm will be disabled before they can enter the uterus. Antisperm antibodies in the cervical mucus reflect a subtle level of Blood stagnation. Adding Blood-regulating herbs to those which reinforce the Kidney Yin will usually reduce the antibody load, allowing sperm to penetrate. Add to Gui Shao Di Huang Tang:

Tao Ren	6 g	*Semen Persicae*
Chuan Xiong	6 g	*Radix Ligustici Wallichii*
Hong Hua	3 g	*Flos Carthami Tinctorii*

CASE HISTORY – TOULA

Toula, 40 years of age, had a 10-year history of infertility. She had every possible investigation, as did her husband. Her tubes were fine, her hormones were fine, the sperm was fine. She noticed no symptoms at midcycle and an ovulation kit showed she ovulated on Day 13/14. BBT charts (Fig. 4.10) indicated the same. The luteal phase temperatures were often slow to rise.

But when a post-coital test (PCT) was carried out it was observed that the sperm were stopped dead in their tracks. The PCT was repeated twice more over a period of a year during her early 30s — each time her husband's sperm were immobilized. The diagnosis was the unfortunate label 'a hostile cervix'. The specialists at the ART clinic suggested intrauterine insemination (IUI). This involves insertion of a sperm sample high in the uterus at midcycle, avoiding the cervix and hopefully the antibodies. This rationale proved to be a good one and after two attempts Toula became pregnant and had a son. Five years on and several more attempts at IUI later Toula still didn't have the much desired second child to complete her family. In TCM the diagnosis of her infertility was Kidney Yang deficiency. This was indicated by her BBT charts and the strong lower back pain she suffered before and during each period. Before a period she was bloated and grumpy and craved carbohydrates and her feet and hands were always cold, indicating a Spleen Qi deficiency. Her pulse was thready and her tongue was dull and dark with a white coat. The tongue made me suspect some Blood stagnation on top of the Yang deficiency and the inclusion of Blood-regulating herbs is an important part of the treatment for antisperm antibodies.

Her treatment began at the beginning of a cycle reinforcing Kidney Yin and Yang and regulating Blood. We hoped to encourage more and better quality fertile mucus.

She took Gui Shao Di Huang Tang in a granulated form plus:

Dan Shen	9g	Radix Salviae Miltiorrhizae
Chuan Xiong	6g	Radix Ligustici Wallichii
Tao Ren	6g	Semen Persicae
Hong Hua	3g	Flos Carthami Tinctorii
Sha Ren	6g	Fructus seu Semen Amomi
Gui Zhi	6g	Ramulus Cinnamomi Cassiae
Tu Si Zi	6g	Semen Cuscatae

Acupuncture points: Ren-4, Ren-2, ST-29, ST-36, SP-6, LIV-5, KI-3.

This did not appear to have any rapid effect on the fertile mucus, i.e., she still saw none. She relied on a urine kit to indicate the time of ovulation.

After midcycle she took Kidney Yang tonics (with Spleen Qi tonics):

Tu Si Zi	9g	Semen Cuscatae
Ba Ji Tian	6g	Radix Morindae Officinalis
Du Zhong	9g	Cortex Eucommiae Ulmoidis
Xu Duan	9g	Radix Dipsaci
Dang Shen	9g	Radix Codonopsis Pilulosae
Bai Zhu	9g	Rhizoma Atractylodis Macrocephalae
Shan Yao	9g	Dioscorea Oppositae
Yi Yi Ren	15g	Semen Coicis Lachryma-jobi
Gui Zhi	6g	Ramulus Cinnamomi Cassiae

Acupuncture points: ST-36, KI-3, Ren-12, BL-23.

During her period she took Xue Fu Zhu Yu Wan in pill form. Her back pain and period cramps were unchanged. We decided to persist for another cycle, making only minor adjustments to the herbal prescriptions. I encouraged her to take larger doses of the herbs and to ensure that she took them twice each day without fail. The next ovulation was a little improved, with a small amount of stretchy discharge apparent at midcycle. The improvement was enough; she conceived and had a trouble-free pregnancy, delivering a large baby boy at term.

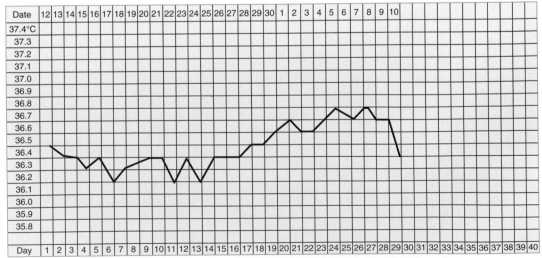

Month   November – December

Figure 4.10 Case history – Toula. The slow, stepwise rise of temperature after ovulation on Day 14/15 indicates a Kidney Yang (and Spleen Qi) deficiency.

Even where there is no Blood stagnation it can be useful to encourage Blood circulation with herbs or acupuncture, as the endometrium is primed after the period and the new lining and blood vessels form. To aid this, add to the guiding formula just one herb:

Dan Shen	9 g	Radix Salviae Miltiorrhizae

Acupuncture Points — Add to points chosen from Table 4.4, additional points to move Blood and Qi:

KI-14	Siman
Ren-3	Zhongji
SP-12	Chongmen
ST-29	Guilai
LIV-5	Ligou
SP-8	Diji

Reducing or regulating techniques are used on these points.

It is generally not a good idea for women to use fertility drugs in these cases and, especially where there is evidence of cysts or tumors on the ovaries or pituitary gland. Acupuncture with its excellent ability to move the Qi and Blood can be very useful in this category. Even where Blood stagnation is not evident, points that circulate the Blood will help the formation of the new endometrium.

Phlegm-Damp Accumulation

Phlegm-Damp accumulation presents us with a clinical challenge. We wish to build Yin to encourage follicle development which may have been retarded by the presence of Phlegm-Damp. However, herbs that enrich Yin create more moisture and are by nature sticky and therefore are not desirable when we want to clear out Damp and stickiness. Similarly, herbs that break up and dispel Phlegm-Damp are drying, which is not really the trend we want to encourage when we need the endometrium to grow and the cervix to start producing more fertile discharge.

Handling such a clinical conundrum requires expert judgment and some juggling. Initially, emphasis remains on building Kidney Yin; however, in this case it is necessary to add Kidney Yang tonics from the early stages as we did with Yang-deficient women. This is because strong Yang Qi prevents Damp accumulation. At the same time, herbs to help clear Phlegm-Damp can be added.

Herbal Formula — Thus, to our guiding formula (Gui Shao Di Huang Tang), we would add herbs such as:

Tu Si Zi	9 g	Semen Cuscatae
Xu Duan	6 g	Radix Dipsaci
Ba Ji Tian	6 g	Radix Morindae Officinalis
Yi Yi Ren	15 g	Semen Coicis Lachryma-jobi
Sha Ren	6 g	Fructus seu Semen Amomi

And Fu Ling will be increased to 15 g.

In severe cases of Phlegm-Damp, or if there is difficulty digesting the herbs Shu Di and Dang Gui in the guiding formula should be replaced with:

Nu Zhen Zi	9 g	Fructus Ligustri Lucidi
Han Lian Cao	9 g	Herba Ecliptae Prostratae
Ji Xue Teng	12 g	Radix et Caulis Jixueteng

Throughout the follicular phase, supplementation of Yin and Yang should be approximately equal. This minimizes some of the risks of using Yin tonics in a Damp environment. As Yin develops, herbs will be added quickly to promote ovulation (i.e., herbs which move Qi and Blood). In cases where there is Phlegm-Damp it is not advisable to wait until Yin is fully expressed (e.g., with copious fertile mucus) before starting to promote ovulation – it may never occur. Thus by Day 9 or 9 of a 28-day cycle, or when there are some initial signs of vaginal discharge or moisture, herbs which move the Qi and Blood (such as those discussed in the next section) will be employed.

Acupuncture Points — Add to the points chosen from Table 4.4:

GB-26	Daimai
SP-5	Shangqui
BL-28	Pangguangshu
Ren-6	Qihai

Use a regulating technique.

Sometimes fertility drugs such as clomifene, which promote ovulation and Kidney Yang, are used with good effect in Phlegm-Damp cases. However, caution must be used if there is evidence of cysts in the ovaries, a not uncommon expression of Phlegm-Damp (see Ch. 5).

MIDCYCLE PHASE – PROMOTING MOVEMENT OF QI AND BLOOD

We have now reached the end of the post-menstrual phase, wherein the Yin and the Blood have been replenished and fortified. The ovary, at the time of fullest Yin, is now ready to release a mature egg. Plentiful stretchy mucus floods the cervical os ready to ferry thousands of sperm upwards and inwards. An egg is poised for liberation from its large ripe follicle when prompted by hormonal messages from the pituitary gland. This is a crucial moment that requires dramatic activity of the Qi and Blood and the switch from Yin to Yang.

The formulas described below for use in promoting ovulation will only be applied once the Yin base is laid, i.e., there must be some fertile mucus or indication of rapidly rising estrogen levels seen in blood tests. Then they can be used twice a day between 3 and 7 days.

Provided that Yin foundation is present we now apply strong herbal treatment to promote ovulation. One way to do this is to use herbs that move the Blood.

Herbal Formula — The formula Cu Pai Luan Tang is a well-known and often-used ovulation formula. In a young or relatively strong woman it will promote an effective ovulation from a sound Yin base. It can be used for around 3 days starting just before the assumed day of ovulation.

Cu Pai Luan Tang (Ovulation decoction)

Dang Gui	9 g	*Radix Angelicae Sinensis*
Chi Shao	9 g	*Radix Paeoniae Rubra*
Chuan Xiong	6 g	*Radix Ligustici Wallichii*
Hong Hua	6 g	*Flos Carthami Tinctorii*
Dan Shen	9 g	*Radix Salviae Miltiorrhizae*
Ze Lan	9 g	*Herba Lycopi Lucidi*
Ji Xue Teng	15 g	*Radix et Caulis Jixueteng*

All seven herbs in this prescription regulate the Blood, ensuring there is no obstruction in the process of ovulation and passage of the egg in the fallopian tube. Circulation in the endometrium as it prepares for an embryo is enhanced also.

This formula should be boiled for a short time only (around 5 min) with the lid on so as not to lose the volatile components which are helpful in provoking Qi and Blood movement. Granulated herbs should be dissolved in hot rather than boiling water for the same reason.

Acupuncture Points — Choose points from (and see Table 4.5):

Local points		Leg channel points	
KI-13	Qixue	LIV-3	Taichong
KI-14	Siman	LIV-5	Ligou
SP-13	Fushe	KI-4	Dazhong
ST-28	Shuidao	KI-5	Shuiquan
ST-29	Guilai	KI-8	Jiaoxin
Zigong		SP-5	Shangqiu
GB-26	Daimai	SP-6	Sanyinjiao
		SP-8	Diji

Arm channel points		Head points
PC-6	Neiguan	Yintang
PC-5	Jianshi	
HE-7	Shenmen	
HE-5	Tongli	

Modifications and Variations

Kidney Deficiency

KIDNEY YIN DEFICIENCY

Herbal Formula — If the woman is not so young (>35 years) or there is Kidney Yin deficiency, some extra herbs need to be added to the basic ovulation formula, Cu Pai Luan Tang. This then becomes Bu Shen Cu Pai Luan Tang and is useful if the Yin levels have not been quite brought up to ideal levels before ovulation or if there is weak Qi and Blood movement.

Bu Shen Cu Pai Luan Tang (Reinforce Kidney Ovulation Formula)

Dang Gui	9 g	Radix Angelicae Sinensis
Chi Shao	9 g	Radix Paeoniae Rubra
Bai Shao	9 g	Radix Paeoniae Lactiflorae
Shan Yao	9 g	Dioscorea Oppositae
Shu Di	12 g	Radix Rehmanniae Glutinosae Conquitae
Nu Zhen Zi	9 g	Fructus Ligustri Lucidi
Mu Dan Pi	9 g	Cortex Moutan Radicis
Fu Ling	12 g	Sclerotium Poriae Cocos
Bu Gu Zhi	9 g	Fructus Psoraleae
Tu Si Zi	9 g	Semen Cuscatae
Wu Ling Zhi	9 g	Excrementum Trogopterori
Hong Hua	6 g	Flos Carthami Tinctorii

Table 4.5   Acupuncture points[a] used in the treatment of infertility – ovulation phase

Treatment goal	Acupuncture point
To regulate the Qi in the area of the ovaries and the fallopian tubes	Choose from: KI-13, KI-14, SP-13, ST-28, ST-29, Zigong
To move the Qi in the Liver channel, which passes through the lateral abdomen region	LIV-3 and LIV-5
To promote ovulation by regulating the Qi and Blood	KI-5 and KI-8
To enhance Kidney function and stabilize emotions	KI-4
To influence activity of the Chong and Ren vessels – especially useful at ovulation time through its influence on the Dai channel, ensuring the fallopian tubes are not obstructed by excess secretions	GB-26
To calm the mind, an important consideration at ovulation; also useful if there is suspicion of tubal obstruction by excess secretions	SP-5
To promote circulation of Blood at ovulation if there is some question of tube patency	SP-8
To promote circulation of Blood and the action of the Spleen as an intermediary between the Heart and Kidneys (i.e., the Bao vessel and Bao channel)	SP-6
To calm the spirit and influence the Bao vessel	HE-5 and PC-5
To further calm the mind	HE-7 and PC-6, Yintang
To regulate the Heart Qi and clear Heat in the Blood which might show as midcycle spotting	PC-4

[a]Use local and leg points with mild reducing method and even method with wrist points. The choice of abdomen or back points can be guided by sensations or pain.

In comparison to Cu Pai Luan Tang, the first priority of this formula is supporting the Kidneys (Shu Di, Nu Zhen Zi, Bu Gu Zhi, Tu Si Zi), Spleen (Shan Yao) and Liver (Bai Shao). Moving the Blood (Wu Ling Zhi, Hong Hua, Dang Gui, Chi Shao, Mu Dan Pi) is secondary. Kidney Yin tonics support ovary function, Kidney Yang tonics promote maturation of the egg and reinforce its energy making capacity and Blood moving herbs promote development of the endometrium and ensure no obstruction to ovulation.

This formula is used for 3–5 days and, if successful, ovulation will occur and the basal body temperature pushed to its high level quickly and efficiently.

Acupuncture Points — Add to the points chosen from Table 4.5:

Ren-4	Guanyuan
KI-3	Taixi
KI-6	Zhaohai

Use reinforcing technique.

KIDNEY YANG DEFICIENCY

Herbal Formula — In cases where there are generalized Kidney Yang deficient or Cold signs and symptoms we use warming and moving herbs to encourage effective ovulation. A formula like Wen Yang Hua Yu Fang can be used as the guiding formula here.

Wen Yang Hua Yu Fang (Warm Yang and transform stasis formula)

Gui Zhi	9 g	*Ramulus Cinnamomi Cassiae*
Hong Hua	6 g	*Flos Carthami Tinctorii*
Dang Gui	9 g	*Radix Angelicae Sinensis*
Chuan Xiong	6 g	*Radix Ligustici Wallichii*
(Huai) Niu Xi	9 g	*Radix Achyranthis Bidentatae*
Ji Xue Teng	15 g	*Radix et Caulis Jixueteng*
Yin Yang Huo	9 g	*Herba Epimedii*
Shu Di	9 g	*Radix Rehmanniae Glutinosae Conquitae*
Zhi Fu Zi*	6 g	*Radix Aconiti Charmichaeli Praeparata*

This formula introduces quite a lot of Heat with herbs such as Zhi Fu Zi and Gui Zhi, and movement of Blood with herbs such as Hong Hua, Chuan Xiong, Ji Xue Teng and Dang Gui. Huai Niu Xi, Shu Di and Yin Yang Huo support the Kidney Yin and Yang.

These herbs are taken for around 3 days at midcycle or from the day of supposed ovulation. If they are used too early they will dry the fertile mucus and the protective mucus lining of the tubes. Because they are very heating it is important to ensure there is no Liver- or Heart-Fire or Yin-deficient Heat present.

Where there is ovulation pain, which is relieved by warmth, add:

Xiao Hui Xiang	6 g	*Fructus Foeniculi Vulgaris*

Acupuncture Points — Add to points chosen from Table 4.5:

Ren-6	Qihai
Ren-4	Guanyuan
ST-29	Guilai
BL-32	Ciliao

Use reinforcing method and moxa.

KIDNEY JING DEFICIENCY

Herbal Formula — A lack of Kidney Jing really needs to be addressed from the beginning of the cycle and there is little more that can be done now we are at midcycle if the Jing Qi is not sufficient, i.e., there will be no eggs ripe and ready for ovulation. However, if the Jing tonic herbs applied early in the cycle seem to be having results, i.e., more fertile mucus is appearing (or blood tests show that estrogen levels are rising adequately), then the guiding formula Bu Shen Cu Pai Luan Tang can be given around midcycle, with the addition of:

Lu Jiao Pian	9 g	*Cornu Cervi Parvum*
Zi He Che**	3 g	*Placenta Hominis*

Acupuncture Points — Add to the choice of points in Table 4.5:

Ren-4	Guanyuan
KI-12	Dahe
ST-27	Daju

Zhi Fu Zi is a restricted herb in some countries.

**Zi He Che is used in Chinese infertility clinics but is restricted in many other countries. Many practitioners prefer not to use human or animal substances in which case this and Lu Jiao Jiao can be replaced with plant substitutes such as Huang Jing (Rhizoma Polygonati).*

Use reinforcing method.

Any rise in the BBT after this treatment must be seen as very encouraging progress, because it indicates that an ovulation has occurred. However, the temperature may drop again quite soon or it may not reach a very high level and it may take many months of treatment before a good ovulation can be produced.

In fertility clinics in China, women are usually advised to establish reliable cycles and good ovulations (i.e., convincing BBT charts) before attempting pregnancy. However, in the case of women with Jing deficiency and a very erratic menstrual history, they will quite understandably want to take advantage of any ovulation at all since they are so few and far between. The risk, of course, is miscarriage, so I do try to persuade these women to wait a few months after commencing treatment before trying to conceive.

Heart and Liver Qi Stagnation

Herbal Formula — It is critical that Liver and Heart Qi remain unobstructed for ovulation to occur, so we must always pay great attention to these at this time of the cycle. Ovulation pain and breast or nipple tenderness alert us to stagnation of Liver Qi at this time. The liver (physiological organ) can be assisted by the following treatments to break down hormones without compromising estrogen production by the ovaries. This will usually be enough to stop symptoms of breast soreness.

In most cases, adding a few herbs to the base formula Cu Pai Luan Tang is enough to facilitate movement of Liver Qi and Heart Blood. For example:

Chai Hu	9 g	*Radix Bupleuri*
Bai Shao	9 g	*Radix Paeoniae Lactiflorae*
Dan Shen	9 g	*Radix Salviae Miltiorrhizae*
Suan Zao Ren	15 g	*Semen Ziziphi Spinosae*

However, if there is marked Heart or Liver Qi stagnation causing emotional disturbance, a stronger approach is necessary. A useful guiding formula is the following:

Yuan Zhi Chang Pu Yin (Polygala Acorus pill)

Yuan Zhi	6 g	*Radix Polygalae Tenuifoliae*
Shi Chang Pu	9 g	*Rhizoma Acori Graminei*
Dang Gui	9 g	*Radix Angelicae Sinensis*
Chi Shao	9 g	*Radix Paeoniae Rubra*
Bai Shao	9 g	*Radix Paeoniae Lactiflorae*
Shan Zha	9 g	*Fructus Crataegi*
Fu Ling	9 g	*Sclerotium Poriae Cocos*
Chai Hu	6 g	*Radix Bupleuri*
Yu Jin	9 g	*Tuber Curcumae*
Dan Shen	9 g	*Radix Salviae Miltiorrhizae*
He Huan Pi	12 g	*Cortex Albizziae Julibrissin*

Yuan Zhi and Shi Chang Pu are combined here to quieten the mind during the ovulation phase. Yu Jin, Dan Shen, Chai Hu and He Huan Pi will support this action by removing Heart or Liver Qi stagnation. Liver and Heart Blood are reinforced with Dang Gui and Bai Shao. Chi Shao ensures that Liver-Heat is cleared and Fu Ling supports the Spleen function in the face of Liver Qi stagnation.

If such emotional instability is occurring in a woman with Kidney weakness (or she is over 35 years old) we should continue Kidney tonic herbs as well. The herbs listed above already include four of the herbs from our Kidney Yin deficiency ovulation formula (Bu Shen Cu Pai Luan Tang) and we could add several more. For example:

Shu Di	9g	Radix Rehmanniae Glutinosae Conquitae
Shan Yao	9g	Dioscorea Oppositae
Xu Duan	9g	Radix Dipsaci
Tu Si Zi	9g	Semen Cuscatae

If the high levels of hormones, which can occur at ovulation (especially where there is Liver Qi stagnation) cause a sensation of fullness or aching in the vulva, then adding herbs to strengthen Spleen Qi is appropriate. Add to the appropriate base formula (Yuan Zhi Chang Pu Yin modified or Cu Pai Luan Tang modified):

| Huang Qi | 12g | Radix Astragali |

Acupuncture Points — Acupuncture is undoubtedly useful at ovulation time and it is worth the patient making an effort to book visits to the acupuncturist's clinic to coincide with this particular time.

Choose points from Table 4.5 which emphasize the movement of Qi in the fallopian tubes and ensure there is no tension or constriction in these fine muscles, i.e., choose local abdomen points and Liver channel points. Additionally, choose points which calm the mind and clear the Bao vessel, i.e., Heart and Pericardium channel points and Yintang and KI-4. Use an even or reducing method.

CASE HISTORY – TORI

Tori (38) had her first child at 32 and had been unable to fall pregnant again. Since that time her cycle had become irregular, varying between 3 and 6 weeks. She kept BBT charts which showed no ovulatory pattern unless she took clomifene. Even on clomifene, which she took for 7 cycles, her cycles were long and irregular and the pattern on her BBT charts was erratic (Fig. 4.11).

At midcycle she felt tense and anxious and experienced crampy abdominal pain for a few days. Her fertile mucus was clear, stretchy and plentiful over 3 or 4 days when she was not taking clomifene. Premenstrually she suffered extreme breast soreness for 2 weeks; she felt very irritable and agitated and tired for 1 week. Sleep was difficult for her before a period. Her period was slightly clotty and painful on Day 1. The flow was quite erratic with a stop-start pattern. Her pulse was wiry except on the Heart position, which was thready. Her tongue was pale on the sides and red on the tip.

The diagnosis of her infertility was Heart and Liver Qi stagnation which was disrupting the regularity of ovulation. There was also some evidence of Heat affecting the Heart (insomnia). Her long period of infertility made me suspect more than just Heart and Liver pathology and treatment therefore included herbs and acupuncture to treat Kidney Yin and Yang function.

The post-menstrual formula concentrated on building Kidney Yin and Blood and regulating Liver and Heart Qi:

Dang Gui	9g	Radix Angelicae Sinensis
Bai Shao	9g	Radix Paeoniae Lactiflorae
Shu Di	9g	Radix Rehmanniae Glutinosae Conquitae
Shan Zhu Yu	9g	Fructus Corni Officinalis
Shan Yao	9g	Dioscorea Oppositae
Mu Dan Pi	12g	Cortex Moutan Radicis
Chai Hu	12g	Radix Bupleuri
Bai Zhu	6g	Rhizoma Atractylodis Macrocephalae
Xiang Fu	9g	Rhizoma Cyperi Rotundi

He Huan Pi	9g	Cortex Albizziae Julibrissin
Suan Zao Ren	12g	Semen Ziziphi Spinosae
Chuan Lian Zi	6g	Fructus Meliae Toosendan

Acupuncture points: LIV-3, LIV-5, KI-3, PC-6, SP-4, Ren-4

As soon as she began to produce fertile mucus (after taking the above formula for 18 days) she switched to the ovulation formula, which she took for 1 week. This formula emphasized the importance of a calm Shen and patent Liver Qi:

Yuan Zhi	6g	Radix Polygalae Tenuifoliae
Shi Chang Pu	9g	Rhizoma Acori Graminei
Dang Gui	9g	Radix Angelicae Sinensis
Chi Shao	9g	Radix Paeoniae Rubra
Bai Shao	9g	Radix Paeoniae Lactiflorae
Shan Zha	9g	Fructus Crataegi
Fu Ling	9g	Sclerotium Poriae Cocos
Chai Hu	12g	Radix Bupleuri
Yu Jin	9g	Tuber Curcumae
Dan Shen	9g	Radix Salviae Miltiorrhizae
He Huan Pi	12g	Cortex Albizziae Julibrissin
Xu Duan	6g	Radix Dipsaci
Tu Si Zi	9g	Semen Cuscatae

Acupuncture points: LIV-3, LIV-5, KI-4, KI-14, PC-5 HE-7, Yin Tang

Her midcycle discomfort was relieved and her breasts less tender. Her BBT chart showed a convincing rise and she continued for the next 10 days with a patent remedy, Jia Wei Xiao Yao San. When her BBT was still elevated 17 days after its ovulation shift, I suggested a pregnancy test, which was positive (Fig. 4.12).

The pregnancy continued happily to 9 months and the birth of a baby girl. It is evident from this rapid result that perhaps Kidney function was not as compromised as I thought. As soon as Liver and Heart Qi were unobstructed conception was easy.

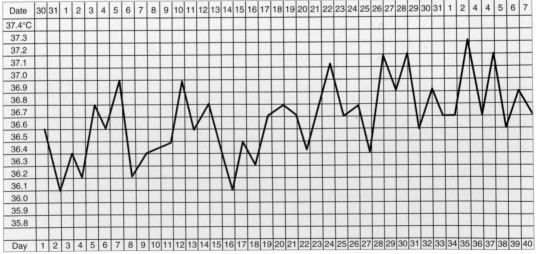

Figure 4.11 Case history – Tori. She ovulated when she took clomifene, but irregularly. In this cycle, which was 41 days long, she probably ovulated around Day 27. Heart and Liver Qi stagnation is evident in the erratic nature of the temperature readings.

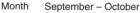

Month   September – October

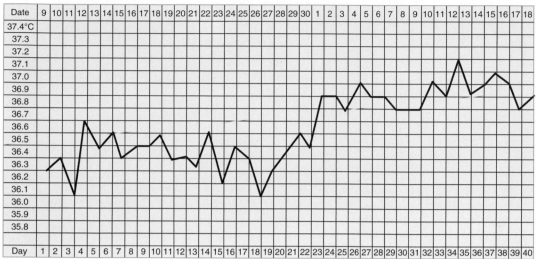

Figure 4.12 Case history – Tori. This chart shows BBT readings during the 1st month Tori took herbs and had acupuncture. The erratic temperature readings stabilized well and ovulation was clearly indicated around Day 18 or 19. She became pregnant during this cycle.

Blood Stagnation

Herbal Formula — The sorts of formulas we use at midcycle already contain Blood-moving herbs. In some cases we might want to add stronger herbs or increase the doses of ones already chosen.

Blood stagnation of the type that will seriously disrupt ovulation might include cysts or endometriomas on the ovary – these are likely to cause pain and therefore demand attention at midcycle. Some forms of tube blockage are caused by Blood stagnation – these are covered in Chapter 6. In the case of substantial obstructions, we usually use Blood-breaking herbs like E Zhu or San Leng although in cycles where conception is attempted these herbs may be too harsh. However in robust young women with significant masses that are obstructing the ovaries or the tubes these herbs may be added for just a couple of days and in small doses.

In the case of cysts or masses in a strong and young woman, Cu Pai Luan Tang can be modified by adding:

Shan Zha (Sheng)	9 g	*Fructus Crataegi*
E. Zhu	6 g	*Rhizoma Curcumae Zedoariae*

and increasing the dose of Wu Ling Zhi to 12 g, and Hong Hua to 9 g.

In the case of endometriomas (and if there is a component of Kidney deficiency) you can modify Bu Shen Cu Pai Luan Tang in exactly the same way.

Acupuncture Points — Consider including among the points chosen from Table 4.5:

ST-28	Shuidao
KI-14	Siman
KI-5	Shuiquan
SP-8	Diji

and add:

ST-29	Guilai
SP-10	Xuehai
LIV-9	Ququan
BL-17	Geshu

Use with reducing method.

Phlegm-Damp Accumulation

Herbal Formula — In most women and in most cycles, herbs which strongly move Qi and Blood to facilitate ovulation are applied only when we get to the point where the Yin is well established and the egg is ready to be launched, i.e., around Day 13 or 14 in a 28-day cycle. However, when Phlegm-Damp is seriously gluing up the works, we need to apply such treatment well before ovulation, otherwise the egg may never be released or, if it is, it will not get very far before being obstructed by excess or pathological mucus secretions in the fallopian tubes.

In women diagnosed with Phlegm-Damp we added to our base formula Yang tonics and Damp-clearing herbs in the early part of the cycle. Once we have some evidence that we have established a good enough basis of Yin (there is fertile mucus or blood tests show rising estrogen levels) we use a more strongly activating formula, even if it is only 1 week past the period. For example, the formula Wen Yang Hua Tan Fang will transform Damp and Phlegm, warm Yang and activate Qi and Blood.

Wen Yang Hua Tan Fang (Warm Yang and Transform Phlegm Formula)

Zhi Fu Zi*	6g	*Radix Aconiti Charmichaeli Praeparata*
Xu Duan	9g	*Radix Dipsaci*
Yin Yang Huo	9g	*Herba Epimedii*
Cang Zhu	9g	*Rhizoma Atractylodes*
Chen Pi	5g	*Pericarpium Citri Reticulate*
Fu Ling	9g	*Sclerotium Poriae Cocos*
Zhi Ke	9g	*Fructus Citri seu Ponciri*
Shan Zha	9g	*Fructus Crataegi*
Hong Hua	6g	*Flos Carthami Tinctorii*
Dan Nan Xing	9g	*Rhizoma Arisaematis*

This formula combines a strong heating element (Zhi Fu Zi) with Yang tonics (Xu Duan and Yin Yang Huo) and herbs which encourage elimination of Damp (Cang Zhu, Fu Ling, Chen Pi, Zhi Ke and Dan Nan Xing). Because it is an ovulation formula, Blood-regulating agents (Shan Zha and Hong Hua) are added. Dan Nan Xing is added here for its ability to dissipate lumps (in this case, obstructions in the tubes).

If the release of the egg from the ovary appears to be obstructed by Phlegm-Damp add:

Zao Jiao Zi	6g	*Fructus Gleditsiae Sinensis*

---

*Zhi Fu Zi is a restricted herb in some countries.

Acupuncture Points — From the points chosen from Table 4.5, emphasize the Spleen channel and Dai vessel points and add:

BL-22	Sanjiaoshu
BL-28	Pangguanshu
GB-27	Wushu
GB-28	Weidao
SP-9	Yinlingquan
KI-7	Fuliu
ST-29	Guilai (with moxa)

Use with even or reducing method.

Midcycle Bleeding

The dramatic peaks and falls of hormone levels (especially estrogen) at midcycle can sometimes provoke some bleeding from the endometrium. This is more likely to occur if the growth and structure of the endometrium has not been established soundly earlier in the follicular phase. In TCM terms, we say the Chong vessel is not consolidated. This can occur in cases of Yin and Blood deficiency or if there is Heat.

Herbal Formula — Rather than simply adding styptic herbs to our midcycle formula, chronic midcycle bleeding must be addressed by treating the imbalance at the early stages of the cycle so the uterine lining can be built after the period. For Yin deficiency with midcycle bleeding add:

Han Lian Cao	15 g	*Herba Ecliptae Prostratae*

and increase Shan Yao and Nu Zhen Zi to 15 g each in post-menstrual and midcycle formulas.

To the midcycle formula add:

Jing Jie Tan	6 g	*Herba seu Flos Shizonepetae tenuifoliae* (charred)

With signs of Heat add:

Zhi Zi	9 g	*Fructus Gardeniae Jasminoidis*

Acupuncture Points — To points chosen from Table 4.4 add:

HE-5	Tongli
LIV-2	Xingjian

PROBLEMS IN THE LUTEAL PHASE OR AT IMPLANTATION

Post-Ovulation Phase – Maintaining Kidney Yang

We now come to that aspect of female functional infertility which concerns problems not with ovulation but with implantation of a fertilized egg. At this time in the cycle we are assuming that ovulation has occurred and that the egg has successfully negotiated the upper reaches of the fallopian tube, has had a productive encounter with a good-looking sperm, and the resulting embryo has arrived in the uterus.

The success of implantation has much to do with the quality of the embryo; thus, treatment focussing on creating healthy gametes and helping them get together should take priority. However, we do know that it is also important to have a healthy and permissive endometrium and that active interaction occurs between the endometrium and the embryo before implantation can occur.

The success of the post-ovulation phase requires implantation in the firm clutches of a receptive uterine lining – in the old Chinese medicine texts they would describe this as a 'warm womb'. To maintain this warmth, the influence of Kidney Yang is important. In Western terms, to maintain a good-quality, receptive, secretory endometrium the progesterone levels produced by the corpus luteum must be high. Blood tests taken in the middle of this phase (mid-luteal phase) give us a good indication of progesterone levels – inadequate progesterone production supports a diagnosis of Kidney Yang deficiency.

The role of Kidney Yang (Fig. 4.13), however, includes more than just maintaining good levels of progesterone. It also includes the active role played by the walls of the uterus as they press inwards, holding the embryo firmly as it burrows in.

We might suspect Kidney Yang deficiency if the menstrual period is accompanied with lower back pain, loose stools, sensation of cold and discomfort in the abdomen and pieces of tissue in the menstrual flow.

Treatment of the fundamental and underlying imbalance is of paramount importance in treating infertility at all stages (called the Ben in TCM). Except in the case of some simple mechanical obstructions in the uterus or tubes, the Ben will always be Kidney Yang deficiency if there is a functional problem in the luteal phase. This applies even when there are other manifestations like Liver Qi stagnation or Damp-Phlegm accumulation (which are called the 'Biao').

Administration of progesterone is one way to approach treatment of Kidney Yang deficiency characterized by low progesterone levels. Generally, however, most specialists consider administration of progestogens (as the drugs are called) not very effective clinically. Although Chinese medicine treatment can be lengthy it gets its result by encouraging the body to do the job itself rather than rely on an external supply of what is missing.

Blood-regulating herbs are used in quite big doses around ovulation time but they are usually withdrawn during the luteal phase. However, keeping in mind the continued growth and tortuous development of the endometrial blood vessels, it makes sense to add small doses of Blood-regulating herbs in the early luteal phase. Their judicious use is even advised during implantation in some infertility clinics in China. Small doses of Dan Shen may be added in the early luteal phase to any of the formulas that follow to encourage microcirculation in the endometrium during implantation. Fertility clinics in the West have recently taken advantage of this idea and recommend women on their programs to take aspirin to thin the blood and improve circulation in the endometrium.

However, once the embryo has burrowed its way into its new home, it is best to let it lie still and avoid the use of herbs (or acupuncture points), which increase movement of Blood.

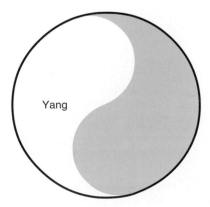

Figure 4.13 The Yang phase.

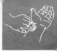

• Timing of Treatment

Back in the clinic, we must adjust our treatment according to the stage of the cycle and to the individual patient's pattern much as we did with treatment applied in the follicular phase. The fundamental approach now is to maintain the high levels of Yang built on the good Yin foundation already established in the previous 2 weeks of the cycle.

Because the menstrual cycle makes such dramatic and fluctuating demands on the Qi and Blood status, and the Yin and Yang balance, approaches to treatment must change all the time. So we will find that our prescriptions may well be quite different now compared to those we were giving just a couple of days earlier. Herein lies the elegance and success of treatment for female infertility.

Herbal Formula — Ai Fu Nuan Gong Wan is the formula recommended in most classics to boost Kidney Yang and warm the uterus in the luteal phase. However, when it comes to raising progesterone levels, other approaches have in more recent times been found to be more effective.[1] One of three basic approaches can be taken, depending upon the tendency to Yin, Qi or Blood deficiency. Often it is the shape of the BBT chart that will help determine which approach should be taken to support Yang in the luteal phase.

Methods to Boost the Yang

We choose a guiding formula which can:

- boost Kidney Yang by supplementing Yin – Method A

- boost Kidney Yang by promoting Qi – Method B

- boost Kidney Yang by nourishing Blood – Method C.

Method A – Boost Kidney Yang by Supplementing Yin

Boosting Yang by supplementing Yin is the most important method clinically for promoting implantation and the survival and nourishment of the embryo. It is an often-used clinical method which acknowledges the interdependence and interconsuming of Yin and Yang that was discussed in Chapter 2.

Herbal Formula — Some of the famous classical Yin or Yang tonic formulas demonstrate the interdependence of Yin and Yang well, e.g., You Gui Wan, which is a well-known Yang tonic formula, contains not only the herbs for building Yang but also three Yin tonics. Therefore, to boost Yang by supplementing Yin, this formula is chosen as the guiding formula. It can be applied in the luteal phase to assist implantation and early fetal development even when there is no marked Kidney deficiency.

You Gui Wan (Restoring the Right pill)

Shu Di	9 g	*Radix Rehmanniae Glutinosae Conquitae*
Shan Yao	9 g	*Dioscorea Oppositae*
Shan Zhu Yu	9 g	*Fructus Corni Officinalis*
Tu Si Zi	9 g	*Semen Cuscatae*
Ba Ji Tian	9 g	*Radix Morindae Officinalis*
Lu Jiao Pian	9 g	*Cornu Cervi Parvum*

This formula includes the first three herbs of Liu Wei Di Huang Tang – Shu Di, Shan Yao and Shan Zhu Yu – which supplement, respectively, the Kidney, Spleen and Liver Yin. Tu Si Zi, Ba Ji Tian and Lu Jiao Pian reinforce Kidney Yang.

Acupuncture Points — In terms of channel activity the emphasis is now moving from the Chong to the Ren vessel. Ren vessel points can be chosen in the days after ovulation to encourage implantation. But once implantation is completed, i.e., in the week before the period, lower abdomen points are used with great caution (or avoided altogether by the less experienced practitioner). The use of Kidney points at this time maintains Kidney Yin and Yang. Choose points from (and see Table 4.6):

Ren-2	Qugu
Ren-4	Guanyuan
Ren-5	Shimen
Ren-7	Yinjiao
Ren-15	Jiuwei
KI-3	Taixi
KI-6	Zhaohai
BL-23	Shenshu

Method B – Boost Kidney Yang by Promoting Qi

Doctors trained in Chinese medicine all recognize the close and dependent relationship between the Yin and the Blood on the one hand, and the Qi and the Yang on the other. Blood nourishes Yin and Yin provides the material basis for Blood. Qi and Yang have a similar relationship, i.e., it is said that Qi is a part of Yang and Kidney Yang is the root of Qi in the body.

When Qi and Kidney Yang are both weak, we see in the clinic a mixture of Spleen Qi deficiency and Kidney Yang deficiency symptoms – some fluid retention, difficult urination, loose stools, abnormal uterine bleeding, etc.

Herbal Formula — Traditionally, this syndrome has been treated with the formula Zhen Wu Tang, which strongly warms Kidney Yang and invigorates Spleen Qi. In gynecology departments, however, the preferred guiding formula is a modified version of Jian Gu Tang.

Table 4.6   Acupuncture points[a] used in the treatment of infertility: luteal phase – boost Kidney Yang by supplementing Yin

Treatment goal	Acupuncture point
To reinforce Kidney Yang	Ren-2
To reinforce Kidney Yin and Yang	Ren-4
To regulate Qi in the uterus and maintain good flexibility in the uterine walls (use only in the first week after ovulation)	Ren-5
To regulate the activity of the Chong and Ren vessels and facilitate the change in their activity at the outset of this time (use just after ovulation)	Ren-7
To calm the mind if there is agitation (shallow needling only)	Ren-15 (the Luo point of the Ren vessel)
To encourage development of Kidney Yang by invigorating Kidney Yin	KI-3, KI-6 and BL-23

[a]Use reinforcing method. Lower abdomen points are avoided (or used with great caution) in the week before the period is due.

Jian Gu Tang modified (Strengthen and Consolidate decoction)

Dang Shen	9 g	Radix Codonopsis Pilulosae
Bai Zhu	9 g	Rhizoma Atractylodis Macrocephalae
Shan Yao	9 g	Radix Dioscorea Oppositae
Yi Yi Ren	15 g	Semen Coicis Lachryma-jobi
Tu Si Zi	9 g	Semen Cuscatae
Ba Ji Tian	9 g	Radix Morindae Officinalis
Lu Jiao Pian	9 g	Cornu Cervi Parvum

In this version of Jian Gu Tang, the primary herbs Dang Shen, Bai Zhu and Shan Yao are employed to invigorate the Spleen Qi. Yi Yi Ren reinforces this action and has the added affect of clearing any Damp that might have accumulated as a result of the Spleen weakness. Tu Si Zi, Ba Ji Tian and Lu Jiao Pian fortify Kidney Yang.

Acupuncture Points — Acupuncture treatment to promote Qi is useful in the 1st week after ovulation to ensure mobility and free passage of the embryo in the proximal part of the fallopian tube.

The process of implantation is a dynamic one which requires vigorous Qi as the embryo binds to the endometrium and then burrows into it. In addition, the uterine walls must be mobile enough to press together and hold the embryo securely as it undergoes implantation.

Choose points from the following (and see Table 4.7):

Ren-4	Guanyuan
Ren-5	Shimen
Ren-6	Qihai
Ren-12	Zhongwan
ST-25	Tianshu
ST-36	Zusanli
SP-6	Sanyinjiao
KI-3	Taixi
BL-20	Pishu
BL-23	Shenshu

Table 4.7   Acupuncture points[a] used in the treatment of infertility: luteal phase – boost Kidney Yang by promoting Qi

Treatment goal	Acupuncture point
To invigorate the Spleen and Stomach Qi	Choose from: Ren-12, Ren-6, ST-36, ST-25, BL-20, SP-6
To support the development of Kidney Yang	Ren-4, KI-3, BL-23
To regulate Qi in the Ren channel and abdomen (use only in 1st week after ovulation)	Ren-5

[a]Use reinforcing method. Points on the abdomen must be avoided or used with great caution in the week before the period is due.

Method C – Boost Kidney Yang by Nourishing Blood

The relationship between Kidney Yang and Blood status is not quite as obvious as its relationship with Kidney Yin or the Qi. It has been noticed in the clinic that Kidney deficiency and Blood deficiency often occur simultaneously in women. Because Blood nourishes Yin and vice versa, it is easy to see how Kidney Yin deficiency develops from Blood deficiency but the connection to Kidney Yang is less direct. Either Kidney Yang is not supported when Kidney Yin is weakened from lack of Blood or it is affected when the Sea of Blood (the Chong channel), with which it has a close relationship, is deficient. There are also some references to the role of the Kidneys in the formation of Blood in the classics. Whichever bit of theory we like to try and make fit the clinical observations, the fact remains that building Blood seems to boost Kidney Yang and vice versa. Certainly, the addition of Blood tonics is important when the endometrial lining is not thick enough or sufficiently secretory.

Herbal Formula — When both Kidney Yang and Blood must be fortified, we use Blood and Qi tonics in combination with Kidney Yang tonics.

Yu Lin Zhu (Fertility Pearls)

Dang Shen	12g	*Radix Codonopsis Pilulosae*
Bai Zhu	9g	*Rhizoma Atractylodis Macrocephalae*
Fu Ling	9g	*Sclerotium Poriae Cocos*
Gan Cao	6g	*Radix Glycyrrhizae Uralensis*
Dang Gui	9g	*Radix Angelicae Sinensis*
Bai Shao	9g	*Radix Paeoniae Lactiflorae*
Chuan Xiong	6g	*Radix Ligustici Wallichii*
Shu Di	9g	*Radix Rehmanniae Glutinosae Conquitae*
Tu Si Zi	9g	*Semen Cuscatae*
Du Zhong	9g	*Cortex Eucommiae Ulmoidis*
Lu Jiao Pian	9g	*Cornu Cervi Parvum*

This formula combines the Qi tonics of Si Jun Zi Tang (Dang Shen, Bai Zhu, Fu Ling and Gan Cao) and the Blood tonics of Si Wu Tang (Dang Gui, Bai Shao, Chuan Xiong and Shu Di) with Kidney Yang tonic herbs (Tu Si Zi, Du Zhong and Lu Jiao Pian).

Acupuncture Points — For successful implantation the endometrium must be both receptive and nourishing (i.e., have good blood circulation). The flow of blood to the endometrium has been shown to be increased by acupuncture.[4] To encourage implantation we choose points which support Kidney function and increase production of Blood and which stimulate blood flow to the uterus (see Table 4.8), such as:

Ren-4	Guanyuan
Ren-12	Zhongwan
ST-36	Zusanli
SP-6	Sanyinjiao
SP-10	Xuehai
KI-5	Shuiquan
BL-17	Geshu

Modifications and Variations

In general, one of these three approaches will adequately cover what is required for most patients at this time of the cycle. However there are times when the chosen formula will need modification to take into account other

Table 4.8   Acupuncture points[a] used in the treatment of infertility: luteal phase — boost Kidney Yang by nourishing Blood

Treatment goal	Acupuncture point
To directly influence Blood formation	BL-17, SP-10
To enhance Blood formation via the Kidney Yang	KI-5
To support the role of the Stomach and Spleen in making and distributing Blood	ST-36, Ren-12 and SP-6
To support the Kidney Yin and Yang and invigorate the Qi and Blood of all the Zang	Ren-4

[a]Use reinforcing method. The lower abdomen and Spleen channel points are generally not used in the week immediately before the period.

traits or symptoms. If there is marked Kidney deficiency, or stagnation of Qi, Blood or Phlegm-Damp, then the following modifications to the guiding formulas just described may be made.

Kidney Deficiency

KIDNEY YIN DEFICIENCY

Herbal Formula — As you know, women with Kidney Yin deficiency often have problems with ovulation. It may be that they ovulate late or irregularly or that the egg released is of poor quality. However, it may also be that they ovulate 'inadequately'. What this means is that the corpus luteum, created after the egg is released, functions poorly, i.e., it secretes inadequate levels of progesterone so that implantation will be unsuccessful. In Chinese medicine terms we say that deficient Kidney Yin cannot produce Kidney Yang.

To address this problem the preferred formula in most gynecology departments in China is a version of You Gui Wan (see method A above). To this can be added further Yin tonics if Kidney Yin deficiency is pronounced. For example, add:

Nu Zhen Zi	9 g	*Fructus Ligustri Lucidi*
Han Lian Cao	9 g	*Herba Ecliptae Prostratae*

Acupuncture Points — Choose points from Table 4.6 and emphasize the points which enhance Kidney Yin and clear Heat. For example:

KI-6	Zhaohai

and add:

KI-2	Rangu

CASE HISTORY – LILLIANE

Lilliane (37) had had many investigations of her infertility and had followed her naturopath's preconception regimen strictly. She charted her cycle and tried actively to conceive for 5 years. Investigations revealed no abnormality but slightly low progesterone in the luteal phase.

A close look at Lilliane and her BBT charts uncovered a diagnosis of Kidney Yang deficiency as the cause of her infertility. Her BBT charts (Fig. 4.14) showed a long cycle with a poor luteal phase.

She experienced lower back pain and abdomen pain throughout her period. She saw little fertile mucus when she ovulated, which was always late. She looked pale and was often tired; she was also quite vague. Both Kidney pulses were very weak; her tongue was pale with a red tip.

It was likely that this Kidney weakness was constitutional, but it certainly wasn't helped by her lifestyle. Her job as a florist required her to get up very early to go the markets and in the evening she studied for her university course. On average, she slept just 5 or 6h a night. All the treatment in the world wasn't going to recover this woman's Kidney Yang if she didn't get more sleep. So on her BBT charts, as well as charting temperature, I asked her to record how many hours sleep she got each night. She worked on getting to bed earlier. While Lilliane's problem with getting pregnant related to events in the luteal phase (implantation of the embryo), she needed to strongly reinforce the Kidney Yin in the follicular phase to provide the necessary base from which to build Kidney Yang later. To this end, she took Gui Shao Di Huang Tang with additions:

Dang Gui	9g	Radix Angelicae Sinensis
Bai Shao	9g	Radix Paeoniae Lactiflorae
Mu Dan Pi	6g	Cortex Moutan Radicis
Dan Shen	6g	Radix Salviae Miltiorrhizae
Shu Di	12g	Radix Rehmanniae Glutinosae Conquitae
Shan Yao	9g	Dioscorea Oppositae
Shan Zhu Yu	9g	Fructus Corni Officinalis
Fu Ling	9g	Sclerotium Poriae Cocos
Tu Si Zi	9g	Semen Cuscatae

This formula had the effect of shortening the follicular phase so that ovulation occurred around Day 18 rather than around Day 25.

After ovulation using the principle of building Kidney Yang from a Kidney Yin base she was prescribed You Gui Wan with additions:

Shu Di	9g	Radix Rehmanniae Glutinosae Conquitae
Shan Yao	9g	Dioscorea Oppositae
Shan Zhu Yu	9g	Fructus Corni Officinalis
Tu Si Zi	15g	Semen Cuscatae
Ba Ji Tian	9g	Radix Morindae Officinalis
Lu Jiao Jiao	9g	Cornu Cervi Parvum
Xu Duan	12g	Radix Dipsaci

Her luteal phase, while still short, improved (Fig. 4.15).

As her cycle became shorter and more regular (around 4{1/2} weeks), some fine tuning could be done at ovulation time. As her fertile mucus increased in quantity, we were able to add Yang tonics to the first formula around Day 12 to further encourage luteal phase function. The BBT charts improved dramatically (Fig. 4.16).

After taking herbs for 5 cycles, Lilliane became pregnant (Fig. 4.17).

She still overexerted herself and when she developed some lower back pain in the very early days of the pregnancy, it was cause for concern. She was prescribed herbs to maintain Kidney Yin and Yang and advised to rest more:

Nu Zhen Zi	9g	Fructus Ligustri Lucidi
Tu Si Zi	15g	Semen Cuscatae
Sang Ji Sheng	15g	Ramulus Sangjisheng
Du Zhong	9g	Cortex Eucommiae Ulmoidis
Xu Duan	9g	Radix Dipsaci
Bai Zhu	9g	Rhizoma Atractylodis Macrocephalae
Gan Cao	3g	Radix Glycyrrhizae Uralensis

Her pulse gradually strengthened and the pregnancy survived. In 9 months she gave birth to a healthy baby boy.

Month   February – March

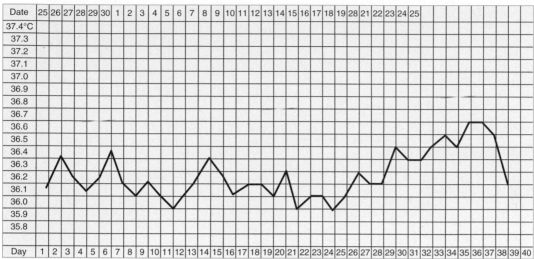

Figure 4.14 Case history – Lilliane. Chart 1: 38-day cycle before treatment.

Month   April – May

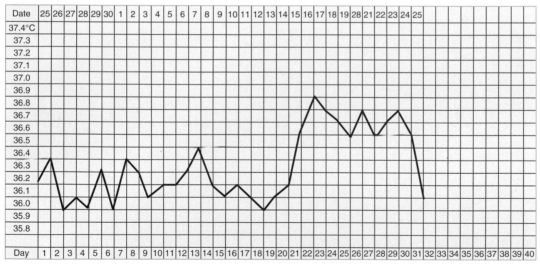

Figure 4.15 Case history – Lilliane. Chart 2: 32-day cycle after 1st month taking herbs.

KIDNEY YANG DEFICIENCY

Herbal Formula — Sometimes we can be completely reassured that Kidney Yin is adequate and yet the Kidney Yang is still showing signs of deficiency. This is demonstrated by BBT charts which rise convincingly from a good Yin foundation to a high temperature straight after ovulation but which fall rapidly thereafter, dwindling to a temperature not much more elevated than those of the first 2 weeks of the cycle. These low temperatures will continue to be recorded throughout the entire luteal phase until the period comes in 2 weeks (see Ch. 3).

A variant on this type of Kidney Yang deficiency is shown in the BBT chart in which the temperature rises minimally after ovulation (also seen in Kidney Yin-deficient pattern) and maintains this low reading until the period (see Ch. 3).

Month   May–June

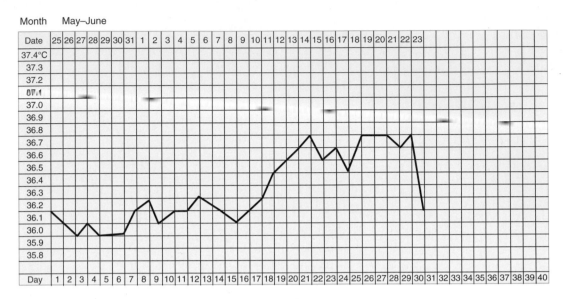

Figure 4.16 Case history – Lilliane. Chart 3: 31-day cycle with improved luteal phase.

Month   June–July

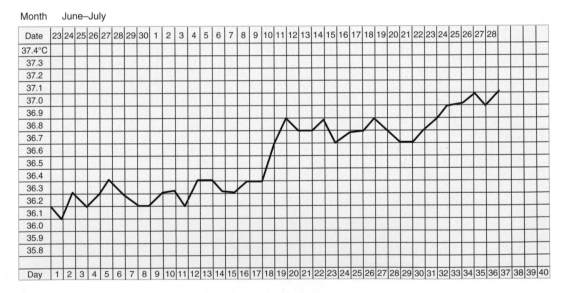

Figure 4.17 Case history – Lilliane. Chart 4: pregnant after 5 months taking herbs.

In this case it is a failure of Qi to promote Kidney Yang, specifically Spleen and Stomach Qi. Clinically, it is common to see Spleen Qi deficiency with Kidney Yang deficiency. The formula Jian Gu Tang (above) is used as the guiding formula in such cases with the addition of more Kidney Yang tonic herbs:

Yin Yang Huo   9 g   *Herba Epimedii*

Acupuncture Points — Choose points from Table 4.6 and apply moxa, especially on Ren-4.

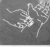

KIDNEY JING DEFICIENCY

Herbal Formula — In most cases of Kidney Jing deficiency the focus of our treatment will be on the post-menstrual phase leading up to ovulation and then during the ovulation event itself. If treatment has been successful and an egg has been sufficiently ripened and then released, it will usually be enough to just maintain the momentum by using a formula like You Gui Wan with the addition of Jing nourishing herbs. For example:

Huang Jing   9 g   *Rhizoma Polygonati*

Acupuncture Points — Choose points from Table 4.6; moxa can be applied to Ren-4.

Heart and Liver Qi Stagnation

As with ovulation, stability of the Heart and Liver are important for implantation. Although instability of the mind usually reveals itself more dramatically on the BBT chart in the follicular phase, it can also produce some swings in the temperature or a sawtooth or saddle pattern in the high or luteal phase (see Ch. 3).

Addition of Blood tonics to strengthen Liver Blood will temper any tendency to Liver Qi stagnation, and building Heart Blood helps to calm the mind. Even more importantly at this time it will help to maintain Kidney Yang levels.

Herbal Formula — The guiding formula to strengthen Kidney Yang and nourish Blood is Yu Lin Zhu (formula given above). For women who are prone to Liver Qi stagnation premenstrually (PMS or premenstrual syndrome), it is advisable to add to this formula herbs to regulate Liver Qi. For example:

Chai Hu   9 g   *Radix Bupleuri*
Chuan Lian Zi   9 g   *Fructus Meliae Toosendan*
Xiang Fu   9 g   *Rhizoma Cyperi Rotundi*

In the case where Liver Qi stagnation gives rise to Liver-Fire, Heat-clearing herbs must be added. The use of strong doses of Kidney Yang tonics for more than 1 week also brings with it the risk of feeding Liver-Fire and exacerbating premenstrual symptoms. If this occurs, the patent medicine Dan Zhi Xiao Yao San is given or some cooling herbs are added to the formula Yu Lin Zhu, such as

Mu Dan Pi   9 g   *Cortex Moutan Radicis*
Zhi Mu   9 g   *Radix Anemarrhena*

The BBT chart is scrutinized closely to see that these herbs do not lower the temperature too much and jeopardize the luteal phase.

The use of Qi- and Blood-regulating herbs is controversial in the luteal phase if the woman is trying to fall pregnant, and some practitioners will avoid such herbs completely. However, as was mentioned earlier, some others find that the inclusion of Qi-regulating and mild Blood-regulating herbs can be useful in facilitating implantation and at the same time can calm the mind. For example:

Dan Shen   6 g   *Radix Salviae Miltiorrhizae*
Yu Jin   6 g   *Tuber Curcumae*
Xiang Fu   9 g   *Rhizoma Cyperi Rotundi*

Once the period is delayed and pregnancy suspected or confirmed, such herbs should be discontinued unless there is significant Blood stagnation.

Table 4.9   Acupuncture points[a] used in the treatment of infertility: luteal phase with Heart and Liver Qi stagnation

Treatment goal	Acupuncture point
To regulate Liver Qi	Choose from all the above Liver channel points
To address Liver Blood deficiency	LIV-3 and LIV-8
To regulate Liver-Fire	LIV-2
To regulate Qi in the uterus	Choose from: LIV-4, LIV-5, LIV-9, LIV-11
To relieve emotional stress	LIV-5
To calm the mind and regulate Liver Qi in the upper body	PC-6, PC-7 and PC-5
To pacify the spirit	HE-5 and HE-7
To regulate Qi in the Ren and Liver channels	Ren-3

[a]Use even or reducing method.

Acupuncture Points — In addition to considering points in Table 4.8, that encourage Liver and Heart Blood formation, choose some points that regulate Liver and Heart Qi (see Table 4.9). For example:

LIV-2	Xingjian
LIV-3	Taichong
LIV-4	Zhongfeng
LIV-5	Ligou
LIV-8	Ququan
LIV-9	Yinbao
LIV-11	Yinlian
PC-5	Jianshi
PC-6	Neiguan
PC-7	Laogong
HE-5	Tongli
HE-7	Shenmen
Ren-3	Zhongji

Blood Stagnation

Herbal Formula — Blood stagnation impacts on ovulation or implantation. When we are considering the effect of Blood stagnation on implantation it is the nature and quality of the endometrium and any disturbances therein which concerns us.

The most obvious impediment to implantation by Blood stagnation is the presence of large fibroids that protrude significantly into the endometrial layer and uterine cavity. If much of the endometrial surface is affected by large or numerous fibroids, then there are limited sites for implantation and development of the placenta. Also, bodies such as polyps inside the uterus can have the effect of an intrauterine device (IUD) and interfere with endometrial development and implantation. Uterine polyps and fibroids can also interfere with implantation if they stick so far out into the uterine cavity to prevent the front and back walls of the inside of the uterus pressing together to help the embryo get a foothold while implanting. Poor circulation, sluggish movement of blood and metabolites, and incomplete development of the spiral blood vessels of the endometrium are all more subtle ways that Blood stagnation might hinder implantation and development of an embryo.

Although Kidney Yang is not implicated so directly here, it is nevertheless important in moving Blood in the lower Jiao. Treatments applied to clear Blood stasis to enhance fertility should also include herbs to boost Yang. Thus, we can use the guiding formula Yu Lin Zhu (see method C above) but modify it to include more Blood-regulating herbs. This formula should be taken in the luteal phase for several menstrual cycles during which time pregnancy attempts must be avoided. Of course, in situations of substantial Blood stagnation, such as large fibroids or polyps, it makes good sense to remove them with surgery (or with strong herbal treatment) and only attempt pregnancy after they are resolved.

Yu Lin Zhu (Fertility Pearls) modified

Dang Shen	12 g	*Radix Codonopsis Pilulosae*
Bai Zhu	9 g	*Rhizoma Atractylodis Macrocephalae*
Fu Ling	9 g	*Sclerotium Poriae Cocos*
Gan Cao	6 g	*Radix Glycyrrhizae Uralensis*
Dang Gui	9 g	*Radix Angelicae Sinensis*
Bai Shao	9 g	*Radix Paeoniae Lactiflorae*
Chuan Xiong	6 g	*Radix Ligustici Wallichii*
Shu Di	9 g	*Radix Rehmanniae Glutinosae Conquitae*
Tu Si Zi	9 g	*Semen Cuscatae*
Du Zhong	9 g	*Cortex Eucommiae Ulmoidis*
Lu Jiao Pian	9 g	*Cornu Cervi Parvum*
San Leng	9 g	*Rhizoma Sparganii*
E Zhu	9 g	*Rhizoma Curcumae Zedoariae*
Pu Huang	9 g	*Pollen Typhae*
Chi Shao	9 g	*Radix Paeoniae Rubra*
Ru Xiang	6 g	*Gummi Olibanum*
Mo Yao	6 g	*Myrrha*

Yu Lin Zhu was described earlier. Additions include San Leng and E Zhu, which strongly break up stagnant Blood.

If a patient is determined to continue attempts to conceive, then Yu Lin Zhu is used with the addition of Blood-moving herbs which are milder. San Leng, E Zhu, Mo Yao, Ru Xiang and Chi Shao will be replaced with:

Dan Shen	12 g	*Radix Salviae Miltiorrhizae*
Yu Jin	9 g	*Tuber Curcumae*
Ji Xue Teng	15 g	*Radix et Caulis Jixueteng*

However, these herbs are unlikely to be effective in reducing large mechanical obstructions.

Acupuncture Points — Choose points from Table 4.8 and add some regulating points (see Table 4.10). For example:

ST-28	Shuidao
ST-29	Guilai
LIV-8	Ququan
SP-6	Sanyinjiao
SP-8	Diji
LIV-5	Ligou

KI-14   Siman
KI-5   Shuiquan
Baliao
Ah Shi points

Treatment of severe Blood stagnation in infertility does not always stop when pregnancy is achieved: often the stagnation must be addressed throughout the pregnancy too.

Table 4.10   Acupuncture points[a] used in the treatment of infertility: luteal phase with Blood stagnation

Treatment goal	Acupuncture point
To regulate Qi and Blood.	ST-28 and ST-29, Ah Shi points
To help the passage of the embryo down the last part of the fallopian tube.	
To facilitate implantation where this may be obstructed by Blood stagnation	
To regulate Blood in the Uterus	LIV-8, LIV-5, KI-14, SP-6 and SP-8
To regulate Blood in the Kidney and Ren channels	KI-5
To help resolve Blood stagnation by strongly regulating Qi in the local area	Baliao

[a]*Use even or reducing method. The abdomen and lower back points are used with caution. In the absence of marked Blood stagnation, do not use them at all.*

CASE HISTORY – SUSAN

Susan (35) had been trying to have a baby for 6 months and was concerned about the bulky fibroids in her uterus. An ultrasound showed four large-to-medium intramural fibroids (the size of an orange, a lemon and two grapes). I recommended that she have them removed surgically then attempt pregnancy. She didn't like my recommendation much and persuaded me to try another tack. I agreed but without too much optimism.

Susan's menstrual cycle was short (18–25 days) with a fresh red period flow, not heavy or clotty. She experienced some aching or dragging period pain. She didn't experience any symptoms at ovulation and had not kept any BBT charts to check when or whether she was ovulating.

She also experienced chronic sinusitis, cough and post-nasal drip and had frequent and loose bowel movements. Her pulse was thready and her tongue was slightly coated and slightly red.

Whereas the fibroids themselves indicate rather substantial manifestations of stagnation, most of Susan's symptoms (namely, dragging period pain, loose stools and tendency to produce Phlegm) indicate Spleen Qi deficiency and accumulation of Phlegm-Damp. The TCM diagnosis of her condition was stagnation of Blood and Phlegm with Qi deficiency.

She was prescribed herbs and acupuncture to reduce fibroids by:

• regulating Blood

• invigorating and regulating Qi

• clearing Phlegm-Damp.

Because of her Qi deficiency, the formula needed to be a little gentler than the Yu Lin Zhu (modified) recommended above. Hence Wu Ling Zhi and Shan Zha were used instead of E Zhu and San Leng. She was advised to avoid conception for 2 months while she took these herbs:

Dan Shen	9g	Radix Salviae Miltiorrhizae
Bai Shao	9g	Radix Paeoniae Lactiflorae
Chi Shao	9g	Radix Paeoniae Rubra
Dang Shen	9g	Radix Codonopsis Pilulosae
Bai Zhu	9g	Rhizoma Atractylodis Macrocephalae
Fu Ling	9g	Sclerotium Poriae Cocos
Chen Pi	6g	Pericarpium Citri Reticulate
Ban Xia	6g	Rhizoma Pinelliae
Shan Zha	9g	Fructus Crataegi
Wu Ling Zhi	9g	Excrementum Trogopterori
Shan Yao	9g	Dioscorea Oppositae
Shen Qu	9g	Massa Fermenta
Gan Cao	6g	Radix Glycyrrhizae Uralensis

Acupuncture points: ST-28, ST-29, SP-10, SP-6, Ren-6, Ren-3

The size of the fibroids were reduced by 50% in just a couple of months using this approach – a surprisingly rapid result.

She then immediately fell pregnant.

However, the hormone levels necessary to establish and maintain a pregnancy caused the fibroids to grow at an alarming rate. The large fibroid (which quickly grew to larger than its original size) was especially worrying both for its size and its position. It was on the posterior wall of the uterus where the placenta was attached. The fibroids were growing much more rapidly than the baby and were causing Susan pain and concern. These considerations led me to begin the judicious use of herbs and acupuncture points which could address the increasing stagnation:

Bai Zhu	9g	Rhizoma Atractylodis Macrocephalae
Tai Zi Shen	9g	Radix Pseudostellariae Heteropyllae
Shan Yao	9g	Dioscorea Oppositae
Bai Shao	9g	Radix Paeoniae Lactiflorae
Tu Si Zi	9g	Semen Cuscatae
Du Zhong	9g	Cortex Eucommiae Ulmoidis
Sha Ren	9g	Fructus seu Semen Amomi
Mo Yao	6g	Myrrha
Ru Xiang	6g	Gummi Olibanum
Gan Cao	6g	Radix Glycyrrhizae Uralensis

Acupuncture points were chosen from: KI-9, ST-27, ST-28, ST-29, Ren-3, ST-36, GB-34, LIV-3, SP-13, KI-14

Abdomen points were selected according to sites of pain. As the uterus grew in size, points chosen were higher on the abdomen.

By week 18, an ultrasound revealed that the fibroids had shrunk dramatically again to pre-pregnancy levels. Susan's abdomen pain was diminished, although she still experienced aches and dragging discomfort. The same ultrasound, however, delivered the unwelcome news that the placenta was positioned over the cervix (grade 4 placenta praevia) and that Susan could expect bleeding from week 28 of her pregnancy, which would then necessitate bed rest and either an emergency or planned cesarean would follow some time after that.

Susan continued treatment with herbs and acupuncture to control the fibroid growth and encourage placental development throughout the pregnancy. She had great faith that this therapy was going to provide the answer to all the challenges her pregnancy was producing. Her instinct was right; as the pregnancy advanced and her uterus grew, the placenta moved away from the cervix and eventually she had a remarkably efficient vaginal delivery of a 10lb baby boy.

Herbal Formula — If Kidney Yang is deficient it is much easier for fluid to accumulate and eventually Phlegm-Damp forms. Whereas the manifestations of Phlegm-Damp can interfere significantly with the processes necessary for a successful pregnancy, they are the Biao and not the Ben, i.e., they are not the fundamental underlying disorder causing the infertility. Treatment will therefore concentrate on building Yang while at the same time clearing Phlegm-Damp.

Most interference by Phlegm-Damp happens on the ovaries (e.g., polycystic ovaries) or in the tubes (tubes obstructed by mucus or fluid). An excessively mucusy or slippery surface on the endometrium may also hamper implantation. For this reason, it is important to maintain some Phlegm-Damp clearing treatment in a woman with a Damp constitution as implantation is being attempted. And it is even more crucial if there is fluid trapped in the tube (a hydrosalpinx), which may flood the uterus just at the time implantation is attempted (see Ch. 5).

To maintain Kidney Yang and clear Phlegm-Damp in the luteal phase, use method B, the Jian Gu Tang method, with the addition of Damp-clearing herbs and replacing Lu Jiao Pian with Yin Yang Huo. Because Phlegm-Damp can cause pronounced obstructions, this formula includes herbs which unblock channels and clear Blood stasis in addition to those which remove Phlegm-Damp.

Jian Gu Tang modified (Strengthen and Consolidate decoction)

Dang Shen	9 g	*Radix Codonopsis Pilulosae*
Bai Zhu	9 g	*Rhizoma Atractylodis Macrocephalae*
Shan Yao	9 g	*Dioscorea Oppositae*
Yi Yi Ren	15 g	*Semen Coicis Lachryma-jobi*
Tu Si Zi	9 g	*Semen Cuscatae*
Ba Ji Tian	9 g	*Radix Morindae Officinalis*
Yin Yang Huo	9 g	*Herba Epimedii*
Shi Chang Pu	9 g	*Rhizoma Acori Graminei*
Dan Nan Xing	9 g	*Rhizoma Arisaematis*
Lu Lu Tong	9 g	*Fructus Liquidambaris Taiwaniae*
Di Long	9 g	*Lumbricus*
Wang Bu Liu Xing	9 g	*Semen Vaccariae*

Jian Gu Tang was used previously in the treatment of Kidney Yang and Spleen Qi deficiency in the luteal phase. This modified version adds herbs which are drying (Yin Yang Huo and Shi Chang Pu) and herbs which can break through Phlegm-Damp obstructions and free the channels (Dan Nan Xing, Di Long and Lu Lu Tong). Wang Bu Liu Xing supports this action by clearing Blood stasis.

Acupuncture Points — Choose points from Table 4.7 which boost Qi and Yang. In addition consider the following points (and see Table 4.11):

Ren-9	Shuifen
Ren-6	Qihai
Ren-3	Zhongji
GB-26	Daimai
GB-27	Wushu
GB-28	Weidao
BL-22	Sanjiaoshu
BL-28	Pangguanshu

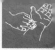

BL-32	Cilaio
SP-9	Yinlingquan
SP-6	Sanyinjiao

Table 4.11   Acupuncture points[a] used in the treatment of infertility: luteal phase with Phlegm-Damp

Treatment goal	Acupuncture point
To transform and distribute accumulation of fluid in the abdomen and specifically the uterus	Ren-9
To resolve Damp by strengthening the Kidney Yang	Ren-3 and Ren-6
To resolve Phlegm-Damp accumulations and help keep fallopian tubes unobstructed for the passage of the embryo	GB-26, GB-27 and GB-28 (Dai vessel points)
To regulate Damp in the pelvic cavity by promoting removal of fluids via the bladder	BL-22 and BL-28
To move fluids by moving Qi in the uterus	BL-32
To support the Spleen in its action of transforming fluids and Damp	SP-9 and SP-6

[a]Use even or reducing method. Care with abdomen and lower back points in the week before the period is due.

CASE HISTORY – MONICA

Monica (30 years) had been trying to become pregnant for 5 years since she married. Her cycle was regular at 26 or 28 days. The period was heavy, with a fresh red flow and was accompanied by mild lower back pain. During the premenstrual week she suffered severe emotional volatility, bloating and general body heaviness. Ovulation was marked by some abdomen discomfort but no fertile mucus. She used a urine ovulation test kit, which indicated that she ovulated on Day 13 or 14 of each cycle. Her BBT showed an early decline in the luteal phase (Fig. 4.18).

A laparoscopy (at age 27) revealed minor endometriosis, which was removed by diathermy. No other abnormality was seen. Her tubes were patent and her uterus normal according to the hysterosalpingogram. The semen analysis was normal.

Frustrated by her lack of success she decided to try an IVF procedure (at age 28). She responded very well to the drugs and produced a large number of eggs, of which 12 fertilized. But neither the embryos transferred in that cycle nor those transferred during three subsequent frozen embryo transfer cycles implanted successfully.

Here we have a young woman who ovulates regularly, has patent tubes and a fertile partner, who has failed to fall pregnant after 5 years and has attempted four ART cycles. If it's not a problem with the ovaries, the tubes, the uterus or the sperm, then chances are it's implantation of the embryo which is failing, i.e., some process is not functioning in the luteal or secretory phase of the cycle. This is the part of the cycle which depends on Kidney Yang. Her BBT charts also indicated a problem of the luteal phase; one we associate with Kidney Yang and Spleen Qi deficiency.

Monica's history revealed past obesity, and even though she had lost some weight she was still overweight. She had a sedentary job and exercised little. Her personality was somewhat phlegmatic and despite a busy job she seldom felt rushed or stressed. Her energy was generally low. She was prone to bloating after eating and before her period. Her pulses were all soft and her tongue was swollen, pale and moist.

The diagnosis of Monica's infertility is Kidney and Spleen Yang deficiency with Phlegm-Damp accumulation.

Treatment aimed to:

- strengthen Kidney Yang

- invigorate Spleen Qi

- clear Phlegm-Damp

- regulate Liver Qi.

By doing this, I hoped we could influence the endometrium and enhance chances of implantation. Strengthening Kidney Yang improves progesterone levels and encourages removal of fluid from the surface of the endometrium at the time of implantation. Accumulation of Phlegm-Damp often causes infertility by obstructing the tubes and the cervix, but in Monica's case, since she had failed to fall pregnant in so many ART cycles, which sidestep the cervix and the tubes, the problem probably lay with the uterine lining itself. During ovulation and premenstrually there were signs that the Liver Qi was not circulating smoothly. She took the following formulas and had acupuncture.

Post-menstrual formula (from Day 4):

Nu Zhen Zi	9 g	Fructus Ligustri Lucidi
Han Lian Cao	9 g	Herba Ecliptae Prostratae
Ji Xue Teng	12 g	Radix et Caulis Jixueteng
Bai Shao	9 g	Radix Paeoniae Lactiflorae
Shan Yao	9 g	Dioscorea Oppositae
Fu Ling	15 g	Sclerotium Poriae Cocos
Cang Zhu	9 g	Rhizoma Atractylodes
Tu Si Zi	9 g	Semen Cuscatae
Xu Duan	6 g	Radix Dipsaci
Ba Ji Tian	6 g	Radix Morindae Officinalis
Yi Yi Ren	15 g	Semen Coicis Lachryma-jobi
Sha Ren	6 g	Fructus seu Semen Amomi

Acupuncture points: Ren-6, Ren-7, ST-28, KI-3, GB-26, ST-40

Ovulation formula (applied earlier than usual, from Day 10)

Xu Duan	9 g	Radix Dipsaci
Yin Yang Huo	12 g	Herba Epimedii
Cang Zhu	9 g	Rhizoma Atractylodes
Bai Zhu	12 g	Rhizoma Atractylodis Macrocephalae
Chen Pi	6 g	Pericarpium Citri Reticulate
Fu Ling	15 g	Sclerotium Poriae Cocos
Gui Zhi	6 g	Ramulus Cinnamomi Cassiae
Zhi Ke	9 g	Fructus Citri seu Ponciri
Shan Zha	9 g	Fructus Crataegi
Hong Hua	6 g	Flos Carthami Tinctorii
Zao Jiao Zi	6 g	Fructus Gleditsiae Sinensis

Acupuncture points: Ren-6, Ren-4, ST-29, SP-6, GB-26, KI-6, LIV-5

Post-ovulation formula (from Day 15):

Dang Shen	9 g	Radix Codonopsis Pilulosae
Bai Zhu	9 g	Rhizoma Atractylodis Macrocephala
Shan Yao	9 g	Dioscorea Oppositae
Yi Yi Ren	15 g	Semen Coicis Lachryma-jobi
Fu Ling	12 g	Sclerotium Poriae Cocos
Tu Si Zi	9 g	Semen Cuscatae

Ba Ji Tian	9g	Radix Morindae Officinalis
Yin Yang Huo	9g	Herba Epimedii
Xian Mao	6g	Rhizoma Curculiginis Orchioidis
Fu Pen Zi	9g	Fructus Rubi Chingii
Shi Chang Pu	9g	Rhizoma Acori Graminei

Acupuncture points: Ren-6, ST-28, KI-3, SP-9, ST-36 (abdomen points were needled with little stimulation).

Her premenstrual symptoms improved in the 1st month but she still had back pain with her period. In the 2nd month she reported more vaginal discharge at midcycle but not the typical stretchy type. Her energy was improving, there was no ovulation discomfort and less bloating. The lower back pain during her period disappeared. In the 3rd month of treatment she saw stretchy mucus at midcycle and this was the month she conceived. Her pregnancy was uneventful and her baby was large and healthy. It took just 3 cycles to sufficiently clear Phlegm-Damp from the cervix and the endometrium to allow conception and implantation.

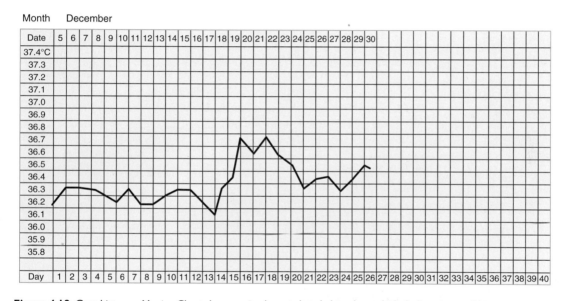

Figure 4.18 Case history – Monica. Chart shows an inadequate luteal phase (one which declines too early).

IN THE CLINIC: PUTTING IT ALL TOGETHER

A summary of treatments for infertility applied at different phases of the menstrual cycle is given in Table 4.12. These protocols, as they are practised in a fertility clinic in China, describe a high level of precise care to maximize chances of conception. As you can see this approach requires frequent clinic visits, frequent adjustments to herbal formulas and detailed understanding of all the processes involved from a western and a Chinese medicine point of view. In this scenario the meeting of a committed patient with a dedicated intelligent practitioner can provide the best possible care and outcomes.

But there are some situations where prescribing treatment by following the menstrual cycle with the sort of minute attention to detail that I have described in this chapter does not suit the patient or the practitioner. In fact, the increasing pace and complexity of life in the West means that this level of intense monitoring and treatment modification is often not possible. There are ways to cut corners.

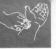

The diagnosis must still be made with great care and accuracy, and of course this means that examining all aspects of the menstrual cycle, the medical history and the constitution cannot be sidestepped. Once this is done, however, one or two general prescriptions might be given which can be taken for half or all of the cycle with certain additions made at key times. The additions might be a Blood-moving formula to be taken during the period, or a Damp-clearing formula or Blood-moving formula before ovulation, or a Shen-calming formula during the follicular phase for example. To simplify treatment, these additions may be patent medicines in pill form, although these are generally not as strong in action as herbs which are decocted or taken as teas made from granules.

In Chapter 11, we discuss ways to simplify treatment protocols even further for patients who need to do IVF and want to prepare in the weeks or months beforehand. For the women with Kidney weakness (and this, once we exclude male factor or tubal infertility, is a majority of women doing IVF) we will focus largely on the post-menstrual formulas which reinforce Kidney Yin and Blood to optimize ovarian function and responsiveness. If the formula is to be taken all month then we shall add some Kidney Yang herbs and for good measure some shen calming herbs. If there is some Blood stasis another formula will be given during the period. Thus we can construct a simple but complete approach that will prepare the woman and her ovaries for the IVF drugs and for pregnancy.

TREATMENT DURING PREGNANCY

Once a positive pregnancy test is announced the patient and practitioner must decide whether treatment should be continued. Pregnant patients must be very cautious of taking medicines of any kind, including herbal medicines. Early pregnancy is a most vulnerable time for the rapidly growing fetus and many pregnant women instinctively reject many foods and flavors. In fact, it is thought that morning sickness evolved from exactly this need to be very cautious of eating plant materials which contain small amounts of toxic chemicals designed to repel insects and animals. The body will therefore be wary of herbal substances and, where morning sickness is pronounced, will reject them outright.

Where there is a history of infertility or previous miscarriage, it is often recommended to take herbs for the first few weeks of pregnancy to help it establish. Chinese herbalists are very careful to use only herbs which are known to be safe for the fetus. They know this not from scientific trials (such trials could never be authorized by an ethics committee) but from the experience of herbalists in China over many hundreds of years. There are a number of Chinese herbs which are forbidden for use in pregnancy (see Appendix 2).

The use of pesticides on cultivated herbs is another issue which causes concern. The main bulk of herbs in our dispensaries in the West come from China where it is sometimes difficult to monitor growing and processing methods. However, now that so many of the herbs grown in China are exported for overseas use, herb suppliers are more open to scrutiny. Some countries like Australia have a requirement that manufactured herbal preparations meet certain standards and conform to the Australian Code of Good Manufacturing Practice (GMP). Thus, the source, quality and consistency of different batches of herbs are examined and required to reach certain standards before the product can be sold in Australia. Herbs are analyzed before and after processing for heavy metals and other contaminants. While these procedures currently apply to Chinese herbs made into pills or powders rather than those sold in large herbal dispensaries for decoction, more and more the original sources and methods of cultivation will be coming under scrutiny of companies wishing to use the herbs for preparations for foreign markets which impose controls.

So we can say that some Chinese herbs can be used safely in early pregnancy and may help to save a pregnancy at risk. For pregnancies not at risk it seems better to let nature do what it does so well when left to its own devices.

A formula commonly given to women who have become pregnant after experiencing a period of infertility is one which boosts Kidney and Spleen function and nourishes Qi and Blood.

Table 4.12 Summary of treatments of infertility applied at different phases of the menstrual cycle

Phase	Guiding formula and suggested points	With Kidney Yin deficiency	With Kidney Yang deficiency	With Kidney Jing deficiency	With Liver or Heart stagnation	With Blood stagnation	With Phlegm-Damp accumulation
Period Regulate Blood	Tao Hong Si Wu Tang SP-10, 6 CO-4 ST-28 KI-14						
Post-period Reinforce and Blood Yin	Gui Shao Di Huang Tang Plus Yang tonics before ovulation Choose from: Ren-4, 7 KI-3, 4, 5, 6, 8, 13 ST-27, 30, 36 BL-23, 32 LIV-3, SP-4, 6, 10	Add Nu Zhen Zi Han Lian Cao Mai Dong Sheng Di Add KI-2	Add Tu Si Zi Rou Cong Rong Add BL-23, Ren-3, Ren-2, BL-32	Add Ze He Che Lu Rong Add KI-12	Add for Liver Qi stagnation Huang Lian Zhi Zi Lian Zi Xin Suan Zao Ren Chuan Lian Zi Mu Dan Pi Or for Heart Qi stagnation Chi Shao He Huan Pi Bai Zi Ren Mu Li Add LIV-2, HE-5, 7, PC-6, 7	Add Yi Mu Cao Chi Shao Shan Zha Tao Ren Hong Hua Wu Ling Zhi Dan Shen Add KI-14, Ren-3, SP-12, ST-29, LIV-5, SP-8	Add Tu Si Zi Xu Duan Ba Ji Tian Fu Ling Cang Zhu Sha Ren Add GB-26, SP-5, BL-28

Continued

Table 4.12 Summary of treatments of infertility applied at different phases of the menstrual cycle—cont'd

Phase	Guiding formula and suggested points	With Kidney Yin deficiency	With Kidney Yang deficiency	With Kidney Jing deficiency	With Liver or Heart stagnation	With Blood stagnation	With Phlegm-Damp accumulation
Ovulation Regulate Qi and Blood	Cu Pai Luan Tang Choose from LIV-3, 5 KI-13, 14, 8, 5, 4 SP-13, 8, 6, 5 PC-6, 5, HE-7, 5 Yintang Zigong GB-26	Bu Shen Cu Pai Luan Tang Add Ren-4 KI-3, 6	Wen Yang Hua Yu Feng Add Ren-6, 4 ST-29	Bu Shen Cu Pai Luan Tang plus Lu Jiao Jiao Ze He Che Add Ren-4, KI-12, ST-27	Cu Pai Luan Tang plus Chai Hu Bai Shao or Yuan Zhi Shi Chang Pu	Cu Pai Luan Tang or Bu Shen Cu Pai Luan Tang plus Shan Zha Add ST-29, SP-10, LIV-8, BL-17	Wen Yang Hua Tan Fang plus Zao Jiao Zi Add choice of: BL-22, 28 GB-27, 28 SP-?, KI-7, ST-29
Post-ovulation Boost Kidney Yang	A You Gui Wan B Jian Gu Tang C Yu Lin Zhu A Ren-2, 4, 5, 7, 15, KI-3, 6, BL-23 B Ren-4, 5, 6, 12 ST-25, 36, SP-6 KI-3, BL-20, 23 C Ren-4, 12, ST-36 SP-6, 10, KI-5 BL-17	You Gui Wan plus Nu Zhen Zi Han Lian Cao **A** points selection plus KI-2	Jian Gu Tang (modified) **B** points selection with moxa	You Gui Wan plus Huang Jing **A** points selection	Yu Ling Zhu plus Chai Hu Chuan Lian Zi Xiang Fu Mu Dan Pi Zhi Mu **C** points selection plus choice of: LIV-2, 3, 4, 5, 8 LIV-9, 11 PC-5, 6, 7 Ren-3	Yu Ling Zhu plus Pu Huang Dan Shen Yu Jin Ji Xue Teng **C** points selection plus choice of: ST-28, 29 LIV-8, 5 SP-6, 8 KI-4, 5 Baliao	Jian Gu Tang modified plus Yin Yang Huo Shi Chang Pu Dan Nan Xing Lu Lu Tong Di Long Ma Bian Cao Wang Bu Liu Xing **B** points selection plus choice of: Ren-3, 6, 9 GB-27, 28, BL-32, SP-6, 9

Yishen Gutai Tang (Nourish Kidney and Protect Fetus) modified

Tu Si Zi	20 g	Semen Cuscatae
Du Zhong	15 g	Cortex Eucommiae Ulmoidis
Xu Duan	15 g	Radix Dipsaci
Sang Ji Sheng	15 g	Ramulus Sangjisheng
Dang Shen	15 g	Radix Codonopsis Pilulosae
Bai Zhu	15 g	Rhizoma Atractylodis Macrocephalae
Huang Qin	9 g	Radix Scutellariae Baicalensis
Gou Qi Zi	12 g	Fructus Lycii Chinensis
Dang Shen	12 g	Radix Codonopsis Pilulosae
Da Zao	3 pieces	Fructus Zizyphi Jujuba
He Shou Wu	12 g	Radix Polygoni Multiflori
Sha Ren	6 g	Fructus seu Semen Amomi

It can be modified if there is any bleeding, with the addition of:

E. Jiao	15 g	Gelatinum Corii Asini
Zhu Ma Gen	9 g	Radix Boehmeriae

However, it cannot prevent the miscarriage of a pregnancy which is not viable.

A formula like this has been used to good effect with IVF patients in trials in China. Women who took Chinese herbs had a significantly lower miscarriage rate than those who did not take it.[5]

MORNING SICKNESS

Debilitating morning sickness is another clinical situation in which Chinese medicine is sometimes recommended. TCM describes morning sickness as the rising of the Qi up the Chong vessel once the Uterus has closed. It affects the Stomach, making its Qi rise also, causing nausea and vomiting. If the woman is still able to eat adequately, then the nausea of pregnancy is not considered pathological. However, if vomiting becomes extreme or the Qi rises along the Chong vessel further to affect the Heart, then treatment is required or the pregnancy may be endangered.

Acupuncture Points — Acupuncture is the treatment of choice for morning sickness and is often very effective, although it may need to be repeated frequently (even daily) in more severe cases. Medical researchers have experimented with applying pressure to the point Neiguan PC-6 on women experiencing morning sickness.[6] Significant and continued reduction of nausea compared to use of a placebo point was reported.

In the acupuncture clinic, we use the following points (and see Table 4.13), which regulate the rising Qi of the Chong channel and encourage Stomach Qi to descend:

ST-36	Zusanli
PC-6	Neiguan
KI-21	Youmen
ST-19	Burong
K-27	Shufu
K-6	Zhaohai

Use with reinforcing or even method.

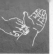

Table 4.13   Acupuncture points[a] used to treat nausea of pregnancy

Treatment goal	Acupuncture point
To strengthen and regulate the Stomach and Spleen, to regulate the Chong channel and to encourage Stomach Qi to descend	ST-36, PC-6, KI-21, ST-19, K-27, K-6
If symptoms are worse with stress	GB-34, LIV-2, LIV-3, LIV-14
If Stomach Qi is weak	Ren-12, Ren-13
If there is vomiting of mucus	ST-40

[a]Use reducing or reinforcing method depending on the action of the point.

If there are emotional or stress-related components add:

GB-34	Yanglingquan
LIV-2	Xingjian
LIV-3	Taichong
LIV-14	Qimen

Use with even or reducing method.

If the Stomach Qi is weak, add:

| Ren-12 | Zhongwan |
| Ren-13 | Shangwan |

Use reinforcing method.

If there is vomiting of mucus, add:

| ST-40 | Fenglong |

Herbal Formula — Herbal remedies for morning sickness are described in Chinese medicine texts but it takes a very strong-minded patient to swallow herbal decoctions when her stomach is rejecting most foods. Even the smell of many Chinese herbal decoctions provokes nausea. Hence, I have included here only one of the many text-listed morning sickness formulas. The following formula addresses most of the causes of severe morning sickness – namely, rising Stomach Qi, accumulation of Phlegm and Liver Qi stagnation. If nausea and vomiting are severe and the fetus is at risk, give this formula in small amounts, in combination with cupping or Gua Sha described below. A granulated form of the herbs can be put in capsules if the smell and taste are too repugnant.

Yi Gan He Wei Yin (Restrain Liver and Harmonize the Stomach decoction)

Zi Su Ye	3 g	Folium Perillae Frutescentis
Huang Lian	6 g	Rhizoma Coptidis
Ban Xia	6 g	Rhizoma Pinelliae
Zhu Ru	6 g	Caulis Bambusae in Taeniis
Chen Pi	6 g	Pericarpium Citri Reticulate

Gou Teng	15 g	Ramulus Uncariae Cum Uncis
Huang Qin	9 g	Radix Scutellariae Baicalensis
Sheng Jiang	3 g	Rhizoma Zingiberis Officinalis Recens

This formula is a variation of Su Ye Huang Lian Tang, a popular morning sickness formula, which harmonizes Liver and Stomach. Zi Su Ye, Ban Xia, Sheng Jiang and Chen Pi all harmonize the center to suppress vomiting. Huang Lian clears Heat, calms the Stomach and prevents vomiting. Gou Teng pacifies the Liver and Huang Qin settles the fetus.

If severe vomiting persists, add:

Wu Mei	3 g	Fructus Pruni Mume
Lu Gen	15 g	Rhizoma Phragmites Communis
(Zhi) Pi Pa Ye	9 g	Folium Eriobotryae

Cupping the point Ren-12 Zhongwan strongly for 15 min will sometimes pacify the rising Stomach Qi long enough to drink and absorb some herbs.

Rubbing the skin, a technique known as Gua Sha, on the points

BL-20	Pishu
BL-21	Weishu
BL-17	Geshu,

each day or every 2nd day can also relieve severe vomiting long enough to ingest small amounts of herbs to resolve morning sickness.

Ginger on its own is a recognized and effective remedy for morning sickness. Even at doses as low as 1 g/day symptoms can be relieved, but the ginger has to be taken a minimum of 48 h up to 4 days before it becomes effective.

There are many pregnancy conditions which respond well to acupuncture and these are covered thoroughly in texts dedicated to obstetric acupuncture.[7,8]

TOWARDS THE END OF PREGNANCY

Acupuncture Points — Acupuncture may be of benefit if the position of the baby is not good for delivery. Seeing very pregnant women at the acupuncture departments of Chinese hospitals is not at all rare. They come any time after 34 weeks if their baby has not turned into a head-down position. Moxa treatment is applied for 15 min each day to just one point:

BL-67	Zhiyin

The treatment may need to be repeated five or more times before the baby turns and adopts a cephalic position. It is most common for the pregnant woman to report increased activity in the womb and sometimes to actually feel the baby turn during the night when she is resting. If there is some physical impediment to its moving (e.g., fibroids or placement of placenta and umbilical cord) then the moxibustion will have no effect. This time-honored technique has recently been assessed favorably in clinical trials.[9,10] The simplicity of the treatment and easy diagnosis of the condition and its outcome without the necessity of a TCM analysis makes this one of the few conditions which is easy to analyze according to the criteria of Western science.

Table 4.14   Acupuncture points[a] used in induction of labor

Treatment goal	Acupuncture point
To open the cervix, increase contractions and encourage descent of the baby	SP-6 and CO-4
To help the baby descend into the pelvic rim and engage either before labor (for first borns) or during labor (for second and later births)	GB-21
To help move Liver Qi where there is stress or tension contributing to failure to start labor	LIV-3
To relieve back pain and stimulate the muscles of the uterus	BL-32

[a]Use reducing method, except with GB-21 which should be needled gently and shallowly.

Midwives often recommend their patients have acupuncture in the month before the due date since this approach appears to significantly reduce the number of medical inductions, epidurals and emergency cesareans.[11] Acupuncture frequency may be increased if the patient is past her due date and is facing medical induction of labor. It has also been shown that electro-acupuncture is just as effective as the use of prostaglandin gel in ripening the cervix. This study also found that there were fewer cesarean deliveries and obstetric complications when acupuncture was used to induce labor.[12]

The main points are (and see Table 4.14):

SP-6   Sanyinjiao
CO-4   Hegu

A gentle electric current is often applied to these points, especially SP-6.

Other useful points are:

GB-21   Jianjing
LIV-3   Taichong
BL-32   Ciliao

And here with the birth of a red squirming baby, ends this chapter!

REFERENCES

1. Xia GC. *Zhong Yi Lin Chuang Fu Ke Xue*. 2nd edn : PRC: Chinese People's Health Publishing; 1996.

2. Odeblad E, Hoglund A. The dynamic mosaic of the human ovulatory cervical mucus. *Proc Nordic Fertil Soc* 1978;January.

3. Stener-Victorin E, Waldenstrom U, Andersson SA, et al. Reduction of blood flow impedance in the uterine arteries of infertile women with electro-acupuncture. *Hum Reprod* 1996;**11**:1314–7.

4. Ko KM, Leon TY, Mak DH, et al. A characteristic pharmacological action of 'Yang-invigorating' Chinese tonifying herbs: enhancement of myocardial ATP-generation capacity. *Phytomedicine* 2006;**13**(9–10):636–42.

5. Ying Liu, Jing-zhi Wu. Effect of Gutai decoction on the abortion rate of in vitro fertilization and embryo transfer. *Chin J Integr Med* 2006;**12**(3):189–93.

6. Werntoft E, Dykes A. Effect of acupressure on nausea and vomiting during pregnancy. A randomized, placebo-controlled, pilot study. *J Reprod Med* 2001;**46**:835–9.

7.   Betts D. *Essential guide to acupuncture in pregnancy childbirth*. Hove: Journal of Chinese Medicine Ltd.; 2006.

8.   West Z. *Acupuncture in pregnancy and childbirth*. London: Elsevier; 2001.

9.   Cardini F, Weixin H. Moxibustion for correction of breach presentation: a randomized controlled trial. *J Am Med Acad* 1998;**280**:1580–4.

10. van den Berg I, Kaandorp GC, Bosch JL, et al. Cost-effectiveness of breech version by acupuncture-type interventions on BL 67, including moxibustion, for women with a breech foetus at 33 weeks gestation: a modelling approach. *Complement Ther Med* 2010;**18**(2):67–77.

11. Betts D, Lennox S. Acupuncture for prebirth treatment: An observational study of its use in midwifery practice. *Med Acupunct* 2006;**17**(3):16–9.

12. Gribel G, Coca-Velarde LG, Moreira de Sá RA. Electroacupuncture for cervical ripening prior to labor induction: a randomized clinical trial. *Arch Gynecol Obstet* 2011;**283**(6):1233–8.

Gynecologic disorders which can cause infertility

5

Chapter Contents

INTRODUCTION

In Chinese medicine clinics in the West, many, if not most, patients will arrive having already had some investigations and sporting a diagnostic label or two. For the TCM doctor, these labels are interesting: they will tell some details about the disorder and perhaps, some idea about prognosis. But the treatment offered by the TCM doctor will be decided largely on the basis of a completely different sort of label, i.e., that determined using Bian Zheng or pattern differentiation according to Chinese medicine diagnostic principles. Keeping this in mind, we now examine some of the labels women bring to an infertility clinic and how they might be reconfigured in the framework of Chinese medicine. All treatments suggested are based on (or modified from) those used in the Jiangsu Province TCM Hospital[1] or other published sources and are intended to be guides only.

140

DISEASES AND DISORDERS WHICH CAUSE OR CONTRIBUTE TO INFERTILITY

• Endometriosis

Endometriosis is a complex disorder which causes disturbing symptoms and can affect fertility in myriad ways from obstruction of the ovaries and tubes, to impaired oocyte development to dysfunction in the uterine lining hindering implantation and normal placenta development. However, unlike the disorders discussed in Part 2 of this Chapter, amenorrhea or polycystic ovary syndrome (PCOS), the ovaries are usually functioning and ovulation is regular most of the time.

This disorder typically involves stagnation of Blood in conjunction with other pathologies. Deficiency of Kidney Yang is often involved, especially if there is also infertility. TCM treatment will follow the menstrual cycle in the fashion discussed in Chapter 4 but more attention is paid to clearing Blood stasis and breaking up masses during the period, moving qi and Blood at ovulation and fortifying the Kidney yang. If there is such severe stagnation that a pregnancy is impossible, then treatment will focus on clearing the stagnation and reducing inflammation throughout the entire menstrual cycle while attempts at conception are postponed.

• Inflammation of Pelvic Organs (Pelvic Inflammatory Disease, Endometritis, Salpingitis)

While not so common in their acute presentations (which are best treated with antibiotics), subtle or chronic manifestations of infection and inflammation of reproductive organs can present in the Chinese medicine fertility clinic. It is important that these are resolved before conception is attempted.

Infections and inflammation are commonly described as Damp-Heat in Chinese medicine. Chronic or persistent Damp-Heat in the lower Jiao can impair fertility by creating an environment that is not conducive to sperm survival, good egg quality, smooth transport of the embryo or endometrial health and implantation. Chronic cases respond well to acupuncture and herbal therapy, which clears Damp and Heat and supports Kidney function.

• Disorders of Ovulation

Part 2 of this chapter covers many of the different reasons that a woman might not be falling pregnant due to ovary dysfunction. She may ovulate very infrequently (oligomenorrhea) or not very well (luteal phase defect). She may not ovulate at all (amenorrhea) due to resistant ovaries or premature menopause or primary ovarian failure.

Many cases of irregular ovulation are related to Kidney Yin and Yang imbalance and the best way to approach treatment of these is promoting the natural trends in the cycle, as we have discussed in Chapter 4. Where there is no ovulation, it may be necessary to purge or resolve a pathogenic factor, or strongly boost Kidney Jing.

• Polycystic Ovary Syndrome

This is one type of ovulation disorder and those women with this syndrome who are having difficulty conceiving usually have some disruption to the function of the Chong and Ren channels. The menstrual cycle is often irregular or infrequent and treatment attempting to follow the usual movements of Kidney Yin and Yang in the follicular and luteal phases is not so easy. The obstruction to the Chong and Ren can arise from accumulation of Phlegm-Damp, or stagnation of Qi. Either may or may not be associated with Kidney deficiency but where there is infertility, Kidneys are likely to be involved. Our treatment will focus on achieving ovulation – this may require clearing Phlegm-Damp and building Yin and Blood all together initially; then, as signs of ovulation develop, Kidney Yang will be strongly boosted to promote successful ovulation. Or we may need to re-establish the circulation of Qi and Blood in the Chong and Ren at the same time as building Kidney Jing. We shall discuss the many different ways to view and apply treatment to this syndrome in Part 2 this chapter.

• Tubal Blockage

This cause of infertility will be discussed in Chapter 6. Doctors in China, in the absence of advanced surgical methods and affordable IVF (in vitro fertilization) technology, have devised ingenious methods for trying to unblock fallopian tubes. The blockage is regarded as a stagnation of Qi and Blood, and treatment includes flushing the tubes with saline and herbal solutions, introducing herbal decoctions per rectum, electrotherapy on the abdomen, various other physiotherapeutic manipulations and, of course, acupuncture. Where the technology exists, microsurgery and IVF procedures offer a good chance of pregnancy in women with blocked tubes.

Part 1 – Endometriosis, Pelvic Inflammatory Disease, Fibroids and Polyps

ENDOMETRIOSIS

Endometriosis is a not an uncommon diagnosis in recent times. This is due in part to the increasing frequency with which diagnostic surgery is carried out but also to deferred child-bearing and to increasing levels of environmental pollutants. The disease is defined by the presence of endometrial tissue somewhere in the pelvic cavity but outside the uterus. Rarely, endometrial tissue can be found in other locations in the body. Adenomyosis is the term used for endometrial tissue appearing in the myometrium (muscle layer) of the uterine wall.

Endometriosis affects approximately 6–7% of all females, 30–40% of whom are infertile. This is two to three times the rate of infertility in the general population. A quarter of the women attending IVF clinics have endometriosis. There is likely a genetic component since patients with an affected mother or siblings are more likely to have severe endometriosis than those without affected relatives. Magnetic resonance imaging (MRI) has revealed a high correlation between endometriosis and adenomyosis in first-degree relatives.[2]

Etiology

The most widely held theory, retrograde menstruation, states that endometriosis occurs when endometrial fragments pass through the fallopian tubes during menstruation and attach to nearby pelvic structures and grow.

Endometrial cells are seen in peritoneal fluid in all women at the time of menses, so it might be expected that endometriosis should develop in all these women. The fact that only some women develop the disease may have something to do with impaired immune surveillance. Immunologic changes have been demonstrated in women with endometriosis, however, researchers are uncertain whether these immunologic findings are responsible for the endometriosis or are a result of the inflammation caused by it. Doctors of Chinese medicine relate impaired immune surveillance to Kidney Yang deficiency, which as we shall see later is an important factor in the etiology of the disease.

Under the influence of menstrual cycle hormones, each month the displaced endometrial tissue grows and sheds blood at the time of menses. Instead of flowing harmlessly outside the body, however, the internal bleeding wreaks havoc in the abdominal cavity.

The resulting inflammation leads to the formation of adhesions which attach to and distort the tubes, ovaries, uterus and other pelvic organs.

To date, laparoscopy is the most reliable way to diagnose endometriosis. During this procedure, the surgeon is able to look inside the pelvic region and see exactly what is there. What the surgeon sees if endometriosis is present is patches (from tiny pinpricks which are hard to see to large lumps which can distort organs in the pelvis) of endometrial tissue. These are commonly located on the back of the uterus, on the tubes, around the ovaries (or as a cyst inside the ovary), on the ligaments which hold the uterus in place or on the bowel or bladder.

Patches of endometrial tissue can be of different appearance, and exhibit different behavior:

- Brown or pigmented endometriosis appears as small dark brown spots. The blood lost from this endometrial tissue during the time of menstruation has nowhere to go and gets trapped and may cause pain, depending on the site of implantation. The old dried blood then gives these spots a dark brown appearance. These peritoneal lesions are most active when they are superficial and hemorrhagic and become less active over time as dead and fibrotic tissue forms.

- Chocolate cyst is the name given to endometriosis which forms a cyst in the ovary. The blood from this tissue is encapsulated in a cyst and becomes thick and dark brown and appears like chocolate.

- Pale pink, white or non-pigmented endometriosis looks like pale lesions on the surface of different parts of the pelvic cavity. These lesions have not yet become brown because they have not developed far enough to bleed, but they seem to be active in secreting substances which inhibit conception. They may also be more active in producing prostaglandins and be associated with more pain than older lesions. It can take 7–10 years for these lesions to become red and then dark as they age and become fibrotic.

Endometriosis tissue not only varies in its appearance but also in how deeply it attaches to the membrane covering the pelvic cavity and the organs. This too influences its effect on the body:

- superficial endometriosis sits on the surface of the membrane and seems to be more implicated in infertility

- deeper endometriosis penetrates a few millimeters into the membrane and the underlying tissues and causes pain.

The Clinical Picture

Endometriosis is a condition which has puzzled doctors for a long time – it is associated with pelvic pain during periods and at other times, pain during intercourse, bowel symptoms, spotting before periods and infertility. But not always so – there are many cases of severe endometriosis discovered by accident during investigation or surgery for something else, or during a hysterectomy, which have never contributed to any difficulty with periods or with conceiving. On the other hand, severe dysmenorrhea and great difficulty falling pregnant are sometimes seen to be associated with almost insignificant amounts of endometriosis seen on laparoscopy. For nearly one-third of endometriosis patients the only symptom is infertility. Premenstrual spotting occurs in the majority of endometriosis cases.

Endometriosis and Infertility

In this text, we are particularly interested in how this disorder reduces fertility. We are aware of several different mechanisms whereby endometriosis might hinder conception; very likely this is still only part of the story.

Distortion of the Position of Tubes or Ovaries

If there is a significant amount of endometriosis in an inconvenient place, near the fallopian tubes or ovaries for example, it is not difficult to see how the distortions it causes could prevent conceptions by preventing the egg and the sperm meeting. Over time, the fallopian tubes may become inflamed and blocked by adhesions. Thus, ectopic pregnancies are more common in women with endometriosis. Even mild endometriosis is associated in most cases with peri-ovarian adhesions which may interfere with ovulation or transport of the egg between ovary and fallopian tube.[3]

Immune Dysfunction

Endometriosis is characterized by a low-grade inflammation in the pelvis, which manifests as an increase in peritoneal fluid, increased number of macrophages and their secretions, i.e. prostaglandins, proteolytic enzymes and cytokines.[4]

Macrophages are large cells which mop up cellular debris and bacteria and other foreign material; one of their jobs is to kill off sperm that swim all the way out of the tubes and into the abdomen. When there is endometriosis present, there are increased numbers of macrophages[5] which become more active and go on their seek and destroy missions with great vigor. Unfortunately, these vigilantes can enter the fallopian tubes and pick off sperm before they have had a chance to meet the egg. In women with partners who have poor sperm counts, this can be quite disastrous, leaving no sperm at all to fertilize the egg. Additionally, the cytokines which macrophages produce are toxic to sperm affecting their mobility and ability to fertilize the egg, providing yet another impediment to fertility.[6,7] Cytokines and chemokines such as tumor necrosis factor-alpha, and interleukins IL-1, IL-6, IL-8, etc. contribute to the pathogenesis of endometriosis by enhancing attachment, angiogenesis and/or proliferation of ectopic endometrial tissues in the pelvis.[8]

The disease is further characterized by impaired T-cell mediated cytotoxicity, natural killer (NK) cell activity and B-cell function.

Production of Secretions which Obstruct Fallopian Tubes

The type of endometriosis that sits superficially on the membrane surrounding the pelvic structures has been shown to have glands similar to that found in the endometrium. These glands secrete mucus. This mucus can coat the fimbriae or the ovary, preventing the transfer of the egg to the tube. Such a phenomenon has been observed in animal studies.[9]

Increased Prostaglandin Production

Endometriosis is associated with increased levels of prostaglandins (PGE_2 and PGF), which may have a deleterious effect on the patency and flexibility of the fallopian tubes. Muscular contractions of the uterus are also increased causing pain and possibly interfering with implantation.[10]

LUFS and Low Progesterone

Endometriosis is associated with a higher incidence of the ovulatory disturbance called luteinized unruptured follicle syndrome (LUFS) and lower progesterone levels in the luteal phase.

Things can go awry just before ovulation if luteinizing hormone (LH) levels are less than adequate. A developing follicle may respond to the extent that it forms a corpus luteum and produces progesterone but there is not enough LH to soften the follicle casing and allow the release of a mature egg. A luteinized unruptured follicle (or LUF) is formed. The amount of progesterone this LUF produces is often less than usual and for fewer days, and is the basis of an inadequate luteal phase or luteal phase defect. Obviously, conception is impossible in such cycles since there is no egg released, and even if there were, the progesterone support is such that implantation and development of an embryo is unlikely. It is estimated that endometriosis results in anovulation in up to 20% of cycles of some patients.

Endometrial Changes and Reduced Implantation Rates

Although appearing histologically normal, the endometrium and inner myometrium (the junctional zone) in women with endometriosis and adenomyosis show marked functional disturbances. The lining has aberrant responses to ovarian hormones such that factors important for implantation are affected.[10,11] Implantation and placentation involve deep invasion of the junctional zone and it may be the failure to do this properly that accounts for the increase in premature births and other adverse pregnancy outcomes seen in women with endometriosis.[12]

Disruption in the deepest layer of the endometrium may also explain functional abnormalities such as hyperperistalsis, dysperistalsis and inordinate smooth muscle proliferation associated with endometriosis and adenomyosis which can affect the way sperm are transported.[13]

Other studies have suggested that there are disruptions to shedding of the uterine lining during menstruation in endometriosis sufferers, which leads to abnormalities in the uterine lining in the subsequent luteal phase.[14]

All of the above possibly contribute to the observed reduced embryo implantation rate.[15]

Reduced Oocyte Quality

Studies with IVF patients receiving donor eggs have shown that success rates were reduced when the oocytes were from women with endometriosis indicating that the disease affected in some way the quality of the donated oocytes.[16]

Ovarian Reserve may be Lower in Endometriosis

Studies on infertile women with mild or minimal endometriosis show reduced ovarian reserve (measured by AMH). Whether this is an association or a cause is not known.[17] Surgical removal of endometriomas can also have a deleterious effect on ovarian reserve (measured by AMH).[18]

Treatment with Western Medicine

Surgery is used to de-bulk severe endometriosis. If it is successfully removed, leaving undamaged tubes and ovaries, then chances of conception may increase dramatically in the months following the surgery, especially if endometriosis was the only cause of the infertility.

If endometriosis is mild and in its early stages, it may be difficult to find and remove all the small non-pigmented lesions. The substances produced by such lesions which interfere with the meeting of egg and sperm and possibly disrupt implantation, continue to be made.

While surgery is the preferred medical option for endometriosis patients trying to conceive, there are a number of different drug regimens which, at different times and in different clinics, have gained popularity. The strategy behind all of them is to prevent ovulation and the flux of hormones associated with a normal menstrual cycle. This is achieved by using drugs which mimic pregnancy – progestogens like Provera (medroxyprogesterone acetate) or Duphaston (dydrogesterone) – or induce temporary menopause – testosterone derivatives such as Danocrine or Danazol or gonadotrophin-releasing hormone (GnRH) analogs such as Zoladex (goserelin) or Synarel (nafarelin) – or by using the oral contraceptive pill continuously. In all cases, the menstrual cycle is halted. Some of these drug regimens produce a wide range of side-effects and are not easily tolerated by all women. The length of treatment varies from 3 to 9 months or more and if it is successful, the endometriosis is 'starved' into shrinking or disappearing. Women are usually encouraged to try to fall pregnant soon after their cycle resumes on the cessation of the drug treatment.

IVF procedures, wherein the meeting of the eggs and the sperm is arranged outside the body, neatly circumnavigate some of the troublesome ways that endometriosis exerts its influence. In cases where mild endometriosis meets a low sperm count, IVF can greatly improve a couple's chances of having a baby. However, endometriosis patients have poorer IVF outcome in terms of reduced pregnancy rate per cycle, reduced pregnancy rate per transfer and reduced implantation rate when compared with women doing IVF for other reasons.[16] It is thought that abnormalities of the uterine lining in endometriosis patients can also negatively impact IVF outcomes.[15,19] The risk of pre-term birth is increased in endometriosis patients who do IVF.[20]

TCM Treatment of Endometriosis

But is there another way to view the treatment of this disease? A way that does not just remove or shrink the manifestations of the imbalance that allowed it to occur but tries to address that imbalance or underlying pathology itself? And if that could be corrected, may be the lesions (especially the pink or superficial type), might become innocuous and no longer produce mucus or attract and activate macrophages. I don't know if Chinese medicine can claim to change the nature and troublesome behavior of the endometriosis lesions but if the basic and underlying imbalance (as the TCM doctor understands it) is addressed, then symptoms and fertility can certainly improve.

Diagnosing Endometriosis

Endometriosis, as you may have gathered, is a multifarious type of disorder which can manifest in many guises. Sometimes, there are no bothersome symptoms at all. Often there is period pain and sometimes there is also pain with intercourse. Infertility is involved in some cases and not in others. And the ways that endometriosis contributes to infertility is at many different levels, the quality of the eggs, the integrity of the uterine lining, the way the tubes and uterus move, the distortion of tubes or ovaries or the inflammation and over-activity of the immune system. Any diagnosis a Chinese medicine doctor comes up with, should keep in mind all these possibilities. Figure 5.1 outlines some of the etiologic relationships relevant to the development of endometriosis.

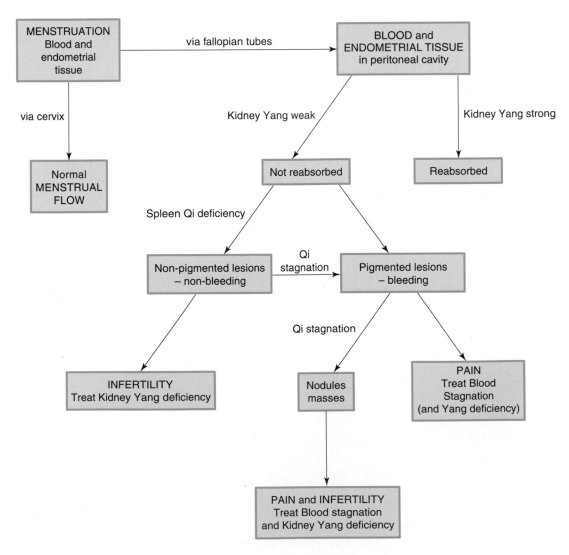

Figure 5.1 Theoretical relationships between different types of endometriosis.

There are some characteristic signs that are recognized by doctors working in infertility clinics in China, which will alert them to the possible presence of endometriosis. These are distinctive patterns on the basal body temperature (BBT) charts (see below) and spotting before periods, which is also recognized by Western doctors as strongly indicative of endometriosis. These two signs, together with some of the clinical symptoms mentioned earlier – especially period pain getting worse with age and accompanied by a bearing-down sensation in the abdomen or palpation of nodules along the sacrospinal ligament – constitute as definite a diagnosis of endometriosis that a doctor working in China without a laparoscope can reach.

It must then be remembered that to a TCM doctor, the unique and individual presentation of each patient is what will determine the appropriate treatment.

BBT Patterns

You will recall from our discussions in Chapter 3 that the typical BBT chart has a low phase, which begins at (or just prior to) the beginning of the period, and a high phase, which begins at ovulation and persists until the next period. The two changes to this pattern which can suggest endometriosis are:

- The temperature does not drop very much when the period comes, or if it does drop it may start to go up again after 1 or 2 days. These patterns indicate that the switch to Yin from Yang has not been on time or complete. One of the factors that both signifies and contributes to the switch from Yang to Yin is the loss of blood and therefore body heat to the outside. In the case of endometriosis, which involves significant bleeding inside the pelvic cavity or in the ovary (if there is an endometrioma) which cannot escape the body, one of the conditions of switching Yin to Yang is not met and the temperature will not drop convincingly (see Ch. 3).

- The temperature of the high phase may rise very slowly after ovulation, or may not rise enough or may fall again after only a few days. These patterns all indicate inadequate Kidney Yang function (see Ch. 3).

Strategies for Treating Endometriosis

Targeting the Lesion

The emphasis of TCM treatment for endometriosis usually involves clearing Blood stagnation. Endometriosis is a Western medical label not a TCM one, but the scientific medical understanding of this disease has contributed to the notion that this is a disease characterized by blood being where it shouldn't and unable to escape the body, i.e., what we call Blood stasis. Symptoms such as severe stabbing period pain, clotty menstrual flow and palpable nodules or masses in the abdomen verify the diagnosis of stagnant Blood.

The mark of a skilful doctor is to keep close sight of exactly what requires changing, maintaining awareness of the constellation in which it appears. In the case of endometriosis the central part of the picture is the lesion which can manifest in various guises:

- superficial and pink/pale red

- deeper, brown and bleeding

- large and bulky (± obstruction to tubes)

- cysts in the ovary.

Table 5.1 lists the theoretical relationship between these different types of lesions and their treatment principles.

Treatment to target implants of endometriosis (Zheng Jia, or masses, in TCM) involves the use of heavy handed 'Blood busting' herbs and those that reduce inflammation by clearing Damp and Heat. Table 5.2 lists some of these herbs and substances. (See also Appendix 2.)

Table 5.1   The theoretical relationship between different types of endometriosis lesions and the appropriate treatment principles

Type of lesion (Zheng Jia)	Action	Treatment
Non-pigmented lesions	Produce secretions which may clog the fimbrial end of fallopian tube and cause infertility	Boost Kidney Yang and invigorate Spleen Qi to remove Phlegm-Damp (or Damp-Heat)
Pigmented lesions	Cause pain, bleeding and inflammation in pelvic cavity and infertility	Resolve Blood stagnation and inflammation with Blood regulating and Damp-Heat clearing herbs and boost Kidney Yang to promote dispersal of stagnation.
Cysts, nodules and masses	Cause pain, inflammation and infertility due to distortion of tubes or ovaries	Resolve Blood stagnation with Blood breaking herbs, clear Damp-Heat and boost Kidney Yang to promote dispersal of stagnation.

Table 5.2   Examples of herbs and other substances employed to break up pelvic endometrial masses

	Action
Herbs and medicinal substances	
San Leng – *Rhizoma Sparganii* E Zhu – *Rhizoma Curcumae*	Resolve Blood stasis, break up implants and relieve pain.
Ru Xiang – *Resina Olibani* Mo Yao – *Resina Commiphorae Myrrhae* Xue Jie – *Resina Daemonoropis*	Resolve Blood stasis, break up implants, stop bleeding, remove old blood and make new tissue
Bai Jiang Cao – *Herba Patriniae* Hong Teng – *Caulis Sargentodoxae* Bai Hua She She Cao – *Herba hedyotidis Diffusae*	Clear Damp-Heat and inflammation and calm immune reactions
Animal products which search and pick out enduring disease	
Wu Ling Zhi – *Excrementum Trogopteri seu Pteromi*	Resolve Blood stasis, dissolve congealed blood and stop pain
Shui Zhi – *Hirudo*	Resolve Blood stasis in the collaterals of the pelvis, dissolve masses.
Tu Bie Chong – *Eupolyphaga Sinensis*	Resolve Blood stasis, reduce fixed palpable masses
Di Long – *Lumbricus*	Clear Heat, promote circulation in the collaterals, break up nodulations and adhesions
Wu Gong – *Scolopendrae*	Pierce congealed accumulations of Qi and Blood

We can incorporate these substances in potent formulas designed to break down endometriosis tissue. Such formulas are only used short term, and often just at or near the time of greatest pain, usually the period. Some of these animal products are toxic and are used in small doses for a specific time for a specific purpose. Wu Ling Zhi, however, is one substance that can be used in the longer term and in women of weak constitutions with Blood stasis. We shall see the use of some of these substances in formulas used during the period.

Treating Infertility Associated with Endometriosis

Most of our discussion of treatment will however be somewhat broader than a narrow focus on breaking down endometriosis tissue. As Western medical researchers discovered more about this disease, so did TCM doctors, who developed their treatment protocols of infertility caused by endometriosis, in different directions. For example, in the infertility clinics in China, doctors found that more pregnancies resulted if treatment of women with endometriosis targeted the Kidneys, with removal of Blood stasis only when and if necessary. Of course, this dovetails neatly with the discovery that some endometriosis lesions contain no extravasated blood at all and that such tissue can produce secretions which clog up the system – Phlegm-Damp we call it in TCM. Treatment which boosts Kidney Yang is generally rather effective at clearing such Phlegm-Damp.

A patient presenting to a TCM clinic with endometriosis will be diagnosed according to her main symptoms and her constitution. When treatment is prescribed as part of an infertility treatment, the doctor will be particularly mindful of reinforcing Kidney Yang and resolving Blood stagnation. Liver Qi stagnation and Spleen Qi deficiency may also contribute and some cases of endometriosis will exhibit elements of Heat or Cold or Damp. To understand the part that Blood stagnation plays it is necessary to explore further our understanding of the way endometriosis is formed and how we relate this to TCM concepts (Fig. 5.1).

Our knowledge about the anatomy and behavior of endometriosis is still limited and so some of these ideas may change or be expanded in the future.

We do know that menstrual blood travels not only downwards from the uterus and out through the cervix but also upwards through the fallopian tubes and out into the peritoneal cavity (retrograde menstruation). This small quantity of blood carries with it bits of discarded endometrium. Women with strong uterine cramps (due to Liver Qi stagnation) are more likely to lose more menstrual flow upwards through the tubes. The blood and the tissue will either be reabsorbed, or will remain and establish itself somewhere in the pelvic cavity. If Kidney Yang is strong, then movement of Qi in the pelvis will mobilize the menstrual debris, which should not be there, and it will be efficiently reabsorbed. A weakness of Kidney Yang, on the other hand, will allow the accumulation of blood and tissue such that it stagnates and creates the basis for Zheng Jia or masses to develop.

The bits of endometriosis tissue which develop in the pelvic cavity will be either non-pigmented (i.e., not bleeding) or pigmented because they contain blood vessels. The non-pigmented lesions can develop into the pigmented ones if they develop the blood vessels and start to bleed during the menstrual phase. The non-pigmented types of endometriosis are associated with infertility for reasons not yet fully understood but possibly because they produce secretions which coat the fimbrial ends of the tubes. The treatment which will most directly address this type of endometriosis is one which will strengthen the Kidney Yang and clear Phlegm-Damp. The development of the non-pigmented types of endometriosis is probably facilitated in Spleen Qi-deficient individuals. In this case, treatment must also address the Spleen Qi to facilitate removal of Damp.

The pigmented endometriosis, containing tissue which responds to the hormonal changes, which makes the uterine lining bleed, is the type more likely to cause pain, especially if it is implanted more deeply than just the surface of the peritoneum. Removal of this type of lesion requires the use of Blood-moving herbs and Kidney Yang tonic herbs. The pigmented lesions, especially under the influence of Qi stagnation, can form substantial Zheng Jia in the form of nodules and masses and scar tissue. In these cases, there may be both pain and infertility: the latter may be absolute if the masses have damaged or obstructed the tubes. Treatment calls for the use of strong Blood-'breaking' herbs backed up with Kidney Yang tonics. Table 5.1 charts these relationships.

The skilful approach to treatment is to appropriately target that lesion with unerring aim – whether with a scalpel, laser or acupuncture treatment or strong eliminating herbs to push out or break up obstructions or with gentle herbs to coax hormone levels to balance – and apply these precise arrows in a context of supports: supports for the Kidney Qi, the Spleen Qi, the Liver Qi or whatever it is an individual patient needs. If the ultimate aim is to push the endometriosis to one side to allow pregnancy to occur, then the ovaries, the follicles and eggs and the endometrium must become the central focus of the treatment plan. Maintaining treatment focus on the menstrual cycle at the same time as clearing the endometriosis lesions will bring greater clinical success and increase fertility.

You may remember from Chapter 4, that following and promoting the natural rhythms of the normal menstrual cycle is the basis of all fertility treatments. Thus, Kidney Yin and Blood are nourished in the first part of the cycle after the period and Kidney Yang is supported during the second half of the cycle.

The treatment of endometriosis as a cause of infertility does not differ from this principle but will place emphasis on certain key factors. First, particular emphasis will be placed on building Kidney Yang, since this is one of the causative factors. Strong Kidney Yang tonics will be applied during the luteal phase and the previous (follicular) phase will be primed appropriately to support the growth of Yang. Remember that Kidney Yang is usually built out of a Yin, Blood or Qi base, depending on the body constitution and the pathologic condition of each patient.

Second, if there are signs of stagnant Blood, such as severe period pain with clotty flow, palpable nodules or masses or laparoscopic evidence of bleeding endometriosis tissue in the abdomen, then Blood-regulating treatments will be employed. If treatment is following the natural rhythm of the cycle, then the time to use these herbs is during the period or around ovulation time. Depending on the degree of stagnation, i.e., whether the endometriosis is just small brown dots on the surfaces in the pelvic cavity or whether it is large substantial masses or endometriomas, we will use herbs which gently move the stagnant Blood or herbs which strongly break up Blood stasis (see Table 5.2 and Appendix 2).

Referring to Figure 5.1, you will see there are a number of places where Qi stagnation contributes to the formation of endometriosis. Any prolonged Qi stagnation will of course eventually lead to Blood stagnation because the Qi can no longer lead the Blood adequately. And Liver Qi stagnation, having its roots in emotional stress, is commonly involved. Qi-regulating herbs play an important part in prescriptions which treat endometriosis.

Similarly, Spleen Qi deficiency is frequently a component of Kidney Yang deficiency syndromes. It is the Spleen Qi deficiency which leads to the dragging-down sensation some women experience in the abdomen during the period and may contribute to the heavy bleeding or premenstrual spotting. When Kidney Yang is deficient, and especially when Kidney Yang and Spleen Qi are both deficient, then Damp accumulation will be a problem. Treatment will therefore often include herbs and acupuncture points which clear Phlegm-Damp and invigorate Spleen Qi. Where Damp obstructions persist, Damp-Heat may form, in which case stronger Heat clearing herbs will be necessary.

Whereas TCM treatment follows and corrects any disturbances of the menstrual cycle caused by endometriosis, Western medicine takes the opposite approach. It stops the cycle completely with the use of hormones which trick the body into thinking it is pregnant or menopausal. When the course of treatment is completed, endometriosis is reduced but frequently reoccurs over the next few months. This is because the cause has not been addressed, only the obvious manifestations. The TCM doctor endeavors to locate the original imbalance which allowed the endometriosis to develop in the first place (namely the Kidney Yang deficiency, Spleen Qi deficiency or Liver Qi stagnation) and to treat that, together with the outward manifestations (stagnant Blood, Phlegm-Damp and Damp-Heat); however, that is not to say that the TCM doctor necessarily has greater success than the Western doctor and his drugs. Endometriosis is a difficult disease to treat in any modality, but if the patient is prepared to pursue TCM treatment over 6–12 months the results are generally very encouraging.

TCM treatment of infertility caused by endometriosis begins at the start of a cycle, i.e., it begins with the maturing of a new egg and the growth of new uterine lining as the period is ending, usually around Day 4 of the new

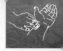

cycle. Our aim, of course, is to reduce or clear the manifestations (the endometrial implants and masses) of the disease, the 'Biao' in TCM. But this can only be done effectively and completely by treating the 'Ben' or the underlying imbalance itself which requires attention to all aspects and functions of the reproductive system during the menstrual cycle. This approach to treatment is especially important if improved fertility is the desired outcome. Treatment of a woman with endometriosis who has no desire to fall pregnant or has already borne children does not need to adhere so strictly to a monthly regimen, although in the opinion of many TCM doctors it is a superior approach.

It is useful to review the guiding formulas and acupuncture protocols for each stage of the cycle, which were presented in Chapter 4:

- Post-menstruation

- Ovulation

- Post-ovulation

- Menstrual period.

Herbs and acupuncture points to specifically address the endometriosis can be added at different stages.

Post-menstruation

At this time, our main aim is to build the Blood and reinforce the Yin. Treatment at this time is particularly important for fertility but is not always so important in a woman who is not trying to become pregnant. The protocols suggested for the stages which follow (ovulation and the luteal phases), however, are considered important in the treatment of endometriosis even if pregnancy is not desired.

In the case of severe endometriosis in which the Blood stagnation is pronounced, Blood-regulating herbs can be added at the early phase of the cycle. However, great caution must be applied at this delicate (for the Yin) stage. Unless the woman's constitution is very strong, there is the risk of damaging Yin with strong Blood movers. Better results are to be obtained by holding them until a later stage of the cycle (i.e., nearer to the period) or until the woman's constitution can be improved. In many cases, however, some mild Blood-regulating herbs (see below) can be safely introduced. If the case of endometriosis involves the type of lesion that does not cause internal bleeding and the main problem is infertility rather than symptoms of Blood stagnation, then treatment will focus simply on following the Yin and Yang stages of the cycle. No additional Blood-moving herbs above those added routinely at ovulation and period time are required although herbs, which clear Damp may be needed.

Herbal Formula — Guiding formula applied from Day 4 of menstrual cycle:

Gui Shao Di Huang Tang (Angelica Peonia Rehmannia decoction)

Shu Di	12g	Radix Rehmanniae Glutinosae Conquitae
Shan Yao	9g	Radix Dioscorea Oppositae
Shan Zhu Yu	9g	Fructus Corni Officinalis
Fu Ling	9g	Sclerotium Poriae Cocos
Mu Dan Pi	9g	Cortex Moutan Radicis
Ze Xie	12g	Rhizoma Alismatis
Dang Gui	9g	Radix Angelicae Sinensis
Bai Shao	9g	Radix Paeoniae Lactiflorae

This is the guiding formula recommended for use in the post-menstrual phase in Chapter 4 and is discussed there.

- **Modifications**

Where Kidney Yang deficiency is present, add Yang tonics:

Tu Si Zi	9g	*Semen Cuscatae*
Rou Cong Rong	9g	*Herba Cistanches*

With Blood stagnation, choose from:

Dan shen	12g	*Radix Salviae Miltiorrhizae*
Chi Shao	9g	*Radix Paeoniae Rubra*
Mu Dan Pi	9g	*Cortex Moutan Radicis*
(Sheng) Shan Zha	15g	*Fructus Crataegi*
Mo Yao	3g	*Resina Commiphorae Myrrhae*

With Damp-Heat add:

Hong Teng	6g	*Caulis Sargentodoxae*
Bai Jiang Cao	6g	*Herba cum Radix Patriniae*
Lian Qiao	6g	*Fructus Forsythiae Suspensae*

With Spleen deficiency add:

Bai Zhu	9g	*Rhizoma Atractylodis Macrocephalae*
Cang Zhu	9g	*Rhizoma Atractylodes*

Acupuncture Points — A selection from the following points creates a basic formula which addresses the requirements of the post-menstrual phase (Table 5.3). Other points can of course be added, according to the individual patient's need at the time:

KI-13	Qixue
Ren-7	Yinjiao
KI-14	Siman
KI-18	Shiguan
Ren-3	Zhongji
Ren-4	Guanyuan
SP-6	Sanyinjiao
LIV-8	Ququan
Ren-12	Zhongwan
ST-30	Qichong

It is during this part of the cycle that we are mindful of the follicular environment and oocyte quality. We know that endometriosis can affect the quality of the follicular fluid, particularly in terms of levels of elevated inflammatory cytokines.[21]

This may be the reason that oocyte or egg quality is diminished in endometriosis sufferers. Chinese herbs have been shown to reduce these levels in follicular fluid of IVF patients with endometriosis. Women who took herbs which addressed Blood stasis and cleared Heat for 3 weeks showed significantly reduced levels of TNF and IL 6

Table 5.3   Acupuncture points[a] used in the treatment of infertility related to endometriosis: post-menstruation phase

Treatment goal	Acupuncture points
To program the Chong and Ren vessels early in the cycle	KI-13 and Ren-7
To move stagnant Blood in the Chong vessel and Uterus	KI-14 and 18, ST-30
To clear stagnant Blood in the abdomen	Ren-3
To reinforce the Kidney Yin	Ren-4 and SP-6
To support the Blood and Yin at the same time as clearing stagnation from the abdomen	LIV-8
To encourage Spleen and Stomach function in making more Blood to replace that lost during the period	Ren-12

[a]Points are reinforced unless they are addressing stagnation, in which case they may be reduced.

in the follicular fluid at the time of egg collection. Thus focusing on boosting Kidney function to maximize ovary function, and resolving stasis and clearing Heat (or Damp-Heat) is a useful way to improve the environment of the growing oocyte, and thereby its quality.[22]

Using acupuncture to synchronize the activity of the Chong and the Ren channels at this important phase, may help the follicles develop normally and help to avoid the heterogeneous follicular cohort development seen in some endometriosis patients.

During this phase, the uterine lining is developing and because we know that uterine environment is affected in endometriosis patients in a way that reduces implantation success (discussed above), the addition of small amounts of herbs which help to circulate blood and build tissue are useful. A foundation of Kidney Yin is required before the Blood can build.

Ovulation

If ovulation is associated with pain, as it is in many endometriosis sufferers, then we shall focus more pointedly now on dispelling any Blood stagnation and/or resolving masses if necessary. Caution must still be applied: in less robust women, very strong Blood breakers can upset the sensitive process of switching Yin to Yang, and therefore the process of ovulation itself. Acupuncture can be very helpful in encouraging the movement of Qi and Blood at this time. At the junction of Yin and Yang, attention must be paid to the rise of Yang, and strong Yang tonics must be employed now to ensure its rapid increase if the endometriosis is to be resolved. If Yang does not rise sharply at this point and the Qi and Blood do not move well, then the egg may not be released (as in luteinized unruptured follicle syndromes, or LUFS), or the tube may not successfully capture it or the luteal phase may be inadequate.

You may remember from Chapter 4, that a typical guiding formula to use at this time is the ovulation formula Bu Shen Cu Pai Luan Tang (below) or Wen Yang Hua Yu Fang (below) both of which reinforce Kidney Qi while moving Qi and Blood. When we are treating endometriosis we will add more Blood-moving and Kidney Yang tonic herbs.

If there is severe Blood stasis, then we need to resolve this but in most cases we reserve the Blood-breaking herbs until another time in the cycle if we want to safeguard the Kidney Yin and Yang and potential fertility. Herbs such as San Leng and E Zhu are usually too strong to use at this time unless there are significant and substantial masses or cysts which must be addressed.

Herbal Formula — Where Kidney Yang deficiency is predominant, use:

Wen Yang Hua Yu Fang (Warm Yang and Transform Stasis formula) modified

Gui Zhi	9 g	Ramulus Cinnamomi Cassiae
Hong Hua	6 g	Flos Carthami Tinctorii
Dang Gui	9 g	Radix Angelicae Sinensis
Chuan Xiong	6 g	Radix Ligustici Wallichii
Chuan Niu Xi	9 g	Radix Cyathulae
Ji Xue Teng	15 g	Radix et Caulis Jixueteng
Xiang Fu	9 g	Rhizoma Cyperi Rotundi
Huang Qi	9 g	Radix Astragali Membranacei
Fu Ling	9 g	Sclerotium Poriae Cocos
Yin Yang Huo	9 g	Herba Epimedii
Shu Di	9 g	Radix Rehmanniae Glutinosae Conquitae
Zhi Fu Zi*	6 g	Radix Aconiti Charmichaeli Praeparata

*Zhi Fu Zi is a restricted herb in some countries.

This formula is described in Chapter 4, although in this case Chuan Niu Xi is used instead of Huai Niu Xi to further reinforce the Blood-moving action of the formula, Xiang Fu is used to promote Qi movement and Huang Qi and Fu Ling are added to support the Spleen and clear Damp.

Where Blood stagnation is present, but not severe, use:

Bu Shen Cu Pai Luan Tang (Reinforce Kidney Ovulation formula) modified

Dang Gui	9 g	Radix Angelicae Sinensis
Chi Shao	9 g	Radix Paeoniae Rubra
Bai Shao	9 g	Radix Paeoniae Lactiflorae
Shan Yao	9 g	Radix Dioscorea Oppositae
Shu Di	9 g	Radix Rehmanniae Glutinosae Conquitae
Nu Zhen Zi	9 g	Fructus Ligustri Lucidi
Mu Dan Pi	9 g	Cortex Moutan Radicis
Fu Ling	9 g	Sclerotium Poriae Cocos
Xiang Fu	9 g	Rhizoma Cyperi Rotundi
Huang Qi	9 g	Radix Astragali Membranacei
Xu Duan	9 g	Radix Dipsaci
Tu Si Zi	9 g	Semen Cuscatae
Wu Ling Zhi	9 g	Excrementum Trogopterori
Hong Hua	6 g	Flos Carthami Tinctorii

This formula is described in Chapter 4. Here we have added Xiang Fu and Huang Qi to reinforce Qi movement and support circulation of Blood.

If more Blood-moving agents are required, add to either formula:

(Sheng) Shan Zha	9 g	Fructus Crataegi
Dan Shen	9 g	Radix Salviae Miltiorrhizae

Table 5.4   Acupuncture points[a] used in the treatment of infertility related to endometriosis: ovulation phase

Treatment goal	Acupuncture points
To regulate Liver Qi in the abdomen	LIV-3, LIV-5
To regulate Liver Qi in the Uterus	LIV-11
To ensure that the movement of Qi in the fallopian tubes and the ovaries is not obstructed	ST-29 and Abdomen Zigong
To regulate Qi and Blood, especially if there is pain or evidence of abdominal masses	SP-12 and SP-13
To regulate the Qi in the Liver, Spleen and Kidney channels as well as the Bao vessel and Bao channel	SP-6
To regulate Qi in the Chong and Ren vessels	KI-8
To regulate Qi in the Chong vessel	SP-4
To calm the Shen, regulate Bao vessel	KI-4, PC-6 and HE-7

[a]Even method is used or reducing method where there is pain.

For inflammation or Damp-Heat add:

| Hong Teng | 9 g | Caulis Sargentodoxae |
| Bai Jiang Cao | 6 g | Herba cum Radix Patriniae |

Where there are abdominal masses and the patient is strong, then add to Cu Pai Luan Tang or Bu Shen Cu Pai Luan Tang or Wen Yang Hua Yu Fang or Wen Yang Hua Tan Fang the following for a few days only:

| San Leng | 6 g | Rhizoma Sparganii |
| E Zhu | 6 g | Rhizoma Curcumae Zedoariae |

In some cases, it will be important to add more herbs that clear Liver Qi stagnation to encourage good flexibility of the fallopian tube. Spleen Qi tonic herbs and Damp-clearing herbs can be added to reduce any mucus obstructions which may be produced by endometrial implants and collected around the fimbriae or in the tube, e.g.

Cang Zhu	9 g	Rhizoma Atractylodes
Qing Pi	6 g	Pericarpium Citri Reticulatae Viridae
Zhi Ke	6 g	Fructus Citri seu Ponciri

And increase the dose of Fu Ling to 12–15 g.

Acupuncture Points — Treatments applied at this time require a selection of points which keep Liver Qi patent in the tubes and abdomen, help move Qi and Blood, clear Damp and calm the spirit (Table 5.4). For example:

LIV-3	Taichong
LIV-11	Yinlian
LIV-5	Ligou
ST-29	Guilai

Abdomen Zigong

SP-12	Chongmen
SP-13	Fushe
SP-6	Sanyinjiao
SP-4	Gongsun
KI-4	Dazhong
KI-8	Jiaoxin
PC-6	Neiguan
HE-7	Shenmen

Smooth movement of Liver Qi, removal of obstructing Blood or Damp stasis and the correct development of Kidney Yin into Kidney Yang, should ensure that ovulation happens and the egg passes unhindered into the tube. A problem in any one of these areas can cause ovulation to be delayed or not occur, e.g., as in LUFS.

Post-ovulation

After ovulation, the aim is to maintain good Yang levels and also to address Spleen Qi deficiency and Damp if that is part of the constitutional picture. Remember that the clinical approach in the second phase of the cycle is to:

- boost Kidney Yang by supplementing Yin

- boost Kidney Yang by promoting Qi

- boost Kidney Yang by nourishing Blood.

These approaches depend on the body constitution and the pathologic condition. In the case of endometriosis, promoting Qi to build Yang is the most commonly used approach.

Herbal Formula — The formula of choice is:

Jian Gu Tang modified (Strengthen and Consolidate decoction) modified

Dang Shen	9 g	Radix Codonopsis Pilulosae
Bai Zhu	9 g	Rhizoma Atractylodis Macrocephalae
Cang Zhu	9 g	Rhizoma Atractylodes
Shan Yao	9 g	Radix Dioscorea Oppositae
Yi Yi Ren	15 g	Semen Coicis Lachryma-jobi
Tu Si Zi	9 g	Semen Cuscatae
Ba Ji Tian	9 g	Radix Morindae Officinalis
Lu Jiao Pian	9 g	Cornu Cervi Parvum
Xiang Fu	9 g	Rhizoma Cyperi Rotundi

This formula is described in Chapter 4. In this case, we have once again added Xiang Fu, to prevent Qi stagnation and Cang Zhu to address Damp accumulation.

To the guiding formula, we may add a couple of Blood-moving herbs where there is Blood stasis. Again, gentler Blood-regulating herbs such as:

Wu Ling Zhi	9 g	Excrementum Trogopterori
Dan Shen	9 g	Radix Salviae Miltiorrhizae
(Sheng) Shan Zha	9 g	Fructus Crataegi

are the herbs of choice because they will not consume Kidney Yang and are safe to use in the short term (in the presence of Blood stasis) if there is a conception.

If the woman is Blood or Yin deficient, a different base formula can be chosen to reinforce Kidney Yang (see Ch. 4).

Acupuncture Points — The following points are used (and see Table 5.5):

Ren-4	Guanyuan
KI-3	Taixi
ST-29	Guilai
BL-23	Shenshu
PC-7	Daling
LIV-2	Xingjian
SP-1	Yinbai
HE-7	Shenmen

Watch for improvements in the luteal phase on the BBT charts. If the luteal phase is maintained well, i.e., the temperature is high and stable for at least 12 or 13 days, then we can be sure that the endometriosis will not be developing. It is in the next phase, the period, that Blood can be moved strongly and endometrial implants reduced.

Chinese herbs have been shown to improve the immune milieu of the endometrium of patients with endometriosis, reducing antigenic and antibody markers.[23]

It is our hope that such improvements can reduce the risks of immune rejection and increase the chance of successful implantation. It is also our hope that our treatment will suppress prostaglandin levels such that contractility of the uterine wall is reduced and it can remain quiescent at this time. Some of the treatment we applied at other times of the cycle, in particular promotion of Blood circulation during the menstrual phase and the post menstrual phase, aimed at encouraging the formation of a well ordered endometrium. During this post-ovulation phase we continue to support function of the endometrium, and by boosting Kidney Yang promote its secretory function and facilitate successful implantation.

The Menstrual Period

Where pregnancy is being attempted, treatment to strongly move Blood stagnation must wait until the first signs of a period or the BBT drops (sometimes the temperature drops a day or even two before the period) or there is a confirmed negative pregnancy test. Some tests are sensitive enough to diagnose pregnancy just 10 days

Table 5.5 Acupuncture points[a] used in the treatment of infertility related to endometriosis: post-ovulation phase

Treatment goal	Acupuncture points
To maintain Kidney Yang	Ren-4, KI-3 and BL-23
To ensure Heat from the Yang tonic herbs does not affect the Liver and Heart	LIV-2, PC-7 and HE-7
To encourage unfettered transport of the egg/embryo in the fallopian tube in the early part of the luteal phase	ST-29 with moxa
To prevent spotting before the period	SP-1 with moxa

[a]Use even method, or reducing method if there is Heat.

after ovulation; these are particularly useful when we want to apply strong Blood-moving treatments before the period but want to exclude a pregnancy first. If there is no pregnancy being attempted (or possible) then herbs or acupuncture points that promote menstrual flow can be commenced well before the period (1 week before). While we used great caution in applying Blood-breaking herbs at other times of the cycle, now we can use them enthusiastically to help remove masses during this phase when endometrial tissue (both inside the uterus and out) is breaking down.

Herbal Formula — This is just one example of a formula used during the menstrual flow with the aim of clearing Blood stasis and stopping pain:

Nei Yi Zhi Tong Tang (Simplified Arrest Pain decoction)

Gou Teng	15 g	*Ramulus Uncariae Cum Uncis*
Zi Bei Chi	9 g	*Mauritiae Concha*
Dang Gui	9 g	*Radix Angelicae Sinensis*
Chi Shao	9 g	*Radix Paeoniae Rubra*
Wu Ling Zhi	9 g	*Excrementum Trogopterori*
Yan Hu Suo	9 g	*Rhizoma Corydalis Yanhusuo*
E Zhu	9 g	*Rhizoma Curcumae Zedoariae*
Rou Gui	3 g	*Cortex Cinnamomi Cassiae*
Quan Xie	1.5 g	*Buthus Martensi*
Wu Gong	1.5 g	*Scolopendra Subspinipes*
Mu Xiang	6 g	*Radix Saussureae seu Vladimiriae*
Xu Duan	9 g	*Radix Dipsaci*

This formula targets the endometriosis lesions and the resulting pain directly by breaking up and moving Blood stasis. The first two herbs relieve spasms and calm the mind – reflecting an ancient wisdom, recently paid much heed by modern medicine, that the degree of pain experienced is influenced greatly by the mind (Liver and Heart in TCM). The other herbs all move Blood, and in the case of Xu Duan support Kidney Yang. Some of these (Yan Hu Suo, Quan Xie, Wu Gong) have been shown to reduce prostaglandin levels and relieve pelvic pain.

If the patient's constitution is strong, and there are masses to be reduced we can further augment the Blood breaking capacity of this formula.

A few of the herbs chosen from the list below (or Table 5.2) may be added as required.

San Leng	9 g	*Rhizoma Sparganii*
Shui Zhi	1.5 g	*Hirudo seu Whitmaiae powder*
Di Long	6 g	*Lumbricus*
Tu Bie Chong	6 g	*Eupolyphaga Sinensis*
Hong Teng	9 g	*Caulis Sargentodoxae*
Bai Jiang Cao	9 g	*Herba Patriniae*
Bai Hua She She Cao	15 g	*Herba hedyotidis Diffusae*
Ru Xiang	3 g	*Resina Olibani*
Mo Yao	3 g	*Resina Commiphorae Myrrhae*
Xue Jie	3 g	*Resina Daemonoropis*

San Leng and E Zhu are commonly used when there are masses to reduce: they invigorate both Qi and Blood. Di Long is a substance which is useful for loosening adhesions in the pelvic cavity and Shui Zhi strongly dissolves masses. Hong Teng, Bai Jiang Cao, or Bai Hua She She Cao may be added to a prescription when the Blood stagnation is complicated with Damp-Heat. Addition of small doses of a resin is useful to aid efficient deconstruction of the endometrial lining so it can be reconstructed correctly.

Animal substances have strong tastes and odors and are often more easily tolerated in powdered or capsulated form rather than in decoctions.

Acupuncture Points — To move Blood strongly if there are masses or signs of stagnation, choose from the following points (and see Table 5.6):

ST-28	Shuidao
ST-29	Guilai
SP-12	Chongmen
SP-13	Fushe
KI-14	Siman
SP-8	Diji
SP-6	Sanyinjiao
SP-10	Xuehai
Ren-6	Qihai
BL-31–34	Baliao
BL-26	Guanyuanshu
BL-28	Pangguanshu
BL-22	Sanjiaoshu
Shiqizhuixia	
LIV-2	Xingjian
LIV-8	Ququan
CO-4	Hegu
PC-5	Jianshi

Table 5.6   Acupuncture points[a] used in the treatment of infertility related to endometriosis: menstrual phase

Treatment goal	Acupuncture points
To move the Qi and Blood locally (choose points according to areas of pain or where masses can be palpated)	ST-28 and ST-29, SP-12 and SP-13 and KI-14
To promote discharge of menstrual blood	SP-6 and CO-4
To remove obstructions to the flow	SP-8
To dispel Blood stagnation but at the same time control heavy blood loss	SP-10
To move and support the Qi to control blood flow	Ren-6
To move stagnation of Blood and relieve back pain	BL-31–34, BL-26, BL-28, BL-22 or Shiqizhui-Xia
To disperse Liver Qi stagnation and facilitate reduction in abdomen masses	LIV-2, LIV-8
To move Liver Qi and calm the mind, and promote unfettered menstrual flow	PC-5

[a]All points can be reduced. Electro-acupuncture is applicable if pain is severe, using abdomen points ST-29 connected to ST-28 or Ah Shi point on same side.

If the treatment is successful, there will gradually be a lessening of the period pain, and the period flow should become smooth and fresh red without clots. Initially, however, the action of the Blood-breaking herbs may provoke more large clots in the menstrual flow. A key sign of good progress is the reduction of premenstrual spotting, reflecting a reduction in the extent of stagnant Blood remaining inside the pelvis.

A Simpler Approach

Sometimes the patient with endometriosis cannot attend the clinic regularly for treatment or finds the regimen described above complex and difficult to follow. Some practitioners may find this the case too, though where practicable following the four menstrual phases as closely as possible when prescribing is ideal. Additionally, there are cases where it is advisable to take a more focused approach attacking the endometriosis itself and leave attempts to conceive aside temporarily. For example, there may be diagnosed endometriosis which has not been able to be removed effectively by surgery, or it is growing back after surgery, or your patient wants to avoid surgery, in which case she should be advised to stop trying to conceive for 2 or 3 months and take strong herbs to try and reduce the lesions.

A formula which focuses on the endometriosis itself will incorporate several of the strong Blood breaking and Damp-Heat clearing herbs we mentioned in Table 5.2.

But if your patient is going to take such a formula for weeks or months, then some herbs to protect the Qi and Blood and Yin and Yang will be required. One example of such a formula is Hua Yu Li Shi Tang (Transform Blood Stasis and Resolve Damp decoction), which we have modified and expanded below.

Hua Yu Li Shi Tang (Transform Blood Stasis and Resolve Damp decoction) modified

San Leng	12g	Rhizoma Sparganii
E Zhu	12g	Rhizoma Curcumae Zedoariae
Pu Huang	9g	Pollen Typhae
Wu Ling Zhi	9g	Excrementum Trogopterori
(Sheng) Shan Zha	9g	Fructus Crataegi
(Zhi) Da Huang	6g	Rhizoma Rhei
Tu Bie Chong	6g	Eupolyphagae seu Opisthoplatiae
Mo Yao	3g	Resina Commiphorae Myrrhae
Dang Gui	9g	Radix Angelicae Sinensis
Dan Shen	9g	Radix Salviae Miltiorrhizae
Bai Jiang Cao	9g	Herba cun radice Patriniae
Lian Qiao	6g	Fructus Forsythiae Suspensae
Hong Teng	9g	Caulis Sargentodoxae
Xu Duan	9g	Radix Dipsaci
Yin Yang Huo	9g	Herba Epimedii
Gui Zhi	6g	Ramulus Cinnamomi
Tai Zi Shen	12g	Radix Pseudostellariae

The main thrust of this formula is to break up accumulations of stagnant Blood (the first 10 herbs) and to clear Damp-Heat (next three herbs) to reduce inflammation. Additional supports for the Kidney Yang and the Qi (final four herbs) aim to ensure that new endometriosis lesions will not form.

This formula can be used in many ways. In a strong patient, it can be used continuously for some weeks or months (although Tu Bie Chong should be removed if it is used for more than a few weeks). Alternatively, it can be used before and during the period and another more nourishing formula used in the follicular phase. If your patient wants to start trying to conceive again, and is doing well with this sort of formula, then it can be taken until ovulation and then switching to the post ovulation formula described above. Close observation of the BBT chart or ovulation signs are necessary to ensure that the strong Blood breaking herbs are not de-railing ovulation. It is only in robust women with significant stagnation that such an approach is taken.

If a slightly gentler approach is needed, for an endometriosis patient who is not so robust, and not attempting to conceive, then the following formula can be used.

Ge Xia Zhu Yu tang (Remove Stasis from Below the Diaphragm decoction) and Bu Shen Qu Yu Fang (Supplement Kidney and Dispel Blood Stasis formula) modified

Yin Yang Huo	9 g	Herba Epimedii
Xu Duan	9 g	Radix Dipsaci
Tu Si Zi	9 g	Semen Cuscatae
Gou Qi Zi	9 g	Fructus Lycii
Huang Qi	9 g	Radix Astragali
Dang Gui	9 g	Radix Angelicae Sinensis
Ze Lan	12 g	Herba Lycopi
Dan Shen	9 g	Radix Salviae Miltiorrhizae
San Qi	6 g	Radix Notoginseng
Yan Hu Suo	9 g	Rhizoma Corydalis
Wu Ling Zhi	9 g	Excrementum Trogopterori
Niu Xi	9 g	Radix Achyranthis Bidentatae
Rou Gui	3 g	Cortex Cinnamomi
Tao Ren	6 g	Semen Persica
Hong Hua	6 g	Flos Carthami Tinctorii
Xiang Fu	9 g	Rhizoma Cyperi Rotundi
Cu San Leng	9 g	Rhizoma Sparganii
E Zhu	6 g	Rhizoma Curcumae Zedoariae

This formula can be applied in much the same way as the one described above.

While this formula still employs many Blood stasis removing herbs (Cu San Leng, E Zhu, Dang Gui, Ze Lan, Dan Shen, San Qi, Yan Hu Suo, Wu Ling Zhi, Niu Xi, Tao Ren) it avoids the stronger animal products and toxic heat clearing herbs. In this formula more emphasis is placed on supporting the Kidneys and warming the Kidney Yang (Rou Gui, Yin Yang Huo, Xu Duan, Tu Si Zi, Gou Qi Zi, Huang Qi) than in the previous one.

In many clinics in China, herbal decoctions are used per rectum (PR) rather than orally if there are large and bulky implants of endometriosis. This technique is described in greater detail when we discuss pelvic infections and blocked tubes later. It is not a technique which has yet gained favor in the West, although its effectiveness is well documented in the Chinese medical literature. When acupuncture and herbal medicine become a more integral part of our hospital clinics, then administration of PR herbal medicine becomes a more practical option for treatment.

Research and General Comments

Much research is done in China investigating the specific action of herbs on endometriosis – too extensive to describe here in detail but typically they show that treatment with Chinese medicine can help symptoms of endometriosis and reduce blood markers of inflammation. We mentioned a couple of specific observations that have been made on the effect of herbs on follicle and endometrium quality above.

In general, the use of formulas that clear Blood stasis (and modified for each patient) will, over a 3-month period, reduce symptoms and markers of endometriosis, namely, pain relief and reduction of prostaglandin levels and increases in Beta endorphin levels.[24]

Programs comparing the use of acupuncture and herbal treatment with hormonal treatment for endometriosis have demonstrated superior results for the former in many aspects of clinical presentation and concurrent reduction of prostaglandins PGE2 and PGF2.[25]

Individual herbs, such as Dang Gui, Bai Shao, Yan Hu Suo, Mo Yao, Ru Xiang, Jiang Huang, E Zhu, Fu Ling, Huang Qin are just some of those that have shown an ability to reduce inflammation and cytokine levels in laboratory and animal studies.[26]

We said at the beginning of this chapter that endometriosis was a Western medical label and not a Chinese medicine one. Similarly cytokines, inflammation and prostaglandins are Western terms. We cannot see or feel raised levels of cytokines in the follicular fluid, or prostaglandins in the blood, or mucus secreted by endometriotic lesions near the tubes, or disordered implantation sites in the endometrium or inflammation and adhesions in the pelvis but we know that these are all physiologic manifestations of endometriosis. We are also starting to discover through research, that appropriate application of Chinese medicine can change these subtle signs as well as the more obviously assessable ones such as pain and infertility. Thus, even though an endometriosis patient might not manifest strong symptoms or signs of Damp-Heat or Blood stasis, if there is a history of long-term endometriosis (and by the time the patient comes to the acupuncture clinic this is usually the case), then it is appropriate to assume some degree of these pathologic states exist, and you should use herbs or acupuncture points accordingly. However, because treatment of endometriosis is long term, matching the treatment to the patient's constitution correctly is particularly important. For example, even if a patient has severe widespread endometriosis and adhesions, strong Blood moving treatment cannot be applied long term if she is very Blood and Qi deficient. Similarly, even if we assume there must be significant inflammation in the pelvis, because of the long history and extent of the endometriosis, we cannot just give unmodified and strong Damp-Heat clearing treatment to someone who is very Yang deficient. Rather, addition of herbs which we know can reduce inflammation (or levels of cytokines or prostaglandins), or can break up Blood stagnation can be added at certain times of the cycle in judicious amounts to a larger formula. And at certain times, more single pointed formulas can be given that target the lesion primarily for a short carefully chosen time.

CASE HISTORY – CECILY

Cecily (28) was considering a hysterectomy to control the pain she experienced from endometriosis. Two years earlier, she had had surgery which removed extensive endometriosis from many sites in her pelvic cavity followed by drug therapy for many months. Any relief from the pain was short lived. Her periods were heavy and painful but it was the knife-like pain that shot through her abdomen and anus at midcycle in debilitating episodes for 4 or 5 days, which she could no longer tolerate.

Her menstrual cycle was short, at 25 days. The flow was heavy and fresh red, with cramping pain which responded well to heat. She complained of low energy generally, and often felt cold.

Her pulse felt tight and thready, especially on the left Kidney position. Her tongue looked fluted and dull.

The nature of Cecily's pain indicated a clear case of Blood stagnation, but her constitution was Kidney and Spleen deficient. A case like this, with significant substantial implants of endometriosis, requires strong breaking up of stagnant Blood but, because her constitution is weak, it must be done cautiously using herbs to protect Kidney and Spleen Yang at the same time. Cecily did not want to become pregnant and could visit Sydney infrequently, so she was given the same prescription to take continuously.

Yin Yang Huo	12g	*Herba Epimedii*
Bu Gu Zhi	12g	*Fructus Psoraleae*

Huang Qi	15 g	Radix Astragali
Ren Shen	9 g	Radix Ginseng
Gui Zhi	6 g	Ramulus Cinnamomi Cassiae
E Zhu	6 g	Rhizoma Curcumae Zedoariae
San Leng	9 g	Rhizoma Sparganii
Tu Bie Chong	9 g	Eupolyphagae seu Opisthoplatiae
Wu Ling Zhi	9 g	Excrementum Trogopterori
Pu Huang	9 g	Pollen Typhae
Yan Hu Suo	6 g	Rhizoma Corydalis Yanhusuo

Acupuncture points: Ren-4, Ren-3, ST-29, SP-8, LIV-5, GB-28

In the first month, there was little significant improvement, but by the second month, the pain was 75% better. She continued the formula with reduced doses of the Blood 'busters' for another 2 months, with the pain further improving. Cecily stopped taking the herbs, no longer feeling the necessity, but within 2 cycles her pain returned. Clearly the stagnation had not been completely resolved. She recommended the same formula, with additional support for the Kidney Yin and Yang and the pain improved again. Our plan is for her to eventually stop the herbs altogether but it may be some time before we can be confident the endometriosis is eradicated.

CASE HISTORY – TERRI

Terri (35) had been trying to fall pregnant for 2½ years. She had been given every test. The blood tests showed that her hormone levels were normal; an X-ray of her tubes showed no abnormality; and her husband's sperm passed all the tests. But her periods were heavy and very painful and it was this plus the premenstrual spotting and stinging pain in her lower back which made endometriosis a suspect.

And, as expected, a laparoscopy revealed moderate endometriosis, which was removed during the surgery. However, 6 months later, she was still not pregnant and although her periods had been lighter and less painful after surgery, the pain was starting to return. Premenstrual irritability and breast swelling and soreness bothered her considerably. Her menstrual cycle was long, she experienced spotting at Day 16 or 17, and she saw little fertile mucus. Her BBT chart (Fig. 5.2) showed a long, slightly erratic follicular phase and a small rise to the luteal phase temperatures.

Her digestion was poor, with a tendency to bloating and constipation. Her tongue was fluted and had a white coat and her pulse felt wiry.

Terri's diagnosis included a bit of everything. The delayed ovulation and the lack of fertile mucus indicate Kidney Yin deficiency, whereas the back pain and poor luteal phase on the BBT chart indicate Kidney Yang deficiency. The Blood stagnation component had been largely removed by the surgery but to prevent it returning, Kidney Yang needed to be boosted quickly. She tended to Spleen deficiency and suffered Liver Qi stagnation symptoms pre-menstrually.

In the clinic, we needed to reinforce Kidney Yin to produce Kidney Yang, to invigorate Spleen Qi and to regulate Liver Qi. Unlike the case of Cecily (above), Terri *was* trying to fall pregnant, so our treatment needed to carefully follow her menstrual cycle to maximize chances of conception. Her treatment began at the beginning of a cycle just after her period. Our focus would be on Kidney Yin and Blood at this time of the month and on the Kidney Yang and Liver Qi later in the month.

Dang Gui	9 g	Radix Angelicae Sinensis
Bai Shao	9 g	Radix Paeoniae Lactiflorae
Shu Di	9 g	Radix Rehmanniae Glutinosae Conquitae
Chuan Xiong	6 g	Radix Ligustici Wallichii
Tao Ren	6 g	Semen Persicae
Shan Zhu Yu	9 g	Fructus Corni Officinalis

Shan Yao	9g	Radix Dioscorea Oppositae
Bai Zhu	12g	Rhizoma Atractylodis Macrocephalae
Chai Hu	6g	Radix Bupleuri
Suan Zao Ren	12g	Semen Ziziphi Spinosae
Tu Si Zi	9g	Semen Cuscatae

Acupuncture points: Ren-6, Ren-4, SP-6, PC-6, LIV-5

After just 1 week taking the above herbs, she produced more fertile mucus than ever before – also a day or two earlier than usual. The herbs were then changed to boost Kidney Yang further:

Tu Si Zi	15g	Semen Cuscatae
Yin Yang Huo	9g	Herba Epimedii
Xu Duan	12g	Radix Dipsaci
Bai Zhu	12g	Rhizoma Atractylodis Macrocephalae
Dang Shen	9g	Radix Codonopsis Pilulosae
Fu Ling	9g	Sclerotium Poriae Cocos
Xiang Fu	9g	Rhizoma Cyperi Rotundi
Chuan Niu Xi	9g	Radix Cyathulae

We planned her next cycle in a similar sequence: stronger Blood-regulating herbs to be taken during the period followed by Kidney Yin and Yang tonics at the right time. But we didn't have the opportunity – she fell pregnant immediately. Clearly in the absence of Blood stagnation (removed by the surgery), all the Kidney energy needed, was a little help.

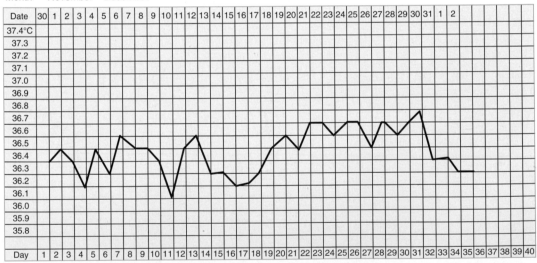

Figure 5.2 Case history – Terri. This chart shows an erratic follicular phase and luteal phase temperatures not much elevated over follicular values.

PELVIC INFLAMMATORY DISEASE

Pelvic inflammatory disease or PID describes inflammation, usually from infection, of the reproductive organs. It can be acute, or long term and chronic. When the infection or inflammation is in the uterus, it is called endometritis. This can cause infertility by disrupting implantation. When the infection is in the fallopian tubes, it is called salpingitis; this causes infertility because the tubes cannot transport egg or sperm due to the inflammation, scarring or fluid accumulation in the tubes (this latter is called hydrosalpinx). Fertility is also decreased because abdomen pain does not predispose to frequent sexual intercourse.

The disease may follow certain procedures, such as insertion of IUDs (intrauterine devices) or curettage of the uterus, or it may be sexually transmitted.

When the condition is acute, there is evidence of severe infection (usually by chlamydial, gonorrheal or streptococcal bacteria) manifesting in symptoms such as fever, purulent discharge from the vagina, dysuria, lower back pain and abdomen pain. Such acute infection must be treated with aggressive antibiotic treatment as rapidly as possible to try and save the tubes from permanent damage and conserve fertility. Usually, intravenous antibiotics are given in hospital.

Chronic PID is an insidious disease which can be unresponsive to antibiotic treatment. Sometimes, it develops from acute PID if it is not treated adequately and sometimes there are no symptoms or only mild intermittent symptoms of lower back and abdomen pain accompanied by a feeling of fatigue or malaise. Microorganisms *T-strain mycoplasma* (Ureaplasma) and *Candida* have been implicated in some cases of chronic PID, as has untreated *Chlamydia*. In the case of chronic PID, treatment with Chinese medicine often offers good resolution and restores fertility.

TCM Analysis of Pelvic Inflammatory Disease

According to TCM the cause of acute PID is invasion of Damp-Heat. Because antibiotic therapy clears Damp-Heat rapidly, it is the treatment of choice in this case where fertility is greatly at risk.

The symptoms of chronic PID develop when acute Damp-Heat is not thoroughly resolved, or when Liver Qi stagnation slows up fluid metabolism such that low-grade Damp-Heat develops. In other words, the vitality and health of the pelvic tissues are compromised due to sluggish metabolism and low-grade infections can more easily become established.

The pathology of chronic PID is complex because it is a mixture of excess pathogens and a deficient body condition. Chronic PID only develops when there is some weakness in the body's constitution. Typically, the weakness is in the Spleen, Kidney, or Liver or a combination of any of these.

Liver Qi is especially important in pelvic pathologies, particularly those of the tubes, because this is where the Liver channel travels. If the Liver Qi is weak and easily obstructed, then Qi, Blood and Body Fluids can stagnate and Phlegm-Damp can accumulate. The Kidney and the Spleen are important in the production of adequate Qi and Blood, so that the Liver does not become weak and allow such stagnation in the pelvis. The Kidney and Spleen also play an important role in maintaining good control of fluids and avoiding accumulation of Phlegm-Damp.

Laid on top of weaknesses in the Kidney, Spleen, or Liver are pathologic influences which then create the symptoms of PID. The pathogens involved are:

- Damp-Heat

- Stagnation of Qi

- Blood stagnation.

The ways these pathogens can combine with the underlying weakness are many and various. The more common clinical presentations are Spleen deficiency with Damp, Kidney deficiency with Blood stasis, or Liver Blood deficiency with stagnation of Qi.

The channels of the abdomen, particularly the Chong and Ren vessels, are disrupted by these imbalances and infertility can result. If the doctor is skilful and can correctly untangle the various aspects of the disease to make the right diagnosis and apply the correct treatment, then good results from TCM treatment can be expected.

Treatment of Pelvic Inflammatory Disease

Because we are looking at a disease which contains Ben and Biao factors, i.e., an underlying weakness (Ben) and an overlaying pathology (Biao) – then the doctor must decide on which is to be addressed first. If the PID is chronic, the underlying weakness is of paramount importance. If the condition of the woman is not so weak and the manifestations of the PID are strong, e.g., significant pain, then treatment of the Biao may take priority.

Treating the Biao

Herbal Formula — A formula which can be used to address all the common Biao of PID – namely, Damp-Heat, stagnation of Qi or Blood – is the following:

Fu Fang Hong Teng Bai Jiang San (Sargentodoxae Patriniae Compound powder)

Dang Gui	9 g	*Radix Angelicae Sinensis*
Chi Shao	9 g	*Radix Paeoniae Rubra*
Bai Shao	9 g	*Radix Paeoniae Lactiflorae*
Hong Teng	15 g	*Caulis Sargentodoxae*
Bai Jiang Cao	15 g	*Herba cum radice Patriniae*
(Sheng) Shan Zha	12 g	*Fructus Crataegi*
Yan Hu Suo	9 g	*Rhizoma Corydalis Yanhusuo*
Chai Hu	6 g	*Radix Bupleuri*
Chen Pi	6 g	*Pericarpium Citri Reticulate*
Mu Xiang	6 g	*Radix Saussureae seu Vladimiriae*
Yi Yi Ren	15 g	*Semen Coicis Lachryma-jobi*
Sang Ji Sheng	12 g	*Ramulus Sangjisheng*

This formula addresses pain and internal sepsis. Hong Teng and Bai Jiang Cao clear Damp-Heat and have proven antibiotic and anti-inflammatory effects. Yan Hu Suo and Shan Zha together with Chi Shao and Dang Gui move Blood stasis to relieve pain. Additionally, Mu Xiang, Chai Hu and Chen Pi help relieve pain by moving stagnant Qi. Bai Shao, with its ability to soothe the Liver Qi, reduces abdominal pain. Finally, Yi Yi Ren and Sang Ji Sheng clear any Damp which may have accumulated. If the abdomen pain is worse for cold and better for heat, then add:

Rou Gui	3 g	*Cortex Cinnamomi Cassiae*
Ai Ye	6 g	*Folium Artemisiae*

If there are palpable masses, add:

San Leng	9 g	*Rhizoma Sparganii*
E Zhu	9 g	*Rhizoma Curcumae Zedoariae*
Tu Bie Chong	6 g	*Eupolyphagae seu Opisthoplatiae*

If diarrhea or loose stools develop, then remove Dang Gui and add:

Sha Ren	6 g	*Fructus seu Semen Amomi*
Bai Zhu	9 g	*Rhizoma Atractylodis Macrocephalae*

Thus, this formula addresses most of the manifestations of PID but it must be used with great caution if there is Spleen, Kidney, or Liver weakness.

Table 5.7   Acupuncture points[a] used in the treatment of acute PID

Treatment goal	Acupuncture points
To regulate Qi to relieve abdomen pain	KI-14, Ren-5, SP-12, SP-13, ST-25 and LIV-4
To move the Qi to clear Damp-Heat from the lower Jiao	GB-26, GB-27 and GB-28 (on the Dai vessel)
To clear Damp-Heat from the Lower Jiao	KI-10, SP-9, LIV-5, LIV-8, Ren-3

[a]Use reducing technique. Deep needling on the abdomen may be appropriate.

Acupuncture Points — Points may be chosen to relieve pain and clear Damp-Heat (Table 5.7). Choose from the following points to construct a treatment or add points chosen from this list to point prescriptions in the following section describing treatment for the underlying condition (Ben):

KI-14	Siman
Ren-5	Shimen
SP-12	Chongmen
SP-13	Fushe
ST-25	Tianshu
LIV-4	Zhongfeng
Ren-3	Zhongji
GB-26	Daimai
GB-27	Wushu
GB-28	Weidao
KI-10	Yingu
SP-9	Yinlingquan
LIV-5	Ligou
LIV-8	Ququan

Treating the Ben

If the Damp-Heat and pain are not so severe, then it is appropriate to address the underlying condition immediately. This is especially so when we want to recover fertility as quickly as possible.

• Liver Qi stagnation predominant

This diagnosis will be made for a clinical picture including abdomen discomfort, breast soreness, irritability and moodiness.

Herbal Formula — The formula of choice is:

Xiao Yao San plus Jin Ling Zi San (Free and Easy powder with Gold Bell powder) modified

Chai Hu	9 g	*Radix Bupleuri*
Bai Zhu	12 g	*Rhizoma Atractylodis Macrocephalae*
Dang Gui	9 g	*Radix Angelicae Sinensis*
Bai Shao	15 g	*Radix Paeoniae Lactiflorae*
Fu Ling	15 g	*Sclerotium Poriae Cocos*

Gan Cao	3g	Radix Glycyrrhizae Uralensis
Sheng Jiang	3g	Rhizoma Zingiberis Officinalis Recens
Bo He	3g	Herba Menthae
Chuan Lian Zi	9g	Fructus Meliae Toosendan
Yan Hu Suo	9g	Rhizoma Corydalis Yanhusuo
Ju He	12g	Semen Citri Reticulatae

Chai Hu, Chuan Lian Zi, and Ju He are the main ingredients to address Liver Qi stagnation. Ju He is particularly indicated for lateral abdomen pain. Yan Hu Suo backs up this action by regulating any Blood stagnation which may have developed. The remaining herbs, constituents of Xiao Yao San, safeguard Spleen Qi.

If Spleen and Stomach function are affected by the Liver Qi stagnation, add:

Dang Shen	9g	Radix Codonopsis Pilulosae
Mu Xiang	9g	Radix Saussureae seu Vladimiriae
Chen Pi	3g	Pericarpium Citri Reticulate

For Damp-Heat, add:

| Bai Jiang Cao | 12g | Herba cum Radice Patriniae |

Acupuncture Points — Points (Table 5.8) are chosen from:

LIV-3	Taichong
LIV-5	Ligou
GB-34	Yanglingquan
Ren-6	Qihai
ST-26	Wailing
GB-28	Weidao

• Spleen weakness predominant

This form of PID presents a clinical picture of dull dragging abdomen ache, sometimes felt in the sides, abdomen bloating, fatigue, poor appetite and sweet or carbohydrate cravings.

Herbal Formula — The formula of choice is:

Xiang Sha Liu Jun Zi Tang (Six Gentlemen decoction) modified

Dang Shen	12g	Radix Codonopsis Pilulosae
Bai Zhu	9g	Rhizoma Atractylodis Macrocephalae
Fu Ling	9g	Sclerotium Poriae Cocos
Gan Cao (zhi)	9g	Radix Glycyrrhizae Uralensis
Chen Pi	6g	Pericarpium Citri Reticulate
Ban Xia	12g	Rhizoma Pinelliae
Mu Xiang	6g	Radix Saussureae seu Vladimiriae
Sha Ren	6g	Fructus seu Semen Amomi
Bai Jiang Cao	15g	Herba cum Radice Patriniae
Yi Yi Ren	20g	Semen Coicis Lachryma-jobi

Table 5.8   Acupuncture points[a] used in the treatment of PID with Liver Qi stagnation

Treatment goal	Acupuncture points
To regulate Qi in the Liver channel	LIV-3 and LIV-5, GB-34
To regulate Qi in the abdomen	Ren-6
Local points to regulate Qi and relieve pain	ST-26 and GB-28

[a]Use reducing technique.

The emphasis of this formula is first to strengthen the Spleen with Dang Shen, Bai Zhu, and Gan Cao (zhi), while Fu Ling and Ban Xia clear any Damp which has accumulated as the result of Spleen weakness. Sha Ren, Mu Xiang, and Chen Pi ensure the Qi keeps moving and Bai Jiang Cao and Yi Yi Ren are added to clear Damp and Heat. Bai Jiang Cao is safer to use than Hong Teng if Spleen Qi is weak.

If there are any signs of Blood stasis (pain becomes more pointed and severe), add:

Yan Hu Suo	9 g	Rhizoma Corydalis Yanhusuo

If there is a lot of Damp evident (e.g., discharges), then more herbs can be added to dry the Damp:

Huo Xiang	9 g	Herba Agastaches seu Pogostei
Cang Zhu	12 g	Rhizoma Atractylodes

Acupuncture Points — Points (Table 5.9) are chosen from:

Abdomen Zigong	
Tituo	
Ren-6	Qihai
Ren-12	Zhongwan
ST-36	Zusanli
SP-5	Shangqiu
SP-9	Yinlingquan
GB-26	Daimai

Table 5.9   Acupuncture points[a] used in the treatment of PID with Spleen deficiency

Treatment goal	Acupuncture points
To support the function of Stomach and Spleen	Ren-6, Ren-12 and ST-36
Local abdomen points which treat dragging down pain	Zigong and Tituo
To aid in clearing Damp	SP-5, SP-9 and GB-26

[a]The points can be used with even or reinforcing method.

• **Liver and Kidney deficiency predominant (complicated with Damp-Heat and Blood stagnation)**

The main symptoms of this type of PID are lower back pain, dizziness, mental restlessness, feeling hot in the evenings, some abdomen discomfort and vaginal discharge. There may be palpable masses or other signs of Blood stagnation such as clotty painful periods.

Primary aim of treatment is to reinforce Liver and Kidney Yin while still paying attention to Damp Heat and Blood stagnation.

Herbal Formula — The formula of choice is:

Gui Shao Di Huang Tang (Angelica Peonia Rehmannia decoction) modified

Shu Di	9 g	Radix Rehmanniae Glutinosae Conquitae
Shan Yao	9 g	Radix Dioscorea Oppositae
Shan Zhu Yu	9 g	Fructus Corni Officinalis
Mu Dan Pi	9 g	Cortex Moutan Radicis
Fu Ling	15 g	Selerotium Poriae Cocos
Bai Shao	9 g	Radix Paeoniae Lactiflorae
Dang Gui	9 g	Radix Angelicae Sinensis
Bai Jiang Cao	12 g	Herba cum Radice Patriniae
Chai Hu	6 g	Radix Bupleuri
Yan Hu Suo	6 g	Rhizoma Corydalis Yanhusuo
Xu Duan	9 g	Radix Dipsaci
Sang Ji Sheng	15 g	Ramulus Sang Ji Sheng

This formula primarily supplements the Kidney and Liver Yin and the Blood, but with the addition of Bai Jiang Cao and Sang Ji Sheng it also clears Damp-Heat. Yan Hu Suo and Chai Hu supply additional impetus to move Qi and Blood, which may have become retarded by Damp. Kidney Yang is supported by Xu Duan.

If Kidney Yang deficiency is marked, add:

Du Zhong	12 g	Cortex Eucommiae Ulmoidis
Lu Jiao Pian	9 g	Cornu Cervi Parvum

Acupuncture Points — Points (Table 5.10) are chosen from:

Ren-4	Guanyuan
SP-12	Chongmen
SP-13	Fushe
ST-28	Shuidao
KI-6	Zhaohai
KI-7	Fuliu
KI-10	Yingu
LIV-8	Ququan
BL-23	Shenshu
BL-28	Pangguanshu

Pelvic inflammation and infection is not uncommon in China and they have done a number of clinical studies examining herbal remedies. Formulas which clear toxic heat and transform static Blood have been shown to effectively reduce symptoms in 90% of cases.[27,28]

Table 5.10 Acupuncture points[a] used in the treatment of PID with Liver and Kidney deficiency (and Damp-Heat and Blood stagnation complications)

Treatment goal	Acupuncture points
To support the Kidneys and clear Damp-Heat	KI-7 and KI-10
To reinforce the Kidneys and clear Yin-deficient Heat	KI-6
To move stagnation and relieve abdomen pain	SP-12, SP-13 or ST-28
To reinforce Kidneys	Ren-4
To supplement Liver Yin and clear stagnation in the lower Jiao	LIV-8
To reinforce Kidneys and clear Damp-Heat and relieve back pain	BL-23 and BL-28

[a]Points are needled with even method or reducing method. Deep but cautious needling on the abdomen over sites of pain increases therapeutic effect.

Abdomen Masses

If there are palpable masses apparent in any of the above types of PID, then the patient is recommended to take appropriate patent medicines along with the main prescription. Because the constitution is weak in the case of chronic PID and the treatment will need to continue a long time, strong Blood-regulating treatment in the form of herbal decoctions is not advisable and most often pill or other preparations, such as the following, will be used:

Gui Zhi Fu Ling Wan (Ramulus Cinnamomi – Poria pill)

Gui Zhi	*Ramulus Cinnamomi Cassiae*
Fu Ling	*Sclerotium Poriae Cocos*
Chi Shao	*Radix Paeoniae Rubra*
Mu Dan Pi	*Cortex Moutan Radicis*
Tao Ren	*Semen Persicae*

This formula contains Blood moving and cooling herbs: Mu Dan Pi, Chi Shao and Tao Ren. Gui Zhi is added to assist these herbs in moving Blood and ensures their effect is not too cooling.

Where the stasis of Blood has been very long term, then a stronger formula may need to be employed to break up the congealed Blood. Again, the pill form will be used for long term use as it is less potent than decoction.

Da Huang Bie Chong Wan (Rheum Eupolyphaga pill)

Da Huang	*Rhizoma Rhei*
Tu Bie Chong	*Eupolyphagae seu Opisthoplatiae*
Tao Ren	*Semen Persicae*
Gan Qi	*Lacca Sinica Exsiccata*
Qi Cao	*Holotrichia*
Shui Zhi	*Hirudo seu Whitmaiae*
Meng Chong	*Tabanus Bivittatus*

Huang Qin	Radix Scutellariae Baicalensis
Xing Ren	Semen Pruni Armeniacae
Sheng Di	Radix Rehmanniae Glutinosae
Bai Shao	Radix Paeoniae Lactiflorae
Gan Cao	Radix Glycyrrhizae Uralensis

This formula contains many strong agents for breaking up long-term Blood stasis (such as Tu Bie Chong, Shui Zi and Meng Chong) and must be used with caution. It cools Heat in the Blood at the same time.

External Treatment

Herbal compresses can also be placed on the abdomen to help ease the pain of PID. The following herbal compress can be used:

Qian Nian Jian	6 g	Rhizoma Homalomenae Occultae
Hong Hua	6 g	Flos Carthami Tinctorii
Mo Yao	6 g	Myrrha
Bai Zhi	6 g	Radix Angelicae
Xue Jie	6 g	Sanguis Draconis
Xu Duan	20 g	Radix Dipsaci
Dang Gui	20 g	Radix Angelicae Sinensis
Fang Feng	20 g	Radix Ledebouriellae Sesloidis
Sang Ji Sheng	20 g	Ramulus Sangjisheng
Wu Jia Pi	20 g	Cortex Acanthopanacis
Tou Gu Cao	50 g	Herba Impatients Balsamina
Ai Ye	50 g	Folium Artemisiae
Chi Shao	20 g	Radix Paeoniae Rubra

This mixture is ground into a powder and put in a bag, which is then steamed for 15 min. The bag is placed on the abdomen and left until it gets cold. This procedure can be repeated two or three times a day. The above amount can be used for 5 days before a new batch needs to be made up.

More formulas for treatment of abdomen masses are described in Volume 3 of the *Clinical Handbook of Internal Medicine*.[29]

In the case where discharge and itching of the vulva are associated with PID, then external washes or sitz baths can be helpful. Herbs which remove Damp-Heat and calm inflamed skin are boiled in a large pot of water for half an hour. This liquid is then transferred to a sitz bath. The genital and abdomen area is soaked by sitting in the bath for 15–20 min or while the solution is still hot. The following external wash can be used:

Huang Bai	15 g	Cortex Phellodendri
She Chuang Zi	15 g	Fructus Cnidii Monnieri (in a muslin bag)
Bai Xian Pi	15 g	Cortex Dictamni Dasycarpi
Ku Shen	12 g	Radix Sophorae Flavescentis
Ai Ye	12 g	Folium Artemisiae
Chuan Jiao	1 g	Fructus Zanthoxyli Bungeani
Bian Xu	15 g	Herba Polygone Avicularis

Another approach, which is gaining favor in Chinese hospitals, is the use of herbal enemas in difficult cases of PID. Such an approach has been found to be particularly helpful for abdomen masses and for blockages in the tubes (see Ch. 6).

Fibroids and Polyps

These masses can be such that they impair implantation of an embryo or cause it to miscarry. They are discussed in Chapter 8. Often these masses will be dealt with by surgery if they are significant. Should a patient want to avoid surgery, then masses can be addressed with Chinese medicine[29] but the length of treatment required is often not compatible with the desire to conceive in the near future.

Dysmenorrhea and PMS

Neither period pain nor premenstrual syndrome are causes or even direct contributing factors to female infertility; however, they can be useful diagnostic components in a clinical picture which includes infertility. That is, they reflect the imbalance which is also the cause of reduced fertility. Most often, they are clear pointers to some stagnation that, in the interests of fertility, must be resolved. Less often, they are pointers to deficiency. Dysmenorrhea and the symptoms of PMS often resolve rapidly when the protocols of Chapter 4 are followed. There may need to be special treatment emphasis on Liver and/or Blood stagnation (or Spleen Qi deficiency) in the luteal phase and Kidney or Blood deficiency in the follicular phase.

Part 2 – Ovulatory Disorders and Polycystic Ovarian Syndrome

AMENORRHEA AND DISORDERS OF OVULATION

A discussion of amenorrhea (no periods) and other disorders of ovulation returns us to an examination of events in the follicular phase (see Ch. 4). In the case of amenorrhea we are looking at the very extreme of the spectrum, i.e., ovulation is not just premature or delayed, it completely fails to occur. You will remember that problems occurring in the follicular phase leading to ovulation most often fall into the Kidney Yin deficient category. It is certainly so in many cases of amenorrhea. Sometimes, however, Kidney Yin is sufficient to develop the egg to some degree but the release of the egg (or its final preparation) is hampered by an obstruction of some kind. Such obstructions are called Phlegm-Damp, Qi or Blood stagnation in TCM and may actually manifest as cysts or tumors on the ovaries or pituitary.

Primary amenorrhea is the term used to describe no periods ever, i.e., puberty has never arrived. It occurs when there is no uterus and vagina or if the ovaries do not function. There are many reasons why ovaries might never start producing eggs or stop producing eggs. They are often quite complex clinical and physiologic pictures. If pregnancy is desired, Western medicine confronts the issue by trying direct stimulation of the pituitary or ovary in the hope of producing an egg or eggs that may then be fertilized directly in an IVF procedure. Chinese medicine approaches the problem by trying to reestablish a regular menstrual cycle. The latter is often much more difficult to achieve than the one-off ovulation that drugs can achieve. If conception is the only aim, then often these drugs will be the first choice. From the point of view of Chinese medicine this may not be such a good step to take. If a woman is not ovulating because she has a profound Kidney deficiency, then the eggs that the drugs stimulate may not be of such good quality (from a Jing perspective). However, if an obstruction (e.g., by Phlegm-Damp or Qi or Blood stagnation) is causing the lack of ovulation then drug treatment may be quite useful.

Western medicine describes a number of disorders which result in no or intermittent ovulation. We shall examine these disorders, and the usual treatment options and then analyze them from a TCM perspective.

Different Types of Ovulatory Dysfunction

- Hypothalamic anovulation

- Hyperprolactinemia

- Premature ovarian failure

- Tumors of the ovary, adrenal or pituitary glands

- Post-oral contraceptive pill amenorrhea

- Polycystic ovary syndrome.

Hypothalamic Anovulation

The hypothalamus fails to give the pituitary the messages necessary for ovulation in circumstances of weight loss, stress, narcotic drug use and extreme exercise like marathon or classical ballet training.

Treatment includes the use of ovulation-inducing drugs (see below) if conception is desired. If pregnancy is not desired, hormones such as those in combined oral contraceptive pills are prescribed to reduce symptoms related to estrogen shortage.

Hyperprolactinemia

High levels of prolactin are produced by the pituitary gland in certain circumstances, causing ovulation to be suppressed. This happens normally in pregnancy to prepare the breasts for lactation and persists while breast-feeding continues. High prolactin levels also occur in abnormal circumstances such as the presence of tumors on the pituitary gland or from the effects of drugs like tranquilizers, heroin, blood pressure medication or drugs for nausea. Treatment of pituitary tumors employs a drug called bromocriptine, which will shrink the tumor and usually allow pituitary function to return to normal.

Where levels of prolactin are elevated only slightly, ovulation may still occur but the corpus luteum function is diminished, causing inadequate progesterone production.

Premature Ovarian Failure (POF) and Resistant Ovary Syndrome

If the menstrual cycle ceases before age 40, it indicates a premature depletion of ovarian follicles. A biopsy taken from the ovary shows few or no follicles. The use of drugs to stimulate ovulation is pointless because there are too few follicles to stimulate. This disorder has a strong genetic component but can also be related to autoimmune conditions or infections or iatrogenic causes. It is sometimes called premature menopause. Women with POF are usually offered the option of donor oocytes should they want to conceive. Another and less common form of ovarian failure is called resistant ovary syndrome. Unlike the previous case, a biopsy of the ovary will reveal plenty of primordial follicles which appear dormant or unstimulated (and are unable to be stimulated by the drugs usually used to induce ovulation). It is thought there may be a receptor block on the surface of the ovary to FSH, or antibodies to FSH or LH that prevent the ovary from responding.

Drug treatment involves giving small amounts of estrogen for 4–6 weeks and at some time during this course progesterone will be added for 2 weeks. A small number of women with resistant ovaries respond to this approach and they will ovulate and conceive.

Tumors in the Ovaries or Adrenal or Pituitary Glands

Tumors in the ovary or adrenal gland, causing a disturbance to ovulation will usually require surgery. Tumors in the pituitary gland are usually discovered when high levels of serum prolactin are investigated, mentioned above.

Post-pill Amenorrhea

In a significant number of women, periods do not return after stopping the oral contraceptive pill. It is thought by gynecologists that one of the above described causes of amenorrhea has developed during the time the pill was being taken and that this is incidental to the effect of the pill. However, some doctors would relate the amenorrhea to the action of the pill (see PCOS, below). Many cases of post-pill amenorrhea resolve by themselves within a year, but where there is evidence of a tumor, medical treatment will be undertaken.

Polycystic Ovary Syndrome (PCOS)

This disorder is an increasingly common cause of amenorrhea or oligomenorrhea. We will discuss this condition later, in another section.

Drugs used to Induce Ovulation

To stir recalcitrant ovaries into action we can stimulate them directly with FSH, the hormone the pituitary produces to ripen follicles, or indirectly by making the pituitary make more FSH. Clomifene does the latter, whereas FSH drug preparations act directly on the ovary.

Clomifene

This drug, sold as Clomid or Serophene, blocks the negative feedback action of estrogen, so that the pituitary is tricked into producing a lot of FSH in an attempt to stimulate follicles. Clomifene is cheap and easier to administer than other ovulation-inducing drugs and so is usually the first drug tried. It is given for 5 consecutive days starting between Day 2 and Day 6 of the menstrual cycle. Where there is no menstrual cycle, a period is created by giving a course of a progestogen. The starting dose of clomifene is 50 mg/day, though this can be raised progressively in subsequent cycles to as much as 200 mg/day if necessary. If the action of the clomifene is successful, it will induce ovulation 9–15 days after the first day it is taken. Most patients ovulate in response to 50 or 100 mg/day and, if conception occurs, it will likely be in the first three ovulatory cycles.

Side-effects are common, especially at the higher doses. They are:

- ovarian enlargement (>6 cm)

- abdominal discomfort

- flushing

- irritability, mood disturbances

- lack of fertile mucus, vaginal dryness

- visual symptoms (blurring, spots or flashes)

- headaches

- thinning of the endometrium

175

- breast tenderness

- nausea and/or vomiting.

From the fertility point of view, the useful stimulation of the follicles that the clomifene achieves is undone to some extent by the deleterious effect it has on the fertile mucus (which is dried up) and the endometrium (which becomes too thin). These unwanted side effects mean that only 50% of patients who do ovulate successfully with clomifene will become pregnant, even with its continued use. Since some of these side-effects (like the thinning of the endometrium) appear to get worse with repeated clomifene cycles, it is not advisable to continue the drug for more than three cycles at a time. In addition, 20% of pregnancies achieved with the use of clomifene will miscarry, a high rate that may also be due to inadequate development of the endometrium or poor embryo quality.

FSH Preparations

The other way to induce ovulation is to bypass the pituitary gland and stimulate the ovaries directly using FSH. The drug form of FSH (Gonal-F, Puregon, Follistim) is a synthesized molecule using recombinant gene technology. It is given by subcutaneous injection every day for around 2 weeks. Once several follicles reach a mature size (around 2 cm diameter), then the FSH stimulation is stopped to allow all but one or two to undergo atresia (die) before a trigger injection is given to make the follicle release its egg. Intrauterine insemination (IUI) is often performed shortly after this.

If many eggs are desired for use in an IVF procedure (see Ch. 10), then larger doses of FSH are continued right up to the trigger injection and egg collection.

Because this treatment acts so directly on the follicles in the ovary, there is little in the way of natural feedback controls or brakes in the process and ultrasounds and blood tests must be used to monitor the response of the ovaries.

Treatment with FSH, while it can have side-effects, is successful in inducing ovulation in more than 90% of the cycles in which it is used. However, the viable pregnancy rate is only 5–25% per cycle, depending on the reason for the ovulatory disturbance in the first place. Miscarriage occurs in 12–30% of these pregnancies, a higher than normal rate, which may reflect defects of the luteal phase or the quality of the embryo.

hCG Preparations

Pregnyl, Novarel, and Profasi are preparations of human chorionic gonadotrophin (hCG) isolated from the urine of pregnant women. Ovidrel is a genetically manufactured product that is identical to the body's hCG. These drugs do not stimulate follicle development but induce ovulation of follicles which have already been stimulated by other drugs. hCG preparations have a physiologic action similar to LH, i.e., they prepare the eggs and the follicles which encase them for ovulation. These drugs are used in IUI and IVF treatment cycles.

Bromocriptine

Bromocriptine (Parlodel) is given for the disorder hyperprolactinemia. It mimics the action of dopamine, the natural inhibitor of prolactin production, and thereby lowers prolactin levels to normal so ovulation can occur. The drug can cause side-effects in the beginning and if these continue it is given as a vaginal pessary rather than an oral medication to minimize its effect on the liver. Ovulation and conception usually occur soon after the administration of bromocriptine unless there are other factors influencing fertility.

Metformin

Metformin (Glucophage, Diaformin, Diabex) is used in the treatment of type 2 diabetes to control blood sugar levels. Such control of blood sugar has proved to be useful in women with polycystic ovary syndrome (PCOS), especially if they are overweight. Ovulation tends to occur more frequently in women with PCOS if they take metformin.

TCM Analysis of Drugs

Clomifene

TCM affords us an interesting perspective on drugs like clomifene – by examining and analyzing the effects it can have we can determine its action in an energetic sense. Clomifene is considered a 'heating' drug and it has been observed to be effective in increasing fertility in cases where there is Kidney Yang deficiency. However, infertility related to Kidney Yang deficiency often develops from or is accompanied by Kidney Yin deficiency. When there is pronounced Yin deficiency and internal Heat, then taking something as heating and drying as clomifene presents more of a risk. From the Chinese medicine point of view, the Yin damaging effects of the drug – namely, the hot flushes, the drying up of the fertile mucus, the thinning of the endometrium and the irritability – are quite worrying. In sensitive individuals, the Liver and Kidney Yin, which are so vital for fertility, can be damaged. At best, in such cases, it produces uncomfortable side-effects and at worst, it damages the ovaries so that they stop functioning altogether.

On the other hand, in a Yang-deficient woman, perhaps with Phlegm-Damp accumulation, its heating and drying effect can be most beneficial.

FSH Preparations

If we analyze what symptoms occur when these IVF drugs (Gonal-F, Follistim, Puregon) are used, we can see that the main side-effect is stagnation of the Liver Qi. Usually this is not severe; symptoms include abdomen swelling and tenderness, breast soreness and a feeling of irritability or emotional volatility.

hCG Preparations

The ovulation trigger – hCG (Pregnyl, Novarel, Profasi) – in assisted reproduction or IVF cycles is added to mimic the action of LH in releasing the egg from the follicle. This is the equivalent of adding a sudden dose of a Yang influence to switch the artificially manipulated cycle from its Yin phase to its Yang phase. At this point, pre-existing Qi stagnation can be greatly compounded. A worst case scenario sees the precipitation of a condition called ovarian hyperstimulation syndrome or OHSS (discussed in Ch. 9), which in its more severe manifestations is associated with abdomen pain and swelling, nausea, dizziness, headaches, and ascites, which are all signs of increasingly significant Liver Qi stagnation. This can further develop into Blood stagnation, resulting in embolism or into Liver Wind, causing stroke or fitting, both potentially life-threatening situations.

Bromocriptine

Once again the side-effects of Parlodel (bromocriptine) tell us which organ system it affects. If too much is given too quickly, then headaches, nausea, and dizziness can develop, indicating that the Liver Qi is disordered.

Metformin

This drug can damage Spleen function, causing diarrhea, bloating, flatulence and nausea in susceptible women. The concurrent use of Spleen tonic formulas can increase tolerance to the drug; however, where any digestive symptoms persist, then it is not advisable to continue the medication.

Knowing how a particular drug affects the balance of the body in an energetic sense gives the TCM doctor a good understanding of whether it is an appropriate drug treatment for any given patient. For example, women who are already quite Yin deficient with internal Heat must use clomifene with great caution. Likewise, women with a tendency to Liver Qi stagnation must be monitored even more carefully than usual if they are administered ovulation-inducing drugs such as Gonal-F, Follistim, Puregon with hCG triggers. Women with Spleen weakness may need to find alternatives to taking metformin.

TCM Analysis of Different Types of Ovulation Disorders and Amenorrhea

Lack of ability to produce eggs is related either to a Kidney or Blood deficiency or to an interruption somewhere in the hypothalamic-pituitary-ovarian axis caused by Heart or Liver Qi stagnation, Phlegm-Damp obstruction or Blood stagnation. These conditions were covered in detail in Chapter 4; we shall cover them again briefly as they pertain specifically to amenorrhea. Some TCM gynecology texts which collect information from many different sources and authors will list anywhere up to 9 or 10 different patterns of amenorrhea. Here, we shall discuss the basic patterns which underlie all the others and those which are seen most often in infertility clinics in China.

Amenorrhea related to deficiency includes Kidney Jing deficiency, Kidney Yin deficiency and Blood deficiency amenorrhea.

Kidney Jing Deficiency Amenorrhea

Kidney Jing or essence deficiency represents a congenital cause of primary amenorrhea, whereby the Tian Gui does not arrive and the Chong and the Ren vessels never function.

Kidney Jing deficiency can also contribute to secondary amenorrhea where, although there may be some Chong and Ren vessel foundation laid, the periods stop. Because the Jing is weak, an important component in the production of Blood from marrow is lacking. Thus there is insufficient Blood to fill the Chong vessel and menstruation ceases. The contribution of the Kidney Jing in the production of Blood is more important than the role of the Spleen and Stomach when we are considering this type of amenorrhea.

If periods never begin (primary amenorrhea) we would say that Kidney Jing is deficient and the Tian Gui never arrived. Other types of amenorrhea such as resistant ovary syndrome and some cases of premature menopause or primary ovulatory failure can also be related to Kidney Jing deficiency, especially if they occur at a young age. The problem in primary ovulatory failure and very premature menopause lies within the ovary itself, i.e., primordial follicles are not present, or what little was there has been depleted. In resistant ovary syndrome there are plenty of primordial follicles but they are resistant to the stimulation that normally turns them into functional follicles which produce ripe eggs. In the Chinese medicine view the Jing is deficient and the action of the Tian Gui is lacking. This is the reason so few women with resistant ovary syndrome have success with hormonal treatment. In these women, a very basic aspect of the Kidney Jing is lacking and the first stages of follicle growth and egg maturation are faulty, i.e., the Tian Gui is not functioning.

Treatment of severe Kidney Jing deficiency is unlikely to be successful. Even the amenorrhea resulting from the less severe forms of Kidney Jing deficiency are difficult to treat successfully although an attempt is worthwhile. To treat this condition, formulas which build Kidney Yin and Yang are often modified with the addition of animal products.

Herbal Formula — The formula of choice is:

Gui Shao Di Huang Tang modified (Angelica Peonia Rehmannia decoction)

Dang Gui	9 g	*Radix Angelicae Sinensis*
Bai Shao	9 g	*Radix Paeoniae Lactiflorae*
Shu Di	9 g	*Radix Rehmanniae Glutinosae Conquitae*
Shan Yao	9 g	*Radix Dioscorea Oppositae*
Shan Zhu Yu	9 g	*Fructus Corni Officinalis*

Mu Li	9 g	Concha Ostreae
Yin Yang Huo	9 g	Herba Epimedii
Lu Jiao Pian	9 g	Cornu Cervi Parvum
Zi He Che*	6 g	Placenta Hominis
Ren Shen	6 g	Radix Ginseng

*Zi He Che is a restricted substance in some countries.

This formula, which is based on the Kidney-strengthening formula Liu Wei Di Huang Tang, is modified by the addition of Zi He Che to strengthen the Jing and Yin Yang Huo and Lu Jiao Pian to boost Kidney Yang. Mu Li calms the mind and consolidates Yin, whereas Ren Shen invigorates the Qi and calms the mind. Gui Ban (Plastrum Testudinis), from a farmed source and with a CITES (Convention on International Trade of Endangered Species) certificate, is sometimes substituted for Mu Li.

If there appears to be any increase of estrogen (determined by blood tests, changes in vaginal discharge or breast or ovary sensations), then the protocol outlined below in the treatment of Kidney Yin deficiency amenorrhea can be followed.

CASE HISTORY – SARI

Sari's periods didn't come until she was 18 years old and even then very half-heartedly, at long intervals. She took the oral contraceptive pill from 19–23 years of age and experienced light bleeds each month.

She stopped the pill and in the following 2 years, had no periods at all. In general, she was healthy and exercised moderately. However, she was an anxious person and reported restless sleep and feeling hot at night. Her amenorrhea was contributed to by anemia, resulting from a strict vegetarian diet since the age of 14.

Her pulse was rapid and thin and her tongue had a little coat. Her diagnosis was Kidney Jing, Yin and Blood deficiency. She was treated with the following herbs and was advised to eat more eggs.

Shu Di	9 g	Radix Rehmanniae Glutinosae Conquitae
Shan Yao	9 g	Radix Dioscorea Oppositae
Shan Zhu Yu	9 g	Fructus Corni Officinalis
Dang Gui	9 g	Radix Angelicae Sinensis
Bai Shao	9 g	Radix Paeoniae Lactiflorae
Bai Zi Ren	12 g	Semen Biotae Orientalis
Mu Li	9 g	Concha Ostreae
Mu Dan Pi	9 g	Cortex Moutan Radicis
Zhi Mu	12 g	Radix Anemarrhena
Fu Ling	12 g	Sclerotium Poriae Cocos
Ze Xie	6 g	Rhizoma Alismatis
Zi He Che	6 g	Placenta Hominis
Tu Si Zi	9 g	Semen Cuscatae

She experienced more vaginal discharge after the herbs and she said she felt the best she had in ages, but after 6 months there was still no menstrual cycle. Recovery of the Tian Gui may not be possible in this case.

Kidney Yin Deficiency Amenorrhea

This is the most common cause of amenorrhea (not related to PCOS). The Yin becomes deficient due to lifestyle factors or a constitutional tendency (see Ch. 2). Yin, as we know, is required for the eggs to ripen, the production of fertile mucus and to provide the precursor to making Blood in order to thicken and nourish the endometrium.

Deficient Kidney Yin symptoms include infrequent or no periods, no fertile mucus, dizziness and lower back pain.

Where Yin deficiency gives rise to Heat, Heart- and Liver-Fire can develop. Both will exacerbate the Yin deficiency and compound the amenorrhea in their own way. Heart- and Liver-Fire, which can cause agitation, irritability and insomnia, can also dry the Blood so the endometrium cannot develop. Dryness also leads to constipation and thirst. Many cases of premature menopause fall into this category and it is the aggressive clearing of Heat which, if there are any follicles left, allows the ovary to function again, for a short time at least.

Another more rare expression of Heat from Yin deficiency is sometimes seen in cases of amenorrhea, and this is Kidney-Fire. This occurs in severe amenorrhea when the Yin and Blood are exhausted (possibly after postpartum hemorrhage or long-term illness). It is very difficult to recover the Yin at this point.

Kidney Yin deficiency will, with time, eventually lead to Kidney Yang weakness, since the two are so interdependent. Then there may be lassitude, vertigo, palpitations, blurred vision, lower back pain and edema accompanying the amenorrhea. This can represent an advanced condition which also can be difficult to treat successfully.

In addition to premature ovarian failure or menopause, Kidney Yin deficiency amenorrhea includes hypothalamic anovulation, (often provoked by weight loss or long-term illness) and some variations of polycystic ovary disease.

Treatment of Kidney Yin amenorrhea is little different from the treatment we described in Chapter 4, addressing Kidney Yin deficiency infertility. The only difference is that we don't have a menstrual cycle to follow and so we attempt to create one.

Our first aim is to reinforce the Yin and nourish the Blood using, e.g., the same guiding formula we used in the post-menstrual phase when treating infertility: namely, Gui Shao Di Huang Tang. Where there is no menstrual cycle at all, this formula (or variations of it) will be used in the long term with the addition every 3 or 4 weeks of a group of herbs which boost the Kidney Yang and encourage movement of the Blood. Thus, we attempt to lay a foundation of Yin and Blood, then promote the transformation of Yin to Yang followed by movement of the Blood downwards. If there is no period after 2 or so weeks of taking the Kidney Yang and Blood-regulating herbs, then go back to the base formula for another 2 or 3 weeks before adding Yang tonics and Blood-moving herbs again. Treatment can continue like this for some months before any result is seen if the Yin deficiency is severe.

Herbal Formula — The formula of choice is:

Gui Shao Di Huang Tang (Angelica Peonia Rehmannia decoction)

Dang Gui	9 g	Radix Angelicae Sinensis
Bai Shao	9 g	Radix Paeoniae Lactiflorae
Shu Di	20 g	Radix Rehmanniae Glutinosae Conquitae
Shan Zhu Yu	15 g	Fructus Corni Officinalis
Shan Yao	12 g	Radix Dioscorea Oppositae
Fu Ling	12 g	Sclerotium Poriae Cocos
Mu Dan Pi	9 g	Cortex Moutan Radicis
Ze Xie	12 g	Rhizoma Alismatis

This formula (described in Ch. 4) nourishes the Blood as well as the Yin. Shu Di and Shan Zhu Yu in this case are used in high doses. Additional herbs which can be added after 3 or 4 weeks, if no signs of ovulation are apparent, are:

Tu Si Zi	9 g	Semen Cuscatae
Ba Ji Tian	9 g	Radix Morindae Officinalis
Chuan Niu Xi	9 g	Radix Cyathulae
Ze Lan	9 g	Herba Lycopi Lucidi

This becomes the formula Gui Shen Tang (Restoring the Kidneys decoction), which encourages the growth of Kidney Yang from Kidney Yin. Two Blood-regulating herbs are added because we hope to promote menstruation.

Where there is Heat, more time must be spent on clearing Heat and recovering Yin before the Yang tonics are added. If there is Yin-deficient Heat, we use another variation of the above base formula: namely, Zhi Bai Di Huang Tang (Anemarrhena Phellodendron Rehmannia decoction). To make this formula, add to Gui Shao Di Huang Tang:

Zhi Mu	9 g	*Radix Anemarrhena*
Huang Bai	9 g	*Cortex Phellodendri*

and delete Dang Gui and Bao Shao.

This formula will clear Kidney-Fire but if Heart-Fire is also evident with pronounced mental restlessness, then add Bai Zi Ren Wan.

Bai Zi Ren Wan (Biota pill) modified

Bai Zi Ren	9 g	*Semen Biotae Orientalis*
Dan Shen	9 g	*Radix Salviae Miltiorrhizae*
Chuan Niu Xi	9 g	*Radix Cyathulae*
Bai Shao	9 g	*Radix Paeoniae Lactiflorae*
Ze Lan	9 g	*Herba Lycopi Lucidi*
Xu Duan	9 g	*Radix Dipsaci*

It is hoped that the Bai Zi Ren and Dan Shen will have the effect of calming Heart-Fire for long enough to allow Yin to grow. Chuan Niu Xi and Ze Lan are included to prevent Blood stagnation in the Heart and promote menstruation. Xu Duan fortifies Kidney Yang but as soon as there is any sign of fertile mucus then more Kidney Yang tonic herbs will be added, e.g.:

Ba Ji Tian	9 g	*Radix Morindae Officinalis*
Tu Si Zi	9 g	*Semen Cuscatae*

In the case that Heart- and Liver-Fire are severe enough or long term enough to have dried the Blood, then Heat must be strongly drained before the Blood can be replenished. The usual approach in this sort of amenorrhea (where Heart-Fire is predominant) is to use the following formula:

San Huang Si Wu Tang (Three Yellows Four Substance decoction)

Shu Di	15 g	*Radix Rehmanniae Glutinosae Conquitae*
Dang Gui	9 g	*Radix Angelicae Sinensis*
Chuan Xiong	9 g	*Radix Ligustici Wallichii*
Chi Shao	9 g	*Radix Paeoniae Rubra*
Da Huang	6 g	*Rhizoma Rhei*
Huang Lian	3 g	*Rhizoma Coptidis*
Huang Qin	9 g	*Radix Scutellariae Baicalensis*

Huang Lian, Huang Qin and Chi Shao clear Heat from the Heart and the Blood and purge it downwards with the help of Da Huang. Shu Di, Dang Gui and Chuan Xiong promote the building of new Blood.

Another formula that is preferred by some infertility specialists is based on Liang Ge San (which clears Heat strongly from the upper Jiao) and Si Wu Tang to make San He Yin.

San He Yin (Dissipate and Harmonize decoction)

Da Huang	9g	Rhizoma Rhei
Mang Xiao	9g	Mirabilitum
Zhi Zi	6g	Fructus Gardeniae Jasminoidis
Huang Qin	6g	Radix Scutellariae Baicalensis
Lian Qiao	12g	Fructus Forsythiae Suspensae
Bo He	6g	Herba Menthae
Gan Cao	6g	Radix Glycyrrhizae Uralensis
Dang Gui	9g	Radix Angelicae Sinensis
Chuan Xiong	6g	Radix Ligustici Wallichii
Shu Di	12g	Radix Rehmanniae Glutinosae Conquitae
Chi Shao	9g	Radix Paeoniae Rubra

The strategy behind this formula is the same as the one just described above but more cooling herbs are included (Mang Xiao, Zhi Zi, Lian Qiao, and Bo He). Thus, it clears marked internal Heat affecting the Heart. This is a strong treatment that can cause diarrhea and some intestinal discomfort. When the Heat is cleared, then Mai Wei Di Huang Tang is begun immediately to rescue and retain the Yin.

Mai Wei Di Huang Tang (Ophiopogon and Rehmannia decoction)

Mai Dong	12g	Tuber Ophiopogonis
Wu Wei Zi	9g	Frucuts Schizandrae Chinensis
Shu Di	20g	Radix Rehmanniae Glutinosae Conquitae
Shan Zhu Yu	15g	Fructus Corni Officinalis
Shan Yao	12g	Radix Dioscorea Oppositae
Fu Ling	12g	Sclerotium Poriae Cocos
Mu Dan Pi	9g	Cortex Moutan Radicis
Ze Xie	12g	Rhizoma Alismatis

This formula is another variation on Liu Wei Di Huang Tang (the often used Kidney Yin tonic formula), with the addition of Mai Dong and Wu Wei Zi to further strengthen and consolidate the Yin. Note the relatively large doses Shu Di and Shan Zhu Yu.

Then begins a careful watch for Yin signs (specifically more vaginal moisture or discharge) before Yang tonic herbs can be added to encourage ovulation. If the Yin has not been too badly damaged, then the removal of the Heat can have quite rapid results and ovulation quickly follows. If it doesn't, Gui Shao Di Huang Tang or Mai Wei Di Huang Tang must be continued for many months.

Where Liver-Heat contributes to the Yin damage more than Heart-Fire does, we can use a different Heat-purging formula:

Yu Zhu San (Jade Candle powder)

Da Huang	9g	Rhizoma Rhei
Mang Xiao	9g	Mirabilitum
Dang Gui	9g	Radix Angelicae Sinensis
Chi Shao	9g	Radix Paeoniae Rubra
Chuan Xiong	6g	Radix Ligustici Wallichii
Sheng Di	15g	Radix Rehmanniae Glutinosae
Gan Cao	3g	Radix Glycyrrhizae Uralensis

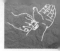

Internal Heat is cleared with the use of Mang Xiao, Sheng Di and Chi Shao. It is expelled from the body with the help of Da Huang. Dang Gui and Chuan Xiong encourage the manufacture of more Blood. Once Heat is cleared, Liver and Kidney Yin can be nourished with Qi Ju Di Huang Tang, i.e., add to the guiding formula Gui Shao Di Huang Wan:

| Gou Qi Zi | 15 g | *Fructus Lycii Chinensis* |
| Ju Hua | 6 g | *Flos Crysanthemi Morifolii* |

and delete Dang Gui and Bai Shao.

When both Kidney Yin and Yang are very deficient, then add to the guiding formula Gui Shao Di Huang Wan, the patent medicine:

Ren Shen Lu Rong Wan (Ginseng Cornu Cervii pill)

Ren Shen	*Radix Ginseng*
Du Zhong	*Cortex Eucommiae Ulmoidis*
Ba Ji Tian	*Radix Morindae Officinalis*
Huang Qi	*Radix Astragali*
Lu Rong	*Cornu Cervi Parvum*
Dang Gui	*Radix Angelicae Sinensis*
Huai Niu Xi	*Radix Achyranthis Bidentate*
Long Yan Rou	*Arillus Euphoriae Longanae*

which further supports Qi, Blood and Kidney Yang.

Where there is definite and observable improvement in the Kidney Yin and it appears that ovulation is successfully being promoted, i.e., there is the appearance of fertile mucus, then a stronger approach to transforming Kidney Yin to Yang and moving Blood may be taken. For example, the formula Bu Shen Cu Pai Luan Tang (Ch. 4) can be taken to more strongly encourage ovulation. If ovulation does occur (the patient would need to be recording her BBT at this point to get this information), then the next formula is one which builds Kidney Yang (see Ch. 4).

Acupuncture Points — Reluctant ovulation is often treated by employing points that regulate the activity of the Chong and Ren vessels (Table 5.11). In the case of absolute amenorrhea where the Chong vessel is not filling at all treatment must consider Blood and Yin status as well. Where Yin and Blood are very deficient, then herbal medicines (and appropriate diet, and lifestyle, see Ch. 9) will be required to nourish these. Once that has been achieved, then acupuncture can promote the functioning of the Chong vessel.

Table 5.11   Acupuncture points[a] used in the treatment of amenorrhea due to Kidney deficiency

Treatment goal	Acupuncture points
To support Kidney Yin	Ren-4 and SP-6
To open the Chong vessel	SP-4 and PC-6, confluent and paired points for the Chong vessel
To regulate the Chong vessel and promote a menstrual cycle	KI-13, Ren-7 and ST-30

[a]Even and reinforcing technique is used.

Table 5.12   Acupuncture points[a] used to promote ovulation

Treatment goal	Acupuncture points
To open and regulate the Ren vessel	LU-7 and KI-6, confluent and paired points for the Ren vessel
To promote Ren vessel activity	Ren-1 and Ren-4
To harmonize and regulate the Qi and Blood in the Ren and Chong vessels	KI-6 and KI-8
To regulate Qi in the pelvis/ovaries	ST-29, LIV-5, Abdomen Zigong

[a]Even technique is employed. Points in the abdomen should be needled deeply. Electric stimulation connecting abdomen points to other abdomen points or to leg points on the same side, can be added at a mild level of intensity at a frequency of 2–10 Hz.

Use some or all of the following points (and see Table 5.11):

SP-4	Gongsun
PC-6	Neiguan
KI-13	Qixue
ST-30	Qichong
Ren-7	Yinjiao
Ren-4	Guanyuan
SP-6	Sanyinjiao

• Promoting ovulation

Some ovulatory disorders may be caused by a problem in the switch of activity from the Chong to the Ren vessel. The mildest expression of this scenario is the lack of synchronization sometimes seen between the production of fertile mucus and the release of the egg. More serious examples include some forms of ovarian dysfunction whereby the follicle ripens somewhat but does not release an egg (as in LUFS, see previous section on Endometriosis, and see PCOS, next section).

Acupuncture treatment requires precise timing to be successful. Using information obtained by careful observation by the patient of her own signs and symptoms can help to determine the maturity of the follicle in the ovary. Specifically, it is the cervical secretions which indicate the degree of ripeness of the follicle and its readiness to ovulate. Other subtle symptoms of abdomen tenderness or breast or nipple tenderness or mood changes can also alert the patient to the presence of a surge of estrogen, indicating the maturation of a follicle. Acupuncture points to regulate Chong and Ren vessel function and support Kidney Yin and Blood (see Ch. 4) can be applied for a time after a period. At the point where it appears that the Chong vessel is approaching fullness (i.e., the cervical secretions increase or the above symptoms are felt) then acupuncture to facilitate the switch to the Ren vessel should be used. Choose from the following (and see Table 5.12):

LU-7	Lieque
KI-6	Zhaohai
Ren-1	Huiyin
Ren-4	Guanyuan

KI-5	Shuiquan
KI-8	Jiaoxin
ST-29	Guilai
LIV-5	Ligou
Abdomen Zigong	

Some studies in China have indicated that acupuncture is most successful in inducing ovulation in women who have normal levels of estrogen and whose sympathetic nervous system is inhibited by the action of acupuncture. This latter is tested by needling CO-4 Hegu and PC-6 Neiguan for 30 min while the patient's hand temperature is measured. An increase in hand temperature indicates the sympathetic nervous system has been inhibited, and this patient can expect a good outcome with acupuncture induction of ovulation.[30]

CASE HISTORY – MARY

Mary (36 years) had been trying to fall pregnant for 12 months before she saw me. She had been diagnosed with premature menopause. The blood test showed her FSH was very high and her estrogen low. Her menstrual cycle, which had always been erratic, was becoming even more infrequent. She felt anxious, agitated, irritable and depressed. Her sleep was very disturbed and she often felt flushed, hot, and thirsty. Headaches were a common feature. There was very little in the way of vaginal secretions and the dryness bothered her. When a period did come, the flow was very scanty and premenstrually she felt 'ready to kill'. Mary began to record her basal body temperature (BBT) when she started trying to fall pregnant. Her charts (Fig. 5.3) revealed for the most part short or long anovulatory cycles, i.e., there was no biphasic pattern.

Her pulse was thready and rapid and her tongue was red and peeled, especially on the sides and the tip.

Here we have a mental picture of severe internal Heat affecting the Liver and Heart. The Heat arises as a result of Kidney Yin deficiency. In addition to giving rise to Liver-Fire (headaches, flushing, irritability) and Heart-Fire (insomnia, agitation, anxiety) the Yin deficiency is starting to cause dryness (vaginal dryness and thirst) and Blood deficiency (scanty periods, depression). A vicious circle is created as the internal Heat dries the Yin and the Blood, which of course allows more internal Heat to manifest. The more the Heat disturbs the Shen or the mind, the harder it is for Yin to recover and grow. To manage the headaches and the insomnia, clearly the Heat in the Liver and the Heart had to be cooled and Liver and Heart Yin had to be strengthened. To address the long and irregular cycles, the Kidney Yin had to be reinforced and the Liver Blood nourished. Purging the empty Heat in an attempt to recover and reactivate what Yin was left was a radical but necessary first step.

Da Huang	9 g	Rhizoma Rhei (boiled 10 min only)
Bo He	9 g	Herba Menthae (boiled 5 min only)
Lian Qiao	9 g	Fructus Forsythiae Suspensae
Sheng Di	12 g	Radix Rehmanniae Glutinosae
Shan Yao	9 g	Radix Dioscorea Oppositae
Shan Zhu Yu	9 g	Fructus Corni Officinalis
Dang Gui	9 g	Radix Angelicae Sinensis
Bai Shao	9 g	Radix Paeoniae Lactiflorae
Mu Dan Pi	9 g	Cortex Moutan Radicis
Dan Shen	9 g	Radix Salviae Miltiorrhizae
Suan Zao Ren	18 g	Semen Ziziphi Spinosae

This formula seemed to do the trick – she immediately started sleeping better and the flushing and her thirst subsided and she felt emotionally much calmer. More significantly, the vaginal dryness improved and secretions returned quite quickly. After 2 days of the purging herbs she began to get diarrhea and we switched to another treatment (based on Mai Wei Di Huang Tang) to quickly capture and maintain the ground gained.

Shan Yao	9g	Radix Dioscorea Oppositae
Shu Di	15g	Radix Rehmanniae Glutinosae Conquitae
Shan Zhu Yu	15g	Fructus Corni Officinalis
Mai Dong	9g	Tuber Ophiopogonis
Mu Dan Pi	9g	Cortex Moutan Radicis
Dan Shen	9g	Radix Salviae Miltiorrhizae
Fu Ling	12g	Sclerotium Poriae Cocos
Yi Yi Ren	15g	Semen Coicis Lachryma-jobi
Wu Wei Zi	9g	Fructus Schizandrae Chinensis
Suan Zao Ren	18g	Semen Ziziphi Spinosae

With these herbs, the vaginal discharge began to thicken and get stretchy (i.e., she started producing fertile mucus) and her libido increased.

Because Mary had the feeling that something had changed markedly, she persuaded her gynecologist to take another blood test. The result of this was so different from those taken previously (namely, the levels of FSH were now in the normal range for the midcycle of an ovulatory cycle) that the diagnosis of premature menopause was retracted. Her estrogen levels, however, were still low and her LH was still a little elevated. It appeared that more nourishment of the Yin and Blood was needed to bring about an ovulation and a period. The following herbs were used, incorporating the principles of building, cooling and moving the Blood and calming the mind. By keeping the mind calm, it was hoped the Yin could build too.

Shu Di	12g	Radix Rehmanniae Glutinosae Conquitae
Sheng Di	9g	Radix Rehmanniae Glutinosae
Bai Shao	9g	Radix Paeoniae Lactiflorae
Chi Shao	9g	Radix Paeoniae Rubra
Shan Yao	9g	Radix Dioscorea Oppositae
Shan Zhu Yu	9g	Fructus Corni Officinalis
Dan Shen	9g	Radix Salviae Miltiorrhizae
Fu Ling	9g	Sclerotium Poriae Cocos
Yi Yi Ren	15g	Semen Coicis Lachryma-jobi
Han Lian Cao	9g	Herba Ecliptae Prostratae
Suan Zao Ren	18g	Semen Ziziphi Spinosae
Huang Lian	6g	Rhizoma Coptidis

After 3 weeks on this formula, she had her first period in 6 months. Her BBT chart looked a whole lot more promising, although the follicular phase still showed signs of lingering Heart-Fire and the short-lived luteal phase indicated her Kidney Yin was not strong enough to promote Kidney Yang (Fig. 5.4).

From this point, we began a program of alternately reinforcing Kidney Yin and (when a basis of Yin was established) Kidney Yang, as described above. Her cycles were never regular or predictable but they did keep coming. Over the following 9 months Mary was deflected from her course occasionally to try fertility drugs but they upset her cycle more than they helped. So she stuck to the Chinese herbs, which eventually helped her to achieve two textbook perfect cycles; on the second of these she was pregnant (Fig. 5.5).

Her large baby was born (not without drama) when she was 37. She tried in vain to have another baby for several years. Chinese herbs managed to keep her ovaries alive intermittently but by 39 years of age, her menopause seemed irreversible. She now takes hormone replacement therapy and is planning to adopt her next child.

Blood Deficiency Amenorrhea

When Blood deficiency causes ovulatory disturbance it is usually associated with Kidney Yin (and sometimes Kidney Jing) deficiency. In some cases, amenorrhea follows loss of large amounts of blood after hemorrhage (e.g., after termination of pregnancy, miscarriage or childbirth) or is a result of a severely compromised Spleen function. Such damage may occur to the Spleen if there is undue physical strain, e.g., young women training intensively in sport, long periods of overwork and/or under-nutrition, or after long-term illness.

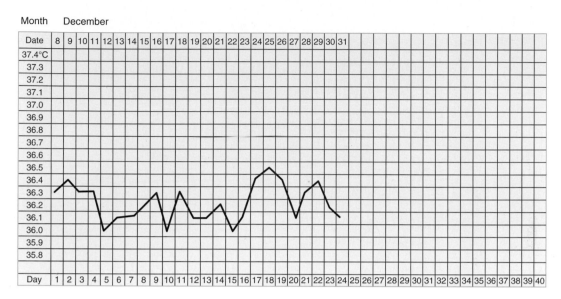

Figure 5.3 Case history – Mary. This 24-day cycle was anovulatory.

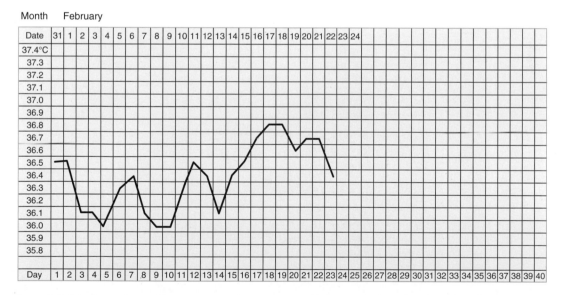

Figure 5.4 Case history – Mary. The short luteal phase indicates Kidney Yang deficiency (from Kidney Yin deficiency).

Treatment principally focuses on diet, with an emphasis on iron-rich and other Blood-building foods (discussed in Ch. 12). A sensible balance between rest and exertion is advised. There are no absolutes here: it depends very much on the individual constitution. However, if it is lifestyle that has contributed to the loss of periods, then the inappropriate behavior must be rectified.

Herbal Formula — The doctor will prescribe Blood-nourishing formulas, e.g., the famous tonic Ba Zhen Tang, to which herbs are often added to strengthen the Kidneys and calm the mind.

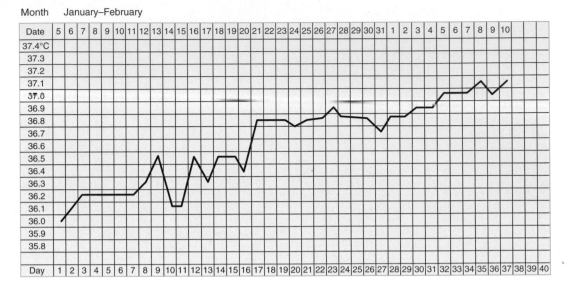

Figure 5.5 Case history – Mary. Once Mary's BBT charts began to reliably show a typical ovulatory pattern, she quickly became pregnant.

Ba Zhen Tang (Eight Precious decoction) modified

Dang Gui	9 g	Radix Angelicae Sinensis
Shu Di	9 g	Radix Rehmanniae Glutinosae Conquitae
Bai Shao	9 g	Radix Paeoniae Lactiflorae
Chuan Xiong	6 g	Radix Ligustici Wallichii
Dang Shen	12 g	Radix Codonopsis Pilulosae
Dan Shen	9 g	Radix Salviae Miltiorrhizae
Bai Zi Ren	9 g	Semen Biotae Orientalis
Bai Zhu	9 g	Rhizoma Atractylodis Macrocephalae
Fu Ling	9 g	Sclerotium Poriae Cocos
Tu Si Zi	12 g	Semen Cuscatae
Sang Ji Sheng	12 g	Ramulus Sangjisheng
Xiang Fu	9 g	Rhizoma Cyperi Rotundi
Gan Cao (zhi)	3 g	Radix Glycyrrhizae Uralensis

The first four herbs constitute the Blood tonic portion of Ba Zhen Tang and to these we add Sang Ji Sheng, because not only does it further nourish the Blood but it also supplements Liver and Kidney Yin. The Kidney Yin supplementing function of Sang Ji Sheng combined with the Kidney Yang boosting function of Tu Si Zi will promote ovulation once Blood levels are sufficient. Dan Shen and Bai Zi Ren are included in the modifications to this formula because the integrity of the Heart Blood is of paramount importance for ovulation. Dang Shen, Bai Zhu, Fu Ling and Gan Cao (zhi) are the Qi tonic portion of Ba Zhen Tang. Xiang Fu is added to encourage movement of the Qi, which is especially important as the ovaries and tubes become functional again. Depending on the severity of the Blood deficiency, treatment may need to continue for 6 months or more. As signs of a menstrual cycle return, the skilful doctor will immediately start subtly altering the formulas to address Kidney Yin and Yang according to the appropriate stage of follicle and endometrium development. The patient will be

Table 5.13   Acupuncture points[a] used in the treatment of amenorrhea due to Blood deficiency

Treatment goal	Acupuncture points
To reinforce Spleen function to produce Blood	Ren-12, ST-36, BL-20 and SP-6
To activate Qi in the Chong vessel	KI-13 and ST-30
To supplement Heart Blood and calm the mind	HE-7

[a]Reinforcing method is applied to all points.

advised to wait until a regular cycle is well established before attempting pregnancy. However, for a woman who has had long-term amenorrhea an opportunity to conceive is very hard to resist.

Acupuncture Points — As was the case with treating amenorrhea due to Kidney Yin deficiency, acupuncture to treat Blood deficiency plays a secondary role to herbal and dietary therapy. Points which regulate the Chong and Ren vessels are useful but only when there are already sufficient Blood resources to fill the Chong vessel. Acupuncture to encourage fertility in these cases is best employed to strengthen Spleen function and calm the mind, e.g. (and see Table 5.13):

Ren-12	Zhongwan
ST-36	Zusanli
SP-6	Sanyinjiao
BL-20	Pishu
KI-13	Qixue
ST-30	Qichong
HE-7	Shenmen

CASE HISTORY – CHLOE

Chloe at 36 years of age had a long history of intermittent amenorrhea. Her periods didn't start until age 21, probably not because of inherent lack of Tian Gui or Kidney Jing but because she was training such long hours as a gymnast throughout her adolescence. When her menstrual cycle finally began it was regular for about 1 year until she traveled overseas to compete. For the next year and a half she had no periods and it was only when she retired from gymnastics (age 24) that her cycle returned. However, it didn't return very convincingly; she had long or short periods of amenorrhea over the next 12 years and never experienced a monthly cycle. This had not really bothered her in the past but now she wanted to have a baby. She had not had a period for 8 months.

She decided to look into the situation further. Her blood tests were normal, so there was nothing her gynecologist could suggest, except fertility drugs. Before trying these, she thought she'd see what Chinese medicine could offer. It was indeed lucky she did; should she have taken clomifene, the chances are that she would have ovulated and fallen pregnant fairly quickly (because Kidney deficiency was not her main problem) but she was not yet in any shape to nourish herself or a baby throughout a pregnancy.

She looked very pale and was thin. She still trained many hours a day, now as a personal trainer. Her diet was strictly vegetarian but she ate regularly. Her sleep quality was poor, very restless and disturbed by too many dreams. She described herself as easily excited and she experienced anxiety.

Her periods, when they came, were preceded by sore breasts, bloating and emotional volatility. The flow was dark and clotty but with little pain, except a backache. She sometimes saw fertile mucus a couple of weeks before she would bleed. Her circulation was poor, causing cold hands and feet. Her digestive system was sensitive and she often felt wind pain. Chloe's tongue was pale and fluted but had a red tip. Her pulses were thready.

Her diagnosis was clearly Blood deficiency amenorrhea. In particular it was deficiency of Heart Blood that caused not only her sleeplessness but also affected the Bao vessel (see later), interfering with ovulation. She took herbs to build her Blood, invigorate her Spleen function and support her Kidney Yang. In addition, it was important she ease back a little on her very demanding schedule of physical workouts and she was encouraged to eat more protein. Acupuncture was administered to regulate the Chong and Ren vessels and support Spleen and Kidneys.

Shu Di	12g	Radix Rehmanniae Glutinosae Conquitae
Dang Gui	12g	Radix Angelicae Sinensis
Bai Shao	12g	Radix Paeoniae Lactiflorae
Dan Shen	6g	Radix Salviae Miltiorrhizae
Dang Shen	9g	Radix Codonopsis Pilulosae
Huang Qi	9g	Radix Astragali
Fu Ling	9g	Sclerotium Poriae Cocos
Sha Ren	6g	Fructus seu Semen Amomi
Bu Gu Zhi	9g	Fructus Psoraleae
Yin Yang Huo	9g	Herba Epimedii
Mu Li	15g	Concha Ostreae
Bai Zi Ren	12g	Semen Biotae Orientalis
Suan Zao Ren	12g	Semen Ziziphi Spinosae

Acupuncture points: Ren-7, Ren-4 and Ren-3, PC-6, HE-7, SP-6

As is often the case where Kidney deficiency is not the prime disorder, a result was achieved quickly. Within 2 weeks she had a period, though the flow was still dark and brownish. Acupuncture will often induce an ovulation in cases where there is minor dysfunction of the Bao vessel, so this was not yet evidence that a regular cycle was returning. However, when another period came 6 weeks later (she had continued with the herbs but had had no more acupuncture), we could feel more confident that her Blood status was improving and that the Bao vessel communication with the Uterus was operating better.

As her periods became more regular and her sleep and emotional state started to stabilize, we added more support for the Kidneys in the form of Gui Shao Di Huang wan and variations of this in preparation for a pregnancy. She started to eat some animal protein in the form of eggs.

Within a few months she was pregnant and carried her baby to a healthy term.

Amenorrhea from obstruction is a result of stagnation of Heart or Liver Qi, Phlegm-Damp accumulation and Blood stasis.

Periods that cease because they are blocked or obstructed in some way tend to stop quite suddenly compared with periods which stop because of deficiency. In this latter case, the periods may become irregular, infrequent or scanty before stopping.

Chinese medicine treatment of obstruction or stagnation affords rapid results if the stagnation is not too long term and hasn't created other pathologies. However, the stagnation which causes amenorrhea often presents what appears to be a complex clinical picture.

Stagnation of Heart Qi Amenorrhea

Heart Qi becomes stagnant if there is undue or prolonged mental stress or anguish. Apart from disturbance of ovulation, symptoms such as insomnia and much dreaming, palpitations, anxiety, fear or sadness and restlessness may manifest. The role of Heart Qi in ovulation was discussed briefly in Chapter 2 and is revisited here in more detail. There are two ways that the Heart is considered of great importance for ovulation.

The first is the fact that the Heart, with the Kidney, is considered to play an important role in maintaining the balance of Yin and Yang. Here we are concerned specifically with Kidney Yin and Kidney Yang. If the

Heart maintains a harmonious relationship with the Kidney, then it is said that Fire and Water are balanced and therefore the Yin and Yang are balanced. It is only in such circumstances that the menstrual cycle, with its constant growth and ebb of Yin to Yang and Yang to Yin operates effectively. If the Heart Qi does not flow freely, then this important regulation of Yin and Yang can be affected. In terms of the menstrual cycle, the transformation of Yin to Yang may be disrupted and ovulation will fail.

The second way that the Heart is thought to influence ovulation is via the Bao vessel, which was discussed earlier (Ch. 2). The Heart Qi must travel to the Uterus to control its opening. If Heart Qi is stagnant, the Uterus will not open – in other words, ovulation does not occur.

Both these aspects of Heart function therefore represent the hypothalamic and pituitary control of the ovarian cycle. Amenorrhea caused by Heart Qi stagnation falls specifically into the Western medical category of hypothalamic anovulation.

Most of the amenorrhea that has an emotional basis will fall into the Heart Qi stagnation category but there are some special cases which are related more to Liver Qi stagnation and some which are related to both Liver and Heart Qi stagnation.

Herbal Formula — To treat and disperse Heart Qi stagnation, calm the mind and regulate menstruation use Bai Zi Ren Wan with extra sedative herbs.

Bai Zi Ren Wan (Biota pill) modified

Bai Zi Ren	9 g	Semen Biotae Orientalis
Dan Shen	9 g	Radix Salviae Miltiorrhizae
Xu Duan	9 g	Radix Dipsaci
Shu Di	9 g	Radix Rehmanniae Glutinosae Conquitae
Chuan Niu Xi	9 g	Radix Cyathulae
Ze Lan	9 g	Herba Lycopi Lucidi
Yu Jin	9 g	Tuber Curcumae
He Huan Pi	9 g	Cortex Albizziae Julibrissin
Yuan Zhi	6 g	Radix Polygalae Tenuifoliae
Fu Ling	9 g	Sclerotium Poriae Cocos

In this formula, the herbs Bai Zi Ren, He Huan Pi and Yuan Zhi calm the spirit. Dan Shen, Yu Jin, Chuan Niu Xi, and Ze Lan, keep Heart Blood moving, Shu Di reinforces the Yin and the Blood while Fu Ling supports the Spleen Qi. Xu Duan boosts Kidney Yang, which will help to promote ovulation.

Acupuncture Points — The following points are used (and see Table 5.14):

PC-5	Jianshi
PC-6	Neiguan
HE-7	Shenmen
KI-19	Yindu
SP-6	Sanyinjiao
KI-3	Taixi
Abdomen Zigong	

Qi Gong, yoga, meditation or stress-reducing techniques are an important adjunct to the treatment. If the Heart stagnation has not caused damage to the Kidney Yin and Yang, then resolution of the stagnation will be enough to re-establish a regular menstrual cycle. In some cases, however, treatment to reinforce Kidney Yin and promote Kidney Yang (see Ch. 4) will be necessary to ensure that the cycle continues in a regular fashion and that fertility is optimal.

Table 5.14 Acupuncture points[a] used in the treatment of amenorrhea due to stagnation of Heart Qi

Treatment goal	Acupuncture points
To calm the spirit, open the Bao vessel and regulate Qi in the chest	PC-5
To calm the spirit and soothe the Heart	PC-6
To regulate Qi around the ovaries	Abdomen Zigong
To calm the spirit and treat dream disturbed sleep	HE-7
To supplement Kidney Yin (Water) to maintain balance between Heart-Fire and Kidney Water	KI-3 and SP-6
To regulate Heart Qi and the Chong vessel	KI-19

[a]All points are used with even or reducing method.

CASE HISTORY – SALLYANNE

Sallyanne's amenorrhea was a combination of Heart Qi stagnation and Kidney deficiency. While puberty came when she had just turned 13, it disappeared just as quickly with the shock of losing her mother in a car accident. Her family life was very difficult after this.

Over the years she had tried many different hormone treatments, none of which provided her with a regular menstrual cycle. Her general health was good, though she showed signs of Heart Qi disturbance. Her sleep was unsettled. She was an anxious and talkative patient who suffered from palpitations. At 29 when she consulted me, she hadn't had a period for some years.

Her pulse was rapid and slightly choppy; her tongue had a red tip.

She was given herbs to nourish Heart Blood, calm the Shen and resolve Heart Qi stagnation and promote Kidney function:

Bai Zi Ren	15 g	Semen Biotae Orientalis
Dan Shen	12 g	Radix Salviae Miltiorrhizae
Shu Di	9 g	Radix Rehmanniae Glutinosae Conquitae
Dang Gui	9 g	Radix Angelicae Sinensis
Bai Shao	9 g	Radix Paeoniae Lactiflorae
Gou Qi Zi	9 g	Fructus Lycii Chinensis
He Shou Wu	9 g	Radix Polygoni Multiflori
Chuan Niu Xi	9 g	Radix Cyathulae
Xu Duan	9 g	Radix Dipsaci
Ba Ji Tian	6 g	Radix Morindae Officinalis
Tu Si Zi	9 g	Semen Cuscatae
Mu Li	15 g	Concha Ostreae
Ye Jiao Teng	15 g	Caulis Polygoni Multiflori
He Huan Pi	9 g	Cortex Albizziae Julibrissin

Acupuncture points: HE-7, PC-6, KI-19, SP-6, KI-3, Abdomen Zigong

She took the herbs and had acupuncture for about 1 month before her periods returned. Her periods came monthly for the following 8 months, during which time she continued to have acupuncture but preferred not to take the herbs. Because the main reason for her amenorrhea was obstruction rather than deficiency, acupuncture proved to be effective therapy. Her menstrual cycle continued regularly when she discontinued treatment.

Stagnation of Liver Qi Amenorrhea

Liver Qi can become stagnant and lead to amenorrhea if there is prolonged frustration, irritability or depression. High levels of stress or life changes such as moving countries or a lot of traveling can cause periods to disappear in prone individuals. Amenorrhea related to Liver Qi stagnation can also occur after long-term breast-feeding (more than 1 year is considered long term if the mother's constitution is not strong). The use of certain drugs, including antipsychotic agents such as chlorpromazine (Largactil) and the oral contraceptive pill, can also precipitate amenorrhea. When the Liver Qi is obstructed, it can give rise to Liver-Fire, weaken the Spleen and Stomach function and exacerbate any underlying Kidney Yin deficiency. If the Liver-Fire invades the Stomach channel, it can force the menstrual Blood upwards, which then appears as milk secretion from the nipples. If the Stomach and Spleen are affected, there may also be anorexia.

The diagnosis of amenorrhea caused by Liver Qi stagnation is indicated if the patient's history includes drug taking or oral contraceptive pill use (see also section on PCOS, below) or if there are abnormal breast secretions and pathology test results indicate high prolactin levels in the blood. The diagnosis of Liver Qi stagnation should be confirmed by the presence of symptoms such as chest stuffiness (sometimes with breast soreness), agitation and irritability and a wiry pulse.

Liver Qi stagnation can contribute to infertility in a number of ways other than disturbing ovulation (see Blockage of the fallopian tubes, Ch. 6). Amenorrhea of the Liver Qi stagnation type includes those in the hyperprolactinemia category, post-pill amenorrhea and that caused by some tumors.

Herbal Formula — The best results in treating Liver Qi stagnation amenorrhea are achieved with a formula which will regulate the Liver Qi, clear Liver-Fire and nourish Liver Yin. The well-known formula, Dan Zhi Xiao Yao San, can be used with the addition of herbs which nourish the Liver.

Dan Zhi Xiao Yao San (Moutan Gardenia Free and Easy powder) modified

Dang Gui	9 g	Radix Angelicae Sinensis
Bai Shao	12 g	Radix Paeoniae Lactiflorae
Fu Ling	12 g	Sclerotium Poriae Cocos
Bai Zhu	9 g	Rhizoma Atractylodis Macrocephalae
Chai Hu	9 g	Radix Bupleuri
Mu Dan Pi	9 g	Cortex Moutan Radicis
Zhi Zi	6 g	Fructus Gardeniae Jasminoidis
Gan Cao	6 g	Radix Glycyrrhizae Uralensis
Shan Zhu Yu	9 g	Fructus Corni Officinalis
Bo He	3 g	Herba Menthae
Sheng Jiang	3 g	Rhizoma Zingiberis Officinalis Recens

Shan Zhu Yu is sour in flavor and therefore is nourishing to the Liver. Bai Shao and Gan Cao also nourish the Liver. Mu Dan Pi and Zhi Zi clear Liver-Fire, Chai Hu regulates Liver Qi. Bai Zhu and Fu Ling support the Spleen and Dang Gui nourishes the Blood. Sheng Jiang and Bo He are envoy herbs which help to prevent Qi rising or being obstructed.

A stronger treatment for Liver Qi stagnation and one which is preferred by specialists in the gynecology department in the Jiangsu Province Hospital is Yi Ru San. This formula is more effective than the above if there is hyperprolactinemia causing lactation.

Yi Ru San (Benefiting the Breast powder)

Chuan Bei Mu	6 g	Bulbus Fritillariae Cirrhosae
Bai Shao	9 g	Radix Paeoniae Lactiflorae

Qing Pi	6 g	*Pericarpium Citri Reticulatae Viride*
Gou Teng	9 g	*Ramulus Uncariae Cum Uncis*
Chuan Niu Xi	9 g	*Radix Cyathulae*
Mu Li	15 g	*Concha Ostreae*
Mai Ya	30 g	*Fructus Hordei*
Chuan Lian Zi	9 g	*Fructus Meliae Toosendan*

This formula, which is based on Hua Gan Jian (Transforming Liver decoction), regulates the Liver Qi and restricts lactation. Chuan Bei Mu has a specific action of relieving Liver Qi constriction affecting the chest and the breasts. Bai Shao nourishes Blood and soothes the Liver. Qing Pi and Chuan Lian Zi help to remove Liver Qi stagnation while Gou Teng pacifies any rising Liver Qi. Mu Li also restrains rising Liver Yang. Mai Ya is used in large doses to suppress lactation and relieve breast distension. Chuan Niu Xi regulates and prevents Blood stagnation and encourages downward movement to help counteract rising Liver Yang.

Acupuncture Points — Acupuncture can be very effective in treating this sort of ovulatory disorder. Choose from the following points (and see Table 5.15):

LIV-2	Xingjian
LIV-8	Ququan
PC-7	Daling
PC-5	Jianshi
LIV-14	Qimen
ST-18	Rugen
ST-36	Zusanli
SP-4	Gongsun
Abdomen Zigong	

Table 5.15 Acupuncture points[a] used in the treatment of amenorrhea (including hyperprolactinemia) caused by Liver Qi stagnation

Treatment goal	Acupuncture points
To regulate Liver Qi and drain Liver-Fire	LIV-2 and LIV-8
To move Liver Qi in the upper body and relieve pent up emotions and irritability	PC-7 and PC-5
To remove stagnation of Qi in the breasts and promote normal breast function (if there is inappropriate lactation)	LIV-14 and ST-18
To support Spleen and Stomach function	ST-36
To regulate Qi around the ovaries	Abdomen Zigong
To activate the Chong vessel	SP-4

[a]Points are needled with reducing or even method.

• Hyperprolactinemia-related anovulation

In the experience of infertility specialists in China, hyperprolactinemia is mainly related to Liver Qi stagnation and rarely to Kidney deficiency. This is one of the few types of infertility where treatment will be directed simply and only at clearing stagnation. Once stagnation is cleared, then it is expected the Kidney Yin and Yang and the Chong and Ren vessels will function to produce a cycle. This is certainly the experience of Western specialists who find drug treatment of hyperprolactinemia anovulation quickly re-establishes a cycle and fertility.

However, for the TCM doctor to really succeed, s/he needs to address not only the prolactin in the blood but also its source. If the source is a substantial tumor in the pituitary gland, then treatment with Chinese herbs and acupuncture may not produce such rapid and effective results as will giving bromocriptine. If it is pregnancy which is the desired outcome, then there is good reason to consider this drug treatment; the ovulation thus achieved is not likely to produce inferior eggs because in most uncomplicated cases of hyperprolactinemia there is no Kidney deficiency. On the other hand, if there is no pituitary tumor or pregnancy is not desired immediately, then trying to establish a cycle by removing the Liver Qi obstruction with formulas and acupuncture points just mentioned may be preferable to administration of bromocriptine.

Better results can be expected in the treatment of Liver Qi stagnation amenorrhea with herbs and acupuncture when there is no Liver-Fire and prolactin levels are not high.

• Post-pill amenorrhea

Post-pill amenorrhea is defined as the failure of a menstrual cycle to return within 6 months of discontinuing the oral contraceptive pill (OCP). The pill interrupts natural body cycles so it is easy to see why the Liver Qi (which is fundamental to regular body rhythms) is affected. In some women, this effect lasts after the pill has been stopped, i.e., the cycles do not easily re-establish themselves. In certain individuals, long term use of the oral contraceptive pill may interfere with some metabolic pathways and contribute to the development of PCOS which only becomes evident after the pill is stopped. We shall discuss this and the effect the OCP has on carbohydrate metabolism and Spleen function when we discuss PCOS below.

Dan Zhi Xiao Yao San modified (see above) is applicable in many cases of simple post-pill amenorrhea with the correct presentation. Additionally, a number of women develop Liver Blood deficiency as a result of the inhibition of natural Liver function. This is another reason that periods do not return for some time.

Herbal Formula — In this case, more Blood tonics could be added to Dan Zhi Xiao Yao San modified, e.g.

Ji Xue Teng	15 g	*Radix et Caulis Jixueteng*
Shu Di	9 g	*Radix Rehmanniae Glutinosae Conquitae*

In Chapter 3, we discussed the effect that the pill has on the production of fertile mucus even after it has been discontinued. The Liver channel's pathway passes through the cervix and stagnation of the Qi can contribute to the disruption of the function of the glands responsible for fertile mucus production.

Acupuncture Points — Acupuncture to move the Qi in the Liver channel is useful in helping re-establish cervical gland function. Choose from the following points (and see Table 5.16):

LIV-1	Dadun
LIV-5	Ligou
LIV-8	Ququan
LIV-11	Yinlian
Ren-3	Zhongji
Ren-1	Huiyin
ST-30	Qichong

Table 5.16   Acupuncture points[a] used in the treatment of post-pill amenorrhea related to Liver Qi stagnation

Treatment goal	Acupuncture points
To regulate Qi in the reproductive tract, especially the cervix	LIV-1, LIV-5 and LIV-8
To regulate Qi in the Uterus	LIV-11
To encourage Qi movement and regulate function of glands in the cervix	Ren-3
To reinforce the movement of Qi in the lower abdomen and genital area	ST-30 and Ren-1

[a]Even method needling is appropriate.

Phlegm-Damp Accumulation Amenorrhea

The pathology and etiology of amenorrhea that results from Phlegm-Damp is complex and will be discussed more in the section on PCOS, below. Phlegm-Damp can arise through poor eating habits, especially of rich and sweet foods, or from an inherited weakness of internal organs or disruption in their function by Qi or Blood stagnation.

Amenorrhea associated with weight gain is always indicative of Phlegm-Damp accumulation. However, determining the origin of the Phlegm-Damp requires diagnostic skill and not all such accumulations will manifest as obvious weight gain. There are three pathologic patterns that are most often associated with Phlegm-Damp-type amenorrhea. The first two of these correspond with patterns seen in polycystic ovary syndrome (PCOS) and will be discussed in detail in the next section.

- *Kidney and Spleen deficiency*: most commonly it is a combination of weak Kidney and Spleen function which allows Damp to accumulate, leading to pathogenic obstruction by Phlegm-Damp. Weight gain often accompanies this pattern.

- *Liver Qi stagnation*: Phlegm-Damp can also accumulate if Liver Qi stagnation leads to obstruction of Qi and Blood flow in the Liver, Chong, Ren or Dai vessels creating the conditions for accumulation of Damp obstructions. Liver Qi stagnation will often compromise Spleen and Stomach function and metabolism becomes inefficient as a result.

Minor weight gain may be noticed or the deposition of Phlegm-Damp may be less obvious if it is just layered around the abdominal organs or the ovaries but does not cause marked increase in waist measurement.

- *Blood stagnation*: this stagnation takes the form of tumors, fibroids or cysts, which can obstruct the normal circulation of Qi and fluids, giving rise to Phlegm-Damp.

For Phlegm-Damp accumulation with Spleen/Kidney deficiency and Phlegm-Damp accumulation with Liver Qi stagnation, see PCOS section below.

• Phlegm-Damp accumulation with Blood stagnation

Amenorrhea in this category can usually be traced to a tumor. In the case that tumors are contributing to (or are the result of) Phlegm-Damp, then surgery is often an efficient solution. Once the tumor is removed, then Phlegm-Damp is addressed with the type of Damp-clearing formulas covered earlier.

Herbal Formula — If surgery is not appropriate, then a formula which combines herbs to move stagnant Blood and Phlegm-Damp can be used.

Cang Fu Dao Tan Tang (Atractylodes Cyperus Phlegm decoction) modified

Cang Zhu	15 g	*Rhizoma Atractylodes*
Xiang Fu	9 g	*Rhizoma Cyperi Rotundi*
Ban Xia	9 g	*Rhizoma Pinelliae*

Fu Ling	15g	*Sclerotium Poriae Cocos*
Chen Pi	6g	*Pericarpium Citri Reticulate*
Dan Nan Xing	6g	*Rhizoma Arisaematis*
Zhi Ke	6g	*Fructus Citri seu Ponciri*
Gan Cao	3g	*Radix Glycyrrhizae Uralensis*
Sheng Jiang	3 slices	*Rhizoma Zingiberis Officinalis Recens*
Shen Qu	6g	*Massa Fermenta*
Chuan Xiong	6g	*Radix Ligustici Wallichii*
Chuan Niu Xi	9g	*Radix Cyathulae*
San Leng	6g	*Rhizoma Sparganii*
E Zhu	6g	*Rhizoma Curcumae Zedoariae*
Ze Lan	6g	*Herba Lycopi Lucidi*

This formula clears Phlegm-Damp and with the additional Blood-invigorating herbs, San Leng, E Zhu and Ze Lan, will also break up accumulations of stagnant Blood.

Acupuncture Points — Points (Table 5.17) are chosen from:

LIV-8	Ququan
SP-10	Xuehai
KI-14	Siman
KI-18	Shiguan
KI-19	Yindu
SP-12	Chongmen
ST-29	Guilai
ST-28	Shuidao
Ren-3	Zhongji
SP-9	Yinlingquan
SP-5	Shangqui
KI-5	Shuiquan

If evidence remains of Qi stagnation or Kidney weakness after the removal of Blood and Phlegm-Damp stagnation, then this must be addressed using the relevant formulas described above.

Table 5.17   Acupuncture points[a] used in the treatment of amenorrhea due to Phlegm-Damp accumulation with Blood stagnation

Treatment goal	Acupuncture points
To clear local stagnation of Blood in the abdomen	ST-28, ST-29 and SP-12
To remove stagnation of Blood in the Chong vessel	KI-14, KI-18 and KI-19
To clear both Blood stagnation and Phlegm-Damp accumulation in the lower Jiao	LIV-8
To facilitate movement of Blood	SP-10
To clear Damp from the lower Jiao	SP-9 and SP-5, Ren-3
To promote ovulation, which is delayed or disrupted due to Blood stagnation	KI-5

[a]Points are needled with reducing or even method.

Blood stasis of the type related to tumors in the ovaries or other glands is not common and is best treated with surgery.

Iatrogenic causes of this type of amenorrhea are less rare, particularly those that result after repeated or over enthusiastic D&Cs, which cause adhesions affecting the lining of the uterus and block menstrual flow (Asherman syndrome). Surgery may be required to remove these obstructions, but Chinese herbs are helpful in recovering the integrity of the endometrium.

Herbal Formula — If there are signs of persistent Blood stagnation type pain (and this is often the case after surgery) then well-known formulas like Xue Fu Zhu Yu Tang or Shao Fu Zhu Yu Tang are used.

Xue Fu Zhu Yu Tang (Decoction for Removing Blood Stasis in the Chest) modified

Tao Ren	12g	Semen Persicae
Hong Hua	9g	Flos Carthami Tinctorii
Dang Gui	9g	Radix Angelicae Sinensis
Chuan Xiong	6g	Radix Ligustici Wallichii
Chi Shao	9g	Radix Paeoniae Rubra
Chuan Niu Xi	9g	Radix Cyathulae
Chai Hu	6g	Radix Bupleuri
Yi Mu Cao	9g	Herba Leonuri Heterophylli
Xiang Fu	9g	Rhizoma Cyperi Rotundi
Zhi Ke	9g	Fructus Citri seu Ponciri
Sheng Di	9g	Radix Rehmanniae Glutinosae
Gan Cao	3g	Radix Glycyrrhizae Uralensis

This formula invigorates Blood circulation, removes stasis and alleviates pain. The first six herbs regulate Blood, while Chai Hu and Zhi Ke ensure there is no Qi obstruction. Sheng Di will clear any Heat in the Blood which might develop as a result of stagnation. By replacing Jie Geng in the original formula with Yi Mu Cao and Xiang Fu, Blood and Qi stasis in the abdomen will be targeted.

Shao Fu Zhu Yu Tang (Lower Abdomen Eliminating Stasis decoction)

Dang Gui	9g	Radix Angelicae Sinensis
Chuan Xiong	9g	Radix Ligustici Wallichii
Chi Shao	9g	Radix Paeoniae Rubra
Xiao Hui Xiang	6g	Fructus Foeniculi Vulgaris
Yan Hu Suo	6g	Rhizoma Corydalis Yanhusuo
Wu Ling Zhi	6g	Excrementum Trogopterori
Mo Yao	6g	Myrrha
Rou Gui	6g	Cortex Cinnamomi Cassiae
Gan Jiang	6g	Rhizoma Zingiberis Officinalis
Pu Huang	9g	Pollen Typhae

This formula also invigorates Blood circulation and alleviates pain, especially that caused by Cold. Dang Gui, Chuan Xiong, Chi Shao, Yan Hu Suo, Wu Ling Zhi, Mo Yao and Pu Huang all have an action on Blood stasis, whereas Rou Gui, Xiao Hui Xiang and Gan Jiang will resolve any Cold contributing to the stasis.

In the case of Asherman syndrome or damage to the uterine lining, then 3g Ru Xiang (Resina Olibani) will be added.

Table 5.18   Acupuncture points[a] used in the treatment of amenorrhea from Blood stasis

Treatment goal	Acupuncture points
To regulate Qi and Blood in the lower abdomen and specifically the uterus	ST-29
To clear Blood stagnation in the Chong vessel	KI-14 and KI-19
To regulate Blood in the uterus	SP-10 and SP-6
Useful in the treatment of all Blood disorders	BL-17

[a]Use reducing technique; ST-29 can also be used with moxa.

Acupuncture Points — Points (Table 5.18) are chosen from:

ST-29	Guilai
KI-14	Siman
KI-19	Yindu
SP-10	Xuehai
SP-6	Sanyinjiao
BL-17	Geshu

CASE HISTORY – RUBY

Ruby (36 years) had had no periods for 2½ years. The amenorrhea dated from a pregnancy which was terminated under great duress and with great distress. She saw another herbalist who gave her strong-tasting Chinese herbs for nearly 6 months. She tried acupuncture and her doctor checked the hormone levels with blood tests, which gave normal readings. She described cyclical abdomen, breast and mood changes and described sharp pain low in her abdomen. She was bothered a lot by skin rashes but otherwise was in very good health. Her pulses were unremarkable but her tongue was pale with a mauve hue. I surmised that the diagnosis of Ruby's amenorrhea was Blood stagnation given her history, and that further investigation was required. A gynecologist ordered a hysterosalpingogram, but when no dye could be inserted, arranged for surgery to remove all the adhesions sticking Ruby's uterus together. Ruby then took herbs to help clear the old menstrual blood that had been unable to escape the uterus and to help build a new endometrium:

Tao Ren	9g	Semen Persicae
Hong Hua	6g	Flos Carthami Tinctorii
Dang Gui	9g	Radix Angelicae Sinensis
Chi Shao	9g	Radix Paeoniae Rubra
Chuan Xiong	6g	Radix Ligustici Wallichii
Shu Di	9g	Radix Rehmanniae Glutinosae Conquitae

Acupuncture points: SP-10, SP-6, ST-29, LIV-2, CO-4

After flushing out a lot of old blood, Ruby's periods returned healthy and regular. Her skin improved too, once the stagnation was removed.

Table 5.19   Correlation of TCM amenorrhea categories and Western medical diseases or conditions

TCM category	Disease or condition
Kidney Jing deficiency	Resistant ovary disease
	Primary ovarian failure
	Polycystic ovary syndrome
Kidney Yin deficiency	Premature menopause
	Long-term illness
	Weight loss
	Severe hemorrhage
	Polycystic ovary syndrome
Blood deficiency	Malnutrition or undernutrition
	Excessive exercise
	Hemorrhage after miscarriage, abortion or childbirth
Heart or Liver Qi stagnation	Shock or extreme stress
	Hyperprolactinemia
	Post-pill amenorrhea
	Drug use
	Polycystic ovary syndrome
Phlegm-Damp accumulation	Polycystic ovary syndrome
	Ovarian cysts
Blood stasis	Asherman syndrome
	Pituitary, ovarian or adrenal tumor

Table 5.19 summarizes and correlates TCM amenorrhea categories and Western medical diseases or conditions.

POLYCYSTIC OVARIAN SYNDROME

Polycystic ovarian syndrome is one of the most common disorders of ovulation that we see in our clinics today. It is a multifaceted disorder affecting endocrine, nervous and cardiovascular systems and has many metabolic repercussions and clinical manifestations. Our understanding of the primary etiology for this disorder is incomplete, however its clinical manifestations and signs are well described. We shall spend some time examining the clinical presentations of PCOS, and what we currently know about its endocrinologic and metabolic basis, so that we can begin to construct a TCM analysis that will give us a framework from which we can design appropriate treatment.

On the one hand, we can approach the treatment of PCOS with the sole aim of trying to increase ovulation frequency (and thus increase opportunities for conception) and on the other hand, with a more thorough analysis, we can attempt a broader approach to treatment that takes into account all the ramifications of this syndrome, including ovary dysfunction. This latter approach may also have a more far reaching impact on the function of the ovaries and the quality of the eggs therein, other than just increasing frequency of ovulation.

Defining PCOS: Clinical Presentation and Diagnosis

Polycystic ovary syndrome (PCOS) is the name given to the syndrome in which the ovaries appear to be covered with many small cysts on ultrasound (and likened poetically to a string of pearls), the menstrual cycles are long or irregular with infrequent ovulations and there are signs, such as more than usual body hair or acne, of excess circulating androgens. The syndrome is also linked with an increased incidence of diabetes and other metabolic disorders and pregnancy complications such as pre-eclampsia. Not all women with polycystic ovary syndrome will present the same way or have the same symptoms or laboratory findings.

This syndrome is the commonest endocrinopathy and the most common cause of anovulatory female infertility in Australia and other developed nations with a prevalence of approximately 9% of Australian women and 21% of Australian indigenous women of reproductive age.[31] Some 9–15% of women in living in Europe have PCOS and an estimated 6–7 million women living in America have PCOS. As these figures attest, PCOS is a common disorder, and the frequency with which it is turning up in fertility clinics appears to be increasing.

Until the etiology of PCOS is clarified, diagnosis is made according to clinical manifestations. To receive a diagnosis of PCOS a woman must have two of the following symptoms or signs (according to the Rotterdam consensus 2003 criteria):

- Polycystic ovary morphology on ultrasound (defined as more than 12 follicles, size 2–9 mm on each or one ovary and/or swollen ovaries measuring more than 9 mL in volume

- Infrequent, irregular or no ovulation – cycles longer than 35 days or fewer than nine periods a year

- Hirsutism (unwanted hair growth), acne, male pattern hair loss, or evidence of elevated androgens on blood test.

Blood tests may reveal elevated levels of insulin, testosterone, dehydroepiandrosterone sulfate (DHEAS), estrogen, luteinizing hormone (LH), inhibin, anti-Mullerian hormone (AMH), fibrinogen and adipokines and reduced levels of sex hormone binding globulin (SHBG) and adiponectin.

The phenotype (expression of the disease) varies from mild to severe. For example, menstrual patterns can vary depending on the severity of the hormone disturbance, from no ovulations at all (amenorrhea or erratic anovulatory bleeding) to slightly irregular ovulations (long cycles or oligomenorrhea).

Some women show polycystic ovaries (PCO) or polycystic appearing ovaries (PAO) on ultrasound but do not manifest the full-blown syndrome described above. Up to 60% of teenage girls have polycystic ovaries on ultrasound and many of their early menstrual cycles are anovulatory. As many as 20–25% of women of reproductive age will have polycystic ovaries on ultrasound, but no symptoms other than slightly irregular menstrual cycles. These women usually have no problem conceiving, although it may take a little longer than usual.

For women having no or very infrequent ovulations however, fertility is seriously diminished and most of our discussion in this chapter will focus on these women diagnosed with the full syndrome.

Etiology

- Genetics, epigenetics and uterine factors

- Androgens and folliculogenesis

- Insulin resistance and obesity

- Stress.

Although we know that PCOS is associated with morbid metabolic, endocrine and cardiovascular features, we do not yet fully understand its etiology. The two most consistent endocrine findings are elevated androgens and insulin. We shall discuss these and inherited and lifestyle factors below.

201

GENETICS, EPIGENETICS, UTERINE AND EARLY LIFE FACTORS

The heterogeneity of clinical and biochemical features in PCOS is likely explained by the interaction of a small number of (as yet unknown) genes with certain environmental factors. Likely candidates include genes that regulate ovarian hormone production or influence body mass index, adiposity or insulin sensitivity.

We see that PCOS tends to run in families and is possibly passed on by the father's genes. It is more likely to occur if there is a family history of type 2 diabetes or if there is early baldness (hyperandrogenism) in the men in the family.[32] In addition to the influence of inherited genes, there may also be predisposing factors operating in the womb during pregnancy (i.e., an epigenetic influence).

Diet during pregnancy may have a profound influence on future health of the adult and this is an area being researched extensively. We know little about dietary triggers in utero for the development of PCOS although some researchers have observed that Vit D deficiency in utero can predispose to the development of PCOS.[33]

In animal studies, offspring of sheep and monkeys exposed to testosterone have more PCOS characteristics and this observation is supported by data from human studies.

This has led some investigators to propose that genetically determined hypersecretion of androgens by the fetal ovary may result in many of the observed clinical and pathologic features of PCOS, and may program the pituitary to favor excess luteinizing hormone (LH) secretion, encouraging the abdominal adiposity that predisposes to insulin resistance.[34,35] Other researchers and clinicians feel that the primary genetic predisposition is to insulin resistance rather than androgen overproduction.[36]

Many women with PCOS were small babies. Such intrauterine growth retardation is in some cases associated with premature puberty in girls with PCOS[37] and may be linked with inherited defects in the theca cells of the ovary, which predisposes them to overproduce androgens.[38] Another factor which increases prenatal androgen levels and premature puberty is exposure in utero to commonly used pesticides.[39] This risk is unfortunately an escalating one in modern and developing nations, and is discussed further in Chapter 9.

Early life exposure to phytoestrogens in the form of soy-based infant formulas, has also been examined as a possible endocrine disruptor acting on ovaries at a very sensitive stage of development. Animal studies would indicate that avoidance of soy formulas and drinks is to be recommended, however human studies are limited and results are as yet not clear cut.[40]

ANDROGENS AND FOLLICULOGENESIS

Little is known about the regulation of pre-antral folliculogenesis in the normal ovary, let alone in the polycystic ovary, however there is emerging evidence of an intrinsic abnormality of folliculogenesis in the ovaries of women with PCOS that affects the very earliest, gonadotrophin independent, stages of follicle development.[41]

The result is lots of immature follicles (primary and early pre-antral follicles); a result of accelerated progression of primordial to primary and early antral follicles and/or a reduced rate of atresia of early antral follicles. Excess androgens are the probable cause of both these phenomena.[35]

INSULIN RESISTANCE

As discussed above, there appears to be genetically determined increased levels of androgens which exert their influence in utero (or prepuberty) and predispose to PCOS and possibly also a genetically determined predisposition to decreased insulin sensitivity. But genetics alone rarely dictates the course of a disease. Environment and lifestyle can also contribute to the development of this syndrome, as we will see when we discuss obesity below. In particular the development of insulin resistance has a major impact.

Humans are still genetically 'wired' to thrive on the habits of our ancestors, who consumed nutrient-rich foods, a diet low in carbohydrates and who sustained greater levels of movement and exercise than we do today. In many ways, our environment and lifestyles have evolved too rapidly for our bodies to keep pace. Unhealthy lifestyles and diet and genetic predisposition can cause the pancreas to overproduce insulin in an attempt to maintain normal blood glucose levels. The muscle cells (and others) are overwhelmed by this excess insulin and protect themselves by reducing the number of insulin receptor sites on their surface. The average healthy person has some 20 000 receptor sites per cell, while the average overweight woman with PCOS can have as few as 6000 on the cells of many of their tissues (Fig. 5.6).

Women with PCOS are thought to possess a selective resistance to insulin (within the liver or muscle tissue), whereas other organs, such as the ovaries, maintain normal sensitivity to insulin. The high levels of insulin in the blood stimulate the theca cells that surround the follicles in the ovary to enlarge and produce more than the usual amount of testosterone which interferes with ovary function and the menstrual cycle. Some researchers believe that hyperinsulinemia and abnormal carbohydrate metabolism not only contributes to ovarian dysfunction but also contributes to poor oocyte quality in those PCOS patients who do ovulate.

As long ago as 1996, the oral contraceptive pill was observed to contribute to deterioration in glucose tolerance and recent studies have confirmed an increased risk of developing insulin resistance in women with or without PCOS after taking the OCP.

For this reason and because of concerns over the metabolic effects of PCOS, it is recommended by many specialists that use of contraceptive pills be limited or avoided if possible. Transdermal and vaginal contraceptives have the same effect and Depo-Provera has a negative effect on weight, often causing up to 10 kg weight gain, which brings its own problems for fertility as discussed below.[42,43]

Insulin resistance and weight gain – apples and pears — The severity of the expression of PCOS can be affected by the percentage of body fat. Specialists in Australia report that at least half of their patients with PCOS are obese. (Obesity in women is defined as a waist measurement of 80 cm.) In Europe, 40–60% of PCOS patients are reported to be obese. In Asia, this percentage is lower and in the USA, the percentage is higher.

There is no doubt that obesity worsens the presentation of PCOS but it is also thought that PCOS itself confers a predisposition to obesity. However, it does not have to be extreme weight or obesity that causes a problem in women predisposed to PCOS. Sometimes it is the weight gain itself (even just 10% of body weight) can be enough to affect the ovaries. Excess weight around the abdomen is the pattern typical of PCOS patients and is the pattern associated with insulin resistance and other metabolic disorders. Waist-to-hip ratios are consistently higher (indicating increased abdominal fat mass) in both over weight or normal weight PCOS patients compared with women without this condition. Overweight women without PCOS tend rather to be heavier in the thighs and buttocks than the abdomen,[44] hence, the apple and pear analogy. Central obesity is an android pattern and likened to an apple shape, while the lower body weight gain is a gynoid fat distribution and likened to a pear shape. So we might ask why should a big stomach be more worrying than a big bottom? Many researchers think the

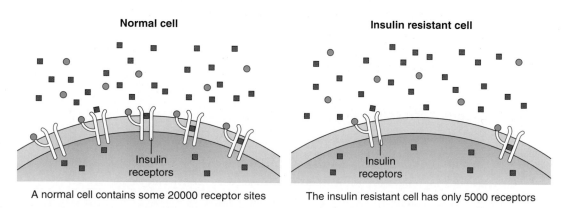

Normal cell

Insulin resistant cell

Insulin receptors

Insulin receptors

A normal cell contains some 20000 receptor sites

The insulin resistant cell has only 5000 receptors

● Insulin
■ Glucose

Figure 5.6 Insulin resistance prevents glucose entering the cells.

culprit is visceral fat, i.e., deposits of fat around the abdominal organs, as opposed to subcutaneous fat, under the skin. Visceral fat is more metabolically active than subcutaneous fat. Visceral fat has been measured by computed tomography X-ray (CT) scans or by dual energy X-ray absorptiometry (DEXA) scans, and shown to be linked to insulin resistance in both overweight and lean women with PCOS in most (but not all) studies.[45–47]

Whether there is abdominal obesity or not, we do know that the fat cells in PCOS patients are significantly larger than in women without PCOS. Also that adipose tissue behaves differently in PCOS, i.e., adiponectin, which is a circulating protein produced by adipocytes is reduced. This appears to be the case in both overweight and lean PCOS patients. These swollen adipocytes are more insulin resistant than regular sized ones, demonstrating how lean women with PCOS are at risk of developing the metabolic effects of the disorder.[48] Losing weight (which we will discuss further below) is a strategy that can bring great benefit to PCOS sufferers.

Finally, it is worth noting that the effects of insulin resistance can be felt well before puberty. In young girls suffering childhood obesity with deposits of visceral abdominal fat, production of excess insulin affects the development of the ovaries. Again this is likely due to raised androgen levels. There is some evidence to show that if this can be prevented early enough (with insulin lowering treatment between 8 and 12 years), then PCOS is less likely to develop compared with other girls with the same risk factors (i.e., obesity and low birth weight), who are not treated before puberty.[49]

In terms of fertility, obesity in PCOS women not only exacerbates ovarian dysfunction but may also negatively affect implantation of an embryo, should a conception occur – these women show significantly altered proteins in the endometrium that are not seen in lean women who do not have PCOS.[50] Additionally we know that obesity markedly changes the follicular environment in a way that is detrimental to the development of the eggs, likely reducing conception rates.[51]

STRESS

Clinicians have observed that stress is a contributing factor in the development of PCOS in some of their patients, notably those who worked 9–14 h a day in professions such as law or finance.[36] And animal studies (both in vivo, and with tissue culture laboratory studies) show that increased stress and sympathetic nervous system activity causes development of PCOS like characteristics and infertility.[52]

In conclusion we can say that there is likely a genetic predisposition in those girls or women who develop PCOS, probably involving genes related to the production of androgens, and possibly those predisposing to insulin resistance. On top of this, events in the womb (including epigenetic changes) and lifestyle factors, during early and middle life can influence the development of the disease. The consequences – including deposits of abdominal or visceral fat – can have deleterious effects on ovary function, follicular environment and the integrity of the endometrium.

PCOS, Fertility and Aging

While lack of regular and predictable release of eggs makes it harder to fall pregnant, the good news is that women with PCOS seem to retain their fertile potential for longer than other women. It appears that the process of ovarian aging may be delayed in women with PCOS and the typical ultrasound features of PCOS appear to diminish with increasing age.

Anti-Mullerian hormone (AMH) is secreted by the primary and preantral follicles and is an indicator of ovarian reserve. It is generally higher and declines more slowly in women with PCOS and it may be the case that their biological clock is not ticking as fast as that of other women. Thus, a greater ovarian reserve is retained in women in their 40s with PCOS and it is possible that they may actually be endowed with a larger ovarian reserve at birth. However, none of this is helpful if the ovaries are not prepared to ripen and release the reserved eggs!

Metabolic Effects of PCOS

So far we have spoken mostly about the effects of PCOS on the ovaries but there are more systemic effects too. Women with polycystic ovary syndrome have a high prevalence of hyperlipidemia, hypertension and progression to type 2 diabetes mellitus. This is similar to the features of the so-called 'metabolic syndrome' or 'syndrome X'. By the age of 40 years, up to 40% of women with PCOS will have type 2 diabetes or impaired glucose tolerance.

The insulin resistance and hyperinsulinemia typical of PCOS stimulates lipid storage, altered lipoprotein and cholesterol metabolism and (possibly) altered steroid hormone metabolism. Women with the syndrome have at least seven times the risk of myocardial infarction and ischemic heart disease of other women.

Risks During Pregnancy

Women with PCOS may suffer increased risks during pregnancy, including higher miscarriage rates, abnormal fetal size for gestational age, pre-term deliveries, gestational diabetes, hypertension and pre-eclampsia.

It is thought that excess androgens, and the related impaired insulin sensitivity, could alter the initial processes of trophoblastic invasion and placentation, leading to some of the above mentioned risks.

However, a high BMI and different PCOS phenotypes may account for some of these obstetric complications, and not all studies have found that PCOS patients have a higher risk of miscarriage.[53,54]

PCOS and Emotions

Women with polycystic ovary syndrome (PCOS) have poorer health-related quality of life (especially psychological) than women in the general population and than patients with other medical conditions such as asthma, epilepsy, diabetes, back pain, arthritis and coronary heart disease. Depression in this group of women is often related to obesity and infertility.[55]

The effects of PCOS at different stages of life is summarized in Table 5.20.[56]

Treatment Strategies (Western Medicine)

The type of treatment offered for patients with PCOS depends on the symptoms and the specific needs at different stages of life.

In young women, this may be reduction of acne, unwanted body hair growth or a desire for regular menstrual cycles. Or management of the health risks associated with PCOS. However, in this text we shall place most emphasis on discussion of treatments that promote fertility.

Table 5.20 The effect of inherited predisposition to PCOS from uterus to middle age

In utero	Peripuberty	Adolescence + adulthood	Middle age
Intrauterine growth retardation Post-term delivery	Increased levels of adrenal androgens and insulin Ovarian hyperandrogenism	PCOS develops Anovulation Hyperandrogenism Cysts on ovaries Obesity Insulin resistance	Metabolic syndrome Diabetes Hypertension Dyslipidemia Cardiovascular disease
→ long-term health effects	→ premature puberty	→ reproductive disorders	→ metabolic effects

LOSING WEIGHT

There is ample evidence that weight loss is beneficial in PCOS. There is also good evidence that weight loss improves fertility in all women whether they have PCOS or not, both in terms of spontaneous conception and IVF pregnancies.[57] Not only does reducing obesity increase ovulation frequency but it improves the very follicular environment in which the eggs themselves mature.[51,58]

However, for women with PCOS, weight loss is not such an easy thing to achieve despite the best of intentions. These women may have an increased susceptibility to weight gain and/or find it harder to lose weight than women who don't have PCOS. High levels of insulin encourage the body to increase fat storage. In a cruel vicious cycle this creates more insulin resistance, which increases blood insulin more and thus there will be even more weight gain.

There is also some evidence that the appetite signals in women with PCOS are disordered – these women produce too much ghrelin which increases appetite and leptin resistance in the brain so that the brain doesn't get the appetite suppression messages. This means there is a higher satiety level and PCOS patients need to eat more to feel satisfied. Elevated androgen levels are linked with increased cravings for carbohydrates.

The good news is that it is a relatively small weight loss and body fat redistribution that is needed to start the ovaries working again. Just 5–10% of initial body weight (or even just 5 kg), enough to change the waist-to-height ratio, will improve metabolic, reproductive and psychological features of PCOS, including hyperandrogenism, insulin resistance, dyslipidemia, glucose tolerance, menstrual function, ovulation, pregnancy, and quality of life. It is the loss of a small volume of critical intra-abdominal fat, which may be only a small percentage of the total body fat, which confers these benefits.

Which diet should be recommended for weight loss in PCOS? This is a large and fascinating topic but we do not have room for detailed discussions of different diets here. Suffice it to say that there is insufficient evidence to date to confidently recommend one specific diet to all women with PCOS. Although some diet types may be more beneficial for metabolic status, individual constitutions and preferences are important so that the diet will be effective and will be maintained. It is important that changes in diet and exercise routine be amenable to the person involved, as a lifetime commitment to these changes will reap the most benefit. Chapter 9 discusses diet in more detail.

In general, high protein, low glycemic index meals are recommended because they are relatively low calorie, they do not raise blood sugar and do not produce as much insulin, and they manage hunger well. The high leucine content of protein contributes to regulation of protein synthesis and insulin signaling pathways. But a variety of approaches, including calorie counting and meal replacements, can be successful for achieving and sustaining a reduced weight.

The inclusion of dietary fiber at each meal (e.g., from whole grains including oats and barley or pulses) or supplemental fiber such as psyllium, also appears to be helpful in controlling insulin levels. The fiber is fermented by microbes in the large intestine creating short chain fatty acids which reduce insulin resistance by mechanisms acting in adipose, liver, and muscle tissue.

Although there is no clear clinical data from human studies, women and girls with PCOS are often advised to avoid soy products so that an extra load of phytoestrogens does not further disrupt the hormonal milieu.

As important as the diet itself, is the ongoing support given as part of a weight loss program. Goal setting, weight monitoring and individualization of the program, follow-up and monitoring by a healthcare practitioner and support from family or friends are crucial in the ongoing success of weight loss programs. Additionally, stress, patterns of eating (including emotional triggers), and self-esteem need to be addressed.

Exercise does not on its own help significantly with weight loss but it is an important part of a program for PCOS patients because it can improve insulin resistance (even without loss of weight). Exercise increases skeletal muscle insulin sensitivity, so that there is less insulin present in the blood, hence less glucose is converted to fat. High intensity interval training has been shown to reduce insulin resistance effectively with a very small time commitment.[59]

Additionally, exercise has been seen to specifically help shrink abdominal fat cells. And another reason that exercise may be important is the associated reduction in the stress hormone cortisol. This hormone specifically promotes visceral fat deposits.

PHARMACEUTICAL

• The Oral Contraceptive Pill

Teenagers and young women with PCOS usually present first to their doctors with acne, which often disturbs them more than the fact that their periods are irregular. Or they may be bothered by increasing hairiness (hirsutism). Western specialists usually respond by prescribing the oral contraceptive pill (OCP) to these young women, thus masking the disease for many years. Missing the diagnosis at this point means an opportunity is lost whereby young women could be advised that lifestyle and weight management is crucial. It is only when a woman stops the OCP when she wants to conceive that the problem is uncovered and properly diagnosed. Even young women who have not been diagnosed with PCOS, who take the OCP for some years, are showing signs of this disorder when they stop the pill. It is an increasingly common observation that these women's periods do not return regularly and the investigations that follow then reveal signs of PCOS.

As we saw above, administration of combined contraceptives appear to increase insulin resistance, increase triglyceride levels and promote inflammation and hence, it is advisable for young women with a predisposition to PCOS to avoid this form of contraception.

• Clomifene Citrate (Clomid, Serophene)

For PCOS sufferers with irregular cycles who wish to conceive, the first step is usually a prescription for drugs that induce ovulation. Clomifene citrate is given as 50 mg dose for 5–7 days just after a menstrual period (the period may first need to be induced with progesterone in a woman who is not having any cycles). The dose can be increased up to 200 mg if necessary. However, as we saw above, this drug has a negative effect on the cervical mucus and the lining of the endometrium, and is usually not continued past 3 cycles or attempts.

Women with PCOS do not respond to clomifene citrate with the same success as other patients with different ovulation disorders. Such failure to respond is correlated with BMI and androgen index. This has been called clomifene resistance and often calls for the addition of insulin lowering medications.

• Metformin (Glucophage, Diaformin)

Metformin is an insulin lowering drug which reduces blood sugar levels, may help weight loss and may increase ovulation frequency. It is prescribed at doses between 1000 and 2500 mg/day and is also used in type 2 diabetes. Common side-effects are diarrhea, nausea, vomiting, abdomen bloating, and flatulence but many of these side-effects diminish with time. Metformin is classed as a Category C drug; it can cause neonatal hypoglycemia at term but is not teratogenic (i.e., it does not cause birth defects). It is usually stopped once pregnancy is confirmed. Other insulin lowering drugs, such as the Glitazones have also been shown to induce ovulation. There is greater concern about the effects on the fetus of these drugs compared with metformin, and they should not be used by women actively trying to become pregnant.

PCOS patients who are reluctant to take pharmaceutical drugs like these can take heart from studies which have shown that exercise and diet can be equally effective in terms of weight loss, increased ovulation and pregnancy rate – and that adding metformin to such a regimen is not necessary since it confers no advantage in terms of pregnancy rates.[60]

• Gonadotrophins

If ovulation cannot be induced by clomifene and/or metformin, then gonadotrophins may be given in small doses. This may be within the context of an artificial insemination (AI) cycle, or an IVF cycle.

Women with polycystic ovary syndrome (PCOS) usually respond to these injectable fertility medications with a degree of success. However, these women are more prone to the problems associated with the use of gonadotropins such as ovarian hyperstimulation syndrome (OHSS) and multiple pregnancy (discussed in Ch. 9).

• Statins

The use of statins, especially in PCOS patients with high cholesterol, is sometimes recommended. This therapy has been shown to reduce testosterone levels. However, women who are attempting pregnancy are not advised to take statins, since they may cause deformities in the baby.

SURGICAL

Ovulation problems in women with PCOS can also be treated by destroying or removing portions of the ovaries. Ovulation often resumes more regularly after this, possibly due to the reduced number of theca cells producing testosterone, and reduced number of resting follicles producing AMH and inhibin.

There have been several surgical methods described for doing this including:

- Wedge resection

- Ovarian drilling or cystectomy

- Ovarian diathermy.

The benefits of surgery include the avoidance of drug side-effects, and these procedures are sometimes offered to those for whom clomifene citrate has not been successful. Skillful drilling with laser or diathermy appears to be as effective in inducing ovulations as clomifene citrate or gonadotrophins. The risks are those associated with any surgery and include damage to ovaries and the formation of adhesions.[61]

PCOS and TCM

Etiology

To understand the origins of ovarian dysfunction in PCOS, the Chinese medicine practitioner needs to consider the effects of both congenital Jing and acquired Jing (also known as Pre-heaven or prenatal Qi and Post-heaven or postnatal Qi).

In terms of congenital Jing, we recognize that there is a genetic or inherited component in PCOS. Other factors (not inherited) operating in the womb can also exert critical influence. This tells us that a deficiency of the prenatal Qi or congenital Jing may set the stage for the development of PCOS long before the function of ovaries is tested in the 2nd 7-year cycle when the Chong and the Ren vessels become active at puberty. The primary influence here is the Kidney Qi or Kidney Jing and reinforcing the Kidney Jing is often the way we address conditions that have their origins in the Pre-heaven Qi. However, PCOS is a complex disorder and the interactions of factors operating postnatally have a large impact and warrant our close attention. This Post-heaven Qi (acquired Jing) is the realm of influence of the Spleen and the Stomach.

Any treatment strategies we devise for the PCOS patient thus needs to take into consideration both Pre- and Post-heaven Qi.

At puberty, the Chong and Ren vessels and the ovaries become active. In some young women, PCOS will manifest at this point, with erratic lengthy menstrual cycles, which do not ever become regular or sometimes may cease altogether. During the process of folliculogenesis in the ovary, whereby egg cells are systematically and repeatedly ripened, there is a spanner in the works; as discussed above, it appears there is an intrinsic fault in folliculogenesis itself. In an ideal world, we would already have identified these at-risk girls and begun treatment before puberty – as we noted above, if some of the manifestations of PCOS like high insulin are addressed early on (from age 8) then the ovaries and folliculogenesis are less likely to be compromised, i.e., the Kidneys, Chong and Ren vessels will be more likely to function normally once puberty arrives.

It is at puberty that part of the Kidney Jing transforms into Tian Gui, which is responsible for initiating and maintaining reproductive function.

Initial recruitment from the pool of resting follicles (the primordial follicles which can be dormant for up to 50 years) to become primary follicles occurs normally in the ovaries of PCOS patients. The function of the Tian Gui, awakening of the follicles, is normal at this stage but then there is a hold up at the next stage of development when primary follicles should develop into secondary follicles and beyond. Hence, large numbers of primary follicles stockpile. This arrest of follicle development, at its root, can be seen as a failure of Kidney Jing, and specifically the Tian Gui, to drive or maintain all the essential steps of folliculogenesis. There may also be some obstruction of the Qi in the Chong and Ren vessels that contributes to this stalling in follicle development. Both these vessels have their roots in the Kidneys.

In many women diagnosed with PCOS, the symptoms do not manifest until some years after puberty (and sometimes after some years on the oral contraceptive pill or other forms of hormonal contraception). In such cases, some other factors have, perhaps in concert with a predisposing Kidney Jing deficiency, caused interruptions in the Chong and Ren vessels. We shall discuss these in detail below.

TCM Analysis and Diagnosis: Analyzing Symptoms and Signs

IRREGULAR PERIODS

A consistent clinical symptom in women with PCOS is the irregular or infrequent nature of their ovulation. This may be mild, i.e., a tendency for menstrual cycles to be 5 weeks or more, or more severe with long periods of amenorrhea. Either way, the Chong and Ren vessels are not functioning optimally.

If amenorrhea (or severe oligomenorrhea) dates from puberty, then we would usually consider this a Kidney Jing deficiency or failure of some aspect of Tian Gui. In the case of more regular but slightly long or irregular cycles, we would look at the relationship between the Liver Qi and the Chong and Ren channels.

WEIGHT GAIN OR A HIGH WAIST-TO-HIP RATIO

There is a clear case to be made for a diagnosis of Phlegm-Damp accumulation in the PCOS patients who present with obesity or a recent weight gain that has affected the menstrual cycle. Even a modest weight gain of 5 kg or so can influence ovarian activity, even though overall physical appearance may be fairly normal. As described above, the sort of weight gain typical of PCOS patients is that around the waist. Dai vessel dysfunction may allow a build-up of Damp and eventually Phlegm-Damp, in this area.

Loss of weight has been seen to improve ovulation frequency. Thus it appears that mobilization of Phlegm-Damp may be all that is required to unblock or to improve the function of the Chong and Ren channels.

The insulin resistance that we discussed above is especially common in PCOS patients who have poor diets and do little exercise. Junk food or rich diets and lack of exercise are associated with sluggish movement of Qi (especially Spleen Qi) and accumulation of Damp. Additionally, those women who are having very infrequent periods are missing the opportunity to expel turbid Damp from the lower Jiao with their menstrual flow and thus it accumulates. As mentioned above, it has been observed that obese women have an altered uterine environment, which is disadvantageous to embryo implantation.[50]

This may be one manifestation of the accumulation of this turbid Damp in the lower Jiao.

ACNE, HAIR LOSS, HIRSUTISM, CARDIOVASCULAR DISEASE

Some of the typical androgenic signs and symptoms of PCOS can be interpreted as Damp or Blood stagnation. For example, acne of the type seen in PCOS will usually be diagnosed as Damp-Heat manifesting in the skin. Both

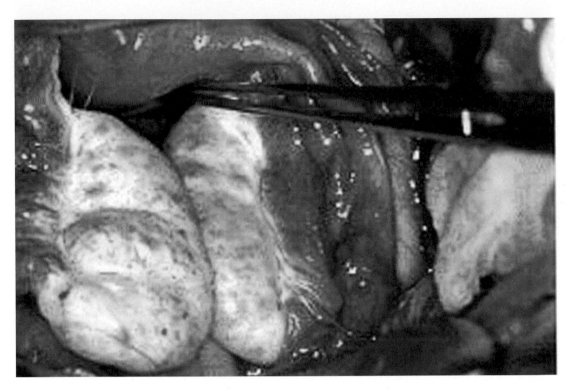

Figure 5.7 Polycystic ovaries appear shiny and swollen.

hair loss on the head and hirsutism on the body are deemed to be a sign of Phlegm-Damp in modern Chinese medicine texts.[62] Many aspects of cardiovascular disease are diagnosed as Blood stagnation.

PRECOCIOUS PUBERTY, SMALL BIRTH SIZE (OR LARGE)

Precocious puberty usually occurs when a young girl is overweight, i.e., there is an excess of Phlegm-Damp. Large size at birth predisposes to excess weight during childhood and beyond. However, a small birth size (also linked to premature puberty and PCOS) is more likely to make us think of Kidney Jing deficiency.

SURGERY, SCANS, AND BLOOD TESTS

TCM diagnosis relies on analysis of clinical symptoms and some signs that are easily evaluated such as pulse and tongue. In some cases, laboratory and surgical investigations can broaden or enhance our diagnostic repertoire. For example, laparoscopic investigations on women with PCOS usually reveal swollen ovaries; the polycystic ovaries themselves look shiny and swollen when viewed during laparoscopy, i.e., they look Damp (Fig. 5.7).

Scans (CT and DEXA) may reveal fat deposits around the central internal organs of women with PCOS even where there is no obesity or weight gain. Similarly, enlarged adipocytes (fat cells) are found in women with PCOS whether they are overweight or not. We would relate these findings to abnormal accumulations of Phlegm-Damp. The pattern of fat deposits or Damp accumulation follows the Dai vessel pathway. The swollen cystic ovaries also lie in the path of the Dai vessel. Even in women where there is no obvious truncal obesity or weight gain, the swelling of the ovaries could indicate smaller localized accumulations in the Dai channel or the Liver channel.

Blood tests that show high levels of clotting factor (fibrinogen) in PCOS patients confirm the increased risk of Blood stagnation in these patients.[63] See Table 5.21 for a summary of this analysis of PCOS signs and symptoms.

Table 5.21   Summary of TCM analysis of PCOS symptom and signs

Symptoms, signs and etiologic factors	TCM analysis
Irregular periods	Chong and Ren channel dysfunction
Swollen shiny ovaries	Phlegm-Damp accumulation
Weight gain around the middle	Phlegm-Damp accumulation
	Dai Channel dysfunction
Visceral fat deposits, enlarged fat cells	Phlegm-Damp accumulation
Losing weight improves ovarian activity	Mobilizing Damp unblocks Chong and Ren channels
Acne	Damp-Heat
Hairiness	Damp?
Prone to cardiovascular disease	Blood stagnation
Increased coagulation factors	Blood stagnation
Precocious puberty	Phlegm-Damp accumulation
Genetic and intrauterine factors	Kidney Jing deficiency
Small birth size	Kidney Jing deficiency

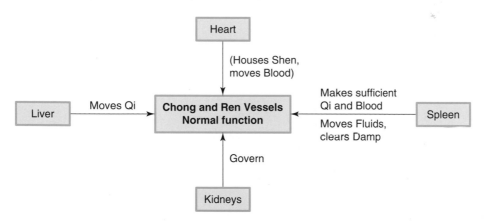

Figure 5.8 Chong and Ren vessels – normal physiology. The Chong and the Ren vessels originate in the Kidneys and are governed by them. The Spleen supplies the Blood and nourishment for them, and clears Fluids and Damp. The Liver moves the Qi and the Heart moves the Blood and houses the Shen.

Making a Diagnosis

Having looked at the PCOS patient's history and analyzed the ways in which she presents in the clinic (and other associated findings), we can now formulate our diagnosis. Irregular or absent periods is the feature that infertile PCOS patients most commonly share. In TCM terms, these women suffer a disturbance of the Chong and Ren vessels.

We know that the foundation of the Chong and Ren vessels is the Kidneys and that the Chong and Ren vessels require nourishment by Qi and Blood and can be obstructed by Phlegm-Damp and stagnation of Qi and Blood (Fig. 5.8).

If we now put the dysfunction of the Chong and Ren vessels at the center of our analysis of women with PCOS who are not ovulating regularly, we come up with this diagrammatic analysis (Fig. 5.9).

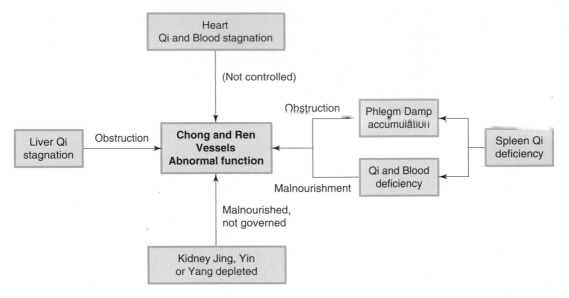

Figure 5.9 Chong and Ren vessels – abnormal physiology in PCOS. When Kidney Jing, Yin or Yang is deficient, the Chong and Ren vessels lose their foundation, are malnourished and no longer properly managed. When Spleen Qi is deficient, Damp and Phlegm-Damp can collect and obstruct the channels, and lack of Qi and Blood can results in a lack of nourishment. If the Liver Qi is stagnant, Qi in the Chong and Ren vessels can become obstructed.

Heart Qi stagnation (and Shen disturbance) may be a reflection or manifestation of long-term Chong and Ren disturbance, but it is less likely to be a causative factor in PCOS. On the face of it, PCOS being an ovulation disorder, we might assume involvement of the Heart and the Bao vessel, as we did in our earlier discussion of amenorrhea, but here the problem lies with the ovary and not with the hypothalamus or pituitary gland, as it did in other instances of ovulation disorder.

While the Chong and Ren vessels are at the center of the problem causing failure to ovulate regularly in PCOS, another extra channel, the Dai vessel is also of interest because of its function of controlling circulation of fluids in the lower Jiao. The Dai vessel is situated around and through the abdomen from the level of the 2nd lumbar vertebrae and extending downwards. Not only is this the precise area where the waist expands in PCOS patients with abdominal weight gain but also includes the part of the body containing fat deposits around the central organs and the swollen ovaries typical of PCOS. Any accumulation in this area is likely to obstruct Dai vessel function. Conversely, Dai vessel dysfunction will allow a build up of Damp and eventually Phlegm-Damp in this area.

The Dai vessel also intersects Ming men and passes through the Kidneys, hence malfunction of the Dai vessel may well be a contributing factor to impaired folliculogenesis and ovary function at a very fundamental stage. Its other important role is to bind the channels running perpendicularly on the abdomen. This includes not only the primary meridians but also the Chong and the Ren, thus Dai vessel disturbances may be reflected here too. Spleen and Liver channels may also be affected.

In addition to the Chong, Ren and Dai vessels, we should mention the Bao vessel and Bao channel (see Ch. 2), which are important in transporting Jing and Tian Gui from the Kidneys, and Blood from the Heart to the Uterus. There are no points on the Bao mai that we use directly, however Heart and Kidney points can indirectly influence its activity.

Our working model for diagnosing PCOS is summarized in Tables 5.22 and 5.23.

A genetic predisposition to PCOS implicating the Kidneys plus a Spleen Qi weakness contributing to weight and blood sugar problems together become the 'Ben' of our diagnosis, combined with an accumulation of Phlegm-Damp, the 'Biao' causing obstruction in the Chong and Ren vessels (Fig. 5.10).

Table 5.22 Diagnosis of PCOS (weight gain)

Organs	Kidneys, Spleen
Pathogen	Phlegm-Damp accumulation
Channels	Chong Ren obstruction
	Dai vessel accumulations

Table 5.23 Diagnosis of PCOS (no obvious weight gain)

Organs	Kidneys, Liver
Pathogen	Qi and Blood stasis (± Phlegm-Damp accumulation)
Channels	Chong Ren obstruction

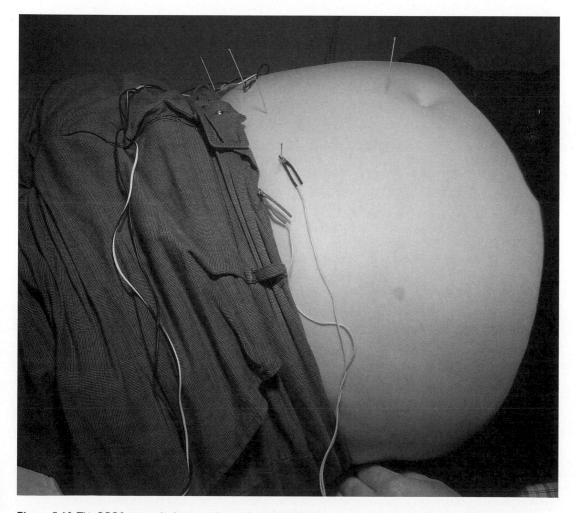

Figure 5.10 This PCOS patient had amenorrhea and weighed 87 kilos – most of her weight was around her stomach.

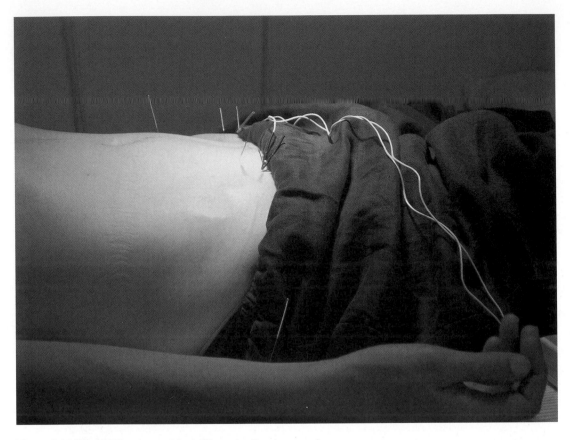

Figure 5.11 This PCOS patient weighed 45 kg, and suffered amenorrhea.

Where weight gain is not a factor, we attribute the obstruction in the Chong and Ren vessels to Qi, Blood, and possible local Phlegm-Damp stasis. The Ben of our diagnosis is the Kidneys (a predisposing factor) but the Biao is the Liver Qi stagnation leading to stagnation of Qi and Blood. Accumulation of Damp is not always apparent, except for the presence of cysts on the ovaries and sometimes deposits of fat around the abdominal organs. Liver Qi stasis can create Phlegm-Damp by disrupting Gall Bladder function. When bile is not produced properly, then fat metabolism is affected, provoking the formation of Phlegm-Damp which may manifest as fat deposits in the abdomen but no apparent weight gain (Fig. 5.11).

Figure 5.12 summarizes some of the ways that different pathologic states can lead to ovulation disorders of the type seen in PCOS. There is a third pattern, Qi and Blood deficiency, which can also affect the Chong and Ren leading to dysfunction due to lack of nourishment; however this is more often a different sort of amenorrhea pattern (not PCOS) and was discussed in an earlier section. This chart also does not include the Blood stasis that sometimes complicates PCOS, particularly long-term disease. It is at its later stages that Blood stasis signs such as cardiovascular disease develop, and the amenorrhea of PCOS is not usually related to Blood stasis alone.

Clinical Progression

Let us now examine how different aspects of the PCOS pathomechanism play out at different times. Specifically, we are interested in how the predisposing Kidney factors interact with Spleen deficiency and Liver Qi stagnation to create the pathology and clinical picture typical of PCOS.

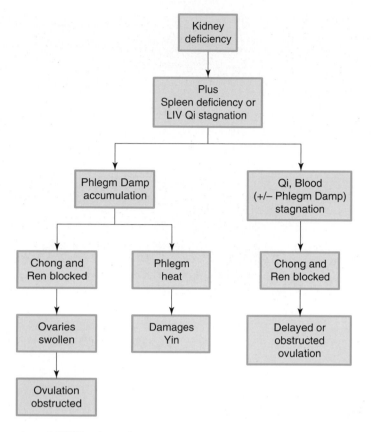

Figure 5.12 Summary chart of PCOS pathomechanism.

Kidney deficiency meets Spleen Qi deficiency or Liver Qi stagnation

- at time of conception

- at time of puberty

- in reproductive years

- in later years.

• At Time of Conception

When there is both Kidney Jing deficiency and compromised Spleen function in the mother (e.g., poor nourishment or inappropriate food) at the time of conception of a baby girl, then that baby may be predisposed to PCOS or blood sugar disturbances. Also intrauterine growth retardation will predispose to PCOS.

• At Time of Puberty

At time of puberty, interaction of Kidneys and Spleen are important to establish the function of the Chong and the Ren cycle. At puberty, or in the second of the 7-year cycles, not only must the Tian Gui flourish but there must also be adequate nourishment and Blood – or the menstrual cycle cannot become well established. Anorexia and bulimia can have very dire consequences at this stage of a girl's development. On the other hand, when nourishment is overdone, and the girl becomes overweight, the 7-year cycle may be advanced and the periods come prematurely, but not regularly. Liver Qi plays a part at this stage too – there are many stresses on young teenage girls, not only academic stresses but social stresses. Early sexual activity can disrupt the Chong vessel activity, as can the use of hormonal contraceptives and the 'morning after' pill.

• In Reproductive Years

The interaction of the Kidney and Spleen later in reproductive years, e.g. 20s and 30s can also lead to disruptions in the Chong and the Ren vessels leading to PCOS. If Spleen function is poor, or the diet is bad and body weight increases, then in susceptible women, Chong and Ren vessels are obstructed and what was a regular cycle may become long or eventually stop. Use of the oral contraceptive pill or other hormonal contraceptives may impair Spleen function, affecting blood sugar metabolism. Hormonal contraception also interrupts the Liver in its function of overseeing cycles in the body and the resulting stagnation can disrupt Chong and Ren function. If stress impacts the Liver Qi sufficiently, this can contribute also to disruption of the Chong and Ren vessels.

• In Later Years

As often happens with long-term disease of any nature, Blood stagnation develops. In the PCOS sufferer this may manifest in cardiovascular disease. Long-term Kidney and Spleen imbalance can lead to diabetes and other manifestations of metabolic syndrome such as hypertension. These are serious disorders which require correct treatment, however in this text we shall keep our focus on the aspects of PCOS which affect fertility.

Treatment with TCM

TCM analyzes pathologic conditions according to how they present in the clinic and as such, we can approach the treatment of PCOS-related infertility as we have been doing all along, gathering information about the menstrual cycle, etc. – however, as we saw with endometriosis, there is a special pathology we need to address in these diseases – in this case, it is the factor inhibiting the growth of the follicles in the ovary and preventing a regular menstrual cycle.

Practically speaking, treatment of PCOS can take two different approaches: one with a single focus on facilitating the release of eggs and conception, and one more complex addressing all the issues inherent in this disease, both Ben and Biao. However, these two approaches are not mutually exclusive.

The PCOS patient who is trying to conceive will generally be more interested in what you can do to help her ovulate regularly than in how you can help her lose weight or prevent heart disease or diabetes in the future. Focussing on ovarian activity and ripening and release of eggs, we use treatments that are aimed primarily at re-establishing function of the Chong and the Ren vessels, with secondary focus on the function of the organs. Acupuncture is particularly useful in this regard but while it may stimulate some ovulations, restoration of a regular menstrual cycle will only be achieved with attention to the underlying organ dysfunction. For a simplified approach to induce ovulation, see the Research section below, where standardized (or largely standardized) point prescriptions were used on PCOS patients in trial settings. The information we have gleaned from these trials has been incorporated into the acupuncture protocols suggested below for treatment of different types of PCOS.

When it comes to treating this condition in the larger context (looking further than ovulation induction), we need to consider several layers of treatment: Kidney or Spleen Qi deficiency or Liver Qi stagnation, with the consequent Phlegm-Damp accumulation or Qi or blood stagnation blocking the Chong and Ren channels. Chinese herbal medicine and acupuncture have a lot to offer in this regard. Lifestyle modification is an important component of any type of treatment a PCOS patient chooses to use.

PCOS with Weight Gain

Resolving Phlegm-Damp to regulate/unblock Chong and Ren Channels

For PCOS patients with weight gain, and Phlegm-Damp accumulation, we can take either of two clinical approaches. First, we can focus on primarily mobilizing the Phlegm-Damp and second, we can focus on supporting Kidneys (or focus on primarily supporting Kidneys and secondarily clearing Damp and Phlegm).

MOBILIZING DAMP AND PHLEGM PRIMARILY

This approach might be chosen for large PCOS patients with stubborn weight gain and who are having few, if any, menstrual cycles per year. The Chong and Ren vessels in this case are seriously obstructed.

Herbal Formula — The combination of a well known formula such as Cang Fu Dao Tan Tang with a more modern formula Bu Shen Hua Tan Tang meets our requirements for these patients. By promoting Spleen function to resolve Damp, expelling Phlegm-Damp accumulation and benefiting Kidneys, we aim to clear Chong Ren obstruction and re-establish ovarian function.

Cang Fu Dao Tan Tang (Atractylodes and Cyperus Guide out Phlegm decoction) with Bu Shen Hua Tan Tang (Decoction for Restoring the Kidney and Removing Phlegm) modified

Cang Zhu	12 g	Rhizoma Atractylodis
Fu Ling	15 g	Sclerotium Poriae Cocos
Ban Xia	9 g	Rhizoma Pinelliae
Sha Ren	6 g	Fructus seu Semen Amomi
Fo Shou	3 g	Fructus Citri Sarcodactylis
Chen Pi	9 g	Pericarpium Citri Reticulate
Dan Nan Xing	6 g	Rhizoma Arisaematis
Zhe Bei Mu	6 g	Fritillariae thunbergii Bulbus
Zao Jiao Ci	9 g	Spina Gleditsiae Sinensis
Shan Yao	9 g	Radix Dioscorea Oppositae
Shu Di	6 g	Radix Rehmanniae Glutinosae Conquitae
Bu Gu Zhi	9 g	Fructus Psoraleae
Yin Yang Huo	9 g	Herba Epimedii
Ji Xue Teng	12 g	Radix et Caulis Jixueteng
Zhi Zi	3 g	Fructus Gardeniae Jasminoidis

Cang Zhu, Fu Ling, Chen Pi and Sha Ren are the main herbs used to clear Damp in this formula. Cang Zhu and Fu Ling strengthen the Spleen to clear dampness. Sha ren augments their action by warming the Middle Jiao, and with Chen Pi and Fo Shou moves the Qi to facilitate the movement of Damp.

Stronger phlegm mobilizing herbs in the form of Fa Ban Xia, Zhe Bei Mu, Zao Jiao Ci and Dan Nan Xing are needed to break up the accumulation of Phlegm — in other words, the shiny swollen theca cells of the ovary and the multiple cysts therein.

To promote ovarian function, we next add Kidney herbs. Shu Di enriches the Kidney Yin and Jing to provide the essential basis for the growth and development of mature eggs in the follicles. It is supported by Shan Yao, which reinforces the Yin of the Spleen and the Kidneys.

Bu Gu Zhi strengthens Spleen and Kidney function and also supports the previous group of herbs by drying Damp. Yin Yang Huo we add to promote maturation of ovarian follicles by boosting Kidney yang function and stoking the fire of Ming Men.

It is hoped that by antagonizing androgens with the action of these herbs, it may be possible to reduce the follicular atresia. Ji Xue Teng is added to promote movement of Blood in the Chong vessel.

Zhi Zi clears Heat arising from accumulated Phlegm-Damp. In some women, this dose will need to be increased. And in the case that Heat has damaged Yin, another herb such as Di Gu Pi would be substituted.

This formula is quite drying, which means we need to carefully monitor the Yin during treatment.

Acupuncture Points — We know that certain acupuncture protocols can help to stimulate ovary function in PCOS patients (see Research section, below), and using these plus points chosen according to our TCM diagnosis,

Table 5.24   Acupuncture points[a] used in the treatment of PCOS with weight gain – Phlegm-Damp accumulation predominant

Treatment goal	Acupuncture points
To invigorate Kidney Yin and Yang	Ren-6 KI-3, SP-6 and BL-23
To promote Spleen function in clearing Damp	SP-5, SP-9, BL-20, ST-40, SP-3, SP-15
To activate the Chong vessel	Ren-3, KI-13 and SP-4
To encourage removal of Damp via the Bladder	BL-28
To encourage removal of Phlegm-Damp obstructing the Dai vessel	GB-26, GB-27/28, GB-41, TH-5
To activate local Qi circulation (around the ovaries)	Abdomen Zigong, K-14, ST-28
To regulate metabolism of fluids in the San jiao	TH-6, TH-9
To clear Heat arising from Phlegm-Damp blockage	CO-11

[a]Reinforcing or reducing technique is used; electro acupuncture can be used on the abdomen or back points and connected to Spleen points on the leg at 10 Hertz 3–5 Amps for 20 min.

provides the basis for treatments applied in the clinic. In the case of the patient with significant Phlegm-Damp, we use Spleen and Stomach points to strengthen the Spleen, Spleen and Dai vessel points to promote clearing Damp and Kidney points to support ovary function.

Acupuncture points (Table 5.24) for the treatment of PCOS with weight gain – Phlegm-Damp accumulation predominant are as follows:

Ren-3	Zhongji
Ren-6	Qihai
SP-6	Sanyinjiao
Sp-9	Yinlingquan
SP-4	Gongsun
SP-5	Shangqiu
KI-13	Qixue
Abdomen Zigong	
BL-23	Shenshu
BL-20	Pishu
BL-28	Pangguanshu
GB-26	Daimai
GB-27	Wushu
GB-28	Weidao
GB-41	Zu Linqi
TH-5	Waiguan
SP-15	Daheng
ST-28	Shuidao
ST-40	Fenglong

SP-3	Taibai
TH-6	Zhigou
TH-9	Tianjing
Co-11	Quchi

SUPPORTING KIDNEYS PRIMARILY

This approach is more likely to be chosen for a PCOS patient with infertility who is not too overweight and who is having some cycles, albeit irregularly indicating that the Chong and Ren, while not functioning well are not as obstructed as in the previous case. Her history of menstrual irregularity may go back as far as puberty.

Herbal Formula — To achieve this, we go back to our primary infertility formula Gui Shao Di Huang Tang that supports Kidneys and the Blood, modifying it with Kidney Yang herbs and Damp clearing herbs.

Gui Shao Di Huang Tang (Angelica Peonia Rehmannia decoction) modified

Dang Gui	9 g	Radix Angelicae Sinensis
Bai Shao	9 g	Radix Paeoniae Lactiflorae
Shu Di	9 g	Radix Rehmanniae Glutinosae Conquitae
Shan Zhu Yu	9 g	Fructus Corni Officinalis
Shan Yao	9 g	Radix Dioscorea Oppositae
Fu Ling	15 g	Sclerotium Poriae Cocos
Mu Dan Pi	9 g	Cortex Moutan Radicis
Ze Xie	15 g	Rhizoma Alismatis
Tu Si Zi	9 g	Semen Cuscatae
Du Zhong	6 g	Cortex Eucommiae Ulmoidis
Sha Ren	9 g	Fructus seu Semen Amomi
Zhe Bei Mu	6 g	Fritillariae thunbergii Bulbus
Zao Jiao Ci	6 g	Gleditsiae Spina

Gui Shao Di Huang Tang, which reinforces Kidney Yin and Blood (described in Ch. 4) is modified here to include herbs (Tu Si Zi and Du Zhong) which supplement Kidney Yang. Sha Ren is added to help the Spleen Qi mobilize Damp. The doses of Fu Ling and Ze Xie are increased to further mobilize Damp.

Alternatively, Gui Shao di Huang tang can be combined with pills to strengthen Spleen Qi and clear the Phlegm-Damp using one of the patent medicines described below.

When the patient starts to notice some stretchy cervical secretions (as distinct from other forms of vaginal discharge which may be present due to the Damp), which indicate the Yin base is being established, then more Kidney Yang tonics can be added to the above formula or to Gui Shao Di Huang Tang:

Ba Ji Tian	6 g	Radix Morindae Officinalis
Bu Gu Zhi	6 g	Fructus Psoraleae
Yin Yang Huo	6 g	Herba Epimedii

These Kidney Yang tonics also provide some support for Spleen Yang and will aid in drying some Damp.

If BBT readings taken at this point indicate that ovulation has been successfully induced, then herbs for the post-ovulatory phase can be given according to the principles outlined in Chapter 4. If ovulation does not occur but secretions from the cervix continue, the doses of the Yang tonics above will be increased: namely,

Ba Ji Tian	9 g	*Radix Morindae Officinalis*
Bu Gu Zhi	9 g	*Fructus Psoraleae*
Yin Yang Huo	9 g	*Herba Epimedii*

Acupuncture Points — Points (Table 5.25) are chosen from:

K-6	Zhaohai
Lu-7	Lieque
SP-4	Gongsun
PC-6	Neiguan
K-13	Qixue
K-14	Simen
Ren-3	Zhongji
Ren-7	Yinjiao
Ren-4	Guanyuan
SP-6	Sanyinjiao
K-5	Shuiquan
BL-23	Shenshu
BL-20	Pishu
GB-27	Wushu
LIV-5	Ligou

To promote weight loss, reduce insulin resistance and encourage ovulation with acupuncture, treatments need to be frequent and regular – preferably 3 times a week. Monitoring of possible ovulation is recommended (with BBT, or in the case of women with reasonably predictable cycles, a urinary LH predictor kit). Once an ovulation has occurred and if the patient has attempted to conceive, the use of electroacupuncture on abdomen and Spleen points should be discontinued for the remainder of that menstrual cycle.

Table 5.25   Acupuncture points[a] used in the treatment of PCOS with weight gain – Kidney deficiency predominant

Treatment goal	Acupuncture points
To invigorate Kidney Yin and Yang and Jing	Ren-4, Ren-6, KI-3, SP-6, KI-6, and BL-23
To promote Spleen function in clearing Damp	SP-5 and BL-20
To activate the Chong vessel/to regulate the Chong and Ren vessels	KI-13 and SP-4 Ren-3, Ren-7, KI-14, K-6, LU-7, PC-6 and KI-5
To regulate Qi in the Dai vessel	GB-27
To activate local Qi circulation (around the ovaries)	Abdomen Zigong and LIV-5

[a]Reinforcing technique is used; moxa is useful on Ren-4. In the case of insulin resistance or elevated testosterone, etc. use electro-acupuncture connecting abdomen points to inner leg points on the same side 10 Hertz, 3–5 Amps, 20 min.

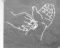

Patent medicines, which can be used concurrently to strengthen Spleen Qi and clear the Damp are:

Yue Ju Er Chen Wan (Gardenia Ligusticum pill)

Cang Zhu	*Rhizoma Atractylodes*
Shen Qu	*Massa Fermenta*
Chen Pi	*Pericarpium Citri Reticulate*
Fu Ling	*Sclerotium Poriae Cocos*
Ban Xia	*Rhizoma Pinelliae*
Xiang Fu	*Rhizoma Cyperi Rotundi*
Zhi Zi	*Fructus Gardeniae Jasminoidis*
Chuan Xiong	*Radix Ligustici Wallichii*

This well-known formula eliminates all types of stagnation, including Phlegm-Damp (Cang Zhu, Ban Xia, Chen Pi, Fu Ling), food (Shen Qu), Qi (Xiang Fu) and Blood (Chuan Xiong) and is especially indicated if there is Heat associated with the stagnation (Zhi Zi).

Cang Fu Dao Tan Wan (Atractylodes Cyperus Phlegm pill)

Cang Zhu	*Rhizoma Atractylodes*
Xiang Fu	*Rhizoma Cyperi Rotundi*
Ban Xia	*Rhizoma Pinelliae*
Fu Ling	*Sclerotium Poriae Cocos*
Chen Pi	*Pericarpium Citri Reticulate*
Dan Nan Xing	*Rhizoma Arisaematis*
Zhi Ke	*Fructus Citri seu Ponciri*
Gan Cao	*Radix Glycyrrhizae Uralensis*
Sheng Jiang	*Rhizoma Zingiberis Officinalis Recens*
Shen Qu	*Massa Fermenta*

This formula (also described above) includes many of the herbs and actions of Yue Ju Er Chen Wan but also includes Dan Nan Xing, which eliminates obstructions caused by Phlegm-Heat. In addition to addressing Phlegm-Damp accumulation in PCOS, this formula can be useful for treating fallopian tubes blocked by Phlegm-Damp.

A third option is:

Xiong Gui Ping Wei San (Ligusticum Angelica Balancing the Stomach powder)

Cang Zhu	*Rhizoma Atractylodes*
Chen Pi	*Pericarpium Citri Reticulate*
Hou Po	*Cortex Magnoliae Officinalis*
Zhi Gan Cao	*Radix Glycyrrhizae Uralensis*
Sheng Jiang	*Rhizoma Zingiberis Officinalis Recens*
Da Zao	*Fructus Zizyphi Jujuba*
Dang Gui	*Radix Angelicae Sinensis*
Chuan Xiong	*Radix Ligustici Wallichii*

This formula attempts to clear Damp by combining herbs that support Stomach and Spleen function with Damp-clearing herbs and Blood tonic herbs. It is more appropriate for women who have a weak constitution.

Treatment of PCOS in women who are overweight must always include some evaluation of diet and lifestyle. Anything we can do to encourage weight loss in these women will enhance ovarian function and fertility. We discussed weight loss and some strategies to achieve this in the previous section.

From a Chinese medicine perspective, one size does not fit all when it comes to diet. (We discuss this in more detail in Ch. 12). When it comes to weight loss most of us look at strategies to boost the action of Spleen Qi in clearing Damp and optimizing metabolism. The typical overweight Damp and Spleen Qi deficient woman is the pear shape we discussed above, i.e., large thighs and bottom, or a low waist-to-height ratio (WHR). While no-one claims to have an easy fix for losing weight, this TCM pattern is at least straight forward to diagnose and treat. And if compliance is good, weight loss will be steady. However, the pattern of obesity that we see in PCOS is a different type, it is more like a male pattern obesity – the large abdomen, or truncal obesity. There may also be fatty deposits around the viscera. The WHR is high. In this case, Damp arising from dietary or lifestyle factors or a genetic propensity is congealed into Phlegm-Damp in particular sites or regions, i.e., the ovaries and the abdominal area. This pattern of obesity can be associated with Heat (e.g., high blood pressure and florid face) and the treatment we apply must take all of this into account not just relying on reinforcing Spleen function.

As mentioned above, it is the first 5–10% of body weight that needs to come off and it is this mobilizing of Damp that appears to make the difference to reproductive function. It is not necessary that a certain number of kilos are lost or that a certain BMI is attained before ovarian function starts to improve. Patients will be heartened to hear that they just have to start the process of mobilization of Phlegm-Damp accumulation. Programs that support PCOS sufferers to lose weight have found that exercise in a group context adds an important psychological component to recovery. Since Damp is an internal environment which can cause sluggishness, low motivation and depression, this sort of encouragement is important.

Exercise, touched on above and also discussed in Chapter 12, is an essential component of a weight loss program, especially where there is insulin resistance. Interestingly, exercise helps weight loss specifically around the abdomen (and reduces visceral fat), whereas calorie restricting diets without exercise tend to encourage more weight loss around the thighs. This tells us that the fat or Damp accumulation around the waist is more stagnant, i.e., more like Phlegm-Damp than just Damp, and targeting this with exercise is particularly important for overweight women with PCOS.

CASE HISTORY – BARBARA

Barbara (39 years) had a long history (all her reproductive years) of oligomenorrhea and amenorrhea, which had only recently been diagnosed as PCOS. She had a weight problem and she wanted to conceive.

Her digestion was sluggish and she tended to bloating and constipation. She suffered constant fatigue, blocked sinuses and was always clearing mucus from her throat. Her tongue was pale and puffy and coated, and her pulse very thready.

The diagnosis of her amenorrhea was a clear-cut case of obstruction by Phlegm-Damp due to Spleen Qi deficiency. To treat this and help her conceive, we needed to strengthen her Spleen and Kidney Yang to clear the Phlegm-Damp.

Taking some of the Damp clearing and Kidney supporting elements of Cang Fu Dao Tan tang and Bu Shen Hua Tan tang, and combining these with Spleen supporting herbs from Si Jun Zi Tang, we made a formula that helped Barbara to mobilize some of the accumulated Damp. Xiong Gui Ping Wei San augmented this action.

Bai Zhu	9 g	Rhizoma Atractylodis Macrocephalae
Dang Shen	9 g	Radix Codonopsis Pilulosae
Shan Yao	9 g	Radix Dioscorea Oppositae
Fu Ling	16 g	Sclerotium Poriae Cocos
Dang Gui	9 g	Radix Angelicae Sinensis
Shu Di	6 g	Radix Rehmanniae Glutinosae Conquitae
Shan Zhu Yu	6 g	Fructus Corni Officinalis
Lu Jiao Pian	9 g	Cornu Cervi Parvum
Tu Si Zi	12 g	Semen Cuscatae
Bu Gu Zhi	9 g	Fructus Psoraleae
Yin Yang Huo	9 g	Herba Epimedii
Zhe Bei Mu	6 g	Bulbus Fritillariae Thunbergii

In addition, she took a patent formula called Xiong Gui Ping Wei San.

Acupuncture points: Ren-4, Ren-6, SP-6, SP-9, ST-25, ST-28, ST-36, ST-40, LU-7

Taking the above herbs and variations on this theme, Barbara's periods returned much more regularly than before (though not faithfully, every 28 days) and her weight dropped somewhat. After 3 periods (and 4 months) she conceived. Her pregnancy was dogged by ghastly nausea and vomiting, thanks to her Spleen deficiency and Damp. The thought of swallowing Chinese herbs was more than she could face, but acupuncture and ginger helped a little.

PCOS without Weight Gain

Regulating Liver Qi to Regulate Chong and Ren Vessel Activity

You will find that there are two main approaches we can take in the clinic for this type of PCOS as well – and I should hasten to say these are very likely not the last word either. As our understanding of this disease grows and clarifies so will the treatment we offer be expanded and finessed.

LIVER QI STAGNATION LEADING TO LOCALIZED DAMP ACCUMULATION

This is a relatively severe clinical picture where ovarian activity is significantly compromised and there are few if any periods. Localized accumulation of Phlegm-Damp manifests as cysts in the ovary and visceral fat deposits.

Where there is significant blockage caused by Liver Qi stagnation, a strong approach incorporating purgatives may be required to eradicate the Phlegm-Damp and any Heat built up with the obstruction. After a short course of our guiding formula (Fang Feng Tong Sheng San), another formula more geared toward maintaining good movement of the Liver Qi can be used.

Herbal Formula

Fang Feng Tong Sheng San (Ledebouriella pills with Magical Effect)

Fang Feng	9 g	Radix Ledebouriellae Sesloidis
Jing Jie	9 g	Herba seu Flos Shizonepetae Tenuifolia
Ma Huang	6 g	Herba Ephedra
Jie Geng	9 g	Radix Platycodi Grandiflori
Bo He	6 g	Herba Menthae
Lian Qiao	9 g	Fructus Forsythiae Suspensae
Huang Qin	6 g	Radix Scutellariae Baicalensis
Zhi Zi	6 g	Fructus Gardeniae Jasminoidis
(Jiu) Da Huang	6 g	Rhizoma Rhei (wine fried)
Shi Gao	9 g	Gypsum
Mang Xiao	6 g	Mirabilitum
Hua Shi	9 g	Talcum
Dang Gui	9 g	Radix Angelicae Sinensis
Chuan Xiong	6 g	Radix Ligustici Wallichii
Bai Zhu	9 g	Rhizoma Atractylodis Macrocephalae
Bai Shao	9 g	Radix Paeoniae Lactiflorae
Gan Cao	6 g	Radix Glycyrrhizae Uralensis
Sheng Jiang	6 g	Rhizoma Zingiberis Officinalis Recens

Table 5.26   Acupuncture points[a] used in the treatment of PCOS from Liver Qi stagnation leading to localized Phlegm-Damp accumulation

Treatment goal	Acupuncture points
To regulate the Liver Qi	LIV-3, LIV-5, LIV-8, LIV-11, LIV-13, BL-18, BL-19
To clear Damp and promote menstruation	SP-6, SP-9, Ren-1, Ren-3,
To open and regulate the Dai vessel which is a conduit for Damp in the lower body	GB-41 and TH-5. GB-27/28, GB-26.
To promote Qi and Blood movement around the ovaries	ST-29, ST-28
To facilitate unblocking the Bao Mai and regulate menstruation	PC-5

[a]Use even or reducing technique. Electroacupuncture can be used, connecting abdomen and Inner leg points 10 Hertz, 3–5 Amps, 20 min.

This formula is not a commonly encountered one in gynecology but it serves our purpose here in clearing Heat and Phlegm-Damp (Lian Qiao, Shi Gao, Huang Qin, Jie Geng) via the bowels (Da Huang and Mang Xiao) and urine (Zhi Zi, Hua Shi). The mild dispersing action (Ma Huang, Fang Feng, Jing Jie, Bo He) it has on the exterior disperses Liver Qi stagnation. Fang Feng has the special attribute of removing Damp blockages by transforming Damp into Yang Qi and lifting the Yang. To protect the Spleen Qi are added Bai Zhu, Gan Cao and Sheng Jiang. To harmonize the Blood are added Dang Gui, Bai Shao and Chuan Xiong.

This formula represents a fairly drastic approach to kick-starting the ovaries again by purging Heat and stagnation. We saw a similar approach when Heat from Liver and Heart Qi stagnation had damaged the Yin, causing amenorrhea, and purgatives were used cautiously to drain Heat and thus recover the Yin. In this case we are dealing with an excess pattern, however, not a deficiency pattern, and can use stronger herbs for longer. Nevertheless, the patient must always be watched carefully to see the response and the formula is used for a limited period of time. Follow-up treatments include formulas such as that mentioned below, which circulate Liver Qi but also reinforce Kidney function.

Acupuncture Points — Points for Liver Qi stagnation leading to localized Phlegm-Damp accumulation (Table 5.26) are chosen from:

LIV-3	Taichong
LIV-5	Ligou
LIV-8	Ququan
LIV-13	Zhangmen
LIV-11	Yinlian
Ren-1	Huiyin
Ren-3	Zhongji
GB-41	Zulinqi
TH-5	Waiguan
GB-26	Daimai
ST-29	Guilai
ST-28	Shuidao
GB-27	Wushu
GB-28	Weidao
BL-18	Ganshu

BL-19	Danshu
SP-6	Sanyinqiao
SP-9	Yinlingquan
PC-5	Jianshi

LIVER QI STAGNATION CAUSING OBSTRUCTION TO QI AND BLOOD FLOW IN THE CHONG AND THE REN VESSELS

Where less drastic measures are called for, or after a course of the above formula, we shall use a formula that promotes movement of Qi and Blood in the Chong and the Ren, at the same time as resolving any local deposits of Phlegm-Damp and reinforcing the Kidneys.

Herbal Formula — Using Xiao Yao San in combination with Bu Shen Hua Tang tang will achieve our aims.

Xiao Yao San (Free and Easy powder) with Bu Shen Hua Tan Tang (decoction for restoring the Kidney and removing phlegm) modified

Dang Gui	9 g	*Radix Angelicae Sinensis*
Bai Shao	12 g	*Radix Paeoniae Lactiflorae*
Chuan Xiong	6 g	*Radix Ligustici Wallichii*
Chuan Niu Xi	9 g	*Radix Cyathula*
Gou Qi Zi	9 g	*Fructus Lycii Chinensis*
Chai Hu	9 g	*Radix Bupleuri*
Xiang Fu	12 g	*Rhizoma Cyperi Rotundi*
Li Zhi He	9 g	*Semen Litchi*
Xia Ku Cao	9 g	*Spica Prunellae Vulgaris*
He Huan Pi	9 g	*Cortex Albizziae Julibrissin*
Tu Si Zi	12 g	*Semen Cuscatae*
Yin Yang Huo	9 g	*Herba Epimedii*
Shu Di	9 g	*Radix Rehmanniae Glutinosae Conquitae*
Shan Zhu Yu	9 g	*Fructus Corni Officinalis*

A variation of Xiao Yao San (the well known Free and Easy powder), combined with elements of the formula Bu Shen Hua Tan tang will move Qi and Blood in the Chong and Ren vessels and aim to restore menstrual regularity.

This formula contains herbs (Bai Shao, Dang Gui, Chuan Xiong, Gou Qi Zi and Chuan Niu Xi) to build the Blood and encourage its movement in the Chong vessel.

These are supported by herbs such as Chai hu, Xiang Fu, Xia Ku Cao and Li Zhe He which move and unblock the Qi in the Liver channel. He Huan Pi is an important addition to relieve constraint in the Liver channel and address emotional stress.

Finally, we add herbs such as Shu Di, Yin Yang Huo, Shan Zhu Yu and Tu Si Zi to tonify Kidneys to encourage normal ovary function.

Acupuncture Points — Points (Table 5.27) are chosen from:

LIV-3	Taichong
CO-4	Hegu
LIV-5	Ligou
Yin Tang	
PC-6	Neiguan

PC-7	Daling
Abdomen Zigong	
ST-29	Guilai
SP-10	Xuehai
SP-4	Gongsun
LIV-8	Ququan
K-13	Qixue
K-14	Siman

Table 5.27   Acupuncture points[a] used in the treatment of PCOS from Liver Qi stagnation causing obstruction to Qi and Blood flow in the Chong and the Ren channels

Treatment goal	Acupuncture points
To regulate the Liver Qi	LIV-3, LIV-5, LIV-8, LIV-11, BL-18, BL-17
To support Spleen	SP-6, SP-10
To build Liver Blood	SP-10, LIV-8
To promote Qi and Blood movement around the ovaries	ST-29, Abdomen Zigong
To pacify mind, relieve stress	LIV-3, LI-4, PC-6 PC-7, Yin Tang.

[a]Use even or reducing technique. Electroacupuncture can be applied connecting abdomen and inner leg points 10 Hertz, 3–5 Amps, 20 min.

CASE HISTORY – EFFIE

Effie was an elegant, young 29-year-old woman who had lost her periods and wanted them back. She wasn't planning on becoming pregnant just yet but was anxious to keep this option open. Plus, she didn't feel right without her periods.

She had started taking the oral contraceptive pill shortly after puberty and continued taking it for 15 years without a break. She stopped the pill and her first natural period came about 6 weeks later; the next was 9 weeks after that and the next was 12 weeks later; then nothing.

At this point, her doctor ordered some tests. An ultrasound revealed polycystic ovaries and her serum testosterone and DHEA levels were slightly elevated. No insulin resistance was evident either on blood tests or with a glucose tolerance test. Her diagnosis was PCOS. Her older sister had also received this diagnosis so an inherited component is likely in this case. Her doctor offered her no treatment since she didn't need Metformin for insulin resistance and didn't want to take clomifene at the time. She decided to look for alternatives and came to my clinic.

Effie appeared to be a slim woman, but she didn't have much of a waist – her waist-to-height ratio was slightly higher than normal. She was not hirsute and despite the occasional breakout, had good skin. She exercised regularly and had a good relatively low carbohydrate diet.

Her job was stressful and involved irregular hours and she described herself as irritable and moody. But she slept well and felt well and energetic.

Her pulse was tight and her tongue slightly coated. Her diagnosis was Liver Qi stagnation, leading to obstruction of Chong and Ren vessels.

Treatment with acupuncture aimed to regulate Liver Qi and regulate Qi, Blood and Phlegm-Damp in the Chong, Ren and Dai vessel, and promote ovulation.

Herbs were prescribed to support Spleen and Kidney function, regulate Qi and Blood.

Acupuncture points: ST-28 and SP-6 with electroacupuncture, GB-27, Ren-3, Ren-7, LIV-5 Co-4

Variations at different times included: SP-4, PC-6, LIV-8, ST-40, ST-36, GB-41, TH-5, SP-9

If we were sure an ovulation had occurred (there were usually clear ovulation signs and Effie's breasts became swollen and sore premenstrually), then we would change to points which moved the Liver Qi and Blood.

For example, LIV-14, LIV-8, SP-10, SP-6, PC-5, ST-29, K-14

Herbal formula

Dang Gui	9 g	Radix Angelicae Sinensis
Bai Shao	12 g	Radix Paeoniae Lactiflorae
Chai Hu	9 g	Radix Bupleuri
Bai Zhu	9 g	Rhizoma Atractylodis Macrocephalae
Fu Ling	9 g	Sclerotium Poriae Cocos
Chuan Xiong	6 g	Radix Ligustici Wallichii
Dan Nan Xing	3 g	Rhizoma Arisaematis
Zao Jiao Ci	6 g	Spina Gleditsiae Sinensis
Xiang Fu	12 g	Rhizoma Cyperi Rotundi
He Huan Pi	9 g	Cortex Albizziae Julibrissin
Bu Gu Zhi	9 g	Fructus Psoraleae
Yin Yang Huo	9 g	Herba Epimedii
Shu Di	6 g	Radix Rehmanniae Glutinosae Conquitae
Shan Yao	9 g	Radix Dioscorea Oppositae

Variations at different times included Tao Ren, Hong Hua, Dan Shen, Chi Shao, Cang Zhu, Sha Ren, Zi Shi Ying.

It was 14 acupuncture treatments (over 3 months) and several formulas later that she got her next period – after 7 months of amenorrhea. I had suggested an intense program of acupuncture would be the best way to get things moving, however her job which entailed a lot of travel did not allow this. Possibly with more intense treatment, the ovarian environment might have changed more rapidly than it did, and she might have ovulated sooner.

Nevertheless, once things got started there was no looking back. Once the Liver Qi was moving (Effie's mood was the first improvement we saw) and obstructions in the Chong, Ren or Dai vessel were cleared, then the ovaries started to function again.

Her next cycle was 7 weeks compared with the previous 7 months, and the next 4 periods followed at precise 6-week intervals, with clearly discernible ovulations signs around Day 28. She continued to have acupuncture weekly or fortnightly throughout this time.

If this continues, and it certainly appears to be a trend, this means Effie will have 8 or 9 cycles per year, which means it may take slightly longer to conceive when she and her partner decide to have a baby, but with the clear predictability of her ovulations hopefully not too long.

Furthermore, the regularity of her cycles now indicate that the Chong and Ren vessels are working although the delayed switch from Kidney yin to Kidney yang in the menstrual cycle indicates there is still some underlying deficiency. This is the inherited component of Effie's condition and may not be able to be changed. She is recommended to continue with herbs and acupuncture from time to time, and certainly if she plans to conceive.

Researchers in various parts of the world have demonstrated that acupuncture can improve ovary function and increase ovulation frequency. Some of these studies have found that levels of LH and testosterone and insulin in PCOS patients were found to be beneficially reduced by course of acupuncture.[64–70] Other studies have specifically looked at the effect of acupuncture in increasing insulin sensitivity.[71]

And several studies have examined the effect of acupuncture on rats with PCOS demonstrating increased ovulations and reduced insulin resistance.[72–75]

These studies used standardized treatments using abdomen and limb points according to segmental innervation of the ovaries in some studies and TCM principles in others. Primary points were chosen from the Ren, Stomach, Spleen, Kidney, Bladder, and Liver channels. Points chosen that relate to sympathetic nervous system segmental innervation of the ovaries (the level of vertebrae T9–L2) were abdomen points Ren-4 and 6, Stomach and Kidney channel points on the abdomen and Bladder channel points on the lumbar region. Points relating to parasympathetic nervous system segmental innervation of the ovaries (the level of vertebrae S2–S4) were sacral points such as BL-27, 28 and medial leg points such as SP-6, SP-9, LIV-3, K-3. Points unrelated to segmental innervation included points such as PC-5, PC-6, TH-6, Co-4, Du-20, etc. Points chosen for their TCM properties include Ren-3, Abdomen Zigong, SP-6, LIV-3, ST-36, ST-40, ST-29 and SP-20. These are summarized in Table 5.28.

Abdomen points were needled deeply and where electroacupuncture was used it was applied with mild to moderate intensity (3–5 mAmps) at low frequency (2–10 Hz) for 20–30 min. Leads were attached from abdomen to leg points on the same side.

The frequency of application of the treatments appears to be important. Some investigators have found that 2–5 treatments per week for 4 months is necessary to return ovary function and regular ovulation. Practically, this is challenging for patients in terms of time and cost, however some clinics have set up programs whereby frequent short treatments at low cost have been provided to great benefit. The mechanism of action of the acupuncture is not yet elucidated although some researchers believe that it is mediated via the sympathetic nervous system.

While a lot of the research emphasis has been on acupuncture for PCOS patients, there have been fewer studies on the effect of Chinese herbs, and most of the trials have been small or not well controlled.[76]

Some trials have compared Chinese herbal preparations with Metformin favorably, e.g., those patients who took the herbs over a 3 months period reported a higher ovulation frequency, greater reduction in testosterone levels and BMI compared with those who took Metformin.[77] We shall discuss the evidence for adding Chinese herbal remedies to a regimen of clomifene below.

Table 5.28   Acupuncture points used in PCOS trials

Segmental innervation of ovaries Sympathetic nervous system	Ren-4 and 6, abdomen Stomach and Kidney channel points, Bladder channel points on lumbar region
Segmental innervation of ovaries Para sympathetic nervous system	SP-6, 9, LIV-3, K-3, Bladder channel points on sacral region
TCM indications	REN-3, Abdomen Zigong, SP-6, LIV-3, ST-36, ST-40, ST-29 and SP-20

Combining TCM and Western medicine

It is likely that many of your PCOS patients will be seeing reproductive specialists or endocrinologists who will have prescribed medications. As we discussed above, the usual pharmaceutical treatment for PCOS patients wishing to fall pregnant includes Metformin (Diaformin) to help reduce insulin and regulate blood sugar levels and clomifene (Serophene) to help induce ovulation.

Looking at these drugs from a TCM point of view we are aware that Metformin can often compromise Spleen Qi (loose stools and nausea) and that Clomid can compromise the Kidney Yin (reduced endometrial thickness and number of endometrial glands and drying of cervical mucus). When our patient is attempting to conceive healthy Kidney Yin and Yang and Spleen Qi are vital, so combining a TCM approach to support Spleen and Kidneys with these drugs is an important consideration.

A large number of trials in China have examined the combined effect of Chinese herbs and Clomid on women who were not ovulating. When they assessed parameters like endometrium thickness, cervical discharge and ovulation and pregnancy rates, typically they show improvement on all counts when they compare with control groups given Clomid alone.[78,79] One trial which compared the ovulation rate induced by acupuncture and herbs compared with that induced by clomifene found they were equally effective, but that a significantly larger number of women conceived using the acupuncture and Chinese herbs.[80] Studies that looked specifically at anovulatory PCOS patients found the same thing, i.e., significantly improved ovulation and pregnancy rates compared to controls.[81] When patients with PCOS proved to be resistant to the effects of clomifene, pre-treatment with Chinese herbs for 2 months overcame this resistance and ovulation could be induced.[82]

A recent review also reports that PCOS patients who take Chinese herbs with Clomid can significantly increase the odds of pregnancy.[83] Studies in PCOS rats have shown that Chinese herbs can improve ovarian function and reduce testosterone levels.[84] Typically the herbs used in the clinical trials are standardized formulas that boost Kidney Yin and Yang, promote Blood and Qi circulation and clear Damp and Phlegm.

Similarly, acupuncture can support the action of Metformin and Clomid in promoting ovulation, while at the same time attempting to ameliorate the undesirable side-effects. If your PCOS patient is not ovulating and is prescribed clomifene (which is appropriate unless they are Yin deficient and dry), then suggesting concurrent treatment with herbs and/or acupuncture has good clinical evidence basis.

In conclusion, we can say that PCOS is one of the most complex and challenging endocrinologic and reproductive disorders that we will see in our clinics. While there is no doubt there are inherited factors in many cases, it is also perhaps caused by what we are doing to our bodies – the OCP, poor diet and too much sugar, adverse influences on female fetuses in utero and the stresses that young girls are subjected to today.

We are well placed with our Chinese medicine sensibilities to find ways to unravel this clinical challenge and find ways to effectively treat it. TCM sits more comfortably with clinical complexity than does Western medicine with its emphasis on analysis and isolation of causative factors.

By gathering all the signs and symptoms (and heeding the information that laboratory and clinical investigations and research have provided us) we can synthesize a known TCM pattern or patterns of disharmony and customize it for each PCOS patient. Thus emerges a clear guiding principle of treatment appropriate for the various presentations of this challenging condition and accordingly, we hope to create effective and holistic ways to help these patients.

REFERENCES

1. Xia GC. *Zhong Yi Lin Chuang Fu Ke Xue*. 2nd edn : PRC: Chinese People's Health Publishing; 1996.

2. Kennedy S, Hadfield R, Westbrook C, et al. Magnetic resonance imaging to assess familial risk in relatives of women with endometriosis. *Lancet* 1998;**352**:1440–1.

3. Campo R, Gordts S, Rombauts L, et al. Diagnostic accuracy of transvaginal hydrolaparoscopy in infertility. *Fertil Steril* 1999;**71**:1157–60.

229

4.   Brosens IA, Brosens JJ. Redefining endometriosis: Is deep endometriosis a progressive disease?. *Hum Reprod* 2000;**15**(1):1–3.

5.   Khan KN, Kitajima M, Hiraki K, et al. Toll-like receptors in innate immunity: role of bacterial endotoxin and Toll-like receptor 4 in endometrium and endometriosis. *Gynecol Obstet Invest* 2009;**68**:40–52.

6.   Khan KN, Kitajima M, Hiraki K, et al. Immunopathogenesis of pelvic endometriosis: role of hepatocyte growth factor, macrophages and ovarian steroids. *Am J Reprod Immunol* 2008;**60**:383–404.

7.   Harlow CR, Cahill DJ, Maile LA, et al. Reduced preovulatory granulosa cell steroidogenesis in women with endometriosis. *J Clin Endocrinol Metab* 1996;**81**:426–9.

8.   Bergqvist A, Bruse C, Carlberg M, et al. Interleukin 1beta, interleukin-6, and tumor necrosis factor-alpha in endometriotic tissue and in endometrium. *Fertil Steril* 2001;**75**:489–95.

9.   Brosens IA. Endometriosis – narrow but deep – important. *Fertil Steril* 1993;**60**:201–2.

10. Noble LS, Takayama K, Zeitoun KM, et al. Prostaglandin E2 stimulates aromatase expression in endometriosis-derived stromal cells. *J Clin Endocrinol Metab* 1997;**82**:600–6.

11. Tseng JF, Ryan IP, Milam TD, et al. Interleukin-6 secretion in vitro is upregulated in ectopic and eutopic endometrial stromal cells from women with endometriosis. *J Clin Endocrinol Metab* 1996;**81**:1118–22.

12. Brosens I, Derwig I, Brosens J, et al. The enigmatic uterine junctional zone: the missing link between reproductive disorders and major obstetrical disorders?. *Hum Reprod* 2010;**25**(3):569–74.

13. Leyendecker G, Kunz G, Wildt L, et al. Uterine hyperperistalsis and dysperistalsis as dysfunctions of the mechanism of rapid sperm transport in patients with endometriosis and infertility. *Hum Reprod* 1996;**11**:1542–51.

14. Palial K, Drury J, Heathcote L, et al. Basement membrane integrity is altered in the late secretory phase in women with endometriosis: implications for the pathogenesis of Endometriosis. *Hum Reprod* 2011;**26**(Suppl 1):i202.

15. Arici A, Oral E, Bukulmez O, et al. The effect of endometriosis on implantation: results from the Yale University in vitro fertilization and embryo transfer program. *Fertil Steril* 1996;**65**(3):603–7.

16. Simón C, Gutiérrez A, Vidal A, et al. Outcome of patients with endometriosis in assisted reproduction: results from in-vitro fertilization and oocyte donation. *Hum Reprod* 1994;**9**(4):725–9.

17. Lemos NA, Arbo E, Scalco R, et al. Decreased anti-Müllerian hormone and altered ovarian follicular cohort in infertile patients with mild/minimal endometriosis. *Fertil Steril* 2008;**89**(5):1064–8.

18. Hwu Yuh-Ming, Wu Frank Shao-Ying, Li Sheng-Hsiang, et al. The impact of endometrioma and laparoscopic cystectomy on serum anti-Müllerian hormone levels. *Reprod Biol Endocrinol* 2011;**9**:80.

19. Chung K, Coutifaris C, Chalian R, et al. Factors influencing adverse perinatal outcomes in pregnancies achieved through use of in vitro fertilization. *Fertil Steril* 2006;**86**:1634–41.

20. Stephansson O, Kieler H, Granath F, et al. Endometriosis, assisted reproduction technology, and risk of adverse pregnancy outcome. *Hum Reprod* 2009;**24**(9):2341–7.

21. Carlberg M, Nejaty J, Froysa B, et al. Elevated expression of tumor necrosis factor alpha in cultured granulosa cells from women with endometriosis. *Hum Reprod* 2000;**15**:1250–5.

22. Lian F, Li XL, Sun ZG, et al. Effect of Quyu Jiedu granule on microenvironment of ova in patients with endometriosis. *Chin J Integr Med* 2009;**15**(1):42–6.

23. Lim CED. Clinical observation of Chinese medicine treatment on secondary dysmenorrhea associated with endometriosis. *Aust J Acupunct Chin Med* 2009;**4**(2):12–7.

24. Yu C-Q, Cai Z-L, Liu Y-H, et al. Study on therapeutic mechanism of Neiyifang in treating endometriosis. *Chin J Integr Med* 2003;**9**:88–92.

25. Yu Fu, Tian Xia. Clinical observation on treatment of endometriosis with acupuncture plus herbs. *J Acupunct Tuina Sci* 2005;**3**(5):48–51.

26. Wieser F, Cohen M, Gaeddert A, et al. Evolution of medical treatment for endometriosis: back to the roots?. *Hum Reprod Update* 2007;**13**(5):487–99.

27. Yang Man-e, Mao Xiao, Wang Pi-yun. Clinical observation of combined acupuncture and herbs in treating chronic pelvic inflammation. *J Acupunct Tuina Sci* 2009;**7**(6):339–42.

28. Bi-fang Peng, Ding Ding. Clinical observations on the treatment of 60 cases of pelvic congestion syndrome with Fu Ke Qian Jin Jiao Nong combined with Ru He San Jie Pian. *Gan Su Zhong Yi (Gansu Chin Med)* 2009;**1**:50–1.

29. Maclean W, Lyttleton J. Abdominal masses. *Clinical Handbook of Internal Medicine*. ;**Vol 3**Sydney: Pangolin Press; 2010, 1.

30. Jin Yu. *Handbook of obstetrics and gynecology in Chinese medicine*. Seattle: Eastland Press; 1998, 70.

31. Moran LJ, Lombard CB, Lim S, et al. Polycystic ovary syndrome and weight management. *Women's Health* 2010;**6**(2):271–83.

32. Carey AH, Chan KL, Short F, et al. Evidence for a single gene effect causing polycystic ovaries and male pattern baldness. *Clin Endocrinol* 1993;**38**:653–8.

33. Segal TR, Dicken CL, Israel D, et al. 2011. In-utero and neonatal vitamin D3 deficiency results in a polycystic ovarian syndrome-like phenotype. *Fertil Steril* 2011;**96**(3):Supplement ASRM abstracts.

34. Abbott DH, Dumesic DA, Franks S. Developmental origin of polycystic ovary syndrome – a hypothesis. *J Endocrinol* 2002;**174**:1–5.

35. Homburg R. Androgen circle of polycystic ovary syndrome. *Hum Reprod* 2009;**24**(7):1548–55.

36. Kidson W. How to treat polycystic ovary syndrome. *Aust Doc* 2011:31–6;June.

37. Ibanez L, Potau N, Marcos MV, et al. Exaggerated adrenarche and hyperinsulinism in adolescent girls born small for gestational age. *J Clin Endocrinol Metab* 1999;**84**:4739–41.

38. Gilling-Smith C, Story H, Rogers V, et al. Evidence for a primary abnormality of thecal cell steroidogenesis in the polycystic ovary syndrome. *Clin Endocrinol (Oxf)* 1997;**47**:93–9.

39. Wohlfahrt-Veje C, Andersen HR, Schmidt IM, et al. Early breast development in girls after prenatal exposure to non-persistent pesticides. *Int J Androl* 2012;**35**(3):273–82.

40. Dinsdale EC, Ward WE. Early exposure to soy isoflavones and effects on reproductive health: a review of human and animal studies. *Nutrients* 2010;**2**(11):1156–87.

41. Francks S. Follicle dynamics and anovulation in polycystic ovary syndrome. *Hum Reprod Update* 2008;**14**(4):367–78.

42. Oelkers W, Foidart JM, Dombrovicz N, et al. Effects of a new oral contraceptive containing an antimineralocorticoid progestogen, drospirenone, on the renin-aldosterone system, body weight, blood pressure, glucose tolerance, and lipid metabolism. *J Clin Endocr Metab* 1995;**80**:1816–21.

43. Puurunen JM, Piltonen TT, Hedberg PS, et al. Combined oral, transdermal and vaginal contraceptives worsen insulin resistance and chronic inflammation in young healthy normal weight women, a randomized study. *Fertil Steril* 2011;**96**(3):S37.

44. Dorte Glintborg, Andersen M. An update on the pathogenesis, inflammation, and metabolism in hirsutism and polycystic ovary syndrome. *Gynecol Endocrinol* 2010;**26**(4):281–96.

45. Lord J, Thomas R, Fox B, et al. The central issue? Visceral fat mass is a good marker of insulin resistance and metabolic disturbance in women with polycystic ovary syndrome. *Br J Obstet Gynaecol* 2006;**113**(9):1203–9.

46. Kirchengast S, Huber J. Body composition characteristics and body fat distribution in lean women with polycystic ovary syndrome. *Hum Reprod* 2001;**16**(6):1255–60.

47. Dolfing JG, Stassen CM, van Haard PM, et al. Comparison of MRI-assessed body fat content between lean women with polycystic ovary syndrome (PCOS) and matched controls: less visceral fat with PCOS. *Hum Reprod* 2011;**26**:1495–500.

48. Manneras-Holm L, Leonhardt H, Kullberg J, et al. Adipose tissue has aberrant morphology and function in PCOS: enlarged adipocytes and low serum adiponectin, but not circulating sex steroids, are strongly associated with insulin resistance. *J Clin Endocrinol Metab 2011* 2011;**96**(2):E304–11.

49. Ibáñez L, López-Bermejo Abel, Díaz Marta, et al. Early metformin therapy (age 8–12 years) in girls with precocious pubarche to reduce hirsutism, androgen excess, and oligomenorrhea in adolescence. *J Clin Endocrinol Metab* 2011;**96**(8):E1262–7.

50. Navaratnarajah R, Sinclair J, Grun B, et al. Proteome investigation in the PCOS endometrium associated with obesity. *Hum Reprod* 2011;**26**(Suppl 1):i65.

51. Norman RJ, Robker R, Xing Y, et al. Components of follicular fluid from obese women induce adverse metabolic defects in cumulus-oocyte complexes. *Hum Reprod* 2011;**26**(Suppl 1):i75.

52. Paredes A, Salvetti N, Diaz A, et al. Sympathetic nerve activity in normal and cystic follicles from isolated bovine ovary: local effect of beta-adrenergic stimulation on steroid secretion. *Reprod Biol Endocrinol* 2011;**9**:66.

53. Palomba S, Falbo A, Russo T, et al. Pregnancy in women with polycystic ovary syndrome: the effect of different phenotypes and features on obstetric and neonatal outcomes. *Fertil Steril* 2010;**94**(5):1805–11.

54. Bagegni NA, Blaine J, Van Voorhis BJ, et al. Risk of early & late obstetric complications in women with polycystic ovary syndrome (PCOS). *Proc Obstet Gynecol* 2010;**1**(2):10.

55. Coffey S, Bano G, Mason HD. Health-related quality of life in women with PCOS: A comparison with the general population using the polycystic ovary syndrome questionnaire (PCOSQ) and the short form-36 (SF-36). *Gynecol Endocrinol* 2006;**22**:80–6.

56. Norman RJ, Wu R, Stankiewicz MT. Polycystic ovary syndrome. *Med J Aust* 2004;**180**(3):132–7.

57. Clark AM, Thornley B, Tomlinson L, et al. Weight loss in obese infertile women results in improvement in reproductive outcome for all forms of fertility treatment. *Hum Reprod* 1998;**13**(6):1502–5.

58. Robker RL, Akison LK, Bennett BD, et al. Obese women exhibit differences in ovarian metabolites, hormones, and gene expression compared with moderate-weight women. *J Clin Endocrinol Metab* 2009;**94**:1533–40.

59. Little JP, Gillen JB, Percival ME, et al. Low-volume high-intensity interval training reduces hyperglycemia and increases muscle mitochondrial capacity in patients with type 2 diabetes. *J Appl Physiol* 2011;**111**(6):1554–60.

60. Tang T, Glanville J, Hayden CJ, et al. Combined lifestyle modification and metformin in obese patients with polycystic ovary syndrome. *Hum Reprod* 2006;**21**:80–9.

61. Lok F, Ledger WL, Li TC, et al. Surgical intervention in infertility management. *Hum Fertil* 2003;**6**:S52–9.

62. Weixin Jin. *Diagnosis of sterility and its traditional Chinese medicine treatment.* : PRC: Shandong Science and Technology Press; 1999, 142.

63. Mannerås-Holm L, Baghaei Fariba, Holm Göran, et al. Coagulation and fibrinolytic disturbances in women with polycystic ovary syndrome. *J Clin Endocrinol Metab* 2011;**96**:1068–76.

64. Lim CED. Acupuncture on PCOS: First World RCT. Abstract. Inaugural Chinese Medicine Academic Conference 20–21 August 2011. Sydney: University of Technology.

65. Stener-Victorin E, Wu X. Effects of electro-acupuncture on anovulation in women with polycystic ovary syndrome. *Acta Obstet Gynecol Scand* 2009;**79**:180–8.

66. Stener-Victorin E, Jedel E, Janson PO, et al. Low-frequency electroacupuncture and physical exercise decrease high muscle sympathetic nerve activity in polycystic ovary syndrome. *Am J Physiol* 2009;**297**(2):R387–95.

67. Pastore LM, Williams CD, Jenkins J, et al. True and sham acupuncture produced similar frequency of ovulation and improved LH to FSH ratios in women with polycystic ovary syndrome. *Endocr Res* 2011;**96**:3143–50.

68. Jedel E, Labrie F, Oden A, et al. Impact of electro-acupuncture and physical exercise on hyperandrogenism and oligo/amenorrhea in women with polycystic ovary syndrome: a randomized controlled trial. *Am J Physiol Endocrinol Metab* 2011;**300**(1):E37–45.

69. Xiaoming MO, Ding LI, Yunxing PU, et al. Clinical studies on the mechanism for acupuncture stimulation of ovulation. *J Trad Chinese Med* 1993;**13**:115–9.

70. Chen BY, Yu J. Relationship between blood radioimmunoreactive betaendorphin and hand skin temperature during the electro-acupuncture induction of ovulation. *Acupunct Electrother Res* 1991;**16**:1–5.

71. Liang F, Koya D. Acupuncture: is it effective for treatment of insulin resistance?. *Diabetes Obes Metab* 2010;**12**:555–69.

72. Feng Y, Johansson J, Shao R, et al. Hypothalamic neuroendocrine functions in rats with dihydrotestosterone-induced polycystic ovary syndrome: effects of low-frequency electro-acupuncture. *PLoS One* 2009;**4**(8):e6638.

73. Yi Zhang Wei, et al. Influence of acupuncture on infertility in rats with polycystic ovarian syndrome. *Chin J Integr Trad Western Med* 2009;**11**:973.

74. Johansson J, Feng Y, Shao R, et al. Intense electro-acupuncture normalizes insulin sensitivity, increases muscle GLUT4 content, and improves lipid profile in a rat model of polycystic ovary syndrome. *Am J Physiol Endocrinol Metab* 2010;**299**:E551–9.

75. Manneras L, Jonsdottir IH, Homang A, et al. Low-frequency electro-acupuncture and physical exercise improve metabolic disturbances and modulate gene expression in adipose tissue in rats with dihydrotestosterone-induced polycystic ovary syndrome. *Endocrinology* 2008;**149**(7):3559–68.

76. Raja-Khan N, Stener-Victorin E, Wu X, et al. The physiological basis of complementary and alternative medicines for polycystic ovary syndrome. *Am J Physiol Endocrinol Metab* 2011;**301**:E1–0.

77. Hou J, Yu J, Wei M. Study on treatment of hyperandrogenism and hyperinsulinism in polycystic ovary syndrome with Chinese herbal formula 'tiangui fang'. *Zhongguo Zhong Xi Yi Jie He Za Zhi* 2000;**20**(8):589–92:[Article in Chinese].

78. Jianan Zhang, et al. *Fujian J. TCM* 2005;**36**(5):9–10:[Article in Chinese].

79. Ma SX, Yin DE, Zhu YL. Yijing Huoxue Cuyun decoction. *Zhongguo Zhong Xi Yi Jie He Za Zhi* 2005;**25**(4):360–2:[Article in Chinese].

80. Jiang DS, Ding D. Clinical observation on acupuncture combined with medication for treatment of continuing anovulation infertility. *Zhongguo Zhen Jiu* 2009;**29**(1):21–4:[Article in Chinese].

81. Shao RY, Lang FJ, Cai JF. Shen and activating blood circulation herbs. *Zhongguo Zhong Xi Yi Jie He Za Zhi* 2004;**24**(1):41–3:[Article in Chinese].

82. Yang YS, Zhang YL. Ganshao capsule. *Zhongguo Zhong Xi Yi Jie He Za Zhi* 2005;**25**(8):704–6:[Article in Chinese].

83. Zhang J, Li T, Zhou L, et al. Chinese herbal medicine for subfertile women with polycystic ovarian syndrome. *Cochrane Database Syst Rev* 2010(9):CD007535.

84. Ma HX, Xie J, Lai MH. Effects of Yangling Zhongyu decoction on the secretion of ovarian granule cells in polycystic ovarian syndrome rat model. *Zhongguo Zhong Xi Yi Jie He Za Zhi* 2012;**32**(1):54–7:[Article in Chinese].

Blockage of the Fallopian Tubes

6

INTRODUCTION

Very fine muscular tubes, called the fallopian tubes, are responsible for transporting the egg (and embryo) from the ovary to the uterus. It is blockage in this passage which is the cause of one-third of cases of female infertility.

CAN CHINESE MEDICINE TREAT FALLOPIAN TUBE BLOCKAGE?

Once a disease has changed or damaged the tissue of the fallopian tube, then acupuncture and herbal medicine can offer limited therapeutic benefit. Western medicine, similarly, offers little to reverse such damage but often has ways of removing or side-stepping the problem. From the point of view of the TCM doctor, blockage of the fallopian tubes is a much more difficult cause of infertility to cure than functional causes. However, from the Western specialist's point of view, this sort of infertility, in the absence of any other complicating factors, is one of the easiest and most satisfying to treat, whether by microsurgery, which removes the damaged portion of the tube, or more commonly by in vitro fertilization (IVF) techniques which circumnavigate the tubes altogether.

Where the structure of the tube is not damaged but its function is impaired, then treatment with Chinese medicine can expect a good outcome.

In determining just how much help a TCM doctor can offer to a woman suffering from infertility due to tubal blockage, we need to know just how much damage has been done and what it is that is causing the obstruction.

DIAGNOSIS OF TUBAL BLOCKAGE

There is no way to test the patency of the tubes other than with rather invasive procedures. A tubal blockage is itself asymptomatic, although a history of pelvic infection will raise suspicion of tubal disease.

A *hysterosalpingo-contrast-sonography* (HyCoSy) is the preferred technique for investigation of Fallopian tube patency. It is a dynamic ultrasound of the uterus and tubes taken while a solution of galactose and 1% palmitic acid (Levovist) – or a mixture of air and saline – is infused into the uterine cavity and observed as it moves through the Fallopian tubes. The bright echoes generated by the solution and the use of color Doppler imaging allow clear visualization of the tubes and their function. The procedure is performed in the first 10 days of the menstrual cycle and after the period has finished. The HyCoSy also allows examination of the other pelvic organs including the ovaries.

A *hysterosalpingogram* (HSG) is an X-ray of the inside of the uterus and tubes, which is achieved by injection of an X-ray opaque medium through the cervix. This dye is forced into the uterus and tubes under pressure until it spills into the pelvic cavity if the tubes are patent.

A degree of discomfort is often experienced by the woman having either the HyCoSy or the HSG. Period pain medication taken before the procedure can lessen the cramps.

The pressure of the fluid passing through the tubes may have the therapeutic function of clearing some tubal obstructions (such as those caused by muscle spasm or mucus secretions).

A *laparoscopy* is a surgical procedure by which a surgeon can see directly into the pelvic cavity by means of a small fiberoptic tube passed down a catheter. The health of the fallopian tubes from the outside can be seen and their patency tested by passing a colored dye up through the cervix and watching for its appearance at the far end of the tube. The patient does not experience the immediate discomfort of the HSG but there will be postoperative discomfort and the after-effects of general anesthesia.

THE STRUCTURE OF THE FALLOPIAN TUBES

Each fallopian tube is a thin, fragile tube about 10 cm long (Fig. 6.1). At the end near the ovaries, it fans out like a hand with fingers (the fimbriae) to catch the egg as it is released from the ovary. The section of tube attached to the fimbria is called the 'ampulla' and is wide and thin-walled. The section of the tube attached to the uterus is called the 'isthmus' and is much narrower and has thicker, more muscular walls. Inside the tube are secretory cells, which produce substances essential for the survival of the egg and the embryo. Also lining the inside of the tube are ciliated cells, so-called for their hair-like projections which push the egg down the tube toward the isthmus with waving motions.

The point where the ampulla meets the narrow isthmus is where the egg waits to meet its sperm, and then where the pre-embryo, if fertilization has occurred, waits to go through its first few cell divisions. The rising levels of progesterone produced by the corpus luteum clear the secretions and relax the muscles in the isthmus to allow the pre-embryo through to the uterus. Although we do not yet know all the secrets of the tube and its relationship with the new embryo, presumably there are special conditions and nutrients provided by the cells lining the tube that are important for the fertilized egg as it completes its first few cell divisions. Two or three days later it will be launched into the uterine cavity to find its nesting spot.

DAMAGE TO THE STRUCTURE OF THE TUBE

Fallopian tubes sustain damage most frequently through infection and inflammation. Chlamydia is one of the most common causes of tubal infection. About 40% of untreated chlamydia infections cause pelvic inflammatory disease (PID), and about 20% of such infected women become infertile. Gonorrhea is the second most common sexually transmitted disease after chlamydia in developed nations, and it also causes PID and consequent infertility. Tuberculosis and yeast infections can also damage the tubes. Intrauterine devices or IUDs have a now infamous history of causing infection, although the subsequent damage is usually isolated to one tube.

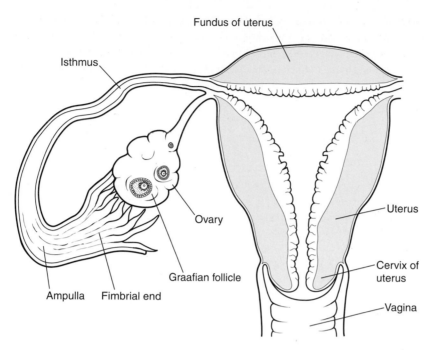

Figure 6.1 Anatomy of the fallopian tube.

If antibiotic therapy is instituted quickly, some of these infections can be controlled in time to prevent damage to the tubes. However, if the infection produces few clinical symptoms and therefore escapes treatment, it often becomes chronic. This leads to chronic salpingitis (chronic inflammation of the tube). In this case, scarring occurs along the inner walls, disrupting the natural function of the cells lining the tube and most often blocking its passage too.

If the blockage occurs near the fimbrial end, the tube can become distended with fluid secretions which cannot escape either from the blocked end or from the isthmus end near the uterus. This creates a hydrosalpinx. In the luteal phase, increasing levels of progesterone relax and clear the isthmus and the fluid is released. The fluid that is released from the hydrosalpinx will flood the uterus and pass out through the vagina, experienced as a watery discharge by the patient. If there has been a conception and an embryo has arrived in the uterus via the other tube (if it is not blocked) or via an IVF transfer procedure, then it is in critical danger of being washed out by this fluid. Therefore, tubes that form hydrosalpinges are usually removed or clipped before IVF procedures.

Microsurgery offers a good treatment option if the tubes are not damaged along too much of their length. If the blockage is in the isthmus near the uterus, then microsurgery is more effective and post-surgery pregnancy rates up to 70% have been reported.[1] If there is extensive damage to the tubes, however, IVF becomes the only option. IVF was developed for exactly these conditions and still obtains its best results in young women who are infertile due to blocked tubes.

Treatment with Chinese Medicine for Early-Stage Structural Blockages

TCM works best if the structure of tissues and organs has not been too damaged by a disease process. In the case of pelvic infections, this means acting as soon as infection is suspected, i.e., giving herbs and antibiotics. In a developing country such as China, where advanced microsurgery techniques or IVF procedures may not be so readily available or affordable for many women, some attempt has been made to develop ways of breaking down blockages in the tubes. The best results are obtained when herbs are administered per rectum in addition to oral administration, and, although clinical research in China is not as scientifically rigorous as in the West, there are a number of reports in their medical literature which indicate encouraging possibilities. Six clinical trials examining fallopian tube blockage are described, which include not only herbs to be swallowed but also herbs used as retention enemas and herbs applied to the abdomen. One paper claims a 72% conception rate in 50 women after 3–6 months treatment; another paper reports a 70% conception rate in 150 women after a year of treatment and a third paper reports a 55% conception rate after 6 months.[2] Until the research is carried out in a regulatory monitored environment, the results should not be accepted uncritically.

Diagnosis

Diagnosis of fallopian tube blockage is based on an understanding of the origins of the disease and the presenting signs and symptoms. Using modern technology is a helpful first step – first, to confirm the blockage itself; then, to determine its extent and site. Prognosis can be helped with this information, e.g.: whether the blockage is an absolute one or one which can be forced open with pressure; whether the tube is extensively damaged and stiff and sclerosed along its length or just in one site; and whether the site of obstruction is near the ovary or the uterus. TCM specialists claim better success with treatment of blockages near the fimbrial end, whereas microsurgeons can treat blockages at the uterus end more effectively.

TCM describes tubal blockage – as it does for any physical tissue damage or obstruction – as Blood stagnation, but in varying degrees and with various complications.

The Blood stagnation in this case can arise from:

- Invasion by Cold

- Heat

- Damp-Heat or Cold-Damp

- Retained products after pregnancy

- Chronic Qi stagnation caused by emotional stress

and is classified as mild (the Blood is retarded) through severe (there is complete Blood stasis).

Blood Stagnation Due to Invasion by Cold

Invasion by Cold of the uterus occurs at times when the uterus is open or vulnerable, i.e. during the period, just after delivery of a baby or after a miscarriage or abortion. Cold is said to congeal the Blood such that its movement is inhibited and local circulation quickly becomes inefficient. Thus, Cold reaching the tubes affects their function and contributes to infertility. There may be a feeling of cold in the abdomen and any period pain or ovulation pain will respond well to warmth. The pulse will be retarded and tight if there is pain, otherwise thready. The tongue may be unaffected if the Cold invasion is recent, or it may be purplish if stagnation has become entrenched.

Herbal formula — If the obstruction of the tube is partial or caused by spasms or contractions, then use of the well-known formula Shao Fu Zhu Yu Tang to warm the lower abdomen and resolve Blood stagnation will be effective.

Shao Fu Zhu Yu Tang (Lower Abdomen Eliminating Stasis decoction)

Dang Gui	9 g	*Radix Angelicae Sinensis*
Chuan Xiong	6 g	*Radix Ligustici Wallichii*
Chi Shao	9 g	*Radix Paeoniae Rubra*

Xiao Hui Xiang	6 g	*Fructus Foeniculi Vulgaris*
Yan Hu Suo	6 g	*Rhizoma Corydalis Yanhusuo*
Wu Ling Zhi	6 g	*Excrementum Trogopterori*
Pu Huang	9 g	*Pollen Typhae*
Mo Yao	6 g	*Myrrha*
Rou Gui	6 g	*Cortex Cinnamomi Cassiae*
Gan Jiang	6 g	*Rhizoma Zingiberis Officinalis*

The addition of warming medicinals (Xiao Hui Xiang, Rou Gui, and Gan Jiang) to a collection of Blood-regulating herbs (Dang Gui, Chuan Xiong, Chi Shao, Yan Hu Suo and Mo Yao) encourages movement of Blood which has been retarded by Cold. Wu Ling Zhi and Pu Huang in combination dissolve any Blood which has congealed and clotted due to the Cold.

If the blockage is complete, add to the decoction 1.5 g of a powder made from grinding:

| Wu Gong | 1 or 2 pieces | *Scolopendra Subspinipes* |
| Quan Xie | 6 g | *Buthus Martensi* |

Acupuncture points — Points (Table 6.1) used in the treatment are:

KI-14	Siman
Ren-4	Guanyuan
ST-29	Guilai
ST-28	Shuidao
SP-13	Fushe
LIV-5	Ligou
SP-6	Sanyinjiao

Blood Stagnation Due to Invasion by Heat

Invasion by Heat to the Uterus causes inflammation and bleeding and eventually Blood stagnation. Endometritis and some forms of acute infection fall into this category. There may be burning pain in the abdomen, thirst and irritability and frequent heavy periods or functional uterine bleeding.

Herbal formula — Combining some herbs from a Blood stagnation formula (Ge Xia Zhu Yu Tang) with one to clear Heat (Dan Zhi Xiao Yao San), addresses the inflammation and the tube obstruction. Antibiotics may also be required in this case.

Table 6.1 Acupuncture points[a] used in the treatment of tubal blockage from Blood stagnation and Cold

Treatment goal	Acupuncture points
To regulate and move Qi and Cold and/or masses in the abdomen	Choose from KI-14, Ren-4, ST-29, ST-28, SP-13
To regulate Qi and Blood in the lateral abdomen	SP-6 and LIV-5

[a]Use even or reducing method and use moxa on the abdomen points.

Ge Xia Zhu Yu Tang plus Dan Zhi Xiao Yao San (Eliminating Stasis below the Diaphragm decoction plus Moutan Gardenia Free and Easy powder)

Dang Gui	9 g	*Radix Angelicae Sinensis*
Chuan Xiong	9 g	*Radix Ligustici Wallichii*
Tao Ren	9 g	*Semen Persicae*
Hong Hua	9 g	*Flos Carthami Tinctorii*
Wu Ling Zhi	9 g	*Excrementum Trogopterori*
Wu Yao	9 g	*Radix Linderae Strychnifoliae*
Yan Hu Suo	6 g	*Rhizoma Corydalis Yanhusuo*
Zhi Zi	6 g	*Fructus Gardeniae Jasminoidis*
Chi Shao	9 g	*Radix Paeoniae Rubra*
Mu Dan Pi	9 g	*Cortex Moutan Radicis*
Xiang Fu	6 g	*Rhizoma Cyperi Rotundi*
Zhi Ke	6 g	*Fructus Citri seu Ponciri*
Fu Ling	12 g	*Sclerotium Poriae Cocos*
Bo He	3 g	*Herba Menthae*
Gan Cao (zhi)	3 g	*Radix Glycyrrhizae Uralensis*

This formula combines herbs to dispel Blood stasis (Dang Gui, Chuan Xiong, Tao Ren, Hong Hua, Wu Ling Zhi, Yan Hu Suo) with herbs to clear Heat (Chi Shao, Mu Dan Pi, Zhi Zi, Bo He) and regulate the Qi (Xiang Fu, Zhi Ke, Wu Yao). Fu Ling helps clear any Damp that might become associated with the Heat and create chronic pelvic disease. Chai Hu is removed from Dan Zhi Xiao Yao San in this combination because of its lifting effect on the herbs; this formula needs to be active in the lower Jiao.

Acupuncture points — Points (Table 6.2) used in the treatment are:

LIV-2	Xingjian
LIV-1	Dadun
SP-10	Xuehai
KI-8	Jiaoxin
KI-13	Qixue

Table 6.2 Acupuncture points[a] used in the treatment of tubal blockage from Blood stagnation and Heat

Treatment goal	Acupuncture points
To clear Heat in the Blood and regulate Qi	LIV-2
To clear Heat in the Blood to stop bleeding and regulate Qi in the lower Jiao	LIV-1
To cool and regulate Blood and dispel stagnation	SP-10
To regulate Blood in the Chong and Ren vessels, clear Heat from the Blood and stop bleeding	KI-8 and KI-13

[a]All points (except LIV-1) are reduced.

Blood Stagnation Due to Accumulation of Damp-Heat

This type of tubal obstruction is associated with pelvic infection which will usually require antibiotic treatment. If any infection or inflammation persists after antibiotic treatment (i.e., chronic PID develops), then further effort is required to clear Heat and Damp and resolve Blood stasis.

Herbal formula — Use the following formula:

Fu Fang Hong Teng Jian (Sargentodoxae Compound decoction)

Hong Teng	30 g	Caulis Sargentodoxae
Bai Jiang Cao	30 g	Herba cum Radice Patriniae
Pu Gong Yin	15 g	Herba Taraxaci Mongolici
Zi Hua Di Ding	15 g	Herba Viola cum Radice
Ru Xiang	6 g	Gummi Olibanum
Mo Yao	6 g	Myrrha
Mu Xiang	6 g	Radix Saussureae seu Vladimiriae
Dang Gui	9 g	Radix Angelicae Sinensis
Chi Shao	9 g	Radix Paeoniae Rubra
Wu Ling Zhi	9 g	Excrementum Trogopterori
Yi Yi Ren	30 g	Semen Coicis Lachryma-jobi

Hong Teng, Bai Jiang Cao, Pu Gong Yin and Zi Hua Di Ding are all used in large doses to clear Heat and pus. Ru Xiang and Mo Yao and Wu Ling Zhi break up Blood stasis and aid in getting the above detoxifying medicinals to the necessary sites in and around the tubes. Dang Gui and Chi Shao also help circulate Blood and Yi Yi Ren dispels Damp. The addition of Mu Xiang ensures movement of Qi in the abdomen and relieves abdomen pain.

Acupuncture points — Points (Table 6.3) used in the treatment are:

LIV-8	Ququan
LIV-5	Ligou
KI-7	Fuliu
GB-26	Daimai
ST-40	Fenglong
SP-12	Chongmen

Table 6.3 Acupuncture points[a] used in the treatment of tubal blockage from Blood stagnation and Damp-Heat

Treatment goal	Acupuncture points
To clear Damp-Heat and Blood stagnation in the lower Jiao	LIV-5 and LIV-8
To clear Damp-Heat	KI-7, GB-26 and ST-40
To regulate Qi and Blood in the tubes	SP-12

[a]All points are reduced.

239

Blood Stagnation Due to Accumulation of Cold-Damp

Obstruction by Cold-Damp manifests as edema of the tube, thick mucus secretions or some adhesions of tubes to the ovary or other organs. Only this latter case (adhesions) represents structural blockage. Blockage caused by mucus or edema will be discussed in the next section on functional blockages.

Herbal formula — If adhesions of the tube are associated with Cold-Damp, Gui Zhi Fu Ling Tang is an appropriate guiding formula.

Gui Zhi Fu Ling Tang (Ramulus Cinnamomi – Poria Decoction)

Gui Zhi	9 g	Ramulus Cinnamomi Cassiae
Fu Ling	9 g	Sclerotium Poriae Cocos
Mu Dan Pi	9 g	Cortex Moutan Radicis
Tao Ren	9 g	Semen Persicae
Chi Shao	9 g	Radix Paeoniae Rubra

This is a famous formula that combines the warming function of Gui Zhi with the Damp-clearing function of Fu Ling to dispel Cold-Damp and allow Blood-regulating herbs like Tao Ren, Chi Shao and Mu Dan Pi to penetrate masses in the lower Jiao.

Acupuncture points — Points (Table 6.4) used in the treatment are:

GB-26	Daimai
ST-28	Shuidao
SP-9	Yinlingquan
SP-6	Sanyinjiao
KI-5	Shuiquan

Blood Stagnation Due to Retention of Pregnancy Products or Placenta

Retention of pregnancy products or placenta after delivery, miscarriage or an abortion represents an acute clinical situation which will usually be addressed by surgical curettage and antibiotic therapy. Chinese herbs and acupuncture can be used adjunctively if appropriate.

Table 6.4   Acupuncture points[a] used in the treatment of tubal blockage from Blood stagnation and Cold-Damp

Treatment goal	Acupuncture points
To clear Damp in lower Jiao	GB-26 and SP-9
To move fluid and Qi in the tubes	ST-28
To clear Damp and Blood stagnation in the lower Jiao	SP-6
To move mucus from the tubes and clear Blood stagnation	KI-5

[a]Use even or reducing method, depending on the nature of the obstruction. Moxa is applicable but used with caution, or avoided, if thick mucus is thought to be blocking the tubes.

Herbal formula — Combine Ge Xia Zhu Yu Tang with Heat-clearing and detoxifying herbs.

Ge Xia Zhu Yu Tang (Eliminating Stasis below the Diaphragm decoction) modified

Dang Gui	9g	*Radix Angelicae Sinensis*
Chuan Xiong	6g	*Radix Ligustici Wallichii*
Tao Ren	9g	*Semen Persicae*
Hong Hua	9g	*Flos Carthami Tinctorii*
Wu Ling Zhi	9g	*Excrementum Trogopterori*
Wu Yao	6g	*Radix Linderae Strychnifoliae*
Yan Hu Suo	6g	*Rhizoma Corydalis Yanhusuo*
Chi Shao	6g	*Radix Paeoniae Rubra*
Mu Dan Pi	6g	*Cortex Moutan Radicis*
Chuan Niu Xi	9g	*Radix Cyathulae*
Xiang Fu	9g	*Rhizoma Cyperi Rotundi*
Zhi Ke	6g	*Fructus Citri seu Ponciri*
Zhi Zi	9g	*Fructus Gardeniae Jasminoidis*
Hong Teng	9g	*Caulis Sargentodoxae*
Gan Cao (zhi)	3g	*Radix Glycyrrhizae Uralensis*

Ge Xia Zhu Yu Tang is a formula which strongly eliminates stasis below the diaphragm with herbs such as Dang Gui, Chuan Xiong, Tao Ren, Hong Hua, Wu Ling Zhi and Yan Hu Suo to regulate Blood and Wu Yao, Xiang Fu and Zhi Ke to regulate Qi. Mu Dan Pi and Chi Shao clear any Heat from the Blood. Added to this formula are Chuan Niu Xi to make descending action more pronounced and encourage expulsion of retained products, and Zhi Zi and Hong Teng to clear Heat and prevent sepsis. Gan Cao (zhi) is added to moderate and harmonize the strong actions of these herbs.

Acupuncture points — Points (Table 6.5) used in the treatment are:

SP-6	Sanyinjiao
SP-8	Diji
ST-29	Guilai
CO-4	Hegu

Table 6.5 Acupuncture points[a] used in the treatment of tubal blockage from retained products and Blood stagnation

Treatment goal	Acupuncture points
To treat stagnation in the Uterus	SP-8 and ST-29
To regulate Qi and Blood in the Uterus	SP-6
To encourage the Uterus to expel its contents in conjunction with SP-6	CO-4

[a]All points will be reduced. If large clots are passed and abdomen pain and fever resolve, reinforcing treatments can be applied.

Lily's story is a long and a rather tortuous one. She had tried for several years in her mid-30s to become pregnant before it was discovered she had blocked tubes. The original cause for this was unknown – probably some silent infection caught in her wild youth. The HSG showed one tube completely closed and the other stiff, scarred and twisted, and barely patent. The specialist pronounced IVF her only option and she started straight away. She completed 2 cycles with transfers of two or three embryos each time but no pregnancy. A friend persuaded her to try Chinese medicine before her third attempt.

Her TCM diagnosis was Liver Qi stagnation with Heat. The evidence for this came from her premenstrual picture of breast-swelling and pain and feeling tense and irritable. Her period was mildly crampy. There were no symptoms accompanying her ovulation and no fertile mucus. Her general health was excellent, though she liked to drink and party which contributed to the Heat in the Liver. She took herbs based on Dan Zhi Xiao Yao San and Gui Shao Di Huang Tang for several months in preparation for the next IVF cycle. Although the structural damage to her tubes represented Blood stagnation, this was not addressed strongly in the prescriptions I gave her, since she intended to use IVF techniques to circumnavigate the stagnation.

Her Liver-Heat subsided and her Liver Qi relaxed enough for her premenstrual symptoms to all but disappear. Her Kidney Yin improved too, evidenced by the appearance of more obvious fertile mucus. She was ready to try again. Happily, she became pregnant with the next IVF cycle; unhappily, her baby was diagnosed with Down syndrome at 10 weeks' gestation. The pregnancy was terminated with a D&C.

But after several months, her periods hadn't returned. Eventually, sensing something was wrong, she went back to the specialist. Investigations revealed that the walls of her uterus had adhered to each other, causing complete obstruction. This condition is called Asherman syndrome and is usually caused by over-zealous curettage (or intrauterine infection). In TCM, the condition reflects severe Blood stagnation. Lily was prescribed estrogen and underwent another bout of surgery to try and separate the uterine walls. Her periods returned after this but the flow was scanty and the blood was very dark, even black. In China, Asherman syndrome is treated with a combination of surgery to remove the adhesions, and Chinese herbs to aid recovery of the endometrium. Formulas which strongly move Blood stasis are given for 3 months. Unfortunately, Lily did not know this and went on to attempt pregnancy with two more IVF cycles. Her ovaries, too traumatized by recent events, did not respond at all. Even if they had, it is unlikely that an embryo would have been able to implant into the damaged endometrium. It is only if healthy periods return that it can be assumed that the lining of the uterus has recovered (i.e. the Blood stagnation has been removed) and pregnancy is possible.

Eventually, Lily returned to my clinic. She was 41 by now and not in good shape. She was tense and anxious and was binge drinking. Signs of Liver-Heat were marked, her tongue was very red on the sides and had some bluish patches near the rear. Her pulse was thready and rapid.

She took herbs to resolve Blood stagnation and was instructed to have no alcohol:

Tao Ren	12g	Semen Persicae
Hong Hua	9g	Flos Carthami Tinctorii
Dang Gui	15g	Radix Angelicae Sinensis
Chuan Xiong	9g	Radix Ligustici Wallichii
Chi Shao	12g	Radix Paeoniae Rubra
Chai Hu	9g	Radix Bupleuri
Yi Mu Cao	9g	Herba Leonuri Heterophylli
Xiang Fu	9g	Rhizoma Cyperi Rotundi
Sheng Di	9g	Radix Rehmanniae Glutinosae
Mo Yao	3g	Myrrha
Ru Xiang	3g	Gummi Olibanum
Di Long	6g	Lumbricus
Zhi Zi	6g	Fructus Gardeniae Jasminoidis
Gan Cao	6g	Radix Glycyrrhizae Uralensis

Acupuncture points: ST-29, SP-10, SP-6, Ren-3, LIV-8, PC-7

She took this formula for a total of 5 weeks (i.e. during two menstrual periods and the month in between). As a result of this treatment, the menstrual flow was bright red and there was more of it, leading us to believe that her endometrium might have recovered sufficiently. What we did not anticipate was that it may have unblocked her tubes as well. It was only when she turned up to start the next IVF cycle and a routine pregnancy test was done before she could start the drugs that the wonderful news was discovered. She was pregnant and the ultrasound showed a strong fetal heart beat.

Blood Stagnation Due to Stagnation of Liver Qi

Stagnation of Liver Qi due to emotional stress can cause spasm and tension in the muscles of the fallopian tubes, causing a functional blockage (discussed below). If the Qi stagnation continues long term, then it can develop into Blood stagnation, i.e., the tubes may become blocked or stiff and sclerosed, effectively making them useless in their function of egg or embryo transport. Liver Qi stagnation also increases the severity of menstrual cramps. When the uterus contracts strongly during a period, it is more likely that some menstrual blood will be forced up into the fallopian tubes. If this happens repeatedly over a long time and the blood is not removed, then Blood stagnation in the tubes may develop.

Herbal formula — Use as a guiding formula:

Chai Hu Tong Liu Ying (Bupleurum Free Lodged Phlegm formula)

Chai Hu	12 g	*Radix Bupleuri*
Dang Gui	9 g	*Radix Angelicae Sinensis*
Chi Shao	9 g	*Radix Paeoniae Rubra*
Yu Jin	9 g	*Tuber Curcumae*
Su Mu	6 g	*Lignum Sappan*
Si Gua Luo	9 g	*Vascularis Luffae, Fasciculus*
Ju He	3 g	*Semen Citri Reticulatae*

Chai Hu and Yu Jin regulate Liver Qi to move stagnant Qi and Blood. Dang Gui and Chi Shao regulate the Blood. Si Gua Luo is used in this context to clear channels (specifically the tubes) and Su Mu to remove obstructions from the tubes; additionally, this herb appears to have strong antibiotic activity in in-vitro tests. Ju He are the seeds of the tangerine from which Chen Pi is made. They help to break up and reduce Qi accumulation and congealed Blood obstructions.

Acupuncture points — Points (Table 6.6) used in the treatment are:

LIV-3	Taichong
LIV-4	Zhongfeng
LIV-5	Ligou
PC-7	Daling
PC-5	Jianshi
SP-13	Fushe
SP-12	Chongmen

Table 6.6 Acupuncture points[a] used in the treatment of tubal blockage from Liver Qi and Blood stagnation

Treatment goal	Acupuncture points
To regulate Qi in the lateral abdomen and the tubes	LIV-3, LIV-4 or LIV-5
To calm the mind and regulate Liver Qi and Blood	PC-7 and PC-5
To regulate Qi and clear stagnant Blood from the tubes	SP-13 or SP-12

[a]Use reducing or even method, depending on the nature and severity of the obstruction.

243

CASE HISTORY – MILLIE

In my clinic in Sydney, I rarely treat structural blockage of the fallopian tubes, simply because IVF usually offers a greater chance of success. Where obstruction is not complete, I may attempt a few months of treatment if the patient is young or if IVF is not desired.

The following case is a patient Dr Xia Gui Cheng saw in my clinic when he was visiting from China.

Millie was 34 and had used no contraception since she was 20 years old, at which age she suffered an acute pelvic infection. As a result of this infection, one of her tubes was blocked by scarring. The other tube was patent, according to examination during laparoscopy, but the fact that she had not fallen pregnant in 14 years, despite an active sex life, indicated that possibly this tube was damaged too. We had no way of knowing if there was damage to the internal walls of the tube. Analysis of the hormones and sperm were normal. Her TCM diagnosis was Blood stagnation (the scarred and blocked tube), Liver Qi stagnation and Kidney Yang deficiency. These were determined by her premenstrual and period picture; she experienced pronounced breast soreness and bloating before her period and was very irritable. The period flow was heavy and clotty and she had strong back pain throughout. Her pulse was wiry and her tongue was normal.

Chai Hu	12 g	Radix Bupleuri
Dang Gui	9 g	Radix Angelicae Sinensis
Bai Shao	9 g	Radix Paeoniae Lactiflorae
Chi Shao	9 g	Radix Paeoniae Rubra
Shan Zhu Yu	9 g	Fructus Corni Officinalis
Mu Dan Pi	9 g	Cortex Moutan Radicis
Yu Jin	9 g	Tuber Curcumae
Su Mu	6 g	Lignum Sappan
Si Gua Luo	9 g	Vascularis Luffae, Fasciculus
Ju He	3 g	Semen Citri Reticulatae
Xu Duan	12 g	Radix Dipsaci
Mu Xiang	6 g	Radix Saussureae seu Vladimiriae

Acupuncture points: LIV-4, LIV-5, PC-5, SP-12, ST-29

This formula was taken after the period for 10 days, followed by Cu Pai Luan Tang. After ovulation, she took the above formula with the addition of more Kidney Yang tonics, namely:

Tu Si Zi	9 g	Semen Cuscatae
Du Zhong	9 g	Cortex Eucommiae Ulmoidis

and Yu Jin, Su Mu and Si Gua Lou were replaced with Wu Ling Zhi and Pu Huang, each 9 g.

Acupuncture points: LIV-5, ST-29 with care, LIV-14, PC-7

The herbal formulas she took for 3 months and, after reporting that her premenstrual symptoms were almost gone, discovered she was pregnant. She miscarried, but a couple of months later was pregnant again. This time her pregnancy went to full term.

FUNCTIONAL BLOCKAGES

Whereas a structural blockage presents an absolute barrier for passage of the sperm to the egg, a functional tubal blockage may obstruct the tube just some of the time. A functional disorder of the tube will usually have the effect of stopping a fertilized egg from reaching the uterus or preventing the embryo from reaching the uterus at the right time. It can also prevent the sperm reaching the egg.

Functional tubal disorders that affect the passage of the embryo include the following.

• Spasm or Stiffness of the Muscles of the Tube Walls

We know that general muscle tension or stress can close the fallopian tubes, because an HSG (which can be a stressful procedure for some women) can sometimes indicate completely closed tubes which, when examined again during a laparoscopy and general anesthetic, prove to be perfectly patent. Women who have been trying to become pregnant for a long time understandably feel some level of stress when attempting to make love at that all crucial time, midcycle, and it is easy to see how tension held in the body and especially in the pelvis might translate into tight or rigid tubes.

In TCM terms, it is when the Qi does not move freely and smoothly that spasms and tension can affect the muscles. When it is the Liver Qi that does not move freely (as a result of emotional factors), then it is in the organs in the pelvis, especially the reproductive organs, that the obstruction will manifest. The main Liver channel traverses the lateral aspect of the inner abdomen wherein lie the fallopian tubes. Obstruction of Qi in this channel quickly damages function and flexibility of the tubes.

Thus, there may be difficulty in releasing the egg and ovulation pain results, the fimbriae may not be nimble enough to catch and guide the egg into the ampulla, and the tube itself may be too rigid or tight to allow smooth passage of the egg or embryo. Stagnation of the Heart Qi can compromise the flow of Qi in the Bao vessel and also the tubes.

• Excess Secretions Blocking the Tubes

During the Yin part of the cycle, when there is plenty of estrogen, the cells lining the tubes will produce ample secretions. These are designed to lubricate the tube and nourish the egg and embryo. In a pathologic situation (Phlegm-Damp accumulation in TCM terms), these secretions may be produced excessively or they may not be able to be mobilized or drained efficiently from the tube, causing congestion and blockage.

• Asynchrony at Ovulation

If you remember the intricate sequence of midcycle events described in Chapter 2, you will appreciate why even small disturbances of synchrony in midcycle events – the release of the egg, fertilization, transport in the tube and the beginning of production of progesterone – can upset development and seriously compromise the future of the embryo right from the outset. The embryo needs to arrive at the uterus at the right point in its development and that of the uterine lining for effective implantation.

If the embryo tarries too long at the isthmus, its stage of development when it reaches the uterus may be inappropriate for implantation. This occurs if the secretions at this part of the tube remain too thick to allow the embryo's passage, a situation that may arise if the progesterone levels grow too slowly. In TCM terms, it is the Kidney Yang function that influences the production of progesterone. If corpus luteum activity is sluggish, then it is Kidney Yang that needs attention.

The embryo may also experience a slow journey down the tube if the ampullary section is not flexible and the cilia are not moving freely. In TCM terms, this is a manifestation of Qi stagnation. Qi stagnation can also retard the release of the egg from the ovary, which may affect its developmental stage at implantation.

On the other hand, if it travels down the tube too fast, the embryo may arrive in the uterus at a stage of development that is too immature for implantation. This might occur if the follicle is luteinized and producing progesterone but the release of the egg is delayed. The secretions of the isthmus may be thinned and dispersed prematurely, allowing the embryo to pass too quickly.

It is important for the correct development of the new embryo that it grows in synchrony with the Yang of the mother's cycle.

Treatment with Chinese Medicine for Functional Blockages

Most cases of functional tubal blockage will be dealt with effectively by correct management of the events approaching ovulation, as described in Chapter 4.

To recap, close attention is paid to the Kidney Yang as ovulation is approached. Herbs to activate Kidney Yang are employed just before midcycle to ensure the production of progesterone at the right time.

This prepares the internal environment of the tube and keeps its internal secretions moving. Malfunction of Kidney Yang can quickly lead to disorders of transportation and nourishment of the egg/embryo while it is in the fallopian tube. Secretions can build up and cause blockage. Such Phlegm-Damp accumulation will be addressed by boosting Kidney Yang, reinforcing Spleen Qi and dispelling Damp.

Attention is also paid to the Liver and Heart Qi, especially where there is emotional stress or symptoms such as ovulation pain, irritability, anxiety or midcycle breast soreness. Herbs which address Liver and Heart Qi stagnation are useful, and acupuncture, particularly around the lower abdomen and on the Liver and Pericardium channels, relaxes muscle tension and encourages flexibility of the tubes. Scheduling appointment times for acupuncture around midcycle is important for cases like these.

When the Liver and Heart Qi move smoothly and the Kidney Yang develops appropriately, then the function of the tubes is assured and functional tube blockages will be avoided or resolved. In addition to the treatment protocols outlined in Chapter 4, some of the herbs or points suggested in the previous discussion of structural blockages related to Cold-Damp obstruction and Qi stagnation will be applicable.

ADDITIONAL TREATMENTS FOR STRUCTURAL BLOCKAGES

Specialists in China, who may not have recourse to microsurgery and IVF, have developed other ingenious ways of dealing with tubal blockages. Most of these treatments are not appropriate or necessary in the West because we have good surgical alternatives but I include them here for interest and, sometimes, some aspects of these treatments might be included in an overall management plan.

Flushing the Tubes

An injection of liquid through the cervix and up through the tubes is carried out in much the same way as the dye is applied for the HyCoSy or HSG, i.e., it is injected through the cervix under gentle pressure. The liquid can be a sterile saline mix containing antibiotics or, if there is definite evidence of structural damage (Blood stagnation), then a saline-diluted decoction of the formula Fu Fang Dang Gui Zhi Shi Ye (below) is injected through the tubes to activate Blood and resolve stagnation. Such flushing must be done soon after the end of the period, so there is time for any reaction or inflammation the injected herbs might cause to settle down before ovulation. The procedure is done once or twice each cycle. If the obstruction is at the distal end of the tube, such therapy achieves better results than if it is at the uterus end. The flushing works in two ways: first, by forcing a passage through an obstruction which is not absolute; second, if the herbal decoction is used, by the action of the active ingredients in the herbs directly on the tissue. In some clinics in China, this procedure has been made more precise with the use of fine catheters introduced into the fallopian tubes and the delivery of small amounts of the herbs direct to the site of the blockage.

Fu Fang Dang Gui Zhi Shi Ye (Angelica Compound Injection fluid)

Dang Gui	15g	*Radix Angelicae Sinensis*
Hong Hua	9g	*Flos Carthami Tinctorii*
Chuan Xiong	9g	*Radix Ligustici Wallichii*

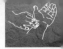

Application of Herbal Medicines Per Rectum

A volume of 100 mL of a decoction of Fu Fang Dang Gui Zhi Shi Ye (above) is introduced per rectum (PR) by enema before going to bed and remains there all night. This is done every second night unless there is abdomen pain, in which case it is done every night. If the blocked tubes are related to pelvic inflammatory disease which is still active, then an enema made from a decoction of Fu Fang Hong Teng Bai Jiang San (see below) may be more effective. The herbs are absorbed through the intestine directly to the inflamed areas. Doctors in China claim much better results with herbal enemas than with oral herbs for such conditions. Pain is controlled more quickly and obstructions resolved more often. Also, herbs which are not so kind to the stomach can be used without concern for damaging the digestion.

Herbal formula — The PR formula of choice is:

Fu Fang Hong Teng Bai Jiang San (Sargentodoxae Patriniae Compound powder)

Dang Gui	9 g	Radix Angelicae Sinensis
Chi Shao	9 g	Radix Paeoniae Rubra
Bai Shao	9 g	Radix Paeoniae Lactiflorae
Hong Teng	15 g	Caulis Sargentodoxae
Bai Jiang Cao	15 g	Herba cum Radice Patriniae
Mu Xiang	6 g	Radix Saussureae seu Vladimiriae
Yan Hu Suo	9 g	Rhizoma Corydalis Yanhusuo
Chai Hu	6 g	Radix Bupleuri
Chen Pi	6 g	Pericarpium Citri Reticulate
Sang Ji Sheng	12 g	Ramulus Sangjisheng
Shan Zha	12 g	Fructus Crataegi
Yi Yi Ren	15 g	Semen Coicis Lachryma-jobi

Dang Gui, Bai Shao and Chi Shao nourish and regulate the Blood. Mu Xiang and Chen Pi regulate the Spleen and Stomach Qi while Chai Hu moves the Liver Qi. Hong Teng and Bai Jiang Cao are herbs used to detoxify and disperse stagnant Blood and reduce inflammation. Yan Hu Suo and Shan Zha also move the Blood. Yi Yi Ren clears Damp. Sang Ji Sheng clears Damp and at the same time supplements Liver and Kidney.

For more Blood-invigorating action, add:

Mo Yao	9 g	Myrrha
Ru Xiang	9 g	Gummi Olibanum

or for badly scarred or obstructed tubes, add herbs which soften and break adhesions:

Lu Lu Tong	9 g	Fructus Liquidambaris Taiwaniae
Su Mu	9 g	Lignum Sappan

If there are palpable masses, add:

Gui Zhi Fu Ling Tang (Ramulus Cinnamomi – Poria decoction)

Gui Zhi	6 g	Ramulus Cinnamomi Cassiae
Fu Ling	9 g	Sclerotium Poriae Cocos
Mu Dan Pi	9 g	Cortex Moutan Radicis

Tao Ren	9 g	*Semen Persicae*
Chi Shao	9 g	*Radix Paeoniae Rubra*

Physiotherapy

Deep tissue massage to the abdomen done two or three times before ovulation is also useful, especially where there are adhesions around the tubes or stiffening of the tubes. In China another form of therapy is sometimes applied with electrodes placed over right and left fallopian tubes. The electrodes are wrapped in gauze and soaked in the above herbal decoction before being placed on the abdomen and attached to an electrical source.

Acupuncture

Acupuncture is a useful therapy for some types of tubal obstruction. A general systemic approach aimed at decreasing muscle tension and increasing the movement of Qi helps some forms of functional blockage. Where there is structural damage to the tubes, and surgery or IVF technology is not acceptable, then it is always worth applying acupuncture to the abdomen with deep but cautious needling to mobilize the Blood and Qi locally. Electrical stimulation can be added, especially if there is pain. This sort of acupuncture treatment can be done in conjunction with herbal enema treatment to good effect.

Choose from the following points (and see Table 6.7):

LIV-5	Ligou
LIV-3	Taichong
LIV-4	Zhongfeng
LIV-8	Ququan
SP-6	Sanyinjiao
SP-8	Diji
KI-14	Siman
ST-29	Guilai
ST-28	Shuidao
SP-12	Chongmen
SP-13	Fushe
Tituo	
Abdomen Zigong	
BL-18	Ganshu
BL-22	Sanjiaoshu
BL-24	Qihaishu
BL-32	Cilaio
PC-5	Jianshi
CO-4	Hegu

Table 6.7   Acupuncture points[a] used in the treatment of functional fallopian tube blockage

Treatment goal	Acupuncture points
To circulate Qi and Blood in the fallopian tubes	LIV-5
Distal points to regulate Qi and Blood in the lower Jiao	LIV-4, LIV-3 or LIV-8
To regulate Qi in the Spleen and Liver channels	SP-6 and SP-8
Local points to regulate Qi	ST-28, ST-29, KI-14 or Abdomen – zigong with moxa if there is Cold obstruction
For pain or discomfort in lateral abdomen at midcycle	SP-12, SP-13 or Tituo
Back points to assist regulation of Qi in the lower Jiao	BL-22, BL-24 and BL-32
To regulate Liver Qi	BL-18
To balance upper and lower body and calm the mind	PC-5 and CO-4

[a]The points on the leg will be needled with even technique or with reducing technique if there is pain. Use even technique on the back and the hand points.

REFERENCES

1.   Jansen RPS. *Getting pregnant*. Sydney: Allen and Unwin; 2003, 188.
2.   Flaws B. *Fulfilling the essence. Colorado.* : Blue Poppy Press; 1993, 155.

Male Infertility

7

Chapter Contents

INTRODUCTION

About one in five Australian couples have difficulty conceiving children. Male infertility is a contributing factor in half of these cases. Extrapolating these figures to the developed world translates into very large numbers of distressed couples seeking medical help for infertility. For example, there are more than 3 million men considered infertile in the USA; these are the ones trying to be fathers already but there are many more who don't yet know their fertility status, because they haven't yet tried to have children.

WHERE AND HOW SPERM ARE MADE

The sperm, known in biological circles as a 'spermatozoon', is a long thin cell with a head which contains the genetic material and a tail which propels the genetic material towards its destiny (Fig. 7.1).

The Sperm Factory

Sperm are made in the male gonads, which are known as the testes or testicles. These organs hang outside the body in the scrotum. The temperature in the scrotum is several degrees lower than that in the abdominal cavity just above it, and this low temperature seems to be important for the function of the sperm-making cells. Just 24 h of raised scrotal temperatures will cause malfunction of sperm production in animal studies.[1]

The sperm form over a period of about 48 days in the tubules in the testes, nurtured by the Sertoli cells, in sequential generations at different stages of development. They then spend 2 or more weeks in the epididymis

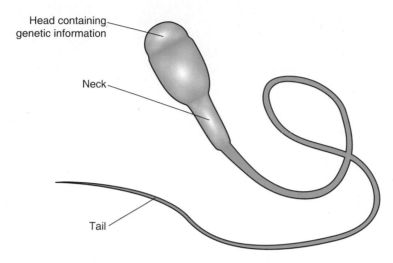

Figure 7.1 Spermatozoon.

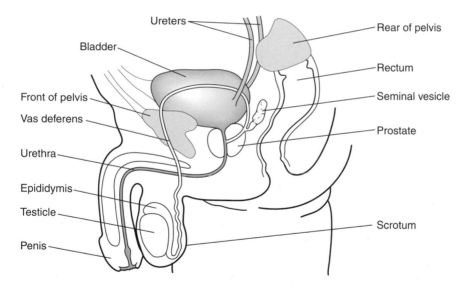

Figure 7.2 Male reproductive system.

(a fine, coiled tube 6 m long and about double the width of a scalp hair) to mature before moving into the vas deferens and the urethra on their way out of the body (Fig. 7.2). The ejaculate contains a mixture of sperm and fluid from the prostate gland and seminal vesicles.

Because of the long development and maturation time of sperm cells, events in a man's life can have far-reaching (in time) effects on the quality of his sperm, e.g., an episode of high fever which wreaks some havoc on the delicate internal machinery of the testes can still influence adversely the quality of the sperm being ejaculated 9 or more weeks later.

To be considered fertile, the male of the human species needs to deposit a minimum of 40 million sperm in the female vagina during intercourse in the hope that just one will have a successful encounter with the egg. Once inside the acid environs of the vagina, few sperm can survive and within just a few minutes, the walls are littered with the corpses of millions. Over the next few hours all but a few are dead. The survivors are the sperm which were able to negotiate a passage through the cervix with the help of the protective cervical mucus and the dipping action of the cervix at orgasm, followed by the contractions of the uterus which propel the sperm into its higher reaches. Once inside the female reproductive tract, the sperm will be lured towards the egg in the tube by chemical signals.

SEMEN ANALYSIS

Male fertility is investigated first by a sperm analysis performed in a pathology laboratory. A sperm test requires the collection, in a sterile plastic jar, of an ejaculation, which is then quickly examined in the laboratory. The sample is usually collected at least 24 h after the previous ejaculation. Doing a sperm test after 5 or more days of abstinence is not helpful because once the sperm have passed through the epididymis and are waiting in the testes for too long, their motility can diminish.

Normal Parameters

Current World Health Organization (WHO) standards[2] for assessing male fertility are:

- Volume: more than 1.5 milliliter (mL)

- Count: more than 15 million sperm per mL

- Motility: more than 50% moving vigorously and purposefully

- Morphology: more than 4% normal forms (i.e., no deformities of the head, midpiece or tail).

'Normal' parameters, as they were defined less than two decades ago, described sperm counts of twice this amount and a much higher percentage of normal forms. The average sperm count has decreased by 1–2% per year from a substantially higher number decades ago.[3] Standards for deposits in sperm banks have thus had to be lowered, or too many donors would nowadays be rejected.

Another way of assessing male infertility is to do retrospective studies of couples achieving or not achieving pregnancy. When a large population of men was studied, those who had succeeded in fathering a child in the previous 2 years had more than 48 million sperm/mL, with more than 63% moving, and more than 12% with normal morphology. Infertility was most likely if a man's sperm count was less than 13.5 million sperm/mL, with less than 32% moving, and less than 9% having a normal shape. Men falling between these two groups had borderline fertility but could still establish a pregnancy.[4]

Sometimes a single ejaculate might give misleading results, especially if the sample was taken when the man was stressed. In such cases, the ejaculate will be a small volume and sperm from the vas deferens may not be ejected into the semen effectively. So, if a single test provides a low count it is always worth repeating the collection of the sample under different circumstances.

On average, we can expect to find about 500 million sperm in one ejaculate of a healthy fertile male. If all these sperm were capable of fertilizing an ovum, theoretically one ejaculate could impregnate all the fertile women of China. In reality, however, the chance of one particular sperm penetrating the egg is less than the chance of winning a million dollar lottery!

Some couples, however, have no trouble getting pregnant with sperm counts lower than normal. Some researchers in the field have gone so far as to say that sperm density tests are not always useful in distinguishing fertile from infertile men and are not useful in diagnosis or in monitoring the progress of treatment for male infertility.[5] Ultimately, all that is really needed is one sperm!

Increasingly, andrology labs are finding that even normal looking sperm may have damage to their DNA. Oxidative stress – stress on the body that is caused by the cumulative damage of free radicals – is the main contributor to sperm DNA damage or fragmentation. A DNA fragmentation test will measure how much breakage there is in the DNA strands of the sperm chromosomes and give a DNA Fragmentation Index (DFI) score to indicate the likelihood of sperm contributing to infertility. The following scores indicate fertility potential for natural conception (or using IUI):

- ≤15% DFI: Excellent to Good fertility potential

- 15–25% DFI: Good to Fair fertility potential

- >25% DFI: Fair to Poor fertility potential.

As many as one-third of men being investigated in the infertility clinic will show significant (>25%) damage to the sperm DNA. Causes include exposure to environmental and occupational pollutants, cigarette or drug use, infections, elevated testicular temperature (from using laptop computers, or frequent use of saunas and hot baths or from a varicocele), chronic diseases such as diabetes, cancer and cancer treatment, and poor diet.

These men are encouraged to avoid pesticides and other environmental toxins, heat sources and smoking, and to increase antioxidant intake. (See Ch. 12 for more discussion.) Frequent ejaculation (i.e. daily) is recommended to reduce the length of time sperm are exposed to reactive oxygen species in the testicular ducts.

More realistic assessment can be made of the working sperm's performance if it is examined in a situation closer to real life, i.e., how the sperm behave in the medium of the mucus produced by the cervix at ovulation, not the confines of a plastic jar or a microscope slide. Now we are looking at the dance of female and male, Yin and Yang, together. A healthy display of flourishing Yin in the form of copious fertile mucus can nourish and enhance the Yang attributes of the sperm, i.e., they can swim and progress better. So, given the right environment, those healthy sperm from among a less impressive or sparse cohort may be selected and transported along by plentiful cervical mucus. However, this test (the post coital or Sims Huhner test) is seldom offered in ART clinics these days.

DECLINING SPERM COUNTS

There has been a lot of press about the precipitous decline in sperm counts over the last few generations. The average male sperm count dropped 45% from 113 million/mL in 1940, to 66 million/mL in 1990. Also the volume of semen dropped, effectively making the reduction in total numbers of sperm per ejaculation 50%. The number of men with low sperm counts (<20 million/mL) has tripled (from 6% to 18%), while the percentage with high sperm counts (>100 million/mL) has decreased. The more recently a man was born, the lower the average sperm count and the greater the number of abnormalities.[6]

Such a trend means that an average 30-year-old man today would have a sperm count about one-quarter the count of that of the average male born in 1925.

Such figures lead some specialists to speculate that if the decrease in sperm counts were to continue at this rate, in a few years we will witness widespread male infertility.[3]

The cause of this decrease appears to be the increased exposure to environmental pollutants, either during the time in the womb or later in life. PCBs (polychlorinated biphenyls), dioxin, phthalates, phenols and several pesticides such as DDT, have been shown to have a harmful effect on sperm as have the solvents used in manufacturing adhesives and printing inks and paints. Pregnancies of the partners of men exposed to damaging substances are also affected, experiencing a higher rate of stillbirth and premature delivery.[7] Many of these substances and other chemicals used in farming or industry act like estrogens or anti-androgens.[8–10] We will revisit this topic in more detail in Chapter 12.

The fact that sperm counts are lower in younger men than older men indicates that some of the damage may be occurring in the womb. It is thought that higher than normal estrogen levels in the womb might limit the number of sperm a man produces in adulthood by inhibiting the development of the Sertoli cells in the forming testicles. Since each of the Sertoli cells (which play an important role in the production of sperm) can only support a fixed number of sperm, the number a male acquires early in life will ultimately limit the quantity of sperm he can produce as an adult.

While the body is able to break down and excrete natural plant estrogens, many of the man-made compounds which act like estrogen resist normal breakdown and accumulate in the body, exposing humans and animals to low-level but long-term exposure. This pattern of chronic hormone exposure is unprecedented in our evolutionary experience and adapting to this new hazard is a matter of millennia not decades.[11]

Prescribed drugs may also be implicated in reduced sperm counts. In some cases, the effects of these drugs last for months after they have been discontinued. Testosterone replacement therapy, anabolic steroid use, cancer medications, certain antibiotics, some blood pressure medications, some ulcer or reflux medication, drugs for ulcerative colitis and some antidepressants have been observed to affect sperm production (Table 7.1).

Table 7.1   Some pharmaceutical drugs and their possible effects on sperm

Class of drug	Effect on sperm
Drugs for high blood pressure:	
e.g., spironolactone	Lowers sperm count
e.g., calcium channel blockers	Interfere with binding of sperm to egg
Drugs for peptic ulcers or reflux:	
e.g., cimetidine	Lowers sperm count
Drugs for ulcerative colitis:	
e.g., salazopyrin (sulfasalazine)	Lowers sperm count
Testosterone and anabolic steroids	Lower sperm count
Some chemotherapy drugs	
e.g., methotrexate	Lowers sperm count
Drugs for epilepsy:	
e.g., phenytoin	Lowers sperm count
Drugs for urinary function:	
e.g., nitrofurantoin	Affects sperm motility
Drugs for gout;	
e.g., allopurinol, colchicine	Lowers sperm count
Antifungal medication:	
e.g., Grisovin and/or Griseostatin (griseofulvin) or ketoconazole	Lowers sperm count and increases abnormal forms
Drugs for depression	
e.g., SSRIs serotonin reuptake inhibitors	May lower sperm count and motility
Some antibiotics	
e.g., tetracycline, erythromycin, gentamicin and nitrofurantoin	Lower sperm count, affect morphology

AGE AND SPERM

It has long been known that a woman's reproductive capacity reduces as she ages. But until recently, it has been assumed that the age of the male partner was irrelevant to the question of fertility – there are plenty of stories of septuagenarians impregnating younger women. It has taken a long time for the researchers to take a hard look at the influence of age on male fertility. The first indications that age might be relevant emerged from studies of miscarriage rates in couples of different ages (see Ch. 8) and, more recently, research has examined the effect of male age on conception rates. This has shown that the older a man is, the longer it is likely to take his partner to conceive, irrespective of her age. The study concluded that in a couple who eventually have a baby, the probability that it will take more than 12 months to conceive nearly doubles, from around 8%, when the man is younger than 25 years, to around 15%, when he is older than 35 years. In other words, men as well as women have a biological clock that starts ticking (though perhaps not so urgently) as they get into their 30s (Fig. 7.3).[12]

IVF outcomes are significantly reduced in couples where the husband is more than 50 years of age.[13] Particularly, it is the morphology and motility that declines with age.[14]

Constriction and Heat

Putting pressure on the testicles reduces sperm motility. Men whose sperm are not swimming so well are advised to stop putting pressure on them by avoiding tight underpants or cycling a lot.[15]

The effect of overheating the testicles with saunas or hot tubs or laptops has also been examined by various groups and it turns out that men with poor sperm quality are better off jumping in the ocean or a swimming pool rather than the hot tub or the sauna.[16]

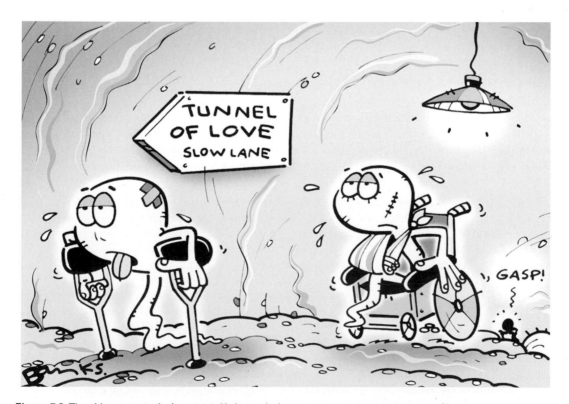

Figure 7.3 The older a man is, the longer it is likely to take his partner to conceive, irrespective of her age.

More discussion of lifestyle and environmental effects on sperm count and quality can be found in Chapter 9.

Antisperm Antibodies, Vasectomies, Varicoceles, and Other Blockages

The organs which make sperm and the tubes that carry them are physically isolated from the body's immune system. If this physical barrier is damaged, then the immune system is likely to tag the sperm cells as foreign and attack them with antibodies. A sperm thus coated with antibodies may die or stop swimming well or stick to its mates or just lose the ability to penetrate the egg.

If there is a blockage in the tubes carrying the sperm, whether this is from an infection or from a vasectomy, the sperm accumulate at the obstruction, causing irritation and inflammation, and an immune response is initiated. Even if this blockage is later removed by surgery, the immune reaction to the sperm persists, which sadly means that most reversed vasectomies are not successful in terms of future pregnancy. Sperm reappear in the semen in about 75% of men who undergo the procedure. Only 25–40%, however, then manage to father children naturally. In addition to the problem of antibodies, it is thought that the repaired epididymis does not adequately perform its function of maturing the sperm. Although of course, the sperm which do appear in the semen after a reversal are able to be used in an IVF cycle combined with intracytoplasmic sperm injection (ICSI).

Sperm which come into contact with the bloodstream of a female partner can also provoke an immune response. Since many sperm reach the abdominal cavity of a sexually active woman (by swimming out the top of the fallopian tubes), it is surprising that there are not more problems caused by women producing antisperm antibodies. But where there is an immune reaction, it is harder for sperm to traverse the fallopian tubes without being knocked out by swarming antibodies.

Another physical impediment impacting on male fertility is the not-uncommon varicocele, which is found in up to 40% of men presenting to an infertility clinic. This is a varicose vein in the scrotum which allows body temperature blood to spill backwards from the abdomen. The raised temperature in the sperm-making cells is one theory behind varicocele-related infertility but defective spermatogenesis in these cases has also been attributed to disturbed hormone status, spermatic venous hypertension, testicular congestion and hypoxia secondary to stasis, and excessive levels of oxidative species.

Surgery to correct varicoceles can often improve pregnancy outcomes, although it is not always a procedure undertaken routinely.[17,18]

Other obstructions in the tubes that carry the sperm can be present from before birth. Such congenital deformities can be the result of exposure to substances such as diethylstilbestrol (DES), which was taken by many pregnant women in the 1950s and 1960s to prevent miscarriage. Another congenital condition which reduces sperm count and quality is undescended testes. This is also dealt with effectively by surgery, especially if it is carried out during boyhood.

Trauma to the testicles or surgery itself can cause bruising and swelling, the effects of which may in some cases have long-term consequences on the delicate tubes. After surgery to the bladder or prostate gland, a condition sometimes develops called absent or retrograde ejaculation. This condition is also sometimes found associated with diabetes or after spinal injury. In such cases, the sperm and seminal fluid are not ejaculated at all or are ejaculated backwards into the bladder. In the latter case, sperm can be isolated from the urine and used with IVF techniques.

DIAGNOSIS OF MALE INFERTILITY IN TCM

Sperm are delivered to the female genital tract in a fluid called semen. This fluid contains constituents important for sperm function and survival and for conditioning the lining of the uterus to accept an embryo containing the father's proteins. Sperm constitutes only about 1% of the semen volume. The dynamic and fast-moving sperm represent the Yang within the moistening and nourishing Yin of the seminal fluid. When doctors of Chinese medicine are treating a sperm disorder, it is important that both the Yin and the Yang aspects are considered, i.e., both the sperm and the fluid containing them. You will see from the examples of treatments given below that both Yin and Yang are treated concurrently, with individual emphasis where necessary.

Male infertility, like female infertility, has everything to do with the Kidneys in TCM terms. As you will be aware, the Chinese medicine term 'Kidney' embraces more functions and areas in the body than does our concept of the kidney organs in Western medicine. Nevertheless, in Western medicine too, it is recognized that kidneys can be related to reproductive function, but this only becomes apparent when kidney function is seriously compromised. For men, renal disease has dire repercussions on fertility and sexuality.[19]

The basic requirement for full reproductive potential is strong Kidney Jing and a normal balance of Kidney Yin and Yang. Most cases of male infertility will be diagnosed as Kidney Yin or Yang deficiency. There appears to be a genetic base for male infertility in about 60% of cases.[20] This alerts TCM doctors to the possibility that Kidney Jing weakness underlies a majority of male infertility cases and will often need to be addressed in treatment protocols alongside the usual treatments for Kidney Yin and Yang. However, where exposure to environmental pollutants in later life has caused a drop in sperm count and quality, we would not assume a Kidney Jing deficiency, although Kidney Yin and Yang function will still play a part in our treatments.

As with female infertility, the exceptions to Kidney deficiency infertility occur if there is mechanical blockage or there is a Damp-Heat condition (although these may overlay a Kidney deficiency). Thus, in the clinic we need to consider the diagnoses:

- Kidney Yin deficiency

- Kidney Yang deficiency

- Damp-Heat

- Blood and Qi stagnation.

The latter two refer to particular clinical conditions and often represent complications of Kidney deficiency.

Kidney Yin Deficiency

Internal Heat is the main cause of poor sperm count in the Yin-deficient man. The slightly raised body temperature means that the sperm-producing cells do not function well and drying of fluids by the Heat means that the quantity and quality of the seminal fluid may be compromised. Internal Heat may cause inflammation of the prostate gland. As with female infertility, this is a common diagnosis of men attending infertility clinics in the West.

The diagnosis is made in the clinic by assessing all the usual sorts of symptoms and signs which indicate Yin deficiency:

- restlessness

- thin wiry body

- hot at night

- thirst

- red face

- red tongue and rapid pulse.

In addition, there may be some Kidney symptoms such as urination frequency, dark scanty urine, poor urine flow, tinnitus, and heel pain. There may be rather a high libido but this is not necessarily accompanied by strong sexual prowess. There may also be premature ejaculation and inability to sustain erections for long.

257

In terms of the sperm test, it is not uncommon to see plentiful sperm but a high percentage have poor morphology and therefore less efficient motility and ability to penetrate the egg.

In the clinic, however, often the only sign to support the diagnosis of Yin-deficient infertility is a red tongue and may be the sort of hectic lifestyle which consumes Yin. The pulse may be rapid and thready, but often in fit men, it is not.

Kidney Yang Deficiency

Kidney Yang deficiency is the main and fundamental disorder of male reproduction. When Kidney Yang fails, not only are the sperm not manufactured properly but also the sexual apparatus does not function either. There will often be:

- impotence or inability to sustain erection

- loss of libido

- chilliness or intolerance for cold

- lethargy

- pale coated tongue and slow soft pulse.

In addition, there may be other Kidney Yang-deficient signs, such as frequent copious pale urine, slight incontinence, lower back and knee pain and puffiness around the lower limbs. The salient feature of the sperm test is usually low numbers of sperm and poor motility.

Damp-Heat

Damp-Heat may accumulate in the lower Jiao generally or in the Liver/Gall Bladder channels specifically. The clinical signpost to a diagnosis of Damp-Heat infertility is an abnormal discharge from the penis or red itchy skin in the genital and groin area. There may be other signs of infection, such as painful urination or tenderness in the scrotum. Prostatitis may be the result of Damp-Heat in the lower Jiao.

As a cause of infertility, this is not so common in Western or developed countries because antibiotics are usually used promptly to address any genitourinary infections. But in China or other developing countries, low-grade untreated infections commonly contribute to the sort of inflammation which does not provide a conducive environment for sperm manufacture. In cases where there is infection in the urogenital tract, antibiotics may be appropriate and studies have shown that sperm counts can improve after such treatment.[21]

The nature of the antibiotic treatment is important, however, as some antibiotics may affect sperm function adversely.[22]

It is also the case that Damp-Heat may contribute to the development of immune infertility, even where there is no obvious infection. Men diagnosed with immune infertility (high antisperm antibody count), especially those who suffer from chronic prostatitis or local skin infections, will fall into a Damp-Heat infertility category in the TCM clinic.

If Kidney Yin or Yang deficiency is complicated with Damp-Heat then the Damp-Heat should be treated first.

Qi and Blood Stagnation

This category of male infertility includes all conditions which obstruct the passage of the sperm, abnormalities of blood circulation, and trauma (including surgery).

Some cases of Damp-Heat (such as gonorrhea) can lead to Blood and Qi stagnation infertility if inflammation in the epididymis causes the walls to stick together, creating an outright barrier to passage of the sperm.

Other obstructions in the tubes which carry the sperm were discussed above.

The varicocele, like other physical defects in the testes, may be treated surgically although this does not improve sperm production in all cases. Any abnormality in the way the blood flows is deemed to be a manifestation of 'Blood stagnation' and it is this underlying pathology that may need to be addressed before varicocele surgery can improve sperm counts.

As we saw above, anti-sperm antibodies often occur in men who have varicoceles and also are common in men who have had vasectomies reversed (or other sorts of testicular surgery or trauma), and men with this diagnosis and history will tend to fall into a Blood and Qi stagnation category. In some cases, there will be a history of inguinal hernia repair.[23]

Blood and Qi stagnation should be addressed before tonification of Kidney Yin and Yang if the stagnation is marked. In mild cases, Qi and Blood regulating herbs can be added to the base formula.

TCM TREATMENT OF INFERTILITY

Many reproductive specialists feel that treatment of male infertility is redundant in the brave new world of assisted reproduction wherein an embryologist can manipulate sperm with almost any sort of disability. However, while IVF with intracytoplasmic sperm injection (ICSI) offers many infertile men a chance to have a baby, it is not a panacea. Our aim should be to maximize the chance of each couple achieving a natural pregnancy while minimizing their health risks and financial costs and as such, increasing numbers of urologists who feel that the treatment of male infertility should not be ignored or sidelined.[24]

Additionally, the doctor of Chinese medicine is concerned with the quality of Kidney Jing the father will pass onto his offspring and will recommend that any men with a less than optimal semen analysis take the time to optimize Kidney Jing before conception attempts, whether using IVF/ICSI or not. If Jing is reflected in the integrity of the chromosomes, then one small study seems to verify that the use of Chinese herbs treating Kidney Jing and other relevant factors can reduce aneuploidy (incorrect chromosomal make-up) in sperm.[25]

Prescribing TCM treatment for male infertility is much simpler than prescribing treatment for female infertility. This is because once the diagnosis is made and the patient appears to tolerate the prescribed herbs, then the same formula (particularly those addressing Kidney Yin and Yang) tends to be continued for a long time, which, for a patient not receiving concurrent acupuncture treatment, reduces the number of clinic visits significantly. Remember that sperm take a long time to form (approx. 3 months) and so treatment should realistically continue for at least 6 months. Reports from China on the treatment of male infertility due to Kidney deficiency typically describe treatment protocols spanning 1 or more years.[26] In China, the infertility clinics are generally dealing with a younger group of people than the infertility clinics in the West, so the long wait is more acceptable. Formulas for men to take over such a long time are often ground up and made into honey pills to make long-term consumption easier.

The other aspect of treatment of male infertility that makes it so simple compared with treatment of female infertility is that formulas can be constructed for long-term use, which address both Kidney Yin and Yang deficiency at the same time. Any formula which treats Kidney Yin or Yang over a long time must always take into consideration the other – as it is said in the classics, Yin and Yang depend on and generate each other. Thus, prescriptions like the guiding formulas shown below (which are used at a large teaching hospital in Guang Dong, China),[26] can be applied to any case of low sperm count, or sperm with poor motility or poor morphology, so long as the diagnosis is Kidney deficiency.

The benefit that Chinese herbs bring to sperm quality has been the subject of a number of clinical trials in China, and include those treating autoimmune infertility.[27–29]

While the benefits are clearly demonstrated the mechanism remains to be elucidated. It is supposed that antioxidant activity in the herbs will contribute to improved DNA integrity and sperm manufacture but this remains to be proved. In one study, levels of the antioxidant superoxide dismutase did not change after administration of Chinese herbs, even though the sperm quality improved.[30]

In the case of autoimmune infertility, it appears that the herbs may influence the balance of T-lymphocyte subpopulations.[31]

Acupuncture treatment, like herbal treatment, is more simple for male infertility than for female infertility, in that the choice of points is not influenced by constantly changing hormone cycles. However, visits to the clinic need to be weekly or more and, if this is inconvenient, then Chinese herbs are often chosen as the preferred treatment for the long term.

Having said that, acupuncture has proven results in improving semen analyses in a number of clinical trials and hence, should be offered to any men with poor sperm quality, especially affecting morphology and motility. Many clinical trials carried out in different countries have shown that acupuncture can significantly improve sperm quality, especially motility and morphology.[32-41]

Most of these trials offered acupuncture over a 5–10 week period using points that addressed Kidney deficiency and mobilized Qi and Blood in local areas. The mechanism of action is not yet clear but we do know that substances in semen called met-enkephalins promote the motility of sperm[42] and that acupuncture can enhance met-enkephalin levels.[43] The level of met-enkephalin is abnormally low in the semen of men with poor motility of sperm but not in those with poor sperm counts. When met-enkephalin is added to the semen of healthy volunteers with normal sperm parameters in vitro, the sperm are able to maintain motility for longer than those without the added met-enkephalin. This may partially explain the observed improvement to motility after acupuncture. Thus, where motility is an issue, acupuncture may be of benefit, possibly even in the short term, e.g., applied at the time of the female partner's ovulation.

Electroacupuncture was seen to improve testicular arterial blood flow, promising the possibility of increased delivery of nutrients, antioxidants and oxygen to the sperm-making cells.[44] These researchers note that particular frequencies of electricity applied to certain acupuncture points provide a stimulus which could improve spermatogenesis by correcting metabolism in the microcirculatory bed and may address the damaged microcirculation associated with varicoceles, and with aging.

Acupuncture was also seen to improve abnormally low sperm counts and to lower elevated (>30.5°C) scrotal temperature in men with signs of genital tract inflammation.[40]

When planning treatment programs for patients with male factor infertility, it is useful to suggest attendance at the clinic for acupuncture at the time of their partner's ovulation (in addition to whatever other regular treatments have been scheduled). A strongly invigorating treatment for the Kidneys can help sexual function at this time when the pressure to perform can be quite defeating. In cases of Kidney Yang deficiency, this treatment may also help to give slow sperm a bit of a hurry up! (See Tables 7.1 and 7.2 for point suggestions).

Kidney Yin and Yang Deficiency

Herbal Formula — The formula of choice is:

Bu Shen Yi Jing Fang (Supplement the Kidneys Benefit the Jing formula)

He Shou Wu	15g	Radix Polygoni Multiflori
Shu Di	15g	Radix Rehmanniae Glutinosae Conquitae
Gou Qi Zi	15g	Fructus Lycii Chinensis
Shan Yao	15g	Radix Dioscorea Oppositae

Shan Zhu Yu	15 g	*Fructus Corni Officinalis*
Tu Si Zi	15 g	*Semen Cuscatae*
Fu Pen Zi	15 g	*Fructus Rubi Chingii*
Nu Zhen Zi	15 g	*Fructus Ligustri Lucidi*
Bai Shao	15 g	*Radix Paeoniae Lactiflorae*
Mu Dan Pi	15 g	*Cortex Moutan Radicis*
Dang Shen	15 g	*Radix Codonopsis Pilulosae*
Huang Qi	15 g	*Radix Astragali*
Yin Yang Huo	15 g	*Herba Epimedii*
Rou Cong Rong	15 g	*Herba Cistanches*
Ba Ji Tian	12 g	*Radix Morindae Officinalis*
Suo Yang	12 g	*Herba Cynomorii Songarici*
Dan Shen	12 g	*Radix Salviae Miltiorrhizae*
Lu Jiao Pian	12 g	*Cornu Cervi Parvum*

Using this guiding formula, herbs can be added or subtracted as required. However, because this formula broadly addresses all the factors at play in Kidney-related male infertility, it can often be prescribed as is, usually in an easy to take honey pill or powdered form. Kidney Yang function is addressed with the herbs Lu Jiao Pian, Ba Ji Tian, Rou Cong Rong, Yin Yang Huo, Tu Si Zi, Fu Pen Zi, and Suo Yang, while Kidney Yin is enriched with the herbs Nu Zhen Zi, Gou Qi Zi, Shan Zhu Yu, and Shu Di. Tonics He Shou Wu and Bai Shao nourish the Blood, He Shou Wu having a special effect on increasing semen quantity. Huang Qi, Dang Shen and Shan Yao invigorate the Qi. Mu Dan Pi regulates and cools the Blood, while Dan Shen regulates the Blood and calms the mind.

Although this excellent formula addresses both Kidney Yin and Yang if there is marked Yin deficiency Heat, then this must be addressed first or in addition. Kidney Yin will not be able to flourish in a dry or hot environment. A formula such as Zhi Bai Di Huang Wan (Eight Flavor Rehmannia pill) can be used initially or the above formula can be modified with these additions;

Table 7.2   Acupuncture points[a] used in the treatment of Kidney Yin deficiency male infertility

Treatment goal	Acupuncture points
To treat Kidney Yin, Yang and Jing[b]	BL-23, KI-3, Ren-4
To clear Yin-deficient Heat	KI-2 and KI-6
For premature ejaculation	BL-52, DU-4, ST-27
For excess libido	SP-6
For spent Jing from excess sexual activity	ST-36, KI-12
For excess nocturnal emissions with dreams	BL-15 and BL-43
To open and regulate the Conception channel	LU-7
To increase blood flow in the testicles[c]	ST-29, SP-6

[a]Reinforcing method is used except in the case of points used to clear Heat, where reducing or even method is used.
[b]Could also be useful at time of partner's ovulation.
[c]Use electroacupuncture (10 Hz) joining SP-6 to ST-29 on the same side for 5–20 min.

Tian Dong	15 g	*Tuber Asparagi*
Huang Bai	12 g	*Cortex Phellodendri*
Zhi Mu	15 g	*Rhizoma Anemarrhenae*
Han Lian Cao	9 g	*Herba Ecliptae Prostratae*

and the removal of Lu Jiao Pian, Yin Yang Huo and Suó Yang and reduction of doses of Ba Ji Tian and Rou Cong Rong.

CASE HISTORY – GUY

Guy and Dinah visited my clinic when he was 38 and she was 42. Guy had few sperm, which swam poorly and had abnormal morphology: what is called triple factor sperm abnormality. His doctor told him that IVF and intracytoplasmic sperm injection (ICSI) were the only way these sperm were going to achieve anything. His wife, who was 40 when they underwent the IVF and ICSI cycle, happily became pregnant first time and gave birth to a healthy baby boy.

But they knew they wanted more than one child and that time was running out. Dinah was now at an age when few IVF procedures are successful, even with perfect sperm. They wanted to know if Chinese herbs could help them with a second baby. I told them it took their chances of a second pregnancy from close to 0 with no intervention at all, to perhaps 5%. This poor prognosis was based on Dinah's age as much as the poor sperm quality. Putting together the disadvantage of older eggs with the not-insignificant impediment of severely compromised sperm, meant the numbers were against them.

Guy's clinical picture was unremarkable. He was apparently very healthy and symptom free. He had good stamina and felt very well. When questioned thoroughly, the only symptom elicited was restless sleep. His lifestyle was a familiar one among the male infertility patients I have seen. He started the day with a breakfast of three coffees and two cigarettes; went to work in the city where he sat at his computer a minimum of 8 h a day; and never exercised. His eating patterns were erratic and he drank a lot of liquid (diet coke). He smoked quite heavily throughout the day. His tongue was very red all over and had little coat. His pulse was thready, especially on the Heart and Kidney positions, and somewhat rapid.

The diagnosis of Guy's infertility was Kidney Yin deficiency with Heat. To address this, I needed to modify the Bu Shen Yi Jing Fang to clear Heat more. I reduced the heating Yang herbs and removed very drying herbs. The Qi tonics were removed and Heat-clearing herbs were added:

Sheng Di	15 g	*Radix Rehmanniae Glutinosae*
Di Gu Pi	9 g	*Cortex Lycii Chinensis*
Chi Shao	9 g	*Radix Paeoniae Rubra*
Dan Shen	12 g	*Radix Salviae Miltiorrhizae*
Huang Bai	9 g	*Cortex Phellodendri*
Zhi Mu	9 g	*Radix Anemarrhena*
Mu Dan Pi	15 g	*Cortex Moutan Radicis*
Bai Shao	15 g	*Radix Paeoniae Lactiflorae*
Gou Qi Zi	15 g	*Fructus Lycii Chinensis*
Shan Yao	15 g	*Radix Dioscorea Oppositae*
Shan Zhu Yu	15 g	*Fructus Corni Officinalis*
Nu Zhen Zi	15 g	*Fructus Ligustri Lucidi*
Han Lian Cao	15 g	*Herba Ecliptae Prostratae*
Tian Dong	15 g	*Tuber Asparagi*
He Shou Wu	15 g	*Radix Polygoni Multiflori*
Tu Si Zi	15 g	*Semen Cuscatae*
Fu Pen Zi	9 g	*Fructus Rubi Chingii*
Rou Cong Rong	9 g	*Herba Cistanches*
Ba Ji Tian	9 g	*Radix Morindae Officinalis*

If Yang deficiency is marked with signs of Cold, add:

| Rou Gui | 6 g | *Cortex Cinnamomi Cassiae* and/or |
| (Zhi) Fu Zi* | 6 g | *Radix Aconiti Charmichaeli Praeparata* |

(Zhi) Fu Zi is a restricted herb in some countries.

If Yang deficiency is marked with poor erectile function, adding more Blood-regulating herbs to increase circulation to the genital organs improves function markedly.[45]
Add:

Chuan Xiong	9 g	*Radix Ligustici Wallichii*
Tao Ren	12 g	*Semen Persicae*
San Qi	6 g	*Radix Pseudo-ginseng*

CASE HISTORY – DON

Don was 35 when he sought treatment for infertility; his wife Beth was also 35. She had fallen pregnant some years earlier but inexplicably, the baby died when almost at term. There was no further pregnancy in the next 2 years. Investigations showed that Don's sperm count was very low, there was a high percentage of abnormal sperm and motility was poor; triple factor sperm abnormality. Blood tests revealed low testosterone levels. He was recommended by a specialist to try IVF with ICSI.

Don had low libido and low energy, both of which were noticeably worse in the winter. He mentioned he had cold hands and feet and said he generally felt the cold more than other people. He suffered from lower back pain, frequent urination, and hay fever. His digestive system could not tolerate heavy or spicy foods. He was often depressed and had difficulty concentrating.

His tongue was pale with a white coat and his pulse was soft.

The diagnosis of Don's infertility was straightforward; Kidney and Spleen Yang deficiency. Seldom are clinical pictures quite so obvious and while Kidney Yang deficiency will definitely have a deleterious effect on male fertility, it is not a diagnosis I come across in the West as often as Kidney Yin deficiency.

Don had tried Korean ginseng and felt better when taking it. I recommended red ginseng and deer horn tablets to treat the Yang of the Kidney. And then he was to take the herbs listed below in decoction form.

In addition, Don was advised to limit sexual activity, including masturbation. This is a specifically Chinese approach to conserving 'Jing'. Jing is lost with every ejaculation and, since Jing is an important precursor to Kidney Yang and full fertile potential, Chinese doctors usually advise sexual abstinence for 3 months in cases where Kidney energy is low. Western doctors are not concerned with conservation of semen. In fact, they often encourage couples to have more sex – one of the contributing factors to low fertility for busy couples in the West is their reduced frequency of sexual intercourse.

Shu Di	24 g	*Radix Rehmanniae Glutinosae Conquitae*
Gou Qi Zi	24 g	*Fructus Lycii Chinensis*
Tu Si Zi	24 g	*Semen Cuscatae*
Du Zhong	12 g	*Cortex Eucommiae Ulmoidis*
Fu Pen Zi	12 g	*Fructus Rubi Chingii*
Ba Ji Tian	12 g	*Radix Morindae Officinalis*
Yin Yang Huo	12 g	*Herba Epimedii*
Xian Mao	12 g	*Rhizoma Curculiginis Orchioidis*

Rou Gui	5 g	Cortex Cinnamomi Cassiae
Wu Wei Zi	3 g	Fructus Schizandrae Chinensis
Lu Jiao Pian	3 g	Cornu Cervi Parvum
Gan Cao	3 g	Radix Glycyrrhizae Uralensis
(Zhi) Fu Zi*	5 g	Radix Aconiti Charmichaeli Praeparata

*(Zhi) Fu Zi is a restricted herb in some countries.

Don took the ginseng and deer horn pills for 2 weeks and then started taking the decocted herbs. He felt improvement straight away, especially when he started the decocted herbs. Everything felt better and it was not so easy to abstain from sex with a renewed libido. In his words: 'I feel rejuvenated, energetic, full of libido, upbeat, my allergies are better, life just seems much more positive.' Exuberant Kidney Yang can make a big difference to a man (and his wife!).

It then got a lot more positive. He and his wife agreed they would limit sexual intercourse to one attempt in the 1st month, at ovulation time. And it worked first time ... Don's wife was pregnant only a few weeks after he started the herbs.

This is an unusually quick result: sperm take many weeks to mature and the action of the herbs is therefore not manifest in the sperm count and morphology for several months. However, the other symptoms of Kidney Yang deficiency can respond very quickly, as Don discovered. And with a lot more Kidney Yang drive behind them, the few sperm that were there got a head start, i.e., presumably their motility picked up substantially enough for one of them to make it to the finishing line!

A healthy baby was born at term.

In addition, Guy's lifestyle needed a radical overhaul. He did his valiant best: stopped the coke, reduced his coffee, tried to include more fresh fruits and vegetables in his diet and he stopped smoking altogether for some months ... it didn't last. He was very diligent with taking the herbs, however, and 6 months later his wife surprised everyone by falling pregnant – and she wasn't even within 'cooee' of an IVF clinic! A healthy and perfect second baby boy was born at term.

Acupuncture Points — Choose from the following points (and see Table 7.2):

Kidney Yin deficiency

BL-23	Shenshu
KI-3	Taixi
Ren-4	Guanyuan
KI-2	Ranggu
KI-6	Zhaohai
BL-52	Zhishi
ST-27	Daju
DU-4	Mingmen
SP-6	Sanyinjiao
ST-36	Zusanli
KI-12	Dahe
BL-15	Xinshu
BL-43	Gaohuangshu

Table 7.3   Acupuncture points[a] used in the treatment of Kidney Yang deficiency male infertility

Treatment goal	Acupuncture points
To treat Kidney Yin, Yang and Jing[b]	BL-23, KI-3, Ren-4 (use deep needling on Ren-4 with moxa), DU-4
To treat Kidney Qi, Yang and Jing	Ren-6
To treat Kidney Yang	GB-25
To regulate genital function and sperm manufacture	BL-30
To warm the lower Jiao	ST-29, Ren-8 (use moxa)
For leakage of sperm	KI-14
For impotence[b]	KI-2, KI-12, Ren-2, BL-52
To increase blood flow in the testicles[c]	ST-29, SP-6

[a]Moxa is applicable to all points, and reinforcing needling method.
[b]Useful at time of partner's ovulation.
[c]Use electroacupuncture (10 Hz) joining SP-6 to ST-29 on the same side for 5–20 min.

Choose from the following points (and see Table 7.3):

Kidney Yang deficiency

BL-23	Shenshu
KI-3	Taixi
KI-6	Zhaohai
Ren-4	Guanyuan
Ren-6	Qihai
Ren-8	Shenque
Ren-2	Qugu
GB-25	Jingmen
BL-30	Baihuangshu
ST-36	Zusanli
ST-29	Guilai
KI-14	Siman
KI-12	Dahe
KI-2	Ranggu
BL-52	Zhishi
DU-4	Mingmen

Damp-Heat

In cases where Damp-Heat complicates Kidney deficiency, it is usually addressed first and the above formula for the Kidney deficiency is taken only when the Damp-Heat is resolved.

Herbal Formula — The representative formula to clear Damp-Heat in the lower Jiao is Bi Xie Fen Qing Yin (Dioscorea separating the Clear decoction) or, if the Damp-Heat is more specifically in the genitals, Long Dan Xie Gan Tang (Gentiana Draining the Liver decoction).

Bi Xie Fen Qing Yin (Dioscorea Separating the Clear decoction)

Bi Xie	12g	Rhizoma Dioscorea
Yi Zhi Ren	9g	Fructus Alpiniae Oxyphyllae
Wu Yao	9g	Radix Linderae Strychnifoliae
Shi Chang Pu	9g	Rhizoma Acori Graminei

Bi Xie drains Damp from the genitourinary system and Shi Chang Pu opens orifices to facilitate this draining. Yi Zhi Ren and Wu Yao warm the Bladder and Kidneys to facilitate efficient excretion of fluids.

Long Dan Xie Gan Tang (Gentiana Draining the Liver decoction)

Long Dan Cao	6g	Radix Gentianae Scabrae
Huang Qin	9g	Radix Scutellariae Baicalensis
Zhi Zi	9g	Fructus Gardeniae Jasminoidis
Ze Xie	9g	Rhizoma Alismatis
Mu Tong	9g	Caulis Mutong
Che Qian Zi	9g	Semen Plantaginis
Sheng Di	12g	Radix Rehmanniae Glutinosae
Dang Gui	9g	Radix Angelicae Sinensis
Chai Hu	9g	Radix Bupleuri
Gan Cao	3g	Radix Glycyrrhizae Uralensis

Long Dan Cao is the main herb in this formula, clearing lower Jiao Damp-Heat and Fire from the Liver channel. Huang Qin and Zhi Zi assist removal of Damp-Heat from the lower body. Chai Hu removes stagnation of Liver Qi and clears any resultant Heat. Mu Tong, Ze Xie and Che Qian Zi act as diuretics to enhance clearance of Damp. Sheng Di and Dang Gui are added to protect the Yin and the Blood and Gan Cao to protect the stomach from the bitter drying action of the above herbs.

Acupuncture Points — Choose from the following points (and see Table 7.4):

KI-7	Fuliu
BL-27	Xiaochangshu
BL-28	Pangguangshu
BL-35	Huiyang
DU-3	Yaoyangguan
Ren-1	Huiyin
Ren-4	Guanyuan
LIV-8	Ququan
LIV-5	Ligou
SP-6	Sanyinjiao
SP-7	Lougu
KI-10	Yingu
GB-27	Wushu
GB-41	Foot Linqi
LI-4	Hegu
LI-11	Quchi
ST-29	Guilai

Table 7.4   Acupuncture points[a] used in the treatment of Damp-Heat male infertility

Treatment goal	Acupuncture points
To strengthen Kidneys and clear Damp-Heat	Ren-4, KI-7, KI-10
To treat discharge from the genitals	BL-27 and BL-28
To clear Damp-Heat and treat impotence	BL-35 and Ren-1
To clear Damp and gently boost Kidney Yang	DU-3
To clear Damp-Heat from Liver channel and lower Jiao	LIV-8, LIV-5, GB-41, GB-27
To support Damp-clearing action	SP-6 and SP-7
To clear Heat, reduce general inflammation	LI-4, LI-11
To increase blood flow in the testicles[b]	ST-29, SP-6

[a]These points can be used with even or reducing manipulation.
[b]Use electroacupuncture (10 Hz) joining SP-6 to ST-29 on the same side for 5–20 min.

Qi and Blood Stagnation

Herbal Formula — Where Qi and Blood stagnation contribute to a problem with healthy sperm production, then formulas such as Xue Fu Zhu Yu Tang or, in the case of simple Qi stagnation, Xiao Yao San (Free and Easy powder) can be used for a course of treatment before the main Kidney tonic formula is applied. For varicoceles or immune issues a formula such as Gui Zhi Fu Ling Wan can be adapted.

Xue Fu Zhu Yu Tang (Decoction for Removing Blood Stasis in the Chest)

Dang Gui	9 g	Radix Angelicae Sinensis
Sheng Di	9 g	Radix Rehmanniae Glutinosae
Chi Shao	6 g	Radix Paeoniae Rubra
Chuan Xiong	6 g	Radix Ligustici Wallichi
Tao Ren	12 g	Semen Persicae
Hong Hua	9 g	Flos Carthami Tinctorii
Chai Hu	3 g	Radix Bupleuri
Zhi Ke	6 g	Fructus Citri seu Ponciri
Chuan Niu Xi	9 g	Radix Cyathulae
Jie Geng	6 g	Radix Platycodi Grandiflori
Gan Cao	3 g	Radix Glycyrrhizae Uralensis

Xiao Yao San (Free and Easy Powder)

Chai Hu	9 g	Radix Bupleuri
Bai Shao	12 g	Radix Paeoniae Lactiflorae
Dang Gui	9 g	Radix Angelicae Sinesis
Bai Zhu	9 g	Rhizoma Atractylodis Macrocephalae
Fu Ling	15 g	Sclerotium Poriae Cocos

Sheng Jiang	3 g	*Radix Rehmanniae Glutinosae*
Bo He	3 g	*Herba Menthae*
Gan Cao	6 g	*Radix Glycyrrhizae Uralensis*

Depending on the severity and nature of the stagnation (i.e, whether it is amenable to treatment with Chinese medicine), the following herbs may be added to Bu Shen Yi Jing Fang even after a course of Qi and Blood stagnation clearing herbs has been completed. For example:

Xiang Fu	9 g	*Rhizoma Cyperi Rotundi*
Wu Yao	9 g	*Radix Linderae Strychnifoliae*
Tao Ren	9 g	*Semen Persicae*
Hong Hua	6 g	*Flos Carthami Tinctorii*

Because the formula is taken for a long period of time, stronger Blood-moving herbs than these are not appropriate.

We can also add to this category more modern formulations which address immune issues.

Where there has been a diagnosis of varicocele or antisperm antibodies then using a formula which expands the actions of Gui Zhi Fu Ling Tang (shown in trials to improve sperm counts in men with varicoceles) can be used.[46]

Gui Zhi Fu Ling Tang (Ramulus Cinnamomi-Poria decoction) modified

Gui Zhi	6 g	*Ramulus Cinnamomi Cassiae*
Tao Ren	6 g	*Semen Persicae*
Mu Dan Pi	9 g	*Cortex Moutan Radicis*
Chi Shao	9 g	*Radix Paeoniae Rubra*
Dan Shen	18 g	*Radix Salviae Miltiorrhizae*
Wang Bu Liu Xing	6 g	*Semen Vaccariae*
Che Qian Zi	9 g	*Semen Plantaginis*
Fu Ling	9 g	*Sclerotium Poriae Cocos*
Pu Gong Yin	12 g	*Herba Taraxaci Mongolici*
Xiao Hui Xiang	3 g	*Fructus Foeniculi Vulgaris*
Ju He	3 g	*Semen Citri Reticulatae*
Chuan Lian Zi	9 g	*Fructus Meliae Toosendan*
Xu Duan	9 g	*Radix Dipsaci*
Huang Qi	18 g	*Radix Astragali*

To the basic therapeutic strategy of Gui Zhi Fu Ling Tang (clearing stasis and Damp), we include additional herbs to clear Qi and Blood stasis to improve circulation and to reduce inflammation. Herbs such as Wang Bu Liu Xing will help this formula target the testicles. And herbs such as Xiao Hui Xiang, Ju He, and Chuan Lian Zi are employed to specifically move the Qi in the testicles, ensuring no hindrance to the blood circulation. Dan Shen and Huang Qi are often employed in rather large doses when addressing autoimmune issues (examined further in Chapter 8).

Because inflammation is often associated with antisperm antibodies, herbs to clear Heat and Damp such as Pu Gong Yin are added.

Studies in China have found that herbal formulas which move the Blood and clear Damp-Heat while supporting Kidney Yin and Yang have a better effect on anti-sperm antibodies than does prednisone.[29]

Acupuncture Points — Choose from the following points (and see Table 7.5):

Ren-1	Huiyin
Ren-2	Qugu
SP-6	Sanyinjiao
SP-10	Xuehai
ST-29	Guilai
ST-30	Qichong
BL-31	Shangliao
BL-32	Ciliao
BL-33	Zhongliao
LIV-1	Dadun
LIV-4	Zhongfeng
K-11	Henggu
PC-6	Neiguan

Also relevant are any of the points, such as those on the Liver and Kidney channels that are indicated for Shan Qi.[47] Shan Qi includes disorders of the testicles which present with pain and swelling.

IVF PROCEDURES

Aside from surgical intervention, infertility specialists in the West offer ART and IVF procedures for inadequate sperm. The onus of the 'treatment' falls largely on the female partner, though the handicap is not hers. Eggs collected from drug-stimulated ovaries can be fertilized in the laboratory with just a few sperm, not the millions per ejaculation required by nature. And in cases where those few sperm do not have enough motility to reach and fertilize the egg, technicians inject them into the egg using a technique called intracytoplasmic sperm injection (ICSI). In a given cycle, typically about two-thirds of the injected eggs are fertilized and about one-quarter to one-third of the women who receive these fertilized eggs will become pregnant – slightly fewer will deliver a full-term baby.

Where there are no sperm being produced at all in the ejaculate, specialists can extract sperm from the epididymis situated on top of the testis (in a procedure called microepididymal or percutaneous sperm aspiration, MESA or PESA) or in cases where there is maturation arrest, immature sperm can be extracted from testicular tissue

Table 7.5   Acupuncture points[a] used in the treatment of Qi and Blood stagnation male infertility

Treatment goal	Acupuncture points
To increase circulation of Qi and Blood in the genitals	Ren-1 and Ren-2, ST-29, SP-6
To encourage circulation of Blood	SP-10, PC-6
To clear stagnation in lower Jiao	ST-30 and BL-31, BL-32, BL-33
To move the Qi (or treat swelling or pain) in the genitals	LIV-1, LIV-4, K-11
To increase blood flow in the arteries of the testicles[b]	ST-29, SP-6

[a]Points are needled with even or reducing technique.
[b]Use electroacupuncture (10 Hz) joining SP-6 to ST-29 on the same side for 5–20 min.

(testicular sperm extraction or TESE). The individual sperm retrieved can then be injected into the egg using the ICSI technique. (We will discuss this further in Ch. 9.)

DIET AND LIFESTYLE

Many aspects of diet and lifestyle are discussed in Chapter 12, but where sperm are concerned, the importance of avoiding damaging chemicals and fumes cannot be repeated too often. Sperm are extremely sensitive to the effects of chemicals in the environment and in food. In Chapter 12, we will explore environmental and dietary factors that might impact sperm quality alongside other aspects of lifestyle and behavior.

REFERENCES

1. Jansen RPS. *Getting pregnant*. Sydney: Allen and Unwin; 2003, 141.

2. Cooper T. World Health Organization reference values for human semen characteristics. *Hum Reprod Update* 2010;**16**(3):231–45.

3. Dindyal S. The sperm count has been decreasing steadily for many years in Western industrialized countries: Is there an endocrine basis for this decrease?. *Internet J Urol* 2004;**2**(1):1–21.

4. Guzick DS, Overstreet JW, Factor-Litvak P, et al. Sperm morphology, motility, and concentration in fertile and infertile men. *N Engl J Med* 2001;**345**(19):1388–93.

5. Badenoch DF, Evans SJ, McCloskey DJ. Sperm density measurement: should this be abandoned?. *Br J Urol* 1989;**64**(5):521–3.

6. Irvine S, Cawood E, Richardson D, et al. Evidence of deteriorating semen quality in the United Kingdom: birth cohort study in 577 men in Scotland over 11 years. *Br Med J* 1996;**312**(7029):467–71.

7. Savitz DA, Whelan EA, Kleckner RC. Effects of parents' occupational exposures on risk of stillbirth, preterm delivery, and small-for-gestational-age infants. *Am J Epidemiol* 1989;**129**(6):1201–18.

8. Colborn T, Myers JP, Dumanoski D. *Our stolen future*. London: Little, Brown; 1996, 70.

9. Hauser R, Meeker JD, Duty S, et al. Altered semen quality in relation to urinary concentrations of phthalate monoester and oxidative metabolites. *Epidemiology* 2006;**17**:682–91.

10. Wu DH, Leung YK, Thomas MA, et al. Bisphenol A (BPA) confers direct genotoxicity to sperm with increased sperm DNA fragmentation. *Fertil Steril* 2011;**96**(3):S5.

11. Colborn T, Myers JP, Dumanoski D. *Our stolen future*. London: Little, Brown; 1996, 81.

12. Ford WCL, North K, Taylor H, et al. and the ALSPAC study team. Increasing paternal age is associated with delayed conception in a large population of fertile couples: evidence for declining fecundity in older men. *Hum Reprod* 2000;**15**(8):1703–8.

13. Frattarelli JL, Miller KA, Miller BT, et al. Male age negatively impacts embryo development and reproductive outcome in donor oocyte assisted reproductive technology cycles. *Fertil Steril* 2008;**90**(1):97–103.

14. Qian-Xi Zhu, Meads C, Lu ML, et al. Turning point of age for semen quality: a population-based study in Chinese men. *Fertil Steril* 2011;**96**(3):572–6.

15. Povey AC, Clyma JA, McNamee R. Modifiable and non-modifiable risk factors for poor semen quality: a case-referent study. *Hum Reprod* 2012;**27**(9):2799–806.

16. Saikhun J, Kitiyanant Y, Vanadurongwan V, et al. The effect of saunas sperm movement characteristics of normal men measured by computer assisted sperm analysis. *Int J Androl* 1998;**21**:358–63.

17. French D, Desai NR, Agarwal A, et al. Varicocele repair: does it still have a role in infertility treatment?. *Curr Opin Obstet Gynecol* 2008;**20**(3):269–74.

18. Daitch J, Bedaiwy MA, Pasqualotto EB, et al. Varicocelectomy improves intrauterine insemination success rates in men with varicocele. *J Urol* 2001;**165**(5):1510–3.

19. Dinulovic D, Radonjic G. Diabetes mellitus/male infertility. *Arch Androl* 1990;**25**:277–93.

20. Jansen RPS. *Getting pregnant*. Sydney: Allen and Unwin; 2003, 140.

21. Cardoso EM, Santoianni JE, De Paulis AN, et al. Improvement of semen quality in infected asymptomatic infertile male after bacteriological cure. *Medicina (Buenos Aires)* 1998;**58**(2):160–4.

22. Hargreaves CA, Rogers S, Hills F, et al. Effects of co-trimoxazole, erythromycin, amoxicillin, tetracycline and chloroquine on sperm function in vitro. *Hum Reprod* 1998;**13**(7):1878–86.

23. Matsuda T, Muguruma K, Horii Y, et al. Serum antisperm antibodies in men with vas deferens obstruction caused by childhood inguinal herniorrhaphy. *Fertil Steril* 1993;**59**:1095–7.

24. Alukal JP, Lipshultz LI. Why treat the male in the era of assisted reproduction?. *Semin Reprod Med* 2009;**27**(2):109–14.

25. Tempest HG, Homa ST, Zhai XP, et al. Significant reduction of sperm disomy in six men: effect of traditional Chinese medicine?. *Asian J Androl* 2005;**7**(4):419–25.

26. Hui Luo Jian. Treatment of male infertility with Chinese herbs. *Pacific Journal of Oriental Medicine* 1996;**7**:40–1.

27. De-Gui Chang, Pei-hai Zhang, Ahi-ping Hu. Effect of Zengjing No.1 capsule on morphology and motility of sperm in patients with oligospermia. *Chin J Integr Trad West Med* 2009;**29**(11):1029–30.

28. Fu B, Lun X, Gong Y. Effects of the combined therapy of acupuncture with herbal drugs on male immune infertility – a clinical report of 50 cases. *J Trad Chin Med* 2005;**25**:186–9.

29. Lu TK, Ouyang HG, Jin GY, et al. Clinical study on the treatment of male immune infertility by. *Huzhangdanshenyin Zhonghua Nan Ke Xue* 2006;**12**(8):750–5.

30. Jin BF, Yang XY, Bian TS, et al. Effects of Jujingwan on nitric oxide and superoxide dismutase in seminal plasma of asthenospermia patients. *Zhonghua Nan Ke Xue* 2007;**13**(1):87–90.

31. Ma HG, Xu JX, Zhang JF, et al. The effect of Chinese medicine yiqihuoxuetang on T-lymphocyte subpopulation in peripheral blood of infertile men with antisperm antibodies. *Zhonghua Nan Ke Xue* 2003;**9**:154–6.

32. Riegler R, Fischl F, Bunzel B, et al. Correlation of psychological changes and spermiogram improvements following acupuncture (article in German). *Urologe A* 1984;**23**(6):329–33.

33. Siterman S, Eltes F, Wolfson V, et al. Effect of acupuncture on sperm parameters of males suffering from subfertility related to low sperm quality. *Arch Androl* 1997;**39**(2):155–61.

34. Siterman S, Eltes F, Lederman H, Bartoov B. Does acupuncture treatment affect sperm density in males with very low sperm count? A pilot study. *Andrologia* 2000;**32**(1):31–9.

35. Zhang M, Huang G, Lu F, et al. Influence of acupuncture on idiopathic male infertility in assisted reproductive technology. *J Huazhong Univ Sci Tech Med Sci* 2002;**22**(3):228–30.

36. Gurfinkel E, Cedenho AP, Yamamura Y, et al. Effects of acupuncture and moxa treatment in patients with semen abnormalities. *Asian J Androl* 2003;**5**(4):345–8.

37. Pei J, Strehler E, Noss U, et al. Quantitative evaluation of spermatozoa ultrastructure after acupuncture treatment for idiopathic male infertility. *Fertil Steril* 2005;**84**(1):141–7.

38. Wang ZQ, Huang YQ, Liang B. Clinical observation on electroacupuncture and Chinese drug for treatment of oligospermia and asthenospermia of the male infertility patient. *Zhongguo Zhen Jiu* 2008;**28**(11):805–7.

39. Siterman S, Eltes F, Schechter L, et al. Success of acupuncture treatment in patients with initially low sperm output is associated with a decrease in scrotal skin temperature. *Asian J Androl* 2009;**11**(2):200–8.

40. Dieterle S, Li C, Greb R, et al. A prospective randomized placebo-controlled study of the effect of acupuncture in infertile patients with severe oligoasthenozoospermia. *Fertil Steril* 2009;**92**(4):1340–3.

41. Chen A, Shen A, Li R, et al. Effect of acupuncture-moxibustion therapy on sperm quality in infertility patients with sperm abnormality. *J Acup Tuina Sci* 2011;**9**(4):219–22.

42. Fujisawa M, Kanzaki M, Okada H, et al. Metenkephalin in seminal plasma of infertile men. *Int J Urol* 1996;**3**(4):297–300.

43. Bensoussan A. *The vital meridian.* Melbourne: Churchill Livingstone; 1990, 112.

44. Cakmak Y, Akpinar IN, Ekinci G, et al. Point- and frequency-specific response of the testicular artery to abdominal electroacupuncture in humans. *Fertil Steril* 2008;**90**:1732–8.

45. Guo J, Kong L, Gao X, et al. A parallel study of the effects in treatment of impotence by tonifying the Kidney with and without improving Blood circulation. *J Trad Chin Med* 1999;**19**(2):123–5.

46. Ishikawa H, Ohashi M, Rayakawa K, et al. Effects of Guizhi-Fuling-Wan on male infertility with varicocele. *Am J Chin Med* 1996;**24**(3–4):327–31.

47. Deadman P, Al-Khafaji M, Baker K. *A manual of acupuncture.* Hove: Journal of Chinese Medicine Publications; 1998, 655–656.

Pregnancy loss, miscarriage, immune infertility, and ectopic pregnancy

8

Chapter Contents

MISCARRIAGE

Healthy fertility does not mean just the ability to conceive. Good fertility means establishing and then nurturing a pregnancy for 9 months to full term. Thus, doctors specializing in the treatment of infertility need to hold clearly in their mind the goal of the birth of a healthy baby and not focus only on the first hurdle, the positive pregnancy test: some of the modern technologies used in assisted reproduction place so much emphasis on achieving that first prize that the integrity of the rest of the pregnancy can be compromised. The quality of that small bundle of just a few cells, the pre-embryo, determines (to a significant extent) the development of the rest of the pregnancy. And the biological integrity of the embryo is directly related to the quality of the gametes that fuse to form it and, of course, the quality of the gametes depends on the health and circumstance of the men and women who make them. Equally, the integrity of the uterine lining and the uterine environment is crucial for successful implantation, development of the placenta and establishment of a viable pregnancy.

So, if we are to approach fertility in the broad view, all aspects of the health of both partners and their gametes must be considered, which means examining all aspects of lifestyle and life stresses before conceiving. It might mean avoiding exposure to certain environmental factors or changing eating patterns or addressing chronic diseases. Many different parts of our lives can have a big impact on fertility and can be reflected not only in ease of conception but also in miscarriage rates (see Ch. 12).

Miscarriage is a common event causing large numbers of women (e.g., a quarter of a million each year in the UK) to experience grief and distress The term miscarriage refers to pregnancy loss after a conception has produced viable quantities of the pregnancy hormone (human chorionic gonadotrophin (hCG) in the blood and urine, or the fetus has developed to the point where either a gestational sac (1 week after a missed menstrual period) or a heart beat is visible on ultrasound (2–3 weeks after a missed period). In its broadest definition, pregnancy loss refers to any fetal loss from conception until the time of fetal viability at 23 weeks' gestation.

In the first part of this chapter, we shall examine pregnancy loss by miscarriage. We shall also look at all the steps that occur between fertilization and a well-established and viable pregnancy and how loss of embryos can happen at any of these stages, even before pregnancy is suspected. After examining all the options for treatment or prevention of miscarriage, the second part of this chapter examines pregnancy loss caused by implantation of the embryo in the wrong place – ectopic pregnancy.

When it comes to treatment, the focus is primarily on the female of the couple, as she is the stage on which the pregnancy is enacted. However, just because the sperm has left the male partner's body and successfully made contact with an egg does not mean that we can ignore its role in the future survival of the fetus. There are many factors affecting both male and female gametes that can influence the future of the fetus and which will be examined in more detail below. Historically, however, in both Western medicine texts and in Chinese medicine texts, the miscarriage spotlight has fallen on the mother-to-be.

Pre- and post-implantation loss

Clinical rates of miscarriage are often reported to be between 10 and 25% – or higher depending on age. However, the loss of embryos after fertilization but before implantation is much higher than that.

Of the potential pregnancies which are lost, 75% are due to implantation failure and are not clinically recognized as miscarriages. If a small (unviable) amount of hCG is measured on an early pregnancy test, it is called a biochemical pregnancy; it has reached implantation stage but gotten no further. In these days of IVF, what used to be occult pregnancy losses are not so occult anymore.

Conceptions, therefore, occur much more frequently than we think but embryos can be lost before the woman even knows she is pregnant, maybe even before the trophoblast (which forms a week or so after fertilization) has started producing hCG to tell the corpus luteum to keep producing progesterone.

Defective embryos reflect faults in the egg (especially if it is older); faults in the sperm (especially if they have been exposed to radiation or toxic chemicals); faults in the fertilization process itself (polyspermia or fertilization by more than one sperm), or may be just a random strike of destiny in the way the embryo itself develops. The technical term for the reason for these failures of implantation or development is chromosomal embryopathy, i.e., a genetic fault exists in the embryo such as to make it unviable, and cell division and development cease. Because the genetic blueprint of each embryo is brand new, it has never been tested and so fatal mistakes are commonplace.

There are some chromosomal embryopathies which unfortunately do not make the embryo unviable enough and these are the chromosomal patterns which produce Down syndrome babies and other genetic syndromes. Ultrasound measurements of the fetus at week 11 or 12 will alert the mother to risk of abnormality. Where there is suspicion of increased risk of genetic abnormalities, tests may be ordered to determine the genetic make-up of the embryo. These tests are done by collecting cells from the newly forming placenta (CVS or chorionic villus sampling) or from the amniotic fluid (amniocentesis); from these cells the chromosomes of the embryo are analyzed.

Once a pregnancy is confirmed by an ultrasound which measures a healthy heartbeat, and there are no symptoms of back or abdomen pain or bleeding, then the risk of miscarriage falls to a low level (approx. 2%).[1]

Miscarriage and age

Advanced age is the primary risk factor for miscarriage. The risk rises sharply and exponentially from age 35 (see Fig. 8.1). While the effect of maternal age on miscarriage is marked, the male partner's age also can impact miscarriage risk. Several studies have looked at the effect of the male partner's age on miscarriage risk, noting that more advanced age (>35–40 years) is associated with more miscarriages.[2–4] This increased risk is especially apparent where the female partner is under 35. The miscarriage rate in younger women with male partners aged ≥35 is double that of women with younger husbands.[5]

What does Chinese medicine say causes miscarriages?

Kidney Jing and Yin deficiency not only mean difficulty in producing gametes in the first place but also difficulty in producing healthy effective gametes (i.e., ones with intact chromosomes and undamaged DNA). Yin deficiency, which exerts its effects more noticeably with age, is a common factor affecting the viability of the gametes. In the case of ova, this viability is measured not only in the integrity of the chromosomes in the nucleus of the egg but also in the mitochondria (the organelles which produce the energy currency the cell needs to carry out all its activities), which have their own DNA. The DNA in a baby's mitochondria is inherited only from the mother.

Although environment and lifestyle can affect the Kidney Jing and Yin (see Ch. 12), it is aging which is the main drain on Kidney reserves, evidenced by the fact that many women who become pregnant in their 40s miscarry (Fig. 8.1). As mentioned above, although the effect of age is not quite so marked in men, presumably because sperm are made afresh constantly, there are nevertheless more miscarriages when the male partner is older. Thus, the Jing-depleting effects of age affect men's fertility too. The difficulty older women and men experience in trying to have children is a control provided by nature to discourage the production of offspring who do not have a strong Jing Qi inheritance. The offspring of parents who pass on poor-quality Jing may suffer the consequences. If the Jing that the new fetus inherits is too deficient, however, nature will ensure it will not survive and miscarriage will follow.

Interestingly, women who have taken the oral contraceptive pill for an extended period of time (≥8 years) have a reduced risk of miscarriage when they are older. In fact, the rate of miscarriage and infertility is half that of other women (≥35 years) who have not taken the pill.[6] Because they have conserved rather than spent the thousands of

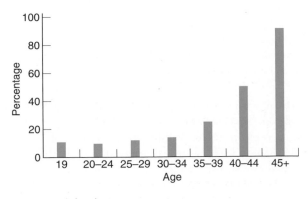

Figure 8.1 Miscarriage risk increases with female age.

eggs which years of menstrual cycles consume, they have a larger store of good-quality eggs and a larger store of Jing later in their reproductive years.

As practitioners of TCM, we can try to apply preventative treatment or measures for the gametes so that they do not develop abnormalities (see Prevention of future miscarriage, later). This might be easier to achieve with sperm than with eggs. Although stem cell science tells us there is a possibility that new oocytes can be produced by ovarian tissue, the fact is that the eggs in a woman's ovaries available for ovulation have been present since before her birth; hence, their genetic integrity has much to do with their age and past history (of radiation, etc.). Certainly no influence can be exerted on the DNA in the chromosomes of these egg cells, but influence can be exerted on the nourishment and development of the follicle (see Ch. 11). Herbal and acupuncture treatment of men diagnosed with Yin deficiency and internal Heat (who often have a high percentage of abnormal sperm forms) can achieve a positive influence on the sperm quality.

Mechanism of embryo loss before implantation

As mentioned before, at least half of the embryos which fall by the wayside before they even implant in the uterus are those that show abnormal development, i.e., there is something wrong with the genetic programing.

For those embryos that do not have a genetic problem, other factors may arrest further development. This may be a lack of energy (ATP) required for cell division in the early embryo (discussed in Ch. 11). In some of these cases, the problem is not so much with the gametes or the embryo itself but with the reproductive tract of the mother; the fallopian tubes or the uterus.

• Tubes – Qi stagnation/Damp

There may be a problem with the tubes such that the pre-embryo does not receive the necessary care and nourishment to take it through the first few cell divisions that occur after fertilization. A fault in the tubes may also mean that the embryo traverses them too rapidly or too slowly, thus it arrives in the uterus at a time when the stage of development of the endometrium does not match its own and implantation is not favored.

The TCM doctor gives treatment around ovulation time and immediately afterwards to regulate the Liver Qi and therefore the passage of the embryo in the tubes. If mucus secretions are suspected to be obstructing or slowing passage in the tubes, treatment to clear Damp will be added. (This has already been discussed in Chapters 4 and 6.)

• Endometrium – Damp or Blood stagnation/Yin, Yang or Blood deficiency

Alternatively, or in addition, there may be a problem with the endometrium. Excess fluid or mucus on the surface can interfere with implantation. In TCM, such a situation represents excess Damp. The aim of treatment will be to clear Damp and Fluids with herbs and acupuncture.

In another situation, the endometrium does not provide a well formed surface with appropriate sites for attachment and implantation. In TCM terms, this may reflect Blood stagnation, deficient Yin or Blood, or a 'Cold womb'. Blood stagnation is best treated during the period to ensure a thorough discharge of the endometrium and smooth remodeling of endometrial tissue to provide a more favorable surface for implantation later on. Blood and Yin deficiency, which lead to a thin or dry uterine lining, is best treated straight after the period with Blood and Yin tonic herbs and foods. A 'Cold womb' is how TCM doctors describe the uterus of a woman who is Yang deficient. Yang deficiency is often manifest in low progesterone levels, which means the lining of the uterus does not secrete sufficient nutrients in the luteal phase to nourish the embryo; thus, it fails to implant or develop.

TCM approach to the treatment of miscarriage

A miscarriage from the Chinese medicine point of view can be nearly as demanding on the body's resources as childbirth, i.e., the physiologic changes experienced by a pregnant body which then suddenly becomes not pregnant are significant and require great adjustments. The hormone levels drop very rapidly after a miscarriage and if there has been significant blood loss, this will leave the body very weak. The recovery is not just physical; in the case of a miscarriage, there is usually emotional distress and this can be considerable if the miscarriage follows a period of infertility.

Chinese medicine texts describe several different clinical approaches to miscarriage, depending on the circumstances.

- *Threatened miscarriage*: trying to save a pregnancy at risk. If a woman who is pregnant starts bleeding, this is called a threatened miscarriage and treatment is employed to 'pacify the fetus' in an attempt to stabilize and save the pregnancy if possible. Since a large percentage of miscarriages are the result of genetic defects in the embryo, such treatment will in many cases, have very limited useful effects. Often, no matter what treatment is given, the miscarriage still occurs. Ideally, the TCM doctor needs to discover whether the fetus is doomed by chromosomal abnormality or whether it is quite healthy and it is the mother's condition which needs to be improved. A master pulse-taker may be able to make such a diagnosis but for many less experienced practitioners, it may be signs of healthy development of the fetus (or not) on the ultrasound that can give us more precise information. In the end, many practitioners will choose to give treatment on a 'lets give it a try, we've got nothing to lose' basis.

- *Inevitable miscarriage and sequelae.* In the event the pregnancy is inevitably doomed, the doctor of Chinese medicine can contribute in quite a different way. Once the fetus has died and has been expelled, or still needs to be expelled, then Chinese medicine can be used to expedite the complete removal of all the contents of the uterus. Subsequently, recuperative treatment will address weakness in the mother due to blood loss and physiologic and psychological stress. When such weakness is made good, treatment to regulate the menstrual cycle again will be appropriate. In most cases, it is only after 2 or 3 healthy cycles that attempting pregnancy again is advised. This is an area in which skillfully applied TCM treatment brings great benefit and may, in the long term, be a sounder approach than the prevailing medical attitude which advises getting back on your feet and trying to conceive again as soon as possible.

- *Recurrent miscarriage*: preventing future miscarriages. If a woman has had two or three or more miscarriages, then it is more likely that a problem exists in one of the would-be parents. The aim of treatment will be to prevent future miscarriages and, in this case, the couple is asked to refrain from attempts to conceive for at least 3–6 months while the male or female partner is being treated.

Chinese medicine can realistically be expected to have a very useful impact on the treatment of recurrent miscarriage because it is the constitution of the would-be parent that is being treated, not the pregnancy or the fetus.

THREATENED MISCARRIAGE

The first signs of a miscarriage are some bleeding and cramping in the abdomen or lower back pain. If the pregnancy is in the very early stages (i.e., the period is late by only 1 week or less), then the woman may just experience what feels like a heavy period. Since the only evidence of pregnancy is the positive blood test for hCG, these are called subclinical miscarriages of biochemical pregnancies. As a rule, the flow of blood will carry all the products of conception out and a surgical procedure like a dilatation and curettage (D&C) to clear out the uterus is not necessary.

Later-stage miscarriages, called clinical miscarriages, occur after the pregnancy has already been well established, i.e., if there has been an ultrasound it reveals the gestational sac and maybe a heart beat. This sort of miscarriage can involve heavy clotty bleeding, pain and cramping, and shock. Where the pregnancy is more advanced, a D&C will often be recommended to resolve the miscarriage and ensure no pregnancy products remain.

If bleeding during pregnancy occurs without pain and examination by a doctor shows the cervix to be firmly closed, then a miscarriage is not inevitable. The bleed may just be reflecting some process in the endometrium as the new placenta starts to form and exchange blood vessel surfaces with those of the mother. A transvaginal ultrasound will usually reveal all; if the gestational sac and the embryo are the normal size for their age and the heart beat is obvious, then there is every likelihood that the pregnancy will develop normally despite some early bleeding. If, however, the gestational sac is too small or the heart beat is absent or too slow at a time when it should be well developed, then a miscarriage will likely follow the bleeding. Most fetuses which miscarry in the 1st trimester (first 3 months) show abnormal development. For the remaining miscarriages in which there is normal development and normal chromosomes, there is likely to be a hormonal, immunological, or emotional cause. Miscarriages occurring for one of these latter reasons are more common among couples who have recurrent miscarriage (described below).

Other causes of a threatened miscarriage (which is not part of a recurrent miscarriage pattern) include isolated events such as a high fever or drug or alcohol abuse, which can cause fetal death.

Causes of threatened miscarriage

Infections, fevers, and accidents

Fever at the time of ovulation can disturb cell division and lead to chromosomal abnormalities, which means, if that particular egg is fertilized the fetus will probably not be viable and miscarriage will follow. Fever during the 1st trimester of the pregnancy can also cause abnormalities in the baby, followed by miscarriage (or in rare cases, a baby with a malformation like a short or absent limb). High fever during pregnancy is usually managed effectively with paracetamol and lots of fluids and bed rest. Chinese herbs to reduce Heat and resolve the causative factor (usually a virus or in TCM terms a Wind-Heat or Wind-Cold attack) can also be useful if applied quickly.

Sometimes, infections are already present in the endometrium before conception and the inflammation they cause (endometritis) can irritate the fetal membranes and cause premature contractions of the uterus. If we are aware of a history of pelvic inflammation or diagnose it from the signs and symptoms the Chinese medicine doctor recognizes as Heat or Damp-Heat, then treatment can be applied to remove the Heat and inflammation and an attempt made to save the pregnancy. Of course it is always preferable to deal with endometritis before conception if possible (see Ch. 5). Sometimes, infections reach the fetus from the outside through the cervix, causing fetal death and a miscarriage. Rapid diagnosis and treatment may be helpful, but often the harm is done before the diagnosis is made.

Other infections which can damage a fetus directly – i.e., by crossing the placenta from the mother's bloodstream – include German measles virus (rubella), the chickenpox virus (herpes zoster), the genital herpes virus (herpes simplex), cytomegalovirus, bacteria such as those causing syphilis and tuberculosis and parasites such as those causing toxoplasmosis and malaria. If the damage to the fetus is serious, then it will miscarry. Sadly, in some cases of rubella and syphilis infection, the baby will survive but be born with serious abnormalities. These infections are not the cause of recurrent miscarriages, because the woman usually develops an immunity to them after the first infection.

Infections in the genitourinary tract which are active at the time of pregnancy increase the risk of 2nd trimester miscarriage about three times over normal.[7]

A history of sexually transmitted disease often causes problems with becoming pregnant rather than with staying pregnant (see Ch. 6).

Accidents such as serious falls or shocks are sometimes blamed for miscarriages. From a TCM point of view, falls and injuries can cause Blood stagnation, which may manifest as a disorder of blood flow in the placenta or endometrium. In addition, the TCM doctor recognizes that shock can affect the Heart and obstruct the Bao vessel, an important channel for controlling Blood to the Uterus and therefore for nourishment of the fetus.

Strain of the lower back associated with lifting heavy loads can also cause a miscarriage. Studies with physiotherapists, kitchen workers, and cleaners show that work which involves lifting and bending can increase the risk of miscarriage more than three times above normal.[8]

Strain and overuse of the lower back damages the Kidney energy which, you may recall from Chapter 4, is a crucial factor from a TCM point of view for a healthy pregnancy.

Alcohol and drugs

Alcohol or drug abuse, if extreme, can create such toxic conditions for the fetus that it cannot survive. Or they damage the mother's health sufficiently that her body is unable to sustain the pregnancy (see also Recurrent miscarriage, below).

In TCM, such agents are usually said to create internal Heat, which at a certain level damages the endometrium. Long-term alcohol or drug abuse is usually accompanied by malnutrition; in TCM terms, this implies insufficient Qi and Blood to nourish a fetus.

Prescription drugs taken in early pregnancy can in some cases present a risk, e.g., there is some evidence that even commonly used drugs such as non-steroidal anti-inflammatory drugs (NSAIDs) can contribute to miscarriage.[9] One study found that the use of NSAIDs (ibuprofen, naproxen, or aspirin) during early pregnancy increased the risk of miscarriage by 80%. The risk was much higher when NSAIDs were taken around conception or were used for longer than a week. It is thought that prostaglandin inhibition by NSAIDs might interfere with implantation.[10] Paracetamol use is not associated with any increased risk of miscarriage.

Other drugs such as Roaccutane (isotretinoin) used to treat resistant acne are well known for their ability to cause defects in the embryo; when these are lethal enough, miscarriage will follow.

There is much more research to be done in this area; meanwhile, drugs should be avoided in early pregnancy if possible.

Hot baths

The use of hot tubs is also a risk factor for miscarriage, especially in the first few weeks of pregnancy. Women who use hot tubs or Jacuzzis (which keep the water temperature high) in early pregnancy are twice as likely to miscarry as those women who do not use them. The use of regular bathtubs does not seem to be a risk factor, but sustained elevation of core body temperature is best avoided, not only because of the risk of miscarriage but also the increase in neural tube defects associated with hyperthermia.[11]

Exposure to chemical agents (e.g., during the preparation of synthetic drugs or use of industrial or domestic cleaners) as either discrete events or on an ongoing basis, can also contribute to miscarriage (such agents are discussed in the Causes of recurrent miscarriage, below).

There has been some debate about the effects of the oral contraceptive pill on pregnancies which closely follow its use. Not all specialists are in agreement about the persisting effects of the pill and, indeed, most claim there is no lingering effect.[12] However, some manufacturers of the pill have advised that it be stopped for 3 or 4 months before attempting pregnancy, claiming an increased risk of miscarriage immediately after using contraceptive hormones.[13] Other surveys have noted that taking the pill for more than 2 years is associated with an increased risk of miscarriage.[14] This may be due to persistent disruption of endometrial function caused by the pill, which can result in implantation difficulties for the embryo, or it may be because oral contraceptive use depletes folic acid stores, which puts at risk the development of the fetus in its first few weeks.

There is much Chinese medicine can contribute to preparing the endometrium and the cervix for a healthy and stable pregnancy after stopping the pill. Following the treatment regimens described in Chapter 4, with a special emphasis on building the Yin (to promote cervical mucus production) and regulating and then building the Blood and boosting Kidney Yang (to promote a healthy endometrium) should facilitate rapid reversal of any undesired effects of the pill.

We will discuss more causes of miscarriage below when we discuss recurrent miscarriages.

TCM treatment of threatened miscarriage

In the event of a threatened miscarriage, TCM intervention can sometimes play a useful role. It is one of those times when Chinese medicine doctors like to be more proactive than their Western medicine counterparts, who view early miscarriages as relatively trivial events from a physiologic point of view (though not from a psychological point of view). If the pregnancy can be saved, the TCM doctor will have something up his sleeve rather than just adopting a fatalistic attitude of wait and see. Obviously in many cases, there is little that can be done and the miscarriage is necessary to expel a defective embryo. But in cases where the problem lies with the mother or the way in which the pregnancy is being established, then timely treatment may save a pregnancy. If there is no lower back pain or bleeding, the pulse is slippery, the tongue is not purple and the abdomen feels warm, then the threatening miscarriage has more chance of being rescued.

Chinese medicine texts describe a threatened miscarriage as 'fetal restlessness' or 'fetal bleeding'. The symptoms are spotting or bleeding in early pregnancy sometimes accompanied by lower back pain and abdomen cramping. If the pregnancy is threatened for reasons other than chromosomal embryopathy, then it is ideal if treatment is administered before bleeding starts. However, this may be difficult to assess. Doctors working in infertility clinics in China will closely supervise the first few weeks of an at-risk pregnancy. 'At risk' in this context means the pregnancy follows a period of infertility, or there has been a history of previous miscarriage. In these clinics, women may be encouraged to continue taking basal body temperature (BBT) readings for the first few weeks after the pregnancy is confirmed; that way, the doctor can determine the vigor of the Kidney Yang by the temperature readings. If the temperature starts to drop at all, Kidney Yang tonics (and Qi tonics) will be administered, or increased if they are already being taken. Similarly, blood levels of hCG and progesterone can be monitored and vaginal ultrasounds can be taken. However, although these tests can give accurate assessments of the progress of the pregnancy, to do them on a frequent basis may be prohibitively costly.

Categories of threatened miscarriage are:

- Kidney deficiency

- Qi deficiency (Blood deficiency)

- Heat in the Blood

- Blood stagnation.

Kidney deficiency

When we constructed treatment protocols for encouraging conception, in Chapter 4, we emphasized Kidney Yin. Once conception has occurred, then treatment of Kidney Yang is emphasized, i.e., the Uterus must be kept 'warm'. It is Kidney Yang deficiency which is the most common cause of early-stage (subclinical) miscarriage and also pre-implantation loss (where there is no chromosomal embryopathy). In the case where a diagnosed pregnancy is threatening to miscarry there will be spotting or bleeding, which may be accompanied by lower back pain, sore legs and frequent urination.

The pulse will be weak and soft. This will be especially notable in the Kidney position, which in a healthy pregnancy should quickly develop a firm, solid and slippery feel. The tongue will be pale or unremarkable.

Herbal formula — The guiding formula in this situation is:

Shou Tai Wan (Fetus Longevity pill)

Tu Si Zi	20 g	*Semen Cuscatae*
Du Zhong	9 g	*Cortex Eucommiae Ulmoidis*
Sang Ji Sheng	9 g	*Ramulus Sangjisheng*
E Jiao	9 g	*Gelatinum Asini*

Tu Si Zi is the most important herb to prevent miscarriage due to Kidney deficiency. It has a strong supplementing effect on the Kidney, combined with an astringent effect; consequently, the dose used is often much larger than usual. However, doses above the level given above are not advised.

Xu Duan can be used instead of Du Zhong in this formula, as they both have the effect of strengthening the Kidney and preventing miscarriage. Sang Ji Sheng supports the Kidneys and with E Jiao nourishes Blood and prevents miscarriage; E Jiao also has the action of stopping bleeding.

More herbs can be added to stop bleeding if necessary, e.g.

Ai Ye tan	9 g	*Folium Artemisiae*
Zhu Ma Gen	15 g	*Radix Boehmeria Nivea*

It is common for Kidney deficiency miscarriage to also show signs of Qi deficiency. In that case, some of the herbs mentioned in the next category (Qi deficiency) will be added to the above guiding formula, e.g.

Huang Qi	20 g	*Radix Astragali*
Bai Zhu	9 g	*Rhizoma Atractylodis Macrocephalae*
Dang Shen	9 g	*Radix Codonopsis Pilulosae*

If there is a history of chronic miscarriage, these Qi tonic herbs will always be used before and after conception to encourage the Spleen Qi to hold the fetus in.

Acupuncture points — Choose from the following points (and see Table 8.1):

Ren-4	Guanyuan
BL-23	Shenshu
Ren-6	Qihai
KI-3	Taixi
KI-6	Zhaohai
Ren-12	Zhongwan
DU-20	Baihui

CASE HISTORY – MORGAN

Morgan's pregnancy was a long time coming – 5 years (between the age of 33 and 38) of trying hard, the last 6 months taking Chinese herbs and having acupuncture. She had almost given up and when she finally conceived, she planned a celebration overseas trip. But by 5½ weeks, she was in trouble. Severe back pain and weakness caused her great discomfort and set off my alarm bells. Everything she did except rest made it worse. In addition, she started spotting a brownish bloody discharge accompanied by aching pain in the abdomen. She felt very irritable. She had no morning sickness. Her Kidney pulse was very weak as was her Stomach and Spleen pulse; the Liver pulse was wiry. Her tongue had a red tip and a yellow coating.

It was all stops out to save this pregnancy and, fortunately, the treatment could be started early. Although we would have felt more reassured had she been experiencing pregnancy-related nausea, at least her strong stomach meant she was able to swallow good doses of herbs regularly.

The diagnosis of her threatened miscarriage was Kidney Yang deficiency with Qi deficiency. Morgan also had a constitutional tendency to Damp-Heat affecting the Liver. Acupuncture at 5–7 weeks of pregnancy:

KI-3, KI-9, DU-20, LIV-3, BL-28, BL-23, DU-4 – all back points with moxa only

Herbal formula

Xu Duan	12 g	Radix Dipsaci
Du Zhong	12 g	Cortex Eucommiae Ulmoidis
Tu Si Zi	15 g	Semen Cuscatae
Bai Zhu	9 g	Rhizoma Atractylodis Macrocephalae
Huang Qi	9 g	Radix Astragali
Sang Ji Sheng	15 g	Ramulus Sangjisheng
Ai Ye tan	9 g	Folium Artemisiae
Huang Qin	9 g	Radix Scutellariae Baicalensis
E Jiao	6 g	Gelatinum Asini

At 7 weeks, the bleeding had stopped, abdomen pain was better and she felt less irritable. However, the most troubling symptom, her lower back pain, was still bad. She had developed mild nausea.

We repeated the acupuncture and moxa, adding PC-6 and ST-36, deleting KI-3. The herbal prescription was also repeated, deleting Ai Ye tan and E Jiao, and increasing Tu Si Zi to 20 g.

At 8 weeks, her lower back weakness and pain were much better, there was no spotting and her nausea became marked. Her right Kidney pulse strengthened, although the left was still weak. The Liver pulse was thin and wiry. At 9 weeks, she experienced vomiting of bile and a chemical taste in the mouth and could no longer tolerate herbs. Her lower back pain returned for 2 days. She was anxious, depressed, and irritable.

We had to rely on acupuncture now: GB-34, LIV-14, Ren-12, PC-6, TB-6, ST-36, KI-21

This was repeated several times over the next 2 weeks.

By 11 weeks, she felt much better. The nausea was mild and manageable and the lower back pain was all but gone. She set off on her overseas trip with confidence (but with lots of warnings about avoiding lifting heavy suitcases). A healthy baby girl was born at term.

Qi deficiency

Qi dropping is another cause of clinical or subclinical (usually the former) miscarriage. The woman will experience abdomen distension, with a bearing down sensation that may spread to the lower back. She will probably feel fatigue and may notice spotting of blood. If the cervix is examined, it may appear to be slightly open. The pulse will be thready and the tongue swollen or pale.

Table 8.1 Acupuncture points[a] used in treatment of threatened miscarriage due to Kidney deficiency

Treatment goal	Acupuncture points
To strengthen Kidneys, especially Kidney Yang	KI-6, KI-3, BL-23 (cautious shallow needling or moxa), Ren-4 (light moxa only)
To reinforce and lift Spleen Qi	Ren-6 (shallow needling or moxa), Ren-12, DU-20

[a]Reinforcing method is used; moxa can be applied on trunk and head points.

Herbal formula — The formula of choice is:

Bu Zhong Yi Qi Tang (Reinforce the Center and Benefit the Qi decoction)

Huang Qi	30 g	*Radix Astragali*
Dang Shen	15 g	*Radix Codonopsis Pilulosae*
Bai Zhu	12 g	*Rhizoma Atractylodis Macrocephalae*
Dang Gui	9 g	*Radix Angelicae Sinensis*
Chen Pi	6 g	*Pericarpium Citri Reticulate*
Sheng Ma	6 g	*Rhizoma Cimicifugae*
Chai Hu	6 g	*Radix Bupleuri*
Gan Cao	6 g	*Radix Glycyrrhizae Uralensis*

Large doses of Qi tonics (Huang Qi, Dang Shen and Bai Zhu) are used to lift the fetus and the Uterus, their tonic effects being moderated by Chen Pi, which regulates Qi. Sheng Ma and Chai Hu both help to lift the fetus. Nourishment of the fetus is very important, especially in Qi and Blood-deficient women. Dang Gui and Bai Zhu are often used together to both nourish the Blood and the Qi and prevent miscarriage. However, Dang Gui does have a slight Blood-moving action, so if there is any bleeding it needs to be replaced with E Jiao. Gan Cao (used here in a smaller dose than regular Bu Zhong Yi Qi Tang formulations) reinforces the Qi and moderates and harmonizes the actions of the other herbs.

If the cervix appears to be opening, add the following astringent herbs:

Jin Ying Zi	9 g	*Fructus Rosae Laevigatae*
Qian Shi	9 g	*Semen Euryales Ferox*

Both these herbs can astringe the Jing, and in these circumstances can help hold in the fetus.

Additionally, one of the following can be added to further the astringing effect:

Sang Piao Xiao	9 g	*Ootheca Mantidis*
Hai Piao Xiao	9 g	*Os Sepiae seu Sepiellae*

Sang Piao Xiao astringes and strengthens the Kidneys and Hai Piao Xiao stops bleeding.

If necessary, more herbs can be added to control bleeding:

Ai Ye tan	9 g	*Folium Artemisiae*
Zhu Ma Gen	15 g	*Radix Boehmeria Nivea*

and replace Dang Gui with:

E Jiao	9 g	*Gelatinum Asini*

and replace Chen Pi with:

Sha Ren	6 g	*Fructus seu Semen Amomi*

If there is lower back pain, add Kidney Yang tonics:

Tu Si Zi	9 g	*Semen Cuscatae*
Bu Gu Zhi	6 g	*Fructus Psoraleae*

Acupuncture points — Choose from the following points (and see Table 8.2):

DU-20	Baihui
Ren-12	Zhongwan
BL-20	Pishu
ST-36	Zusanli
Ren-6	Qihai
KI-3	Taixi

Blood deficiency

Blood deficiency is not a direct cause of threatened miscarriage, but it can compromise the health and development of the fetus. This may be more apparent in the later stages of pregnancy, after the first 2 or 3 months. If the mother is anemic, or the ultrasound shows that the fetus is small-for-dates, then the addition of Blood tonics is timely and useful. Diet and rest are also important considerations for the mother and she will need iron supplements if her diet is inadequate. Symptoms include fatigue, palpitations and pallor. The pulse will be weak and the tongue pale.

Herbal formula — The formula of choice is:

Dang Gui Shao Yao San (Angelica Peonia powder) modified

Dang Gui	9 g	*Radix Angelicae Sinensis*
Bai Shao	15 g	*Radix Paeoniae Lactiflorae*
Fu Ling	9 g	*Sclerotium Poriae Cocos*
Bai Zhu	9 g	*Rhizoma Atractylodis Macrocephalae*
Ze Xie	9 g	*Rhizoma Alismatis*
Dan Shen	6 g	*Radix Salviae Miltiorrhizae*
(Zhi) Gan Cao	3 g	*Radix Glycyrrhizae Uralensis*

This modified formula, originally designed to treat abdomen pain in pregnancy, stimulates blood production with tonics such as Dang Gui and Bai Shao and encourages its supply to the fetus via the placenta. Dan Shen encourages circulation in the endometrium and placenta. Studies in China have shown that if fetal growth is retarded it can, in some circumstances, be accelerated with the use of Dan Shen, although of course this herb must be used very cautiously. Chuan Xiong has been removed from this version of Dang Gui Shao Yao San because in combination with Dang Gui, it has been shown to initiate uterine contractions. Bai Zhu, Fu Ling and Ze Xie work together to support Spleen function in production and circulation of Qi and fluids. (Zhi) Gan Cao

Table 8.2 Acupuncture points[a] used in the treatment of threatened miscarriage due to Qi deficiency

Treatment goal	Acupuncture points
To support the Spleen Qi	Ren-12, BL-20 and ST-36
To lift the Qi	DU-20 and Ren-6
To support the Kidneys	KI-3

[a]Reinforcing method is used.

harmonizes the various actions of these herbs. If there is any bleeding (in the absence of Blood stagnation), then Dang Gui and Dan Shen should be replaced with:

| E Jiao | 9 g | *Gelatinum Asini* |
| He Shou Wu | 9 g | *Radix Polygoni Multiflori* |

Blood tonics like Shu Di are too greasy for most women to digest in early pregnancy and may severely exacerbate any nausea they are experiencing. If Shu Di is prescribed then it is wise to add Sha Ren.

If the Spleen Yang and Kidney Yang of the mother are weak, this can also contribute to a small-for-dates fetus because nutrients from food will not be satisfactorily extracted and distributed and Blood production will be compromised. Also, the fundamental support (the Kidneys) for fetal development will be inadequate.

In such cases, add the Kidney and Spleen tonics:

Du Zhong	12 g	*Cortex Eucommiae Ulmoidis*
Tu Si Zi	9 g	*Semen Cuscatae*
Dang Shen	9 g	*Radix Codonopsis Pilulosae*

Acupuncture points — Choose from the following points (and see Table 8.3):

Ren-12	Zhongwan
ST-36	Zusanli
ST-29	Guilai (moxa only)
KI-13	Qixue
KI-5	Shuiquan
KI-3	Taixi

CASE HISTORY – TONI

Toni (37) was having difficulty conceiving her second child. Her first child was already 10 years old. Toni's periods were irregular and infrequent. When she did have them, they were fairly scanty and pale pink. Toni actually came for treatment of her varicose veins, which were becoming painful. The treatment of Spleen Qi to improve her circulation also encouraged more Blood production and her menstrual cycle improved in frequency. In not too many months she was pregnant.

During Toni's first pregnancy, she had been hospitalized for 6 weeks of bed rest because the baby was failing to grow. The rest helped placental function, and although her baby was small at birth he was healthy. So, now in her second pregnancy, when an ultrasound indicated that her baby was small-for-dates, she immediately rested, had a series of acupuncture treatments and took Chinese herbs for the last 2 months of the middle trimester:

Dang Gui	9 g	*Radix Angelicae Sinensis*
Bai Shao	15 g	*Radix Paeoniae Lactiflorae*
Fu Ling	9 g	*Sclerotium Poriae Cocos*
Bai Zhu	9 g	*Rhizoma Atractylodis Macrocephalae*
Ze Xie	9 g	*Rhizoma Alismatis*
Dan Shen	6 g	*Radix Salviae Miltiorrhizae*
(Zhi) Gan Cao	3 g	*Radix Glycyrrhizae Uralensis*
Dang Shen	9 g	*Radix Codonopsis Pilulosae*

Acupuncture points: ST-36, Ren-12, ST-29 (mild moxa), KI-3

Hospitalization was unnecessary this time and her second baby boy was a healthy 3.2 kg at birth.

Table 8.3   Acupuncture points[a] used in the treatment of threatened miscarriage due to Blood deficiency

Treatment goal	Acupuncture points
To reinforce Spleen function to manufacture Blood	Ren-12 and ST-36
To harmonize the Qi and Blood in the Chong and Ren channels	KI-5 and KI-3
To encourage local blood supply and nourish the fetus; these points are used if there is no bleeding and the cervix is firm but ultrasound indicates that the baby is not growing	ST-29, KI-13 (light moxa)

[a]Use reinforcing method and on the lower abdomen points use moxa.

Heat in the Blood

The Heat responsible for a threatened miscarriage usually arises from Yin deficiency and may threaten the pregnancy in its early stages, especially if it dries the endometrium and forces blood from the uterine blood vessels. Other factors which can contribute to creating a critical level of Heat in the Blood are anger (Liver-Fire) and a very pungent spicy diet. If the Heat affects the Heart, then there is a high risk of miscarriage because the Heart-Uterus connection via the Bao vessel can be disturbed. TCM theory posits that the Heart Qi has much to do with 'opening' of the Uterus and, when its Qi is disturbed (e.g., by Liver-Fire), the disruption in the Bao vessel may precipitate an untimely opening of the Uterus. For this reason, the cautious doctor is ever mindful of the Heart and Kidney relationship in early pregnancy. What this means is that the mental and emotional state of the newly pregnant woman can influence the pregnancy and a skillful doctor will take measures to safeguard the fetus by using acupuncture or herbs to calm the woman's mind if she is excessively anxious or agitated.

A third factor which may contribute to Heat in the Blood is infection, most commonly in the endometrium itself. In the case of bacterial infection, antibiotics are usually given with Chinese herbs. And in the case of high fever, paracetamol is given to bring the temperature down until the herbs can effectively clear the Heat. Examination of the BBT readings taken after pregnancy is confirmed may show consistently and unusually high readings (e.g., 37.4°C or 98.8°F and up) and the woman may feel restless, thirsty, and hot. She may also be constipated with dry stools and the urine may appear dark. Uterine bleeding will be fresh red. The pulse will usually be rapid, while the tongue appears red. In this case, the Heat must be quickly cleared from the Blood (and Liver and Heart), while the Uterus must remain warm enough to nourish the fetus.

Herbal formula — The formula of choice is:

Bao Yin Jian (Protecting the Yin decoction)

Sheng Di	20 g	Radix Rehmanniae Glutinosae
Shan Yao	12 g	Dioscorea Oppositae
Bai Shao	9 g	Radix Paeoniae Lactiflorae
Huang Qin	9 g	Radix Scutellariae Baicalensis
Huang Bai	9 g	Cortex Phellodendri
Xu Duan	9 g	Radix Dipsaci
Gan Cao	3 g	Radix Glycyrrhizae Uralensis

A large dose of Sheng Di cools the Blood to protect the Yin, while Huang Bai and Huang Qin remove Heat and Damp (infection) from the Blood and the lower body. Xu Duan ensures herbs do not cool the Uterus too much and protects the Kidney Yang. Bai Shao soothes the Liver Yin and Shan Yao, the Spleen Yin.

285

To protect Yin further, add:

Nu Zhen Zi	9 g	Fructus Ligustri Lucidi
Han Lian Cao	9 g	Herba Ecliptae Prostratae

To stop bleeding, add:

Bai Mao Gen	9 g	Rhizoma Imperatae Cylindricae
Di Yu (tan)	9 g	Radix Sanguisorbae Officinalis
Qian Cao Gen	10 g	Radix Rubiae Cordifoliae

Acupuncture points — Choose from the following points (and see Table 8.4):

SP-1	Yinbai
SP-10	Xuehai
KI-2	Rangu
LIV-2	Xingjian
PC-3	Quze
KI-8	Jiaoxin
HE-5	Tongli
PC-6	Neiguan

The patient must be advised to avoid heating foods such as curries and drink such as alcohol and coffee. Also, she should be kept as calm as possible.

CASE HISTORY – CHERYL

Cheryl (36 years) had a long history of functional uterine bleeding. This occurred mostly in the luteal phase of her cycle or after sex. No medical investigations, surgical or Chinese medicine treatments made significant or lasting changes to this pattern. She suffered also from mouth ulcers, eczema, tinnitus, and constipation. She was very emotional and easily upset. Her diagnosis was Yin deficiency with Heat. The Heat affected the Heart and the Bao vessel such that the Uterus did not close effectively between ovulation and the period. Treatment which cleared Heat from the Heart and the Blood helped most of her symptoms but not the spotting. I anticipated that pregnancy might be difficult for Cheryl.

At 35, she decided it was time to start a family and when she didn't conceive after some months, investigations were ordered. The biggest surprise was that her husband's test showed no sperm at all. Even the IVF clinic's biopsies were unsuccessful and Cheryl enroled in the donor insemination program at the hospital. She fell pregnant on the first attempt – but experienced spotting (with clotty tissue) continuously from 5 days after the insemination. The blood was a watery fresh red and she felt distending crampy pain in the abdomen. There was no lower back pain and no nausea but her sleep was disturbed by palpitations. She felt very agitated. The outlook was not good – evidently Heat was disturbing the Heart and the Chong vessel was open. Treatment aimed to clear Heat from the Blood, calm the Shen and stop the bleeding.

Sheng Di	20 g	Radix Rehmanniae Glutinosae
Han Lian Cao	12 g	Herba Ecliptae Prostratae
Shan Yao	12 g	Radix Dioscorea Oppositae
Tu Si Zi	6 g	Semen Cuscatae
Xu Duan	6 g	Radix Dipsaci
Huang Qin	9 g	Radix Scutellariae Baicalensis
Mu Li	12 g	Concha Ostreae
Di Yu (tan)	9 g	Radix Sanguisorbae Officinalis
Di Gu Pi	9 g	Cortex Lycii Chinensis

Acupuncture points: KI-8, KI-6, PC-6, HE-5, HE-8, YT

The bleeding stopped almost immediately and the agitation and sleep also improved. She still woke frequently but fell asleep again easily.

At 6 weeks, she had most of the normal signs of early pregnancy: fatigue, intolerance of strong smells, full and heavy breasts. But her pulses and tongue still indicated the presence of Heat; the pulse was rapid and thin and slightly floating and her tongue had a marked red tip and sides. She had no mouth ulcers and her tinnitus was mostly absent. While stopping bleeding was no longer a priority, ensuring that the Yin was consolidated and Heat cleared from the Blood and the Heart was still necessary to secure this pregnancy.

Shu Di	6 g	Radix Rehmanniae Glutinosae Conquitae
Sheng Di	15 g	Radix Rehmanniae Glutinosae
Huang Qin	9 g	Radix Scutellariae Baicalensis
Han Lian Cao	12 g	Herba Ecliptae Prostratae
Nu Zhen Zi	9 g	Fructus Ligustri Lucidi
Shan Yao	9 g	Radix Dioscorea Oppositae
Mu Li	9 g	Concha Ostreae
Xuan Shen	6 g	Radix Scrophulariae
Xu Duan	9 g	Radix Dipsaci

Acupuncture points: KI-6, KI-2, LIV-2, HE-7

Despite this approach, her pulse did not improve markedly and I asked her to have an ultrasound. Sadly, this revealed a blighted ovum – a sac with no resident embryo. After another week with some more spotting but no real bleeding, Cheryl took three doses of Sheng Hua Tang to encourage the expulsion of the uterine contents. This happened effectively with 1 or 2 days of follow-up bleeding. This case indicates the usefulness of ultrasound in discovering something which herbal treatment may have obscured (see Missed abortion, below). Cheryl (and I) feel confident that when she decides to attempt another pregnancy, Chinese medicine will effectively deal with any Heat and (providing there is no chromosomal abnormality) prevent a miscarriage.

Blood stagnation

This cause of threatened miscarriage may occur after a fall or accident has caused some trauma or bruising to the uterus. It may also occur after IVF procedures. There are also some situations where Blood stagnation has preceded the pregnancy (e.g., endometriosis, endometritis, polyps and fibroids), and is contributing to

Table 8.4   Acupuncture points[a] used in the treatment of threatened miscarriage due to Heat in the Blood

Treatment goal	Acupuncture points
To cool the Blood and stop bleeding	SP-1 and SP-10
To clear Yin-deficient Heat	KI-2
To clear Heat and stop bleeding	KI-8
To clear Heart-Fire, Heat in the Blood and safeguard the Bao vessel	HE-5
To clear Liver-Fire	LIV-2
To clear Heat from the Blood	PC-3
To calm the spirit	PC-6

[a]Reducing or even method is used on these points, except SP-10 and KI-8, which should be needled cautiously with little manipulation.
Moxa is used on SP-1.

bleeding from the uterus during the pregnancy. Sharp or gnawing crampy abdominal pain will accompany the bleeding, which may be dark or clotty. The tongue may appear purplish and the pulse will have a choppy feel.

Treatment of such a condition is not without risk. Treatment must aim to clear the Blood stagnation but without dislodging the fetus. Some doctors prefer a conservative approach first, and will apply treatment to strengthen the Kidneys and to lift the Qi before initiating any other treatment. However, if this is not successful, then a careful approach can be taken using herbs.

Herbal formula — The formula of choice is:

Jiao Ai Si Wu Tang (Gelatinum Asini Artemesia Four Substances decoction) modified

E Jiao	9 g	*Gelatinum Asini*
Ai Ye	9 g	*Folium Artemisiae*
Dang Gui	9 g	*Radix Angelicae Sinensis*
Bai Shao	9 g	*Radix Paeoniae Lactiflorae*
Dan Shen	9 g	*Radix Salviae Miltiorrhizae*
Wu Ling Zhi	9 g	*Excrementum Trogopterori*
Pu Huang	9 g	*Pollen Typhae*
Gan Cao	6 g	*Radix Glycyrrhizae Uralensis*
Xu Duan	9 g	*Radix Dipsaci*

Dang Gui, Dan Shen, Wu Ling Zhi, and Pu Huang regulate the Blood. The latter two herbs have been found to be particularly safe in clinics in China in terms of fetus stability. Most other Blood-regulating herbs are too risky to use in early pregnancy. As with the formula Dang Gui Shao Yao San mentioned earlier, Chuan Xiong has been removed because in combination with Dang Gui it can initiate uterine contractions. E Jiao and Ai Ye stop bleeding and Xu Duan, used in this particular context, not only protects the Kidney Yang but also helps invigorate the Blood. Wu Ling Zhi can be a difficult herb to take in decoction if there is much morning sickness because of its smell, so it is recommended this formula be dispensed in granules which are put into capsules.

Acupuncture points — Choose from the following points (and see Table 8.5):

DU-20	Baihui
Ren-12	Zhongwan
PC-6	Neiguan
ST-29	Guilai
SP-10	Xuehai

Table 8.5 Acupuncture points[a] used in the treatment of threatened miscarriage due to Blood stagnation

Treatment goal	Acupuncture points
To regulate Blood and remove stasis and relieve abdomen pain	PC-6, ST-29 and SP-10
To hold the fetus secure while stagnation is being addressed	DU-20 and Ren-12

[a]Reinforcing technique is used for DU-20 and Ren-12; even method needling for others. Particular care (i.e. no manipulation) must be taken with ST-29 and SP-10.

CASE HISTORY – ANASTASIA

Anastasia (41) became pregnant on her seventh attempt at the IVF clinic, after taking herbs to reinforce Liver and Heart Blood and clear stagnant Blood. However, at 7 weeks, she began to bleed heavily with severe, sharp cramping pain. The blood was bright red with large clots. She was also experiencing nausea and severe anxiety. She managed to take some granulated herbs once a day when her nausea allowed. I felt reluctant to do acupuncture in this case.

Xu Duan	9 g	Radix Dipsaci
Tu Si Zi	9 g	Semen Cuscatae
Huang Qin	9 g	Radix Scutellariae Baicalensis
Pu Huang	9 g	Pollen Typhae
Dan Shen	9 g	Radix Salviae Miltiorrhizae
E Jiao	9 g	Gelatinum Asini
Han Lian Cao	9 g	Herba Ecliptae Prostratae
Mu Li	9 g	Concha Ostreae
Long Gu	9 g	Os Draconis
Bai Shao	9 g	Radix Paeoniae Lactiflorae
Gan Cao	3 g	Radix Glycyrrhizae Uralensis

This formula stopped the pain immediately; the bleeding persisted a few days longer, then stopped. An ultrasound showed that the fetus had survived. However, 2 weeks later, the strong pain returned with more heavy bleeding. The herbs were repeated and once again the bleeding subsided.

Blood stasis was the diagnosis of this threatened miscarriage, reflecting either a pre-existing condition or one caused by the IVF procedures themselves.

When baby Bob was born, the placenta hemorrhaged and showed scarring from the earlier bleeds.

Western medical treatment for threatened miscarriage

In Western gynecology clinics, the hormone progesterone may be given in a short course (as progestogens) to try to prevent a threatened miscarriage, although it is generally recognized not to be very effective. From a TCM point of view, progestogen is seen to have warm and Qi raising activity. Viewed like this, the hormone may be of some use in the Kidney Yang deficiency or the Qi deficiency type of threatened miscarriage (used over the long term, however, this drug can harm Kidney Yang and Qi). For threatened miscarriage related to Blood deficiency, Heat or stagnation progestogens have no theoretical application. Progestogens also tend to exacerbate Damp accumulation and would be contraindicated in women of Damp constitution.

INEVITABLE MISCARRIAGE

If the fetus has stopped growing or is abnormal and has died in the 1st trimester of pregnancy (a missed abortion), the TCM doctor will apply treatment on the basis of the following procedures.

Ensuring expulsion of all pregnancy products

This is achieved by using herbs and acupuncture which move stagnant Blood.

Herbal formula — The formula of choice is:

Sheng Hua Tang (Generating and Dissolving decoction)

Dang Gui	25 g	Radix Angelicae Sinensis
Chuan Xiong	9 g	Radix Ligustici Wallichii
Tao Ren	9 g	Semen Persicae
Pao Jiang	3 g	Rhizoma Zingiberis Officinalis
(Zhi) Gan Cao	3 g	Radix Glycyrrhizae Uralensis

Large doses of Dang Gui and other herbs to move stagnant Blood are used for a limited time (usually 2–5 doses) to ensure the expulsion of the fetus, at the same time regenerating new Blood. Pao Jiang warms the channels and moderates the effect of the Blood-moving herbs so that there is no excessive blood loss.

Acupuncture points — Acupuncture treatments which encourage expulsion of all the uterine contents include abdomen points on the Chong, Spleen and Stomach channels such as the following (see also Table 8.6):

KI-14	Siman
KI-18	Shiguan
ST-29	Guilai
ST-28	Shuidao
SP-12	Chongmen
SP-13	Fushe

Two or three of these abdomen points should be chosen (perhaps according to sites of pain if relevant) and can be combined with:

SP-6	Sanyinjiao
CO-4	Hegu

to expel all the contents of the uterus.

CASE HISTORY – PHILLIPA

Phillipa became pregnant at 41 with her second child. The pregnancy started well, the ultrasound at 7 weeks showed a viable fetus and the morning sickness was not as severe as her previous pregnancy. She was very fatigued, however, and resting with a toddler in the house was difficult. By 10 weeks, her energy had improved, but at 11 weeks, she started spotting with a dark discharge. An ultrasound showed that the fetus had not survived beyond 9 weeks. The spotting continued but very faintly.

Phillipa was reluctant to have a D&C if she could possibly avoid it and decided to try Chinese herbs. She took Sheng Hua Tang and the bleeding became a little more constant but it wasn't until the 3rd day of taking the herbs that she experienced strong contractions similar to labor and passed a white jelly-like mass with a lot more fresh red blood. After that, bleeding ceased. A follow-up ultrasound revealed that all the pregnancy products had been expelled and that a D&C was unnecessary.

Table 8.6   Acupuncture points[a] used in the management of inevitable miscarriage to ensure expulsion of all pregnancy products

Treatment goal	Acupuncture points
To move Blood and Qi in the Chong vessel	KI-14 and KI-18
To regulate Blood in the Uterus	ST 28 and ST-29
To regulate Qi and Blood in the abdomen and relieve pain	SP-12 and SP-13
To effect a downward and clearing movement	SP-6 and CO-4

[a]Reducing technique is used on all points.

Control the amount of blood lost

Herbal formula — The formula of choice is:

Tao Hong Si Wu Tang with Shi Xiao San (Persica Carthamus Four Substances decoction with Return the Smile powder) modified

Dang Gui	9 g	Radix Angelicae Sinensis
Chuan Xiong	6 g	Radix Ligustici Wallichii
Shu Di	12 g	Radix Rehmanniae Glutinosae Conquitae
Bai Shao	9 g	Radix Paeoniae Lactiflorae
Tao Ren	6 g	Semen Persicae
Hong Hua	3 g	Flos Carthami Tinctorii
Pu Huang tan	9 g	Pollen Typhae
Wu Ling Zhi	6 g	Excrementum Trogopterori
Qian Cao Gen	6 g	Radix Rubiae Cordifoliae
San Qi	6 g	Radix Pseudoginseng

When herbs are used to stop bleeding in cases like this, we must be careful not to prescribe those which can exacerbate Blood stagnation. Examples of safe styptic herbs, which stop bleeding but do not cause Blood stasis, are San Qi, Qian Cao Gen and Pu Huang. Dang Gui, Shu Di and Bao Shao nourish Blood in an attempt to replace what has been lost. Tao Ren, Chuan Xiong, Wu Ling Zhi and Hong Hua are used in small doses to clear Blood stasis.

Acupuncture points — Controlling blood loss can be achieved with acupuncture treatments similar to those used for heavy periods with Blood stagnation. Use the following points (and see Table 8.7):

SP-10	Xuehai
Ren-6	Qihai
LIV-1	Dadun

These points are added to some abdomen points chosen from the list given in Table 8.6. SP-6 and CO-4 will not be used if the bleeding is heavy.

291

Table 8.7   Acupuncture points[a] used in the management of inevitable miscarriage to control blood loss (in conjunction with points in Table 8.6)

Treatment goal	Acupuncture points
To regulate Blood stagnation and stop bleeding	SP-10
To stop bleeding	LIV-1
To reinforce the Qi to control heavy bleeding	Ren-6

[a]Even or reinforcing technique is employed.

Recover the Qi and Blood

Even early-stage miscarriages are draining on the woman's energy, and this needs to be addressed as soon as the products of the miscarriage are expelled and bleeding is controlled.

Herbal formula — The formula of choice is:

Ba Zhen Tang (Eight Precious decoction)

Shu Di	15 g	*Radix Rehmanniae Glutinosae Conquitae*
Dang Gui	9 g	*Radix Angelicae Sinensis*
Bai Shao	9 g	*Radix Paeoniae Lactiflorae*
Chuan Xiong	6 g	*Radix Ligustici Wallichii*
Dang Shen	12 g	*Radix Codonopsis Pilulosae*
Bai Zhu	9 g	*Rhizoma Atractylodis Macrocephalae*
Fu Ling	9 g	*Sclerotium Poriae Cocos*
Gan Cao	3 g	*Radix Glycyrrhizae Uralensis*

This well-known formula combines four Blood tonics (Dang Gui, Bai Shao, Chuan Xiong, Shu Di) with four Qi tonics (Dang Shen, Bai Zhu, Fu Ling, Gan Cao). In pill form, it is known as Women's Precious Pills and is used in many situations that require tonics.

Acupuncture points — Choose from the following points (and see Table 8.8):

ST-36	Zusanli
Ren-12	Zhongwan
SP-6	Sanyinjiao
Ren-6	Qihai
BL-20	Pishu
BL-17	Geshu
SP-10	Xuehai

Late-stage miscarriage

In the case of the inevitable miscarriage which happens later in the pregnancy (after week 10 or 12), a dilatation and curettage (D&C) will usually be performed. Herbs and acupuncture can be used to reinforce the clearing out

Table 8.8   Acupuncture points[a] used in the recovery from miscarriage

Treatment goal	Acupuncture points
To stimulate Spleen and Stomach function in producing Blood	ST-36, Ren-12, BL-20, SP-6
To reinforce Qi	Ren-6
To supplement Blood	BL-17, SP-10

[a]Points are needled with reinforcing technique.

CASE HISTORY – CATHERINE

Catherine (29) had a traumatic miscarriage when she was 10 weeks pregnant. It began quite suddenly, and continued, with deluge bleeding. She was bundled off to the emergency department and wrapped in towels but nothing could staunch the flow. An emergency D&C was performed and her bleeding was brought under control. For the next 3 weeks, however, she continued to bleed lightly. She was dizzy and weak from the blood loss, a situation exacerbated by the fact that her sleep had become restless since the miscarriage. She took (along with iron pills) a modified Ba Zhen Tang:

Shu Di	15 g	Radix Rehmanniae Glutinosae Conquitae
Dang Gui	9 g	Radix Angelicae Sinensis
Bai Shao	9 g	Radix Paeoniae Lactiflorae
Chuan Xiong	6 g	Radix Ligustici Wallichii
Suan Zao Ren	9 g	Semen Ziziphi Spinosae
Mu Li	12 g	Concha Ostreae
Huang Qi	15 g	Radix Astragali
Dang Shen	12 g	Radix Codonopsis Pilulosae
Bai Zhu	9 g	Rhizoma Atractylodis Macrocephalae
Fu Ling	9 g	Sclerotium Poriae Cocos
Zhi Gan Cao	3 g	Radix Glycyrrhizae Uralensis

The bleeding stopped quite quickly, and after 3 weeks of taking these herbs twice a day she began to feel like her old self again. When we added some acupuncture treatments, her menstrual cycle returned.

Acupuncture points: ST-36, Ren-12, Ren-6, Ren-3, SP-6, HE-7

---

of the uterus (although in most cases I think this is unnecessary). In the event that some products of pregnancy remain after a D&C, then the formula Sheng Hua Tang (see above) with additions of more Blood-moving herbs such as:

Hong Hua	6 g	Flos Carthami Tinctorii
Yi Mu Cao	12 g	Herba Leonuri Heterophylli

can be administered for several days.

Acupuncture treatments applied with strong reducing technique to points such as those described in Table 8.6 encourage expulsion of any retained tissue.

Because miscarriages are very weakening to the body, especially if there has been a significant amount of blood lost, treatments such as those described above need to be applied with caution and the patient's response watched closely. Treatments which strongly move Blood and Qi can be damaging to the Zheng Qi (the upright Qi) of the body. It will be important in cases where such strong treatments are applied to quickly follow-up with recovery treatments as soon as all the pregnancy tissue is expelled from the uterus. Ba Zhen Tang (above) is a good guiding formula. If there has been significant blood loss, more Blood tonics can be added. Such tonics should be continued until the periods return.

The next stage of recovery from miscarriage involves the re-establishment of a healthy menstrual cycle. This is done using the methods we have described in Chapter 4 once the period returns. If a lot of blood has been lost, this may take some time. As the new cycle is established again, so is the mind gradually healed of its grief, and confidence in the ability to create a new pregnancy returns. Attempts to conceive again can resume in a couple of cycles if recovery is rapid and the circumstances are favorable.

RECURRENT MISCARRIAGE

Prevention of future miscarriage

Recurrent miscarriage is so defined after three consecutive miscarriages. However, investigations, and treatment if applicable, should be initiated after two miscarriages if the couple is worried or not so young. Or if the miscarriage occurs after a period of infertility, investigation may be initiated immediately because there is a chance that the miscarriage was caused by whatever is causing the infertility.

Chinese medicine has always recognized that it is often the same sorts of imbalances that can cause difficulty in becoming pregnant and difficulty in staying pregnant. You will see that the types of diagnoses a Chinese medicine doctor makes in the case of recurrent miscarriages are very similar to those that describe different categories of infertility.

Having a miscarriage is not such an uncommon event; it occurs in 10–25% (or more in older women) of all diagnosed pregnancies. However, only 1–3% of couples will suffer recurrent miscarriages. Women who already have a history of miscarriage are more likely to have miscarriages in the future (unless a treatable cause is addressed).[15,16] Clearly, there are persisting risk factors in a number of recurrent miscarriers; discovering and treating these is what this section is about.

Western gynecologists can track down reasons for recurrent miscarriages in some cases and can administer appropriate treatment for a few of these, e.g., physical problems in the uterus and cervix. However, miscarriages can result from some unknown factor in a complex series of interactions between the mother's womb and fetus and environment.

Researchers have noted that the lining of the womb is capable of recognizing and responding to developmentally abnormal embryos but only when adequately prepared (decidualized) for pregnancy.[17] And that the ability of the endometrium to decidualize is grossly defective in women suffering from recurrent miscarriages.[18]

Some researchers have called this the 'non fussy' uterus, i.e., one which is not selective enough about the embryos it accepts. These women fall pregnant all too easily. It appears a filter that the properly prepared uterus offers is not operating.

It is often difficult to isolate just one cause of repeated miscarriage, and it can be even more difficult to provide effective treatments. Medical specialists have tried many remedies for miscarriage; some, like thalidomide and DES (diethylstilbestrol) had devastating effects and some have no proven effects (namely progesterone and hCG).

Similarly, through the ages, claims have been made for many herbal and other remedies to stop miscarriages – but controlled clinical trials are generally lacking. One trial looked at a number of women who conceived via IVF and then took Chinese herbs or progesterone. The miscarriage rate in the group who took the Chinese herbs was significantly less (13%) than that in the progesterone group (23%).[19]

Another group of researchers looking for adverse effects of chinese medicine treatments for threatened miscarriages found none and also found that such interventions were more effective than Western medicine ones.[20] However, the main proof we have that TCM treatment for recurrent miscarriage offers some valid outcome is its performance in the living People's Laboratory of China, where it has been employed for thousands of years and is still in use today, even in areas where modern pharmaceuticals are available. Eventually, Chinese medicine will be tested in the scientific laboratories of the West and, if valid and ethical experimental protocols can be put in place, interesting results should emerge. Until then, the practitioners of Chinese medicine have at their disposal the advice and wisdom distilled over many hundreds of years of doctors treating women who have suffered miscarriages. If the treatments these doctors have repeatedly applied over such a long period of time did not work, then they would not have stayed in the TCM repertoire.

Causes of recurrent miscarriage

Below are listed the known causes of recurrent miscarriage or pregnancy loss. Some of these are easily remedied, others not so easily. Genetic, endocrine or autoimmune causes are found in the majority of couples who suffer from repeated miscarriages. Other causes include structural and environmental factors.

Cervical incompetence and uterine malformations

If the cervix is unable to stay firm and closed because it has been weakened by previous obstetric or surgical trauma, then it can shorten and open sometime after the 14th week of pregnancy. The incompetent or insufficient cervix, as it is called, then releases the contents of the uterus with a gush of fluid and the pregnancy comes to an abrupt end. In women where an incompetent cervix is suspected, a suture can be added to hold the cervix closed, but where it is not suspected, the miscarriage happens suddenly and without warning other than some back pain and possibly some discharge. The use of a suture is the treatment of choice where cervical incompetence is suspected. The Chinese medicine practitioner can offer treatment to aid the lifting of the uterus and the fetus, i.e. take the pressure off the cervix, but this treatment is adjuvant to a surgical aid.

Other abnormalities such as large fibroids causing uterine distortion or congenital abnormality of the uterus may also contribute to the loss of a normally developing fetus. Ironically, women whose mothers took DES to prevent a miscarriage have double the rate of miscarriage themselves due to deformities of the uterus.[21] In addition to increased risk of pregnancy loss, the incidence of fetal malposition and pre-term labor are higher in women with uterine abnormalities.

For serious uterine deformity, the advice of an experienced surgeon is essential. There are many different ways a uterus can be deformed, some of them congenital and some of them acquired from previous surgical procedures. Some of these deformities can be corrected surgically and some are better left alone, despite the higher miscarriage rates.[22]

Chinese medicine offers little in the way of treatment for serious malformations of the uterus.

Hormonal causes

OVARY

The ovary, or more precisely, the corpus luteum, is responsible for producing the progesterone which maintains the first few weeks of the pregnancy until the placenta can take over. While low progesterone levels are commonly associated with pregnancies which miscarry, giving women progesterone in early pregnancy does not improve pregnancy outcome.

This is because low progesterone levels reflect the fact that the pregnancy has not implanted successfully in the first place and this usually relates to the quality of the egg and the embryo.

If there are problems with ovarian function, e.g., in polycystic ovary syndrome (PCOS) or resistant ovaries disease or premature menopause, which contribute to infertility, there is a strong chance the same problem will increase the risk of miscarriage should a pregnancy occur.

The mechanisms for this are not clearly understood from a Western medicine point of view. However, the TCM doctor will be able to make a diagnosis for miscarriages which occur repeatedly during early pregnancy due to lack of hormonal support from the ovary. Often simply rectifying a Kidney Yang weakness (and supporting Kidney Yin) before conceiving, will reduce miscarriage risk in this category.

PLACENTA

The placenta makes hCG, which stimulates the ongoing function of the corpus luteum, particularly its production of progesterone. Failure of the placenta to make this hCG means failure of the corpus luteum to produce progesterone and the pregnancy will not survive. Administration of hCG does not help for the same reason that administration of exogenous progesterone does not help.

For miscarriages due to placental dysfunction, Chinese medicine will approach diagnosis and treatment in the same way as for ovary dysfunction, focusing on strengthening Kidney function before conception.

THYROID

See Thyroid disorders, below.

Genetic or inherited disorders

Chromosomal studies of couples who have suffered recurrent miscarriage sometimes reveal constitutional genetic abnormalities, i.e., abnormalities in the chromosomes which they have been born with and which exist in all their cells in all parts of their bodies but which have not affected them in any damaging way. For example, one of the partners might carry a balanced translocation, which means a part of one chromosome has become transferred to another. This causes no problem to the partner with the translocation but can cause problems during gametogenesis when their chromosomes are divided in half to make the eggs or the sperm. Such gametes have a high degree of chromosomal abnormality and lead to abnormal conceptions, many of which are unviable and will miscarry or, more tragically, lead to the birth of children with multiple abnormalities. There is no treatment offered by allopathic medicine or by traditional Chinese medicine, which can change the genetic make-up of the prospective mother or father; however, in cases of balanced translocations, the couple can be reassured that not all conceptions will be doomed and that hopefully one day, they will conceive a normal baby – an unenviably fraught wait-and-see approach. Genetic analysis of embryos, preimplantation genetic diagnosis (PGD), before they are transferred to the uterus in an IVF protocol, provides a solution for some couples.

Genetic counsellors play an important role for someone diagnosed with a chromosomal abnormality. All the risks and possible outcomes can be explained by the genetic counsellor and an appropriate plan constructed.

THROMBOPHILIAS

Recurrent miscarriages occur in some women who have inherited conditions which increase their blood clotting tendency. Factor V Leiden; prothrombin gene mutations (in the gene that codes for MTHFR, an enzyme involved in folate metabolism); antithrombin III and plasminogen activator inhibitor-1 (PAI-1) are genetically determined factors that may increase the risk of miscarriage. If blood clots occur in the blood vessels of the placenta, the risk of 2nd trimester miscarriage or a small-for-dates baby is increased.

Some autoimmune diseases (this means making antibodies to your own cells) and some alloimmune diseases (making antibodies to foreign cells) are associated with increased incidence of miscarriage. The term immune infertility refers to an inability to conceive or maintain a pregnancy because some aspect of the immune system prevents it. It has been proposed that there may be a syndrome in which the presence of various immune factors (natural killer (NK) cells, antiphospholipid antibodies, thyroid antibodies, etc.) increase the likelihood of an immune reproductive disorder. Examples are autoimmune conditions such as Grave's disease, Hashimoto's disease, systemic lupus erythematosus, antiphospholipid syndrome, scleroderma, psoriasis and Sjögren syndrome.

The mechanisms behind immune disorder pregnancy loss are not fully understood, although we do know that the antiphospholipid antibodies in acquired thrombophilias (also the proteins made by genes in inherited thrombophilias), prevent the placental cells from properly attaching to the uterine lining. These antibodies prevent the formation of the syncytiotrophoblasts which have an important role in the establishment and function of the placenta. With each pregnancy loss, there is an increased chance that the mother will develop antibodies to phospholipid molecules. For the doctor of Chinese medicine, this is evidence that miscarriages themselves can increase the risk of Blood stagnation.

Elevated levels of NK cells have been shown to impede successful implantation or establishment of pregnancy, as have activated T lymphocytes.[23] On the other hand, the actions of some T cells and NK cells are necessary to promote a favorable environment for implantation.[24] It is largely through the secretion of signaling agents called cytokines released by these immune cells, that the intricate processes of implantation and creating a placenta can be either facilitated or stymied. Figure 8.2 summarizes the immune and clotting factors which can contribute to an increased risk of miscarriage.

In other cases, an overactive immune system may attack the gametes themselves, as is the case when excess macrophages phagocytize sperm in the female reproductive tract.

Miscarriages later in the pregnancy can be caused by clots in the blood vessels of the placenta blocking blood supply.

Medical treatment includes administration of low molecular weight Heparin to dissolve blood clots, steroids to dampen overactive NK cell activity and progesterone for its anti-inflammatory properties. These treatments are still the subject of controversy and research, e.g., studies of women with recurrent miscarriage have found little benefit for the use of aspirin or anticoagulants, even in women with known clotting tendencies.[25] However, this medication is widely prescribed to women diagnosed with such factors.

Antibodies to the thyroid gland (thyroid autoimmunity is the most common autoimmune condition) double the chances of miscarriage even when the thyroid function appears to be normal.[26,27] There is no current medical treatment to reduce thyroid antibodies but where this is associated with elevated TSH, small doses of thyroid hormone will be given.

There are some recent findings which indicate that endometriosis shows some characteristics of an autoimmune disease too. Again, there is no medical treatment which addresses this aspect of endometriosis directly, but Chinese medicine treatment of endometriosis will certainly take into account its inflammatory (Damp-Heat) and internal bleeding (Blood stasis) aspects.

Research examining the influence of acupuncture on the immune system is revealing interesting effects – the exact mechanisms are not yet clear and may turn out to be as intricate and as involved as the immune system itself. However it is the anti-inflammatory or immunosuppressive actions of acupuncture are of particular interest in the field of immune related pregnancy loss. Women with autoimmune disorders tend to have an imbalance between T helper 1 cell derived (pro-inflammatory) and T helper 2 cell derived (anti-inflammatory) cytokines. Correcting this Th1/Th2 balance has been a key strategy in the treatment of various immune disorders. One study has shown that this ratio may be reset by acupuncture which corrected an imbalance in Th1/Th2 derived cytokines TNF-α and IL4 (and also decreased pro-inflammatory cytokine interleukin IL1).[28]

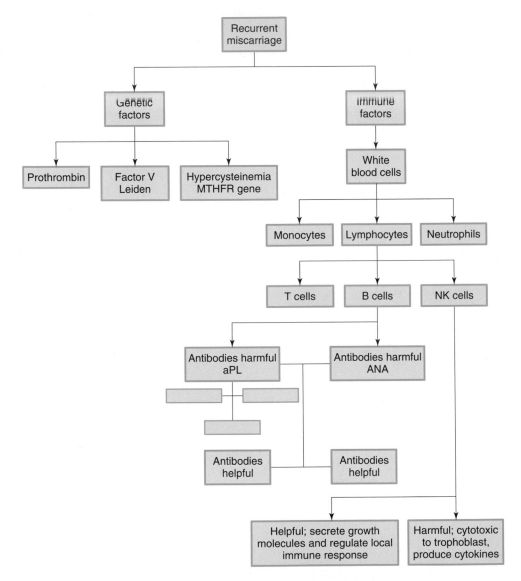

Figure 8.2 Clotting and immune factors which contribute to recurrent pregnancy loss.

Herbal formulas known to be helpful in reducing the risk of miscarriage related to Kidney and Spleen deficiency, have also been shown to correct a Th1/Th2 imbalance (in this case by increasing Interleukin 10 and decreasing Interleukin 2).[29] Recent reviews on the effect of acupuncture on the immune system have concluded that appropriate and frequently applied acupuncture treatment can provoke sustained anti-inflammatory activity, without stimulation of pro-inflammatory cells.[30,31] We know that stress affects the immune system, elevating levels of activated T cells which can reduce implantation rates of embryos. We also know that high resting levels of cortisol are linked with elevated markers of inflammatory processes in the body which may affect successful implantation of the embryo.[32] Fortunately, acupuncture has been shown to exert a beneficial modulatory effect on such immune imbalances caused by anxiety and stress. In one study, the maximum effect on the immune system of women suffering heightened anxiety was measured 72 h after they received acupuncture and the effects of a course of acupuncture were still evident 1 month after it was completed.[33] It is thought that the immunomodulatory effect of acupuncture may result from the increase in levels of endogenous opioids: endorphin, met-encephalin, leu-encephalin, and serotonin, all of which increase with acupuncture treatment. These neurotransmitters create a sense of relaxation and have immunomodulator effects on the immune system.[34]

In general, most research on treatment of autoimmune disorders with Chinese herbal remedies centers around the concepts of clearing Heat, reinforcing Yin, supporting Qi and resolving Blood stasis. One of the factors that is traditionally considered important at the time of early placental development is warm and flourishing Kidney Yang. Interestingly, deficiency of Kidney Yang and Wei Qi is thought by some Chinese Medicine scholars to contribute to disorders of the immune system.

Inflammatory markers are also affected by diet and weight loss,[35] which is one reason that treatment for women diagnosed with immune system disorders will be advised to pay attention to their diet and take supplements such as omega-3 fatty acids, vitamin E and antioxidants which decrease inflammatory markers.

Alloimmune (distinct from autoimmune) origins of pregnancy loss occur when the mother rejects fetal tissue as foreign, which of course it is! Nature has devised schemes whereby the mother learns to tolerate the fetus, but if something goes wrong with this scheme, the mother produces antibodies to the fetus and miscarriage can follow. Some forms of immunotherapy have been devised by specialists, but clinical trials have produced conflicting results. Chinese medicine infertility specialists do not talk in terms of the immune system; however, several of the possible diagnoses for recurrent miscarriage will include immune system disorders, e.g. Kidney Yin deficiency with Heat or Blood stagnation.

Gynecological disorders

There is an increased chance of miscarriage with just about every cause of relative infertility or subfertility. In other words, most gynecological disorders which lower fertility will increase miscarriage risk.

ENDOMETRIOSIS

Pregnancies have been thought to be more at risk of miscarriage if there is active endometriosis at the time of conception. The exceptions are pregnancies achieved with IVF. Possibly, the high levels of hormones given during the IVF procedures help the stability of the pregnancy in the early days, so miscarriages are not unusually frequent.[36]

From a TCM perspective, most cases of endometriosis are associated with Kidney Yang deficiency and Blood stagnation (see Ch. 5), both of which can be associated with an increased risk of miscarriage. Treatment should be applied to correct these conditions well before pregnancy is attempted.

POLYCYSTIC OVARY SYNDROME

PCOS is a complex condition which affects ovary function. Small cysts accumulate in the ovaries and the release of an egg may be sporadic rather than monthly. Those eggs which are released are not always mature or of good quality and, if fertilization is successful, the fetus may be compromised and the risk of miscarriage elevated. Similarly, because the hormonal environment is abnormal in PCOS, conditions in early pregnancy are not always optimum. Women with PCOS who conceive with IVF have been reported to have higher than normal miscarriage rates.[37]

There are many reasons, including Kidney deficiency and obstruction to the Chong and Ren vessels which may account for the observed increase in miscarriages in PCOS patients (see Ch. 5).

ENDOMETRITIS

Infection in the endometrium causes inflammation (called endometritis), which can increase risk of miscarriage by irritating the fetal membranes and causing premature contractions of the uterus. If there is a history of pelvic inflammation or infection (pelvic inflammatory disease or PID), then vigorous and persistent treatment must be applied to correct the condition before it contributes to future pregnancy loss. In cases of low-grade but chronic PID, antibiotics have limited effectiveness; acupuncture, especially the use of abdomen points, and strong Damp-Heat clearing herbal formulas, on the other hand, are usually quite effective (see Ch. 5).

AMENORRHEA

Clearly amenorrhea and anovulation contribute in a very obvious way to infertility and sometimes the conditions which inhibit ovulation can also compromise a pregnancy should one occur (perhaps as a result of drug treatment to induce ovulation). For example, amenorrhea caused by extreme weight loss is often associated with significant under-nutrition. If an ovulation and a pregnancy should happen to occur in these circumstances, then the ability of the mother to sufficiently nourish her baby may be inadequate. From a TCM point of view, this situation would be described as Blood and Qi deficiency, a common cause of a small-for-dates fetus and sometimes of fetal death and miscarriage. Loss of periods related to drug use might create similar conditions and any closely following pregnancy will be at risk of miscarriage. The hormonal imbalances which lead to amenorrhea indicate a Kidney disorder in TCM terms (see Ch. 5) and until this is corrected, any pregnancies which might eventuate will be precarious.

BLOCKED TUBES

Damage to the tubes which causes absolute obstruction creates sterility, but if this is overcome using IVF technology, the tubal pathology will have little impact on the outcome of the pregnancy and generally, the risk of miscarriage is lower in this category than in other types of IVF patients.

Other types of blockages in the fallopian tubes caused by mucus or secretions can be dealt with in a number of ways, including the mechanical clearing of the tubes, which occurs during a tube X-ray (HSG) or ultrasound (HyCoSy), or the application of acupuncture and the use of Damp-clearing herbs. However, if the Damp is not cleared adequately (e.g., if the tubes are cleared mechanically and there is no systemic treatment), then there is an increased risk of pre-implantation loss of the embryo because the endometrium may be too 'slippery' or fluid from the fallopian tubes may wash the embryo off the endometrial surface.

FIBROIDS AND POLYPS

Fibroids which are large or numerous enough to occupy a significant part of the uterine cavity reduce the chances of falling pregnant and increase the risk of miscarriage if pregnancy does occur. This is because the available area for implantation of the embryo or adequate placental development on the uterine wall is reduced. Some late-stage miscarriages are attributed to the failure of placental development due to obstruction by fibroids. In the case of large and numerous fibroids, specialists will often recommend their removal before pregnancy is attempted. This sort of surgery is major and requires long recovery time, but in a young and healthy woman, will usually increase fertility and certainly reduce the risk of miscarriage. Some women choose to use Chinese medicine to address the problem of fibroids, with mixed results. If the woman has a strong constitution, has plentiful Qi and Blood, then strong Blood-moving treatment can be applied to encourage fibroid necrosis and shrinkage. Even if this is successful, the risk of the fibroids growing again during pregnancy is a real one.

If uterine polyps are discovered on ultrasound, they will usually be removed surgically before conception is attempted. There is some evidence that size of a polyp, especially as it approaches 2 cm, may be associated with increased miscarriage. Polyps may contribute to uterine inflammation which can have an IUD sort of effect and prevent implantation or successful placental development. Hysteroscopic polypectomy is a simple procedure, which carries little risk and may improve reproductive outcome in cases of women trying to conceive or undergoing ART.[38]

This is generally a quicker and simpler solution than using Chinese medicine, which in the case of removing pedunculated polyps, has limited success.

Other conditions associated with recurrent miscarriages

DIABETES

Diabetes is a disease that has classically been associated with recurrent pregnancy loss. However, it is only when there is poor blood sugar control in an insulin-dependent female diabetic that there is any increased likelihood of miscarriage. It appears that levels of blood sugar need to be stable at the time of ovulation and conception. If they are not, there is an increased risk of chromosomal abnormalities in the fetus or developmental abnormalities.[39]

Fortunately, these days, diabetes is usually adequately treated and thus is not a frequent contributor to miscarriages in the developed world.

Gestational diabetes is a more insidious form of diabetes, which becomes apparent only after the pregnancy is established. Even when it has resolved completely after the pregnancy, it is important to ensure blood sugar is well-regulated before considering another pregnancy: otherwise, there may be a persisting increased risk of a malfunction during cell division at ovulation, and the risk of creating an embryo with a chromosomal abnormality. Women with a history of gestational diabetes, are advised to follow a good diet before conceiving again.[40]

The same factors in diabetes which can put at risk cell division and create chromosomal defects in the fetus also operate in the male. Poorly-controlled blood sugar can affect cell division in the testes, leading to abnormalities of the sperm that result in infertility or increased miscarriage risk.[41]

Miscarriages associated with diabetes will, according to TCM analysis, often fall in the Kidney Yin Xu category. Mild blood sugar abnormalities are sometimes associated with PCOS and treatment of Spleen Qi deficiency and Damp accumulation may be relevant.

THYROID DISORDERS

Both infertility and miscarriage are more common when the thyroid gland is hypo- or hyperactive. Higher miscarriage rate, more frequent pre-term deliveries, increased hypertension, diabetic complications, higher risk for placental abruption, and adverse fetal effects have all been reported with thyroid dysfunction in pregnancy.

During pregnancy, a 30–40% increased need for thyroid hormones is the result of increased placental uptake, higher thyroid-binding globulin levels, and greater blood volume. Those with subclinical hypothyroidism and/or high-normal TSH levels at the beginning of pregnancy may not be able to meet these needs and may show signs of thyroid insufficiency during pregnancy. It is usually recommended that these women (and those with diagnosed hypothyroidism before they become pregnant) be treated prior to and during pregnancy.[42]

Uncontrolled hyperactivity of the thyroid during pregnancy is rare but can increase the risk of miscarriage.[43] The mechanism is unknown but high levels of thyroid hormones increase body metabolism and temperature which might compromise the endometrium's structure and function.

In TCM terms, we relate this increased metabolism to internal Heat from Yin deficiency. In Yin-deficient women, the endometrium is typically thin and not well nourished; thus, the embryo fails to develop and thrive. Strong Heat-clearing herbs given with Yin-nourishing herbs can often remedy this.

Women who are significantly hypothyroid (underacting thyroid) have more difficulty conceiving, but if they do there is a two-three times increased miscarriage risk.[44]

Early intervention with thyroid hormone medication (before pregnancy) reduces the risk, as do preventative measures taken with Chinese herbs and acupuncture to strengthen Kidney and Spleen Yang over a period of some months.

There is no conclusive evidence that thyroid disease in the male partner contributes to increased miscarriage rates; however, thyroid disease, especially hypothyroidism, has been shown to have a negative effect on semen quality.[45]

This and the fact that thyroid function is so important for controlling cell metabolism and cell division means that ensuring healthy thyroid function is an important part of preconception care in men and especially so if there have been previous miscarriages.

Hypothyroidism is a clinical condition which is often encountered as part of a Kidney Yang deficient picture in TCM terms. In men, Kidney Yang deficiency lowers libido, causes difficulty with erections, and is often related to poor sperm production or production of sperm that have defective motility.

Thyroid antibodies were discussed above in immune disorders.

INTESTINAL DISORDERS

Disorders of the gut such as irritable bowel syndrome, celiac disease, Crohn's disease, ulcerative colitis and candidiasis can compromise nutritional status by interfering with absorption of nutrients through the intestinal wall. Some nutrients are known to be important for fertility or fetal health and if intestinal disorders prevent adequate absorption, then supplementation may be important to prevent recurrent miscarriage.

Additionally, the drugs used to treat some of these diseases can affect fertility or the fetus. Some of these drugs suppress the immune system and some can damage the DNA.[46]

Either of these categories can cause damage to the gametes or the fetus. Such drugs must be withdrawn or replaced before pregnancy is attempted.

Celiac disease (a severe intolerance to gluten) seems to be in some cases related to hormonal abnormalities which are not found in other gut disorders. Many men with celiac disease have smaller than average testicles, low fertility, sexual dysfunction and partners with a history of miscarriage. It is not uncommon for celiac disease to first be diagnosed after recurrent miscarriages.[47]

Candidiasis is an overgrowth in the gut by *Candida albicans*, a benign yeast organism and normal gut inhabitant, which mutates to a fungal form and proliferates and invades the intestines and intestinal walls. According to Foresight, a British association which promotes pre-conception care, *Candida* infection is implicated in infertility, miscarriage and premature birth.[48,49] Dietary interventions will be advised before conception for these disorders.

RENAL DISEASE

When renal disease is chronic, risk of miscarriage is increased. Treatment of Kidney Yin and Yang until the disease is cured or stabilized is advisable before conception is attempted.

CARDIOVASCULAR DISEASE

Women with a family history of ischemic heart disease are more at risk of miscarriage.[50] And conversely, women who suffer recurrent miscarriages are more likely to develop heart problems when they are older. In early pregnancy, the cardiovascular system must do a great deal to ensure that the pregnancy continues and part of preconception planning should be to ensure the cardiovascular system is in as good a shape as possible.

Treatment offered by TCM practitioners in early pregnancy often focuses on the Heart (to treat the Shen and the Bao vessel) and the Pericardium (which helps cardiovascular function).

Excess or low body weight

A relationship has been observed between obesity and miscarriage rates of pregnancies achieved with IVF.[51] Weight loss is an important and low cost measure which is non-invasive and managed by patients themselves. Hence, IVF clinics with their patient's interests at heart will insist that patients with unfavorable BMIs lose weight before attempting IVF. (See Chapter 5 (PCOS) and Chapter 9 for more discussion on weight loss and the role Chinese medicine can play.)

On the other hand, very low body weight is also considered a risk factor for miscarriage and dietary and lifestyle modification should address this before conception.[52] Women with Yin deficiency and internal Heat fall into this category; appropriate lifestyle and treatment measures were discussed in Chapter 4.

Lifestyle and environmental factors can contribute to infertility and to miscarriage and the impact of both of these needs to be considered for both female and male partners. Scientific evidence indicates extreme sensitivity of embryos and fetuses to environmental and occupational chemicals compared with adult responses.[53]

STRESS

The way we live our lives not only affects fertility but also has an impact on how a pregnancy develops, e.g., stress is related to higher miscarriage rates.[54] The effects of stress are discussed further in Chapter 12 (and also Ch. 11).

DIET

Diet is discussed in more detail in Chapter 12, however, we should note here that eating a good diet of fresh foods and taking supplements is associated with a lower miscarriage rate.[53]

CHEMICAL EXPOSURE

• Men

Historically, the fault for miscarriages always fell on the woman, i.e., it was thought she couldn't 'hold on to the baby', and this is reflected in both Chinese and Western medical texts.

Then we came to understand the primary causative role chromosomal abnormality played in fetal loss and research showed how genetic abnormalities in the sperm, and not just the egg, are often implicated in miscarriages, especially if the male partner works in certain trades. For example, men who work with glues, solvents, and paints produce sperm which create fetuses that are two–three times more likely to miscarry than normal.[5]

Sperm can be affected by exposure to toxic chemicals at any time, but miscarriages are most likely if the sperm exposure happened in the 6 months before conception.[55]

• Women

It has also been clearly demonstrated that chemical exposure affects women too, both in their ability to conceive and to hold on to the pregnancy. The chromosomes of the egg are vulnerable to damage by toxic chemicals during the time of maturation of the egg, and especially after it is released from the safe haven of the ovary at the time of ovulation, or at the time of conception and formation of the embryo.

Pharmacists or nurses who handle antineoplastic agents before or when they become pregnant are more likely to miscarry.[56] Similarly, nurses who are exposed to sterilizing chemicals have a higher miscarriage rate.[57] Female veterinarians who are exposed to anesthetics and pesticides have twice the miscarriage rate of the general population.[58]

Some other confirmed environmental causes of miscarriage include lead, mercury, organic solvents, and ionizing radiation.[59,60]

Household cleaners are also a cause of concern (see Ch. 12 for more discussion on the effect of environmental toxins).

CAFFEINE

Caffeine consumption during early pregnancy is clearly related to an increased risk of miscarriage of normal karyotype embryos, especially once daily intake reaches 200 mg (roughly 1.5 cups of coffee, 3 cups of tea or 5 sodas).[61,62]

Caffeine can easily cross the placental barrier. A fetus cannot metabolize caffeine, particularly in the early stages of pregnancy, so it has a direct effect on cells and tissues and may interfere with development. We know that high doses of caffeine have a vasoconstrictive effect and this could possibly reduce blood flow to the placenta and to the fetus.

Many women who have prepared for pregnancy with pre-conception programs will have already eliminated or reduced caffeine consumption before they conceive. If not, then cutting caffeine out (or down) is a sensible strategy for at least the first 3 or 4 months of pregnancy. Those women who suffer from pregnancy nausea will usually not need any persuading to eliminate coffee.

ALCOHOL

The effects of drinking during pregnancy are well known and are significant enough to deter most women from drinking.

But women who are attempting to conceive should be encouraged to avoid even very early exposure to alcohol. There is good evidence that even moderate alcohol consumption is associated with an increased risk of miscarriage.[63]

SMOKING

Several studies have shown that women who smoke have a modest increase in their risk for miscarriage,[64] hence women planning to conceive would be well advised to quit. Marijuana is thought to add to inflammatory processes that can contribute to early pregnancy loss, though this has not been confirmed in human studies.[65]

MYCOTOXINS

Mold contamination of food and environment is widespread. Some mycotoxins such as zearalenone mimic estrogen and have been described in connection with a number of reproductive disorders including miscarriage in animal studies.[66] This and other mold toxins are common in our environment – either in our houses if they are damp or in our kitchens if food (especially grains) is kept for too long. While the effect of mycotoxins is unlikely to be a major concern for women who suffer repeated miscarriages, in the interests of improving the internal hormone environment eating fresh foods and not keeping foods for too long (in or out of the fridge) is to be recommended.

Patients living in damp houses could think about installing dehumidifiers if other more drastic measures, such as moving house or installing damp courses, are not practical.

ELECTROMAGNETIC FIELDS (EMF) AND RADIATION

EMFs are impossible to avoid in modern daily life, but advice to women in the early stages of pregnancy to avoid excessive exposure is important. Miscarriage risk is increased two-fold by exposure to peak levels of $\geq 1.6\,\mu T$. The researchers speculate that EMF spikes (rather than overall exposure) could cause miscarriages by subtly disrupting cell-to-cell communication. The EMF load can be lessened by reducing exposure to such spikes from household gadgets in the early weeks of pregnancy. Vacuum cleaners, food mixers, and hairdryers can produce strong alternating magnetic fields; generally, those with strong motors are the worst culprit, so handing over some of the household chores for the 1st trimester might be an option many women would desire.[67]

X-rays of the abdomen or back in women increases the miscarriage rate, although the effect does not extend over several years, as it does with men. Early embryos are particularly sensitive, since their rapidly dividing cells are easily damaged by ionizing radiation. If genetic damage results, the embryo will not develop properly and will miscarry. A history of either abdominal or lower back X-rays on men increase risk of miscarriage in subsequent pregnancies.[5]

Clearly, assessing the environment at home and at work is important when investigating recurrent miscarriage. Ongoing exposures to chemicals at work, at home or related to hobbies or renovations must be discontinued well before pregnancy is attempted again. And exposure to radiation and EMFs limited where possible.

Psychological factors

A number of workers in this field feel that emotional traumas, leading to low self-esteem or feelings of guilt, may underlie some cases of recurrent miscarriage. There may be a history of incest or sexual assault. Previous abortions may also contribute to a tendency to miscarry if the woman felt ambivalent about the abortion and, especially, if the aborted pregnancy was with the same partner with whom she now wanted to have a baby. Severe stress or domestic abuse have also been linked with increased miscarriage.[68]

Population studies in China have observed that those who do 'mental' work have a higher rate of miscarriage than those who don't; 38% compared with 15%.[69]

Chinese medicine describes a central role of the Heart when it is talking about emotional imbalance. The Heart is said to be the house of the spirit and when it is damaged, there can be many psychological manifestations – some of them deep in the subconscious, some of them manifesting in high levels of anxiety and a number of other clinical symptoms. As described in Chapter 2, the Heart also has a direct link with the Uterus and in fact, is of key importance in controlling the 'opening and closing' of the Uterus. Disturbed Heart Qi during pregnancy can lead to inappropriate opening of the Uterus and miscarriage.

Treatment to prevent miscarriage should always be mindful of the Heart and settling or calming the mind. Counseling or psychotherapy are usually effective methods of addressing unresolved issues from the past and acupuncture can be helpful in changing deeply held or unconscious body–mind patterns and in calming anxiety. Once a patient with a history of miscarriage becomes pregnant, regular acupuncture to calm the mind is recommended. Some research has indicated that just the act of monitoring early pregnancy seems to help reduce miscarriage rates in women with a history of pregnancy loss.[70]

TCM diagnosis and treatment of recurrent miscarriage

Once physical uterine and cervical disorders, inherited genetic disorders, sperm and ova defects due to occupational toxic exposure and complications from other diseases or medications are all ruled out, then the Chinese medicine practitioner can apply his diagnostic skills and determine if there is another, perhaps more subtle, reason for recurrent miscarriage.

Acupuncture and Chinese herbs have been used for many centuries in the treatment of recurrent miscarriage. Of course, if pregnancy loss is recurrent, then it is reasonable to think that there is a persistent factor in one or both of the would-be parents. Thus, recurrent miscarriage lends itself a little more to the sort of treatment that TCM offers (i.e., preventative treatment ahead of the fact) than does a miscarriage, which is already threatening and which in many cases is due to a lethal chromosomal defect.

The TCM doctor would traditionally diagnose the nature of the recurrent miscarriage according to the constitution of the female partner. Nowadays, in the light of new knowledge, the male partner will be assessed too.

The categories into which TCM divides recurrent miscarriage are the same as those for threatened miscarriage with subtle differences. The clinical approach, however, is quite distinct in the two cases. In the former, we have an acute situation with little time in which to make a difference. Treatment must be applied to address the disorder and at the same time, calm the fetus. If the disorder is serious, then there may be little chance of saving the pregnancy. However, in the case of recurrent miscarriage, we can allow plenty of time (preferably ≥6 months) to correct the problem before conception is attempted again. Herbs which calm the fetus are not necessary and, more importantly, we do not have to avoid herbs or points which are contraindicated in pregnancy.

Categories of recurrent miscarriage are as follows:

• Kidney deficiency

• Qi and Blood deficiency

• Heat in the Blood

• Blood stagnation.

Kidney deficiency

Kidney deficiency is the most common pathology underlying both infertility and miscarriage. For threatened miscarriage due to Kidney deficiency, Kidney Yang was our prime treatment target. In the case of recurrent miscarriage, we will treat both Kidney Yin and Yang if necessary. Kidney Yin deficiency is a prime cause of infertility and women with Kidney Yin deficiency may have as much difficulty becoming pregnant as they do staying pregnant. Treatment of such women is necessarily quite long term – the Yin must be recovered so that the egg develops well and the endometrium is thick and secretory. This can take time in the case of a woman who is very Yin-deficient and, since this happens more often in older women, we are confronted with a dilemma. Older women (and Yin-deficient women with Yin-deficient Heat) are impatient to conceive and it is often a difficult task for the practitioner to persuade them of the wisdom of preparing their body first. In cases of recurrent miscarriage due to Kidney Yin deficiency, pregnancy attempts should be avoided for at least three or four menstrual cycles to give time to build the Yin. Most women can understand that risking having repeated miscarriages is very damaging, but the pressure of time ticking by is strong once the woman is already in her late 30s or has turned 40.

For most women who miscarry more than once, it is important to build and balance the Kidney Yin and Yang before the next attempt to conceive. This is achieved best by following a simplified version of the protocols described in Chapter 4. Thus, building Kidney Yin is emphasized in the pre-ovulatory or post-menstrual phase and Kidney Yang in the post-ovulatory phase.

Post-menstrual phase

Herbal formula — The formula of choice is:

Gui Shao Di Huang Tang (Angelica Peonia Rehmannia decoction)

Dang Gui	9 g	*Radix Angelicae Sinensis*
Bai Shao	9 g	*Radix Paeoniae Lactiflorae*
Shu Di	9 g	*Radix Rehmanniae Glutinosae Conquitae*
Shan Zhu Yu	9 g	*Fructus Corni Officinalis*
Shan Yao	9 g	*Radix Dioscorea Oppositae*
Fu Ling	12 g	*Sclerotium Poriae Cocos*
Mu Dan Pi	6 g	*Cortex Moutan Radicis*
Ze Xie	9 g	*Rhizoma Alismatis*

This is the well-known formula for strengthening Kidney and Liver Yin, Lui Wei Di Huang Wan, with the addition of two Blood tonics Dang Gui and Bai Shao. (It is explained in Ch. 4.)
To reinforce the Yin further, add:

Nu Zhen Zi	12 g	*Fructus Ligustri Lucidi*
Han Lian Cao	9 g	*Herba Ecliptae Prostratae*

Where Kidney Yang is constitutionally weak (sore lower back, frequent urination), add:

Tu Si Zi	9 g	*Semen Cuscatae*

Acupuncture points — Choose from the following points (and see Table 8.9):

Ren-4	Guanyuan
KI-13	Qixue
Ren-7	Yinjiao

ST-27	Daju
KI-3	Taixi
KI-5	Shuiquan
LIV-8	Ququan
KI-6	Zhaohai

Post-ovulation phase

Herbal formula — The formula of choice is:

Bu Shen Gu Chong Tang (Reinforce the Kidneys, Consolidate the Chong Channel decoction) modified

Xu Duan	9 g	*Radix Dipsaci*
Ba Ji Tian	9 g	*Radix Morindae Officinalis*
Du Zhong	9 g	*Cortex Eucommiae Ulmoidis*
Tu Si Zi	9 g	*Semen Cuscatae*
Dang Gui	9 g	*Radix Angelicae Sinensis*
Shu Di	9 g	*Radix Rehmanniae Glutinosae Conquitae*
Gou Qi Zi	12 g	*Fructus Lycii Chinensis*
Dang Shen	12 g	*Radix Codonopsis Pilulosae*
Bai Zhu	12 g	*Rhizoma Atractylodis Macrocephalae*
Da Zao	3 pieces	*Fructus Zizyphi Jujuba*
Sha Ren	3 g	*Fructus seu Semen Amomi*

Xu Duan, Ba Ji Tian, Du Zhong, and Tu Si Zi all support the Kidney Yang, whereas Shu Di and Gou Qi Zi reinforce Kidney and Liver Yin and with Dang Gui, the Blood. Dang Shen, Bai Zhu, Da Zao, and Sha Ren are added to invigorate Spleen Qi. This formula can be continued during the first few weeks of pregnancy.

Acupuncture points — Choose from the following points (and see Table 8.10):

Ren-4	Guanyuan
BL-23	Shenshu
KI-3	Taixi
KI-4	Dazhong
LIV-2	Xingjian

Table 8.9   Acupuncture points[a] used in the treatment of recurrent miscarriage due to Kidney weakness, post-menstrual phase

Treatment goal	Acupuncture points
To reinforce Kidney Yin	Ren-4 and KI-3
To reinforce Kidney Yin and clear Heat	KI-6
To regulate the activity of the Chong and Ren vessels	Ren-7, KI-5 and KI-13
To influence Kidney Jing	ST-27
To supplement Liver Yin and Blood	LIV-8

[a]Reinforcing or even method is used.

307

Table 8.10   Acupuncture points[a] used in the treatment of recurrent miscarriage due to Kidney deficiency, post-ovulation phase

Treatment goal	Acupuncture points
To supplement Kidney Yang	Ren-4[b], BL-23 and KI-3
To support the Kidney and stabilize the emotions	KI-4
To clear Liver-Heat	LIV-2

[a]Points are reinforced with the exception of LIV-2, which is reduced.

[b]Ren-4 is used only before and at midcycle in cycles where pregnancy is attempted. In other cycles, it can be used with no restriction.

Watching clinical markers such as the quality of the cervical mucus, the shape of the BBT chart and the nature of the period can help us to assess progress. Of course, the vitality and well-being of the woman will also tell us about improved Kidney energy.

Women with Kidney deficiency tend to miscarry early in the pregnancy. In the case of Kidney Yang failing, this can be so early, as to seem like a slightly late period and the miscarriage may only be detected if BBT charts have been kept.

It may also be the case that there is significant preimplantation loss in women with Kidney deficiency; some of these women may have been told they have a luteal phase defect (see Ch. 4). We prescribe the herbs discussed above to help prepare the endometrium for successful implantation and establishment of a pregnancy. Whether this is by promoting upregulation of implantation factors or modulation of immune factors or increasing progesterone levels, we don't yet know. Studies of some Kidney tonic formulas have reported significant increases in the expression of growth factors and receptors and suggested that these could promote implantation and reduce risk of pregnancy loss.[71]

CASE HISTORY – ARIELLA

Ariella (38) said she fell pregnant as soon as she looked at a double bed. But just as soon as she got the positive test result, she would start bleeding. Once she got as far as 7 weeks, but then the bleeding came again. After four miscarriages, she was emotionally wrung out and terrified of becoming pregnant and miscarrying again. All her blood tests showed nothing wrong, and her chromosomes did not seem to be incompatible with her husband's.

Ariella agreed to not 'look at a double bed' for 3 months, while we fortified her Kidney Yang. Her cycle was short and her BBT charts showed a low and short luteal phase. Her health, however, was for the most part, excellent. Occasionally, she felt some period pain but this was mild, and slightly loose stools before her periods was the only clear symptom of Kidney Yang deficiency. In situations like this, the BBT chart (Fig. 8.3) plays an essential role in diagnosis.

She took herbs to increase her Kidney Yang throughout her menstrual cycle and by the 3rd month, her BBT chart showed a convincing luteal phase (Fig. 8.4). This type of recurrent miscarriage (or infertility) is one of the most rewarding to treat because results usually come quickly, unlike problems with Kidney Yin deficiency.

Dang Gui	9 g	*Radix Angelicae Sinensis*
Bai Shao	9 g	*Radix Paeoniae Lactiflorae*
Shu Di	9 g	*Radix Rehmanniae Glutinosae Conquitae*
Shan Zhu Yu	9 g	*Fructus Corni Officinalis*
Shan Yao	9 g	*Radix Dioscorea Oppositae*
Fu Ling	12 g	*Sclerotium Poriae Cocos*
Mu Dan Pi	6 g	*Cortex Moutan Radicis*
Ze Xie	9 g	*Rhizoma Alismatis*
Ba Ji Tian	6 g	*Radix Morindae Officinalis*
Tu Si Zi	9 g	*Semen Cuscatae*

This formula she took each month before ovulation.

Dang Gui	9 g	Radix Angelicae Sinensis
Shu Di	9 g	Radix Rehmanniae Glutinosae Conquitae
Gou Qi Zi	12 g	Fructus Lycii Chinensis
Dang Shen	12 g	Radix Codonopsis Pilulosae
Bai Zhu	12 g	Rhizoma Atractylodis Macrocephalae
Shan Yao	9 g	Radix Dioscorea Oppositae
Ba Ji Tian	6 g	Radix Morindae Officinalis
Tu Si Zi	15 g	Semen Cuscatae
Du Zhong	9 g	Cortex Eucommiae Ulmoidis
Xu Duan	9 g	Radix Dipsaci
Da Zao	3 pieces	Fructus Zizyphi Jujuba
Sha Ren	3 g	Fructus seu Semen Amomi

This formula she took each month after ovulation.

Ariella fell pregnant soon after, and took more herbs to prevent miscarriage:

Tu Si Zi	15 g	Semen Cuscatae
Sang Ji Sheng	15 g	Ramulus Sangjisheng
Du Zhong	9 g	Cortex Eucommiae Ulmoidis
Xu Duan	9 g	Radix Dipsaci
Bai Zhu	9 g	Rhizoma Atractylodis Macrocephalae
E Jiao	6 g	Gelatinum Asini

Her pregnancy held firm and she gave birth at 9 months.

Qi deficiency

If Spleen Qi deficiency is seriously compromised, there may be a problem with the uterus dropping and the cervix not staying firmly closed and holding the pregnancy. Cervical incompetence usually causes a problem after about 14 or 15 weeks of pregnancy, when the fetus is starting to grow larger and the Uterus to stretch. Several months of treatment to lift and strengthen the uterus prior to conception may help in future pregnancies. However, the

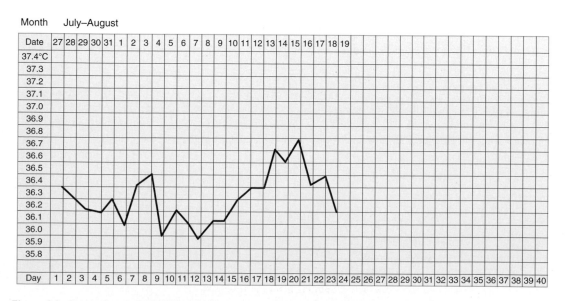

Figure 8.3 Case history – Ariella. This chart shows a slow rise to a short luteal phase.

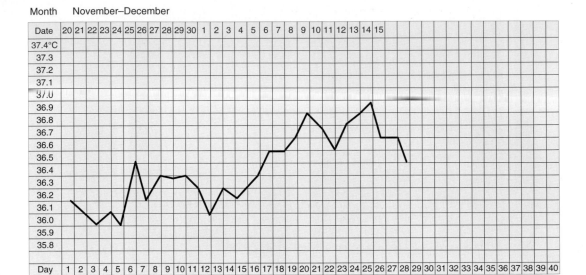

Figure 8.4 Case history – Ariella. This chart shows an improved luteal phase after having treatment for 3 cycles.

woman with a history of cervical incompetence would always be well advised to get a suture in the cervix as well, once she was 14 weeks into a pregnancy.

Herbal formula — The formula of choice is:

Bu Zhong Yi Qi Tang (Reinforce the Center and Benefit the Qi decoction) modified

Huang Qi	15g	Radix Astragali
Dang Shen	12g	Radix Codonopsis Pilulosae
Bai Zhu	9g	Rhizoma Atractylodis Macrocephalae
Dang Gui	9g	Radix Angelicae Sinensis
Chen Pi	6g	Pericarpium Citri Reticulate
Sheng Ma	6g	Rhizoma Cimicifugae
Chai Hu	6g	Radix Bupleuri
Gan Cao	3g	Radix Glycyrrhizae Uralensis
Wu Zei Gu	9g	Os Sepia seu Sepiellae

Dang Shen, Bai Zhu, and Gan Cao invigorate the Spleen Qi, Huang Qi, Sheng Ma, and Chai Hu lift the Uterus, and Chen Pi keeps the Qi moving. Dang Gui and Bai Zhu are often used together to both nourish the Blood and the Qi to help prevent further miscarriages. Wu Zei Gu provides an astringent action to prevent leakage and opening of the Uterus.

To concurrently reinforce the Kidneys, add:

Tu Si Zi	9g	Semen Cuscatae
Bu Gu Zhi	9g	Fructus Psoraleae
Shan Yao	9g	Dioscorea Oppositae

Tu Si Zi builds Kidney Yin and Yang and the Spleen, Bu Gu Zhi builds both Spleen and Kidney Yang, and Shan Yao reinforces Spleen Qi and Yin and the Kidneys.

Table 8.11   Acupuncture points[a] used in the treatment of recurrent miscarriage due to Qi deficiency

Treatment goal	Acupuncture points
To lift the Qi and the organs, in this case the Uterus	DU-20
To reinforce the Spleen Qi	ST-36, Ren-12, Ren-6
To supplement the Kidney Yin and Yang	Ren-4[b]
To regulate the Qi in the Spleen, Liver and Kidney channels	SP-6

[a]Reinforcing or even method is used.
[b]Ren-4 and SP-6 are used only before and at midcycle in cycles where pregnancy is attempted. In other cycles, they can be used with no restriction.

Acupuncture points — Choose from the following points (and see Table 8.11):

DU-20	Baihui
Ren-6	Qihai
Ren-12	Zhongwan
Ren-4	Guanyuan
ST-36	Zusanli
SP-6	Sanyinjiao

CASE HISTORY – JULIANNE

Julianne (36) had a tragic history. Her pregnancies never got past 20 weeks; four times she had lost babies to premature labor when her cervix gave way. Even the suture the surgeon placed in her cervix to keep it closed failed to hold her pregnancies. She could hardly face the thought of going through the trauma again and had started to avoid her husband even though she wanted children more than anything. The treatment she received in my clinic was more related to emotional and physical recovery than to future pregnancies.

Her pulses were thready, her tongue swollen and her digestion weak, indicating a diagnosis of recurrent miscarriage from Qi deficiency. For 4 months she took Bu Zhong Yi Qi Tang with various additions and had regular acupuncture to reinforce her Spleen's holding function.

Huang Qi	15 g	Radix Astragali
Dang Shen	12 g	Radix Codonopsis Pilulosae
Bai Zhu	9 g	Rhizoma Atractylodis Macrocephalae
Dang Gui	9 g	Radix Angelicae Sinensis
Chen Pi	6 g	Pericarpium Citri Reticulate
Sheng Ma	6 g	Rhizoma Cimicifugae
Chai Hu	6 g	Radix Bupleuri
Gan Cao	3 g	Radix Glycyrrhizae Uralensis
Wu Zei Gu	9 g	Os Sepia seu Sepiellae
Tu Si Zi	9 g	Semen Cuscatae
Ye Jiao Teng	6 g	Caulis Polygoni Multiflori

Acupuncture points: DU-20, Yin Tang, Ren-6, SP-6, ST-36

Eventually she felt emotionally strong enough to attempt pregnancy again. Julianne conceived the first time she tried and continued to take the herbs for the first 7 months of the pregnancy. She went to bed and stayed there from early in the 2nd trimester until near to term, and she had a suture placed in her cervix. This time she made it – a full-term baby born at 39 weeks.

If Yin deficiency leads to Blood deficiency, then the endometrium will be thin and may not be conducive to effective implantation, or may not be able to nourish a fetus adequately if implantation is successful. If Qi deficiency is accompanied by Blood deficiency, then the fetus may fail to grow and thrive and will appear small-for-dates on ultrasound tests.

Herbal formula — Give Gui Shao Di Huang Tang (Angelica Peonia Rehmannia decoction) for Yin and Blood deficiency or give the following guiding formula for Blood deficiency with Qi deficiency:

Ba Zhen Tang (Eight Precious decoction)

Dang Gui	9 g	*Radix Angelicae Sinensis*
Bai Shao	9 g	*Radix Paeoniae Lactiflorae*
Chuan Xiong	6 g	*Radix Ligustici Wallichii*
Shu Di	9 g	*Radix Rehmanniae Glutinosae Conquitae*
Dang Shen	12 g	*Radix Codonopsis Pilulosae*
Bai Zhu	9 g	*Rhizoma Atractylodis Macrocephalae*
Fu Ling	12 g	*Sclerotium Poriae Cocos*
Gan Cao	3 g	*Radix Glycyrrhizae Uralensis*

This formula was mentioned above, where it was prescribed for recovery after miscarriage with an increased dose of Dang Gui.

When treating recurrent miscarriage, it is appropriate to add more Kidney tonics to the formula, e.g.:

Huang Jing	9 g	*Rhizoma Polygonati*
Tu Si Zi	9 g	*Semen Cuscatae*
Sang Ji Sheng	15 g	*Ramulus Sangjisheng*
Shan Zhu Yu	9 g	*Fructus Corni Officinalis*

Huang Jing reinforces Qi and Kidneys; Tu Si Zi reinforces Kidney Yin and Yang; Sang Ji Sheng nourishes the Blood, Kidneys, and Liver; Shan Zhu Yu nourishes Kidney Yin and Jing, and provides an astringing action to prevent leakage from the uterus.

Acupuncture points — Choose from the following points (and see Table 8.12):

BL-17	Geshu
BL-20	Pishu
BL-23	Shenshu
Ren-12	Zhongwan
ST-36	Zusanli
Ren-4	Guanyuan
ST-28	Shuidao

As was the case for threatened miscarriage, the Heat which causes repeated miscarriages mostly arises from Kidney Yin deficiency. In some cases, it comes from severe mental agitation, causing Liver- or Heart-Fire; this latter can interfere with the normal 'opening and closing' functions of the uterus. The timing of ovulation and periods may be affected, as well as the ability of the uterus to hold a pregnancy. We can use the same guiding formula here as we used for a pregnancy under threat by Heat in the Blood, but because we are applying

Table 8.12   Acupuncture points[a] used in the treatment of recurrent miscarriage due to Blood deficiency

Treatment goal	Acupuncture points
To strengthen Spleen and Stomach and encourage Blood production	BL-17, BL-20, BL-23, Ren-12, ST-36
To build Blood in the uterus	Ren-4[b]
To regulate Blood in the uterus	ST-28[b]

[a]Reinforcing or even method is used.

[b]Ren-4 and ST-28 are used only before and at midcycle in cycles where pregnancy is attempted. In other cycles, they can be used with no restriction.

preventative treatment, we can expand on the formula and use acupuncture points we may have been hesitant to use on a pregnant woman.

Herbal formula — In the case of long-term endometritis or PID causing the Heat, a combination of herbal medicine, acupuncture and allopathic medicine may be necessary.

Bao Yin Jian (Protecting Yin decoction) modified

Sheng Di	9 g	Radix Rehmanniae Glutinosae
Xuan Shen	9 g	Radix Scrophulariae
Shan Yao	12 g	Radix Dioscorea Oppositae
Bai Shao	9 g	Radix Paeoniae Lactiflorae
Huang Qin	6 g	Radix Scutellariae Baicalensis
Huang Bai	6 g	Cortex Phellodendri
Di Gu Pi	9 g	Cortex Lycii Chinensis
Nu Zhen Zi	9 g	Fructus Ligustri Lucidi
Han Lian Cao	9 g	Herba Ecliptae Prostratae
Suan Zao Ren	15 g	Semen Ziziphi Spinosae
Gan Cao	3 g	Radix Glycyrrhizae Uralensis

Sheng Di and Xuan Shen cool the Blood; Di Gu Pi clears Yin deficient Heat, while Huang Bai and Huang Qin are used to remove Heat and Damp specifically from the pelvic area. Bai Shao and Suan Zao Ren soothe the Liver; Nu Zhen Zi and Han Lian Cao protect the Yin, and Shan Yao the Spleen.

Acupuncture points — Choose appropriate points from the following (and see Table 8.13):

SP-10	Xuehai
KI-6	Zhaohai
KI-2	Rangu
LIV-2	Xingjian
HE-5	Tongli
PC-3	Quze
CO-11	Quchi
KI-3	Taixi

If Heat in the Blood is contributed to by diet, then this should be adjusted in the ways suggested in Chapter 9. If Heat in the Blood is contributed to by emotional factors, then steps to reduce stress should be taken. Even where emotional

Table 8.13   Acupuncture points[a] used in the treatment of recurrent miscarriage due to Heat in the Blood

Treatment goal	Acupuncture points
To cool the Blood	SP-10 and CO-11
To clear Yin-deficient Heat from the Uterus	KI-6 and KI-2
To clear Liver-Fire	LIV-2
To clear Heart-Fire and Heat in the Blood and safeguard the Bao vessels	HE-5
To cool the Blood and calm the spirit	PC-3
To harmonize Heart and Kidney	KI-3

[a]Reducing or even method is applied except in the case of KI-6, which is reinforced.

factors are not the initial cause of Heat in the Blood, they should be considered in women who suffer recurrent miscarriages because there will always be a degree of anxiety and fear. Restlessness and anxiety can be particularly marked in this pattern due to the Heat but should respond favorably to acupuncture and herbal treatment.

Blood stagnation

Women with a history of endometriosis, endometritis, fibroids, cysts, and abdominal surgery are likely to have a degree of Blood stagnation. Sometimes, this can impact unfavorably on pregnancy, especially if there is obstruction, scarring or damage to the endometrium which interferes with placental attachment. If large fibroids are deemed to be a risk for implantation, then surgery is often recommended, as is also the case for polyps. In the case of endometriosis, in which Kidney Yang is frequently a contributing factor, pregnancies may be at risk from inadequate corpus luteum function, increased inflammation, immune system disturbance and disordered blood supply to the endometrium, all of which can impede successful implantation and development of the placenta and therefore increase the risk of miscarriage.

Herbal formula — Our guiding formula in this case can be stronger than that employed for threatened miscarriage with Blood stagnation. While the following herbs are being consumed, it is important that pregnancy is avoided.

Shao Fu Zhu Yu Tang (Lower Abdomen Eliminating Stasis decoction)

Dang Gui	9 g	*Radix Angelicae Sinensis*
Chi Shao	6 g	*Radix Paeoniae Rubra*
Chuan Xiong	6 g	*Radix Ligustici Wallichii*
Yan Hu Suo	9 g	*Rhizoma Corydalis Yanhusuo*
Mo Yao	6 g	*Myrrha*
Pu Huang	9 g	*Pollen Typhae*
Wu Ling Zhi	6 g	*Excrementum Trogopterori*
Xiao Hui Xiang	6 g	*Fructus Foeniculi Vulgaris*
Gan Jiang	3 g	*Rhizoma Zingiberis Officinalis*
Rou Gui	3 g	*Cortex Cinnamomi Cassiae*

Dang Gui, Chi Shao, Chuan Xiong, Yan Hu Suo, Mo Yao, Pu Huang, and Wu Ling Zhi all help to invigorate the Blood. Xiao Hui Xiang, Gan Jiang, and Rou Gui warm the uterus and expel Cold: in cases where this formula is too heating for a patient, these last three herbs will be reduced or removed.

This formula should be administered before and during the period to regulate Blood stagnation. If there are symptoms of Blood stagnation (i.e., pain) at other times of the cycle, it may be administered then too. At other times, Kidney tonic formulas should be given (see Kidney deficiency, above) or, alternatively, Kidney tonic herbs can be added to Shao Fu Zhu Yu Tang, namely:

Nu Zhen Zi	9 g	Fructus Ligustri Lucidi
Xu Duan	12 g	Radix Dipsaci
Tu Si Zi	9 g	Semen Cuscatae

In the case of large submucosal fibroids (where surgery is not appropriate or desired), with little complication by Kidney deficiency, consider a variation of Gui Zhi Fu Ling Wan.

Gui Zhi Fu Ling Tang (Ramulus Cinnamomi-Poria decoction) modified

Dang Gui	12 g	Radix Angelicae Sinensis
Bai Shao	12 g	Radix Paeoniae Lactiflorae
Chuan Xiong	6 g	Radix Ligustici Wallichii
Yi Mu Cao	9 g	Herba Leonuri Heterophylli
San Leng	12 g	Rhizoma Sparganii
E. Zhu	12 g	Rhizoma Curcumae Zedoariae
Tao Ren	6 g	Semen Persicae
Gui Zhi	6 g	Ramulus Cinnamomi Cassiae
Fu Ling	15 g	Sclerotium Poriae Cocos
San Qi	9 g	Radix Pseudoginseng
Wu Ling Zhi	6 g	Excrementum Trogopterori

This is a strong formula for reducing fibroid size and should not be taken at the same time as trying to conceive. Gui Zhi Fu Ling Wan, a well known formula for the treatment of masses, disperses Blood stasis and Phlegm Damp accumulation. Stronger stasis moving herbs in the shape of San Leng and E Zhu are added alongside additional Blood moving herbs San Qi, Yi Mu Cao, and Wu Ling Zhi. This formula can also be considered if other factors such as endometriosis, endometritis, or polyps are contributing to recurrent miscarriage.

See also formulas discussed for endometriosis in Chapter 5.

Acupuncture points — Choose points from the following (and see Table 8.14):

ST-28	Shuidao
ST-29	Guilai
SP-10	Xuehai
SP-8	Diji
SP-6	Sanyinjiao
KI-14	Siman
KI-18	Shiguan
KI-5	Shuiquan
Ren-4	Guanyuan
Ren-6	Qihai
PC-5	Jianshi
CO-4	Hegu

These acupuncture points are applied just before and during the period or when there is pain. Applying moxa to abdomen points can facilitate the moving of Qi and Blood stagnation, providing there is no Heat (inflammation).

Table 8.14   Acupuncture points[a] used in the treatment of recurrent miscarriage due to Blood stagnation

Treatment goal	Acupuncture points
To clear stagnant Blood in the Chong vessel	KI-14[b] and KI-18
To regulate the Blood in the Chong and Ren vessels	KI-5
To move Blood stagnation from the Uterus, especially if it is associated with Cold	ST-28[b] and ST-29[b]
To reinforce Kidney function	Ren-4[b] and Ren-6
To regulate Blood in the Uterus	SP-8 and SP-10
To regulate Qi and Blood in the Bao vessel	PC-5
To release the menstrual flow if it is obstructed and painful	CO-4 with SP-6

[a]Points are used with reducing method to clear stagnation and stop pain.
[b]Used with caution and no manipulation after ovulation in cycles where conception is attempted.

CASE HISTORY – GERALDINE

Geraldine (29) had endometriosis, diagnosed on laparoscopy. It was a mild case according to the surgeon who removed some of the lesions and, he explained, it was probably the reason she hadn't succeeded in becoming pregnant. She had been trying for 2 years: 1 year before and 1 year since the surgery. Her cycle was long and irregular; premenstrually, she experienced breast soreness and abdomen distension; her periods were heavy and clotty and associated with strong pain in the back and abdomen. After the surgery, her periods were less heavy but still somewhat clotty and painful. She had been recording her BBT for the last 9 cycles and a disturbing pattern was evident. In four of the nine charts, her luteal phase was between 19 and 21 days long before a period arrived, indicating early miscarriage (Fig. 8.5). Geraldine didn't register this possibility because her cycle had always been irregular and her premenstrual symptoms mimicked pregnancy ones.

Her pulse was wiry and choppy. Her tongue was normal, except for slight dark discoloration on the right side.

TCM treatment aimed to clear Blood stagnation, regulate Liver Qi, and boost Kidney Yang. She agreed to avoid attempts at pregnancy for 2 cycles, during which time she took strong herbs to remove any endometriosis.

This formula she took for several days before and during the period:

Gou Teng	15g	Ramulus Uncariae cum Uncis
Zi Bei Chi	9g	Mauritiae Concha
Dang Gui	9g	Radix Angelicae Sinensis
Chi Shao	9g	Radix Paeoniae Rubra
Wu Ling Zhi	9g	Excrementum Trogopterori
Yan Hu Suo	9g	Rhizoma Corydalis Yanhusuo
E. Zhu	9g	Rhizoma Curcumae Zedoariae
Rou Gui	3g	Cortex Cinnamomi Cassiae
Quan Xie	1.5g	Buthus Martensi
Wu Gong	1.5g	Scolopendra Subspinipes
Mu Xiang	6g	Radix Saussureae seu Vladimiriae
Xu Duan	9g	Radix Dipsaci

The following formula Geraldine took after her period, until after she ovulated (i.e., her temperature rose on the BBT chart):

Shu Di	12g	Radix Rehmanniae Glutinosae Conquitae
Shan Yao	9g	Radix Dioscorea Oppositae
Shan Zhu Yu	9g	Fructus Corni Officinalis
Fu Ling	9g	Sclerotium Poriae Cocos

Mu Dan Pi	9g	Cortex Moutan Radicis
Ze Xie	12g	Rhizoma Alismatis
Dang Gui	9g	Radix Angelicae Sinensis
Bai Shao	9g	Radix Paeoniae Lactiflorae
Tao Ren	6g	Semen Persicae
Hong Hua	6g	Flos Carthami Tinctorii
Wu Ling Zhi	6g	Excrementum Trogopterori
Tu Si Zi	6g	Semen Cuscatae
Rou Cong Rong	6g	Herba Cistanches
Xu Duan	6g	Radix Dipsaci

The next formula she took for a week after ovulation:

Dang Gui	9g	Radix Angelicae Sinensis
Chi Shao	6g	Radix Paeoniae Rubra
Chuan Xiong	6g	Radix Ligustici Wallichii
Dang Shen	12g	Radix Codonopsis Pilulosae
Tu Si Zi	9g	Semen Cuscatae
Lu Jiao Pian	9g	Cornu Cervi Parvum
Mo Yao	6g	Myrrha
Pu Huang	9g	Pollen Typhae
Wu Ling Zhi	6g	Excrementum Trogopterori
Rou Gui	3g	Cortex Cinnamomi Cassiae

After two cycles, Geraldine once again tried to conceive, so the first formula (above) with the strong Blood-moving herbs was used only when the period arrived. In addition, we added another prescription to be taken for a few days just before and after ovulation:

Dang Gui	9g	Radix Angelicae Sinensis
Chi Shao	9g	Radix Paeoniae Rubra
Bai Shao	9g	Radix Paeoniae Lactiflorae
Shan Yao	9g	Radix Dioscorea Oppositae
Shu Di	9g	Radix Rehmanniae Glutinosae Conquitae
Nu Zhen Zi	9g	Fructus Ligustri Lucidi
Mu Dan Pi	9g	Cortex Moutan Radicis
Fu Ling	9g	Sclerotium Poriae Cocos
Xu Duan	9g	Radix Dipsaci
Tu Si Zi	9g	Semen Cuscatae
Wu Ling Zhi	9g	Excrementum Trogopterori
Hong Hua	6g	Flos Carthami Tinctorii
(Sheng) Shan Zha	9g	Fructus Crataegi
Dan Shen	9g	Radix Salviae Miltiorrhizae

She took these four different formulas at the appropriate time for the next 4 cycles. Her cycle was now a regular 29 days. The 5th month she fell pregnant and stayed pregnant. Her herbs were changed again:

Xu Duan	9g	Radix Dipsaci
Ba Ji Tian	9g	Radix Morindae Officinalis
Du Zhong	9g	Cortex Eucommiae Ulmoidis
Tu Si Zi	9g	Semen Cuscatae
Dang Gui	9g	Radix Angelicae Sinensis
Shu Di	9g	Radix Rehmanniae Glutinosae Conquitae
Gou Qi Zi	12g	Fructus Lycii Chinensis
Dang Shen	12g	Radix Codonopsis Pilulosae
Bai Zhu	12g	Rhizoma Atractylodis Macrocephalae
Da Zao	3 pieces	Fructus Zizyphi Jujuba
Sha Ren	3g	Fructus seu Semen Amomi

And a healthy baby was born at term.

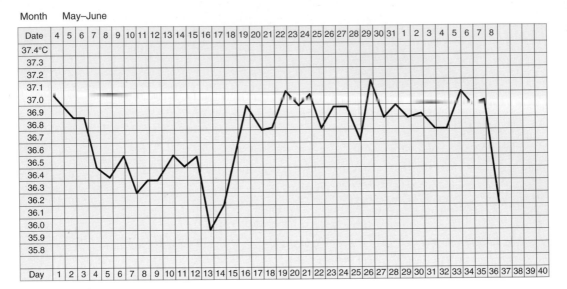

Figure 8.5 Case history – Geraldine. The luteal phase on Geraldine's BBT charts was sometimes as long as 21 days.

IMMUNE-RELATED MISCARRIAGES

Women who are diagnosed with immune factors that might contribute to recurrent miscarriages, will fall into one or more of the TCM categories described above.

However, that said, clinicians working with autoimmune disorders have tended to focus primarily on clearing Blood stagnation or nourishing Yin and clearing Heat.

If your patient has received a diagnosis of clotting factors called antiphospholipid antibodies (the two main ones are anticardiolipin antibodies and lupus anticoagulant), or of genetic factors predisposing to making blood clots (e.g., factor V Leiden, MTHFR or prothrombin mutations), or of autoimmune conditions that we associate with poor placentation (e.g., systemic lupus erythematosus), you can consider using a formula such as Kang Mian Er Hao below, as a guiding formula.[72] This is the sort of formula we could also consider for a patient with a history of recurrent miscarriage who has signs of Blood stagnation from a TCM point of view such as pain, clotty menstrual flow, or a history of endometriosis, whether or not there has been a diagnosis of clotting factors.

Blood stagnation refers to a continuum of states of poor or obstructed blood circulation – from congestion, in which drainage or supply of blood is poor and the blood flow sluggish, to actual stasis, in which the blood circulation at some locale has ceased and a physical obstruction has formed. The sort of impediments we are looking at with clotting factors contributing to miscarriage is at the milder end of the spectrum compared with the substantial Blood stasis of endometriosis and fibroids, etc. At this level of microcirculation, we may not see a lot of obvious clinical symptoms of Blood stasis. The sorts of herbs we will choose will therefore be ones that circulate (and thin) the Blood rather than those that disperse or break up stasis.

Herbal formula — Kang Mian Er Hao is a formula used for autoimmune reproductive issues, which promotes circulation of blood to remove stasis:

Kang Mian Er Hao (Immunity formula for helping pregnancy #2)

Dang Gui	9 g	*Radix Angelicae Sinensis*
Bai Shao	9 g	*Radix Paeoniae Lactiflorae*

318

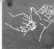

Chuan Xiong	9 g	Radix Ligustici Wallichii
Tao Ren	9 g	Semen Persicae
Hong Hua	9 g	Flos Carthami Tinctorii
Yan Hu Suo	9 g	Rhizoma Corydalis Yanhusuo
Dan Shen	30 g	Radix Salviae Miltiorrhizae
Yi Mu Cao	18 g	Herba Leonuri Heterophylli
Gui Zhi	6 g	Ramulus Cinnamomi Cassiae
Xu Chang Qing	9 g	Radix Cynanchi Paniculati
Yin Yang Huo	15 g	Herba Epimedii
Tu Si Zi	9 g	Semen Cuscatae
Huang Qi	30 g	Radix Astragali
Gan Cao	9 g	Radix Glycyrrhizae Uralensis

The majority of the herbs in this formula have an action of clearing stasis. Some do this by thinning the blood, others by cooling the blood and others by simply promoting blood flow. Many of these herbs have been shown to have anti-inflammatory activity in addition to their function of facilitating blood flow.

It is typical of formulas which address autoimmune factors to have large doses of both Dan Shen and Huang Qi. Yi Mu Cao is used in a high dose in this formula too.

Dan Shen is the main herb in this formula for preventing clotting. It is known for its blood thinning and anti-inflammatory effects. This herb is particularly potent at improving microcirculation. It prevents thrombocyte aggregation and clears stasis right down to the tiniest blood vessels and dissolves obstructions at the level we need it most, in the implantation sites of the endometrium and the newly forming placenta.

Patients with a history of miscarriage related to clotting factors will benefit from taking this formula before trying to conceive again. Once pregnant, these patients are often prescribed low molecular weight Heparin and should be cautioned against taking this formula concurrently.

The other approach is a formula Kang Mian Yi Hao, said to restore Kidneys and reinforce Yin and enrich Jing.[72] Where inflammation is suspected to play a role (e.g., in SLE, rheumatoid arthritis, Sjögren syndrome, scleroderma, excess NK cells, Grave's disease, psoriasis), or if there is a diagnosis of Heat (or Damp-Heat), then cooling herbs will be used alongside Yin tonics.

Kang Mian Yi Hao (Immunity formula for helping pregnancy #1)

Sheng Di	12 g	Radix Rehmanniae Glutinosae
Shan Zhu Yu	9 g	Fructus Corni Officinalis
Mai Dong	9 g	Tuber Ophiopogonis
Bai Shao	9 g	Radix Paeoniae Lactiflorae
Han Lian Cao	12 g	Herba Ecliptae Prostratae
Mu Dan Pi	9 g	Cortex Moutan Radicis
Dan Shen	30 g	Radix Salviae Miltiorrhizae
Huang Qi	30 g	Radix Astragali
Gui Ban	30 g	Plastrum Testudinis
Bie Jia	30 g	Carapax Amydae Sinensis
Huang Qin	9 g	Radix Scutellariae Baicalensis
Huang Bai	9 g	Cortex Phellodendri
Yu Zhu	15 g	Rhizoma Polygonati Odorati
Xu Chang Qing	9 g	Radix Cynanchi Paniculati
Zhi Gan Cao	9 g	Radix Glycyrrhizae Uralensis

The Heat clearing action of this formula soothes inflammation and reduces autoimmune effects in Yin-deficient women. This is strongly backed up by large doses of heavy Yin tonics in the form of Gui Ban and Bie Jia. Provided a certified farmed source is verified, you can dispense these substances to quickly and effectively nourish Yin and promote body fluids. At these high doses, this formula should not be continued for too long, and it is recommended that Shu Di replaces Gui Ban and Bie Jia if the formula is used for more than a few weeks.

Women in this category are sometimes recommended to take steroids, but since the use of these are controversial, and there are some undesired side-effects, herbs which reduce Heat and inflammation are a good alternative.

Acupuncture points — Treatments for recurrent miscarriage related to immune factors will follow the above guiding point prescriptions according to the TCM diagnosis.

EARLY PREGNANCY

Once a woman with a history of recurrent miscarriage conceives, it is important that she continues with treatment which safeguards Kidney function and nourishes Qi and Blood. A commonly used guiding formula is Yishen Gutai Tang (below), which can be modified to address the original cause of the recurrent miscarriages.

Herbal formula — The formula of choice is:

Yishen Gutai Tang (Nourish Kidney and Protect Fetus) modified

Tu Si Zi	20 g	*Semen Cuscatae*
Du Zhong	15 g	*Cortex Eucommiae Ulmoidis*
Xu Duan	15 g	*Radix Dipsaci*
Sang Ji Sheng	15 g	*Ramulus Sangjisheng*
Dang Shen	15 g	*Radix Codonopsis Pilulosae*
Bai Zhu	15 g	*Rhizoma Atractylodis Macrocephalae*
Huang Qin	9 g	*Radix Scutellariae Baicalensis*
Gou Qi Zi	12 g	*Fructus Lycii Chinensis*
Da Zao	3 pieces	*Fructus Zizyphi Jujuba*
He Shou Wu	12 g	*Radix Polygoni Multiflori*
Sha Ren	6 g	*Fructus seu Semen Amomi*

This formula is an expanded version of Shou Tai Wan, used above for Kidney deficiency threatened miscarriage. It strongly reinforces the Kidney and Spleen Qi, and nourishes Blood. Huang Qin quietens the fetus. If there is Heat in the Blood, Sheng Di can be added, and Shu Di in the case of Yin deficiency. Sheng Ma will be added in the case of Spleen Qi deficiency, causing a bearing down sensation. For anxiety, add Suan Zao Ren and for nausea, Sheng Jiang, Zhu Ru, or Zi Su Ye. (Ch. 4 discusses the treatment of pregnancy nausea further.)

Acupuncture points — Acupuncture is particularly useful to relieve anxiety and is strongly recommended for the first few weeks of pregnancy in a woman who has a history of miscarriage. The reassurance she receives from hearing that her pulse is strong and gliding and the calming effect of the acupuncture help to maintain integrity of the Bao vessel and the uterus closed.

Choose from the following points (and see Table 8.15):

Yin Tang
DU-20   Baihui
PC-6   Neiguan
KI-9   Zhubin
KI-6   Zhaohai
ST-36   Zusanli
REN-12   Zhongwan
HT-7   Shenmen
LIV-3   Taichong
GB-34   Yanglingquan
KI-27   Shufu
KI-21   Youmen

MISSED ABORTION

Finally, there is another type of miscarriage called a missed miscarriage or missed abortion. It occurs if a pregnancy, in which the fetus that is not growing normally or dies, continues. The fetus should have miscarried but hasn't. Sometimes it is the use of prescribed progesterone which encourages such a situation, making the abnormal pregnancy tissue stay in the uterus longer than it should. In this case, the operation necessary to remove it (D&C) can be more difficult than usual to perform because the tissue becomes hardened.

I am frequently asked if the herbs prescribed to help prevent miscarriage might do the same thing – or worse, allow a pregnancy to go to term when the fetus is developing abnormally and should under normal circumstances miscarry.

It is important to remember that Chinese medicine usually works in a very different way from allopathic medicine, i.e., it tries to address the source of problems rather than their manifestation. However, during treatment for threatened miscarriage, we are – due to the urgent nature of the situation – addressing both the source of the miscarriage and trying to secure the pregnancy with herbs whose sole aim is to stop bleeding and 'calm the fetus'. In most cases where a pregnancy is already threatened and the woman is experiencing

Table 8.15   Acupuncture points[a] used in the first few weeks of pregnancy

Treatment goal	Acupuncture points
To calm the Shen and regulate the Bao vessel	HT-7 PC-6
To calm the Shen and the mind	Yin Tang, DU-20
To support the Spleen in making Qi and Blood	ST-36, REN-12
To support Kidneys	KI-6, KI-9
To relieve nausea and regulate Qi in the Chong channel	KI-27, KI-21, KI-6, PC-6, LIV-3
To regulate Liver Qi and relieve indigestion	GB-34, LIV-3

Points are used with even method. Abdomen and lower back points are avoided.

bleeding and pain, a miscarriage will follow and it is very unlikely that the herbs prescribed in this case will lead to a missed abortion. However, the herbs to enhance fertility, which are prescribed during the cycle in which conception is attempted may – in the case of someone who has a history of miscarriage – be continued for some weeks after a successful conception to help the body adjust to and maintain the pregnancy. The action of some of these herbs is supposed to encourage the function of the corpus luteum to continue to make progesterone. This is different from supplying exogenous synthetic progesterone and does not usually make a pregnancy persist when the fetus is abnormal. There have been reported cases, however, where large doses of herbs have been taken in an attempt to make a pregnancy stick and they have masked a fetal death for a couple of weeks. It would take an extremely skilled Chinese doctor to detect such a situation on the pulse (because the classically slippery pregnant pulse reflects the changes in the arterial wall provoked by progesterone), although a master pulse-taker may be able to detect fetal death even when progesterone levels remain elevated. But for most TCM doctors, the diagnosis would depend on an ultrasound. Fetal death that is not followed by expulsion of the fetal tissue is not a desirable situation, whether it is created by exogenously administered progesterone or by the action of herbs prescribed after conception or by other unknown factors. TCM practitioners need to be aware of this risk, and where large doses of herbs are being prescribed to maintain a pregnancy which is at risk of miscarriage, it may be appropriate to monitor it with ultrasound or blood tests for hCG levels.

Chinese medicine treatment for missed abortion follows the same principles as that for clinical miscarriage. A D&C will have been performed and, if this is successful, reinforcing the Qi and Blood and regulating the menstrual cycle will be the aim. Since it is harder to remove products of a pregnancy which stopped progressing some time earlier but have been retained in the uterus, there may be a place for adding herbs which can assist the D&C procedure. The same herbs as those used for retained products after a D&C would be used.

MALE FACTOR TREATMENT

In no TCM textbooks will you find treatment of male factors for recurrent miscarriage, but we now know that the condition of the sperm is as important as the condition of the egg in creating a viable pregnancy. Most disorders which cause male infertility do so by compromising sperm quality and, as we know, fertilization with faulty sperm can create embryos likely to miscarry.

You may recall from Chapter 7 that the main patterns of male infertility are Kidney Yin or Yang deficiency (as they are for female infertility). These patterns are sometimes complicated with Damp-Heat or Blood stagnation.

It is the Kidney Yin-deficiency pattern that is most often associated with an increased percentage of abnormal sperm. These are abnormalities which we can see under the microscope and which make it hard for sperm to swim to the egg or to fertilize it effectively if it does get there. But there are also other abnormalities in the chromosomes which we don't see under the regular microscope, because they are deep within the genetic code in the DNA in the chromosomes. Their invisibility, however, does not diminish their potency in contributing to infertility and especially to miscarriage. As mentioned earlier, recent research has shown that exposure to radiation and toxic chemicals increases miscarriage by causing damage to the sperm. Specifically, in TCM terms, radiation dries and damages the Yin, whereas the action of toxic chemicals can manifest in various ways: they can damage Wei Qi and Kidney Yang or Kidney Jing, or create Damp-Heat.

Treatment of the male partner to prevent miscarriage therefore requires exactly the same approach as treatment for infertility and is covered thoroughly in Chapter 7. Clinically, in most cases of recurrent miscarriage due in part or in total to the male partner, tonifying the Yin and clearing Heat is required. Additionally, attention should be paid to lifestyle factors and exposure to fumes in the workplace and at home. Exposure needs to be avoided for several months prior to attempting pregnancy.

CONCEPTION TIMING AND MISCARRIAGE

An interesting study looked at frequency of miscarriage according to how close the day of ovulation was to sexual intercourse and subsequent conception. If women had a history of pregnancy loss, their chances of miscarrying again were much reduced if they attempted conception on the day of ovulation or the day before ovulation compared with pregnancies resulting from attempts at less optimal times. For women who had no history of miscarriage, conception which was not optimally timed produced pregnancies which had no greater risk of miscarrying than those achieved right at midcycle.[73]

Other studies in both animals and humans have indicated that if conception occurs outside the optimal time, a trisomic conception is more likely.[74]

Such a chromosomal abnormality greatly increases the likelihood of miscarriage. If an egg survives more than its usual viable lifetime (>24h) and is fertilized, faulty cell divisions, an abnormal fetus and then a miscarriage, are likely to follow. This is because an aging egg can no longer maintain the same integrity of the cytoplasmic tubular elements. These are the scaffolding elements of the cell which control movement of the chromosomes during cell division. An over-ripe egg also loses some of the integrity of its outer layer and more easily allows entry of more than one sperm at fertilization – a situation which usually creates an unviable fetus.

Eggs will generally be over-ripe and difficult to fertilize if the sperm does not arrive until some time after ovulation. However, there is also the possibility that the egg is released from the ovary late, after it has ripened. This may occur due to illness or hormonal disturbance.

The above research implies that women with a history of even one miscarriage (or a history of infertility) could benefit from charting their cycle and monitoring the exact day of ovulation with cervical mucus observation or by using urine ovulation testing kits. Thus, they can attempt to conceive right at midcycle, at a time when the newly released egg has a firm intracellular structure and the sperm are fresh and vigorous.

ECTOPIC PREGNANCY

Ectopic pregnancies represent a special type of pregnancy loss, one in which the fetus may be completely normal and may have implanted successfully but unfortunately in the wrong place. Implantation can occur in areas such as the outer part of the tube (most common) or the inner narrow part of the tube, or the place where the tube joins the uterus, and occasionally in the ovary or the cervix.

Symptoms include pain in the lower abdomen, usually on one side, accompanied by irregular bleeding, or a long period, or no period. Two blood tests 2 or 3 days apart will indicate whether hCG levels are doubling, as they should in a normal pregnancy, and a transvaginal ultrasound will locate either the pregnancy itself or blood in the abdominal cavity.

Sometimes the doomed embryo is dislodged and expelled out the distal end of the tube (a tubal abortion) and the pregnancy terminates naturally with no intervention. Other ectopic embryos just stop growing and die and the fetal tissue gets absorbed. If the fetus keeps growing, however, the tube can rupture, creating internal bleeding, shock, and a surgical emergency. Ideally, surgery can be performed by laparoscopy, during which the tube is split open and the embryo and surrounding tissues removed. The tube is then left to heal naturally. If there is much internal bleeding, then a laparotomy will be performed during which the ectopic pregnancy is removed or the whole tube is removed. Whether the tube is saved or not depends on its condition and also on whether the other tube is in good enough shape to allow future pregnancies.

If an ectopic pregnancy is diagnosed early and causes few distressing symptoms, it is sometimes left to resolve on its own (under careful observation), or its demise and reabsorption is hurried along by using drugs which are toxic to the embryo and kill it. An example of such a cytotoxic drug is methotrexate.

323

Chinese medicine takes a similar approach to a diagnosed ectopic pregnancy that does not immediately require surgery. Herbs are used to dislodge the embryo and encourage its absorption by the body. This includes the Blood stagnation clearing herbs which we were very careful to avoid using during fertility treatment at a time when there was a chance the patient might become pregnant.

Herbal formula — The formula of choice is:

Huo Luo Xiao Ling Dan (Remove Channel Obstructions formula)

Mu Dan Pi	9g	Cortex Moutan Radicis
Dan Shen	9g	Radix Salviae Miltiorrhizae
Chi Shao	9g	Radix Paeoniae Rubra
Wu Ling Zhi	9g	Excrementum Trogopterori
Shan Zha	9g	Fructus Crataegi
Chuan Niu Xi	9g	Radix Cyathulae
Yu Jin	6g	Tuber Curcumae
Ru Xiang	3g	Gummi Olibanum
Chen Pi	6g	Pericarpium Citri Reticulate
Gan Cao	6g	Radix Glycyrrhizae Uralensis
Di Long	3g	Lumbricus
Wu Gong	3g	Scolopendra Subspinipes

The action of Wu Gong, Di Long, and Chuan Niu Xi is to kill the fetus. The other Blood-regulating herbs all support this action and, in addition, help expulsion or reabsorption of the pregnancy tissue.

This is a strong formula with a powerful clearing action. The patient should be kept under close observation and the formula taken for no longer than 4 or 5 days.

In a patient with Qi deficiency, add:

Huang Qi	9g	Radix Astragali
Dang Shen	9g	Radix Codonopsis Pilulosae

Since methotrexate is a strong chemotherapeutic agent which can affect kidney, lung, liver and bone marrow function, Chinese herbs offer a sound alternative to this drug. Herbs are not without potential toxicity themselves, particularly in people with liver disease. Nevertheless, all the herbs named here have been used for some thousands of years without ill effect. Diarrhea and flatulence are the most disturbing immediate side-effects and if these occur, then the formula is modified.

If the ectopic pregnancy does not resolve or in cases where there is risk of rupture of the tube and consequent shock, hospitalization and surgery are necessary.

Preventing ectopic pregnancies

To think about ways to prevent tubal pregnancies, we need to ask what makes them happen and can we prevent these factors from operating. Tubal pregnancies are caused by:

- kinks, blockages and obstructions of the tube due to scarring from previous infections

- inadequate protection of the lining of the fallopian tube by secretions, either because not enough protective mucus is produced or because it has been lost by the thinning action of progesterone

- mucus plugs

- tension in the fine muscles of the tube.

The incidence of scarring of the tubes as a result of infection has increased significantly in the last few decades and with that, the incidence of ectopic pregnancy. In Chapter 6, we covered in detail the causes and possible treatments for obstructions in the tubes and, if there is a history of infection and positive evidence from a laparoscopy or HSG of tubal obstruction, this treatment should be applied before conception is attempted.

The inside of the fallopian tube is lined with special secretions which are designed to nourish it and the embryo, to facilitate the movement of its cilia, and hence the passage of the embryo, and to protect it from the invasive burrowing instincts of the embryo seeking a home. In normal circumstances, the mucus coats the tubes adequately until a couple of days after ovulation when the progesterone levels have risen to a level that causes the mucus to thin and disappear (i.e., the tube is progestogenized). By this time, the embryo has nearly completed its journey down the tube and implantation will take place in the uterus. But sometimes there are factors operating which mean that the embryo is still in the tube when the protective lining is thinned and dissipated, placing the now-vulnerable tube at risk of invasion. These factors include scarring or constrictions in the tube such that the passage of the embryo is slowed or blocked, a late release of the egg from the ovary or excess progesterone in the system from an exogenous source.

Blockages or constrictions in the tube (caused by scarring, thick mucus secretions or muscle spasms) are dealt with using microsurgery, physiotherapy, Chinese herbal medicine, acupuncture, or massage, depending on the nature and site of the obstruction. Chapter 6 discusses all these possibilities. A retarded release from the ovary, if it happens on a regular basis, can be readily treated with acupuncture applied at the appropriate time. Also, there are herbs which specifically facilitate release of the egg from the ovary (see Ch. 4). In this scenario, a tardy release from the ovary does not refer to an egg which is slow to ripen but rather to one which does not escape the ovary on cue at midcycle. You will remember from Chapter 2, where we covered the processes of the menstrual cycle in detail, that movement of Qi and Blood is considered of prime importance at the time of ovulation. If the Qi and Blood do not move smoothly at this time, then the egg may not be released from the ovary; clinical symptoms which might indicate Qi and Blood stagnation are abdomen pain, breast soreness, or headaches which occur at midcycle. Thus, ensuring that Qi and Blood stagnation is treated before pregnancy is attempted is one way of preventing ectopic pregnancies. Incidentally, such an approach also treats spasm of the muscles of the fallopian tube caused by emotional factors or stress.

Progestogenized tubes also occur in women taking progestogen-based contraceptives. In the rare case that the contraception fails, there is an increased risk of ectopic pregnancy. Practitioners prescribing Western or Chinese herbs should also be mindful of prescribing at ovulation time those herbs which contain progestogens or which increase progesterone synthesis. For example, Kidney Yang tonics, which promote progesterone production should not be prescribed in large quantities until later in the cycle when the embryo is safely in the uterus. The same caution applies to vigorous use of Damp-clearing herbs before ovulation. The trend these days among naturopaths and doctors to prescribe synthesized progesterone creams should also be considered carefully, especially if there is a history of ectopic pregnancy or reason to be concerned about the state of the fallopian tubes.

CASE HISTORY – HELEN

Helen (28) had been trying to conceive for nearly 4 years when she came to my clinic. In that time, she had become pregnant only once and that was an ectopic pregnancy in the right tube, which required surgery. The tube was able to be repaired, however, and a subsequent HSG indicated it and the left tube were patent.

Her cycle was more or less regular (4–5 weekly); however, when she began to keep BBT charts, it became apparent that she did not ovulate every cycle and/or her luteal phase was inadequate (Fig. 8.6).

At midcycle, she sometimes experienced a sharp and grabbing pain on the right side where the ectopic pregnancy had occurred and she didn't see any signs of fertile mucus. During her period, she had only 1 day of menstrual flow, which was of a dark hue and was accompanied by abdomen and lower back pain. Her general health was good but she was overweight and had poor circulation. Her pulse was thready and her tongue was swollen, with fluted sides and had a dull mauve hue.

The lack of regular and effective ovulation indicated Kidney deficiency, this was compounded by Damp accumulation as a result of Qi deficiency. Since the ectopic pregnancy, there were signs of Blood stasis.

The first treatment priority was to reinforce Kidney function and second, to clear Blood stasis. In the post-menstrual phase, building Kidney Yin and Blood was emphasized. Her Spleen Qi was supported at the same time.

Shu Di	9g	Radix Rehmanniae Glutinosae Conquitae
Nu Zhen Zi	9g	Fructus Ligustri Lucidi
Bai Zhu	12g	Rhizoma Atractylodis Macrocephalae
Cang Zhu	15g	Rhizoma Atractylodes
Dang Shen	12g	Radix Codonopsis Pilulosae
Dang Gui	9g	Radix Angelicae Sinensis
Chuan Xiong	6g	Radix Ligustici Wallichii
Ji Xue Teng	9g	Radix et Caulis Jixueteng
Xiang Fu	9g	Rhizoma Cyperi Rotundi

During the ovulation phase, emphasis was placed on Qi and Blood circulation, clearing Damp and supporting Kidney Yang. In addition, she had abdominal massage at this time. To the above formula were added:

Hong Hua	3g	Flos Carthami Tinctorii
Yan Hu Suo	9g	Rhizoma Corydalis Yanhusuo
Xian Mao	6g	Rhizoma Curculiginis Orchioidis
Yin Yang Huo	6g	Herba Epimedii
Yu Jin	6g	Tuber Curcumae

In the post-ovulation phase, building Kidney Yang, clearing Damp and invigorating Qi were emphasized.

Bai Zhu	12g	Rhizoma Atractylodis Macrocephalae
Cang Zhu	15g	Rhizoma Atractylodes
Fu Ling	12g	Sclerotium Poriae Cocos
Yin Yang Huo	9g	Herba Epimedii
Xian Mao	6g	Rhizoma Curculiginis Orchioidis
Xiang Fu	9g	Rhizoma Cyperi Rotundi
Mu Xiang	9g	Radix Saussureae seu Vladimiriae
Bai Shao	9g	Radix Paeoniae Lactiflorae
Shan Yao	9g	Radix Dioscorea Oppositae

As quickly as the 1st month of treatment, the fertile mucus increased and Helen's period pain and lower back pain disappeared. Her right-sided pain persisted but episodes did not come so often, or last so long. In the next 3 cycles, she ovulated well (Fig. 8.7).

On the third of these, she conceived. However, she still had a normal period (this is not unusual in ectopic pregnancies). Her pulses were abnormally full and her BBT remained high (Fig. 8.8).

The joy of a positive pregnancy test was dashed when she developed left-sided pain and an ultrasound showed a mass in the left tube and nothing in the uterus. The diagnosis was an ectopic pregnancy, which had miscarried. Helen took Sheng Hua Tang, which provoked the discharge of two large clots followed by fresh red blood, which stopped after a couple of days.

Helen was very despondent after this second loss of a pregnancy. I asked her to think seriously about trying IVF because the risk of another ectopic pregnancy was now very high. She was reluctant to pursue that option, so I referred her to a microsurgeon. He performed intricate and expert surgery to mend her scarred tubes and a few months later, she was pregnant again – this time in the right place, the uterus. Her pregnancy was uneventful. She gave birth to a large and healthy baby boy 9 months later.

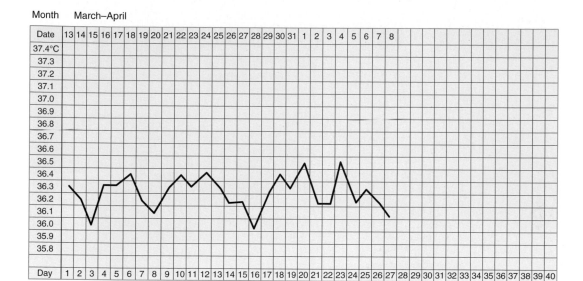

Figure 8.6 Case history – Helen. Some of Helen's BBT charts indicated that she was not ovulating.

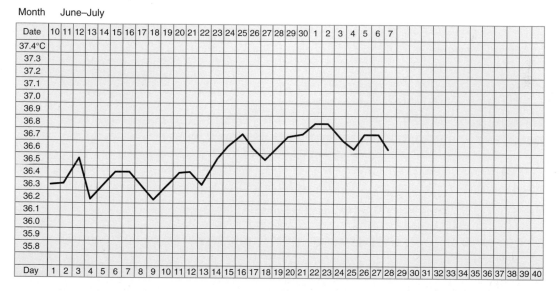

Figure 8.7 Case history – Helen. When Helen took Chinese herbs, the BBT pattern improved, indicating she was ovulating more regularly.

Other ectopic pregnancies

Other locations of ectopic pregnancies are more rare but can happen, e.g., an egg may be fertilized while still in the ovary and get stuck there. Surgical management usually means removal of the ovary; however, if treatment can be instituted early enough, the same approach as was used for tubal pregnancy can be taken. That is, herbs (or cytotoxic drugs) are used to kill the fetus, and encourage reabsorption of dead tissue. From the Chinese medicine practitioner's point of view, special attention will need to be paid to the ovary in future cycles, especially at ovulation time. Any scarring from the ectopic might cause Qi stagnation and ovulation pain. Stagnation of the Qi at ovulation time also raises the risk of inhibited release of the egg and another ectopic pregnancy.

327

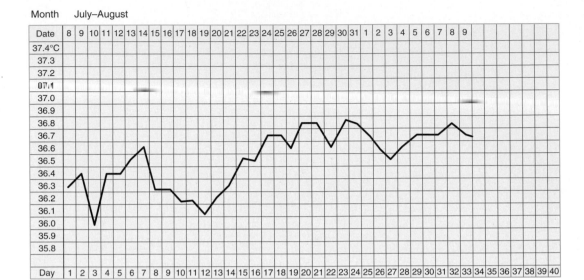

Month   July–August

Figure 8.8 Case history – Helen. Helen fell pregnant this cycle; the luteal phase was 21 days when she did the pregnancy test.

Rarely, an embryo will implant in the cervix and is very difficult to excise surgically because of the cervix's extensive blood supply. Once a diagnosis is sure (usually from a biopsy to distinguish it from malignancy), treatment may be attempted with cytotoxic drugs or Chinese herbs.

CONCLUSION

In summary, we should attempt to minimize the risk of pregnancy loss well before the pregnancy even starts. Preconception care can make a profound difference in the health and viability of the gametes. If women and men take the time and care to optimize their Kidney Qi (with appropriate lifestyle, diet, supplements, and herbs, etc.), then the gametes likewise will be in good shape. We know from previous discussions that good gametes make good embryos and that good embryos develop into good fetuses which tend not to miscarry. In the case that the mother is weak when she conceives and the pregnancy is thus at risk, even though the fetus is a viable one, Chinese medicine has relevant therapy to offer.

We can summarize an appropriate approach in the clinic when faced with a patient having a threatened miscarriage or suffers recurrent miscarriages. Ask yourself …

- Is the Kidney energy strong enough to hold and grow a pregnancy? It is especially Kidney Yang that is responsible for a warm womb, successful implantation and support of early pregnancy.

- Is the Spleen Qi adequate to hold the fetus in and up, hold the blood in the vessels and provide the essential nourishment in the early part of pregnancy that is crucial for everything that happens later in that child's life?

- Are there any signs or symptoms of Damp or Heat – this might be associated with autoimmune factors.

- Are there any signs or symptoms of Blood stasis, or a diagnosis of clotting factors associated with autoimmune or genetic factors.

- Finally, and very importantly, how is the Heart and the Shen? – Crucial for the integrity of the Bao vessel and the uterus and inevitably challenged in recurrent or threatened miscarriage.

Careful consideration of these questions will lead you to the best and correct treatment of the patient at risk of miscarriage.

1. Tong S, Kaur A, Walker SP, et al. Miscarriage risk for asymptomatic women after a normal first-trimester prenatal visit. *Obstet Gynecol* 2008;**111**:710–4.

2. Kleinhaus K, Perrin M, Friedlander Y, et al. Paternal age and spontaneous abortion. *Obstet Gynecol* 2006;**108**:369–77.

3. Slama R, Bouyer J, Windham G, et al. Influence of paternal age on the risk of spontaneous abortion. *Am J Epidemiol* 2005;**161**:816–23.

4. Belloc S, Cohen-Bacrie P, Benkhalifa M, et al. Effect of maternal and paternal age on pregnancy and miscarriage rates after intrauterine insemination. *Reprod Biomed Online* 2008;**17**(3):392–7.

5. Ford JH, MacCormack L, Hiller J. Pregnancy and lifestyle study. *Mut Res* 1994;**313**:153–64.

6. Ford JH, MacCormack L. Pregnancy and lifestyle study: the long-term use of the contraceptive pill and the risk of age-related miscarriage. *Hum Reprod* 1995;**10**:1397–402.

7. Oakeshott P, Hay P, Hay S, et al. Association between bacterial vaginosis or chlamydial infection and miscarriage before 16 weeks' gestation: prospective community based cohort study. *BMJ* 2002;**325**(7376):1334.

8. Florack EI, Zielhuis GA, Pellegrino JE, et al. Occupational physical activity and the occurrence of spontaneous abortion. *Int J Epidemiol* 1993;**22**(5):878–84.

9. Nielsen GL, Sørensen HT, Larsen H, et al. Risk of adverse birth outcome and miscarriage in pregnant users of non-steroidal anti-inflammatory drugs: population based observational study and case-control study. *BMJ* 2001;**322**:266–70.

10. Li DK, Liu L, Odouli R. Exposure to non-steroidal anti-inflammatory drugs during pregnancy and risk of miscarriage: population based cohort study. *BMJ* 2003;**327**(7411):368.

11. Li DK, Janevic T, Odouli R, et al. Hot tub use during pregnancy and the risk of miscarriage. *Am J Epidemiol* 2003;**158**(10):931–7.

12. Farrow A, Hull MG, Northstone K, et al. Prolonged use of oral contraception before a planned pregnancy is associated with a decreased risk of delayed conception. *Hum Reprod* 2002;**17**(10):2754–61.

13. Billings E, Westmore A. *The Billings method*. Melbourne: O'Donavan; 1998, 90.

14. García-Enguídanos A, Martínez D, Calle M, et al. Long-term use of oral contraceptives increases the risk of miscarriage. *Fertil Steril* 2005;**83**(6):1864–6.

15. Cowan B, Seifer D, editors. *Clinical reproductive medicine*. Philadelphia: Lippincott-Raven; 1997. p. 240.

16. Carp HJA, Toder V, Torchinsky A, et al. and the Recurrent Miscarriage Immunotherapy Trialists Group. Allogenic leucocyte immunization after five or more miscarriages. *Hum Reprod* 1997;**12**:250–5.

17. Teklenburg G, Salker M, Molokhia M, et al. Natural selection of human embryos: decidualizing endometrial stromal cells serve as sensors of embryo quality upon implantation. *PLoS One* 2010;**5**(4):e10258.

18. Salker M, Teklenburg G, Molokhia M, et al. Natural selection of human embryos: impaired decidualization of endometrium disables embryo-maternal interactions and causes recurrent pregnancy loss. *PLoS ONE* 2010;**5**(4):e10287.

19. Liu Ying, Wu Jing-zhi. Effect of Gutai decoction on the abortion rate of in vitro fertilization and embryo transfer. *Chin J Integr Med* 2006;**12**(3):189–93.

20. Li L, Dou LX, Neilson JP, et al. Adverse outcomes of Chinese medicines used for threatened miscarriage: a systematic review and meta-analysis. *Hum Reprod Update* 2012;**18**(5):504–24.

21. Cowan B, Seifer D, editors. *Clinical reproductive medicine*. Philadelphia: Lippincott-Raven; 1997. p. 242.

22. Jansen RPS. *Getting pregnant*. Sydney: Allen and Unwin; 2003, Chs 8 and 18.

23. Coulam CB, Roussev RG. Increasing circulating T-cell activation markers are linked to subsequent implantation failure after transfer of in vitro fertilized embryos. *Am J Reprod Immunol* 2003;**50**(4):340–5.

24. Miko E, Manfai Z, Meggyes M, et al. Possible role of natural killer and natural killer T-like cells in implantation failure after IVF. *Reprod BioMed Online* 2010;**21**:750–6.

25. Kaandorp SP, Goddijn M, van der Post JA, et al. Aspirin plus heparin or aspirin alone in women with recurrent miscarriage. *N Engl J Med* 2010;**362**(17):1586–96.

26. Chen L, Hu Renming. Thyroid autoimmunity and miscarriage. *Clin Endocrinol* 2011;**74**(4):513–9.

27. Toulis KA, Goulis DG, Venetis CA, et al. Risk of miscarriage in euthyroid women with thyroid autoimmunity undergoing IVF: a meta-analysis. *Eur J Endocrinol* 2010;**162**:643–52.

28. Song C, Halbreich U, Han C, et al. Imbalance between pro- and anti-inflammatory cytokines, and between Th1 and Th2 cytokines in depressed patients: the effect of electroacupuncture or fluoxetine treatment. *Pharmacopsychiatry* 2009;**42**(5):182–8.

329

29. Liu F, Luo SP. Effect of Chinese herbal treatment on Th1- and Th2-type cytokines, progesterone and beta-human chorionic gonadotropin in early pregnant women of threatened abortion. *Chin J Integr Med* 2009;**15**(5):353–8.

30. Zijlstra FJ, van den Berg-de Lange I, Huygen FJ, et al. Anti-inflammatory actions of acupuncture. *Med Inflamm* 2003;**12**(2):59–69.

31. Kim SK, Bae H. Acupuncture and immune modulation. *Auton Neurosci* 2010;**157**:38–41.

32. Gallinelli A, Roncaglia R, Matteo ML. Immunological changes and stress are associated with different implantation rates in patients undergoing in vitro fertilization–embryo transfer. *Fertil Steril* 2001;**76**(1):85–91.

33. Arranz L, Guayerbas N, Siboni L, et al. Effect of acupuncture treatment on the immune function impairment found in anxious women. *Am J Chin Med* 2007;**35**(1):35–51.

34. Cabioglu MT, Eren Cetin B. Acupuncture and immunomodulation. *Am J Chin Med* 2008;**36**:25–36.

35. Sharman MJ, Volek JS. Weight loss leads to reductions in inflammatory biomarkers after a very-low-carbohydrate diet and a low-fat diet in overweight men. *Clin Sci (Lond)* 2004;**107**:365–9.

36. Geber S, Paraschos T, Atkinson G, et al. Results of IVF in patients with endometriosis: the severity of the disease does not affect outcome, or the incidence of miscarriage. *Hum Reprod* 1995;**10**:1507–11.

37. Balen AH, Tan SL, MacDougall J, et al. Miscarriage rates following in-vitro fertilization are increased in women with polycystic ovaries and reduced by pituitary desensitization with buserelin. *Hum Reprod* 1993;**8**(6):959–64.

38. Lass A, Williams G, Abusheikha N, et al. The effect of endometrial polyps on outcomes of in vitro fertilization (IVF) cycles. *J Assist Reprod Genet* 1999;**16**:410–5.

39. Moley KH, Chil MM-Y, Knudson CM, et al. Hyperglycemia induces apoptosis in pre-implantation embryos through cell death effector pathways. *Nat Med* 1998;**4**(12):1421–4.

40. Ford JH. *It takes two*. Adelaide: Environmental and Genetic Solutions; 1997, 97.

41. Dinulovic D, Radonic G. Diabetes mellitus and male infertility. *Arch Androl* 1990;**25**:277–93.

42. Negro R, Schwartz A, Gismondi R, et al. Increased pregnancy loss rate in thyroid antibody negative women with TSH levels between 2. 5 and 5. 0 in the first trimester of pregnancy. *J Clin Endocrinol Metab* 2010;**95**:E44–8.

43. Anselmo J, Cao D, Karrison T, et al. Fetal loss associated with excess thyroid hormone exposure. *JAMA* 2004;**292**(6):691–5.

44. Cowan B, Seifer D, editors. *Clinical reproductive medicine*. Philadelphia: Lippincott-Raven; 1997. p. 243.

45. Buitrago JM, Diez LC. Thyroid disease affects semen quality. *Andrologia* 1987;**19**:37–41.

46. O'Morain C, Smethurst P, Dore CJ, et al. Reversible male infertility due to sulphasalazine: studies in man and rat. *Gut* 1984;**25**(10):1078–84.

47. Gasbarrini A, Torre ES, Trivellini C, et al. Recurrent spontaneous abortion and intrauterine fetal growth retardation as symptoms of coeliac disease. *Lancet* 2000;**356**(9227):399–400.

48. Naish F, Roberts J. *The natural way to better babies*. Sydney: Random House; 1996.

49. Hay P, Czeizel AE. Asymptomatic trichomonas and candida colonization and pregnancy outcome. *Best Pract Res Clin Obstet Gynaecol* 2007;**21**(3):403–9.

50. Smith G, Wood AM, Pell JP, et al. Recurrent miscarriage is associated with a family history of ischaemic heart disease: a retrospective cohort study. *BJOG* 2011;**118**:557–63.

51. Wang JX, Davies MJ, Norman RJ. Obesity increases the risk of spontaneous abortion during infertility treatment. *Obes Res* 2002;**10**(6):551.

52. Maconochie N, Doyle P, Prior S, et al. Risk factors for first trimester miscarriage – results from a UK-population-based case–control study. *BJOG* 2007;**114**(2):170–86.

53. Kumar S. Occupational, environmental and lifestyle factors associated with spontaneous abortion. *Reprod Sci* 2011;**18**(10):915–30.

54. Maconochie N, Doyle P, Prior S, et al. Risk factors for first trimester miscarriage – results from a UK-population-based case–control study. *BJOG* 2007;**114**(2):170–86.

55. Ford JH. *It takes two*. Adelaide: Environmental and Genetic Solutions; 1997, 73.

56. Valanis B, Vollmer WM, Steele P. Occupational exposure to antineoplastic agents: self-reported miscarriages and stillbirths among nurses and pharmacists. *J Occup Environ Med* 1999;**41**(8):632–8.

57. Lawson CC, Rocheleau CM, Whelan E, et al. Occupational exposures among nurses and risk of spontaneous abortion. *Am J Obstet Gynecol* 2012;**206**(4):327.

58. Shirangi AL, Fritschi L, Holman CD. Maternal occupational exposures and risk of spontaneous abortion in veterinary practice. *Occup Environ Med* 2008;**65**:719–25.

59. Gardella JR, Hill JA. Environmental toxins associated with recurrent pregnancy loss. *Semin Reprod Med* 2000;**18**:407–24.

60. Gerhard I, Waibel S, Daniel V, et al. Impact of heavy metals on hormonal and immunological factors in women with repeated miscarriages. *Hum Reprod Update* 1998;**4**(3):301–9.

61. Weng X, Odouli R, Li DK. Maternal caffeine consumption during pregnancy and the risk of miscarriage: a prospective cohort study. *Am J Obstet Gynecol* 2008;**198**(3):279.

62. Cnattingius S, Signorello L, Annerén G, et al. Caffeine intake and the risk of first-trimester spontaneous abortion. *N Engl J Med* 2000;**343**:1839–45.

63. Kline J, Shrout P, Stein Z, et al. Drinking during pregnancy and spontaneous abortion. *Lancet* 1980;**2**:176–80.

64. Hughes EG, Brennan BG. Does cigarette smoking impair natural or assisted fecundity?. *Fertil Steril* 1996;**66**:679–89.

65. Aisemberg J, Vercelli C, Wolfson M, et al. Inflammatory agents involved in septic miscarriage. *Neuroimmunomodulation* 2010;**17**:150–2.

66. Zinedine A, Soriano JM, Moltó JC, et al. Review on the toxicity, occurrence, metabolism, detoxification, regulations and intake of zearalenone: an oestrogenic mycotoxin. *Food Chem Toxicol* 2007;**45**(1):1–8.

67. Li DK, Odouli R, Wi S, et al. A population-based prospective cohort study of personal exposure to magnetic fields during pregnancy and the risk of miscarriage. *Epidemiology* 2002;**13**(1):9–20.

68. Webster J, Chandler J, Battistutta D. Pregnancy outcomes and health care use: effects of abuse. *Am J Obstet Gynecol* 1996;**174**:760–7.

69. Huang Zhi Ying. The relationship between mental work and threatened abortion. *J Huaihai Med* 2002(Issue 1).

70. Liddell HS, Pattison NS, Zanderigo A. Recurrent miscarriage – outcome after supportive care in early pregnancy. *Aust New Zealand J Obstet Gynaecol* 1991;**31**(4):320–2.

71. Wu RJ, Zhou FZ. Effect of Yangjing Zhongyu decoction on expression of insulin-like growth factor II and its receptor in endometrium of women with unexplained infertility. *Zhongguo Zhong Xi Yi Jie He Za Zhi* 2002;**22**(7):490–3.

72. Weixin Jin. *Diagnosis of sterility and its traditional Chinese medicine treatment*. : Shandong Science and Technology Press; 1999.

73. Ronald H, Gray RH, Simpson JL, et al. Timing of conception and the risk of spontaneous abortion among pregnancies occurring during the use of natural family planning. *Am J Obstet Gynecol* 1995;**172**:1567–72.

74. Ford JH. *It takes two*. Adelaide: Environmental and Genetic Solutions; 1997, 178.

SECTION 3

Combining Chinese And Western Medicine

Assisted reproduction technology and in vitro fertilization

9

Chapter Contents

INTRODUCTION

The previous chapters of this text have examined in detail the TCM approach to infertility as it is practiced in clinics in China (and increasingly in clinics in the West). Let us now look at how assisted reproduction technology (ART), and specifically in vitro fertilization (IVF), approaches the treatment of infertility, and see where the two modalities can complement or influence each other. ART is a term used to include a variety of medical procedures used to bring eggs and sperm together without sexual intercourse. IVF is the most common and technologically sophisticated of these procedures. We shall summarize the different options offered in specialist reproductive medicine clinics below.

IVF, so controversial in the quite recent past, has rapidly gained public acceptance and its jargon has become everyday language. The IVF clinic is now frequently the first port of call for many couples who do not become pregnant as quickly as they would like. The strident voices of ethicists and feminists and moral arbiters have been all but silenced by the overwhelming momentum of this science, which has grown rapidly to meet the demands of modern population groups with dwindling fertility.

In humans, most babies are born as a result of in vivo fertilization but 1% (and rising) of all babies in the Western world are born through ART. In some countries, the rate is even higher and in Australia, where infertility patients receive significant government reimbursement, IVF is responsible for approximately 3% of all live births.[1] Worldwide, IVF babies are numbered in their millions.

Social commentators have remarked that IVF could separate procreation and sex, in the way that the oral contraceptive pill separated sex and procreation in an earlier generation, a view shared by some IVF researchers who predict that in the future sex will be for fun, and IVF for procreation.[2]

In many countries, IVF is used more and more frequently by impatient couples who might not have significant fertility issues. One study done on nearly 1400 women between 28 and 36 with unexplained infertility, found that of those who pursued an ART solution, 53% had a baby, but so did 44% of the women who did not use ART.[3]

IVF STATISTICS

The reported success rates of assisted fertility treatment have edged upwards over the past 2 decades as new methods have been introduced and as techniques have improved. Ways of reporting success rates however, are far from standard.

Countries might report their IVF live birth rates as an overall figure, e.g., the national IVF live birth rate from all IVF cycles in Australia and NZ in 2009 was 17.2% per cycle.[4]

Or they may report birth rates according to the age range. For example, the national IVF live birth rate per cycle in the USA in 2009 was given as: 41.4% under age 35; 31.7% age 35–37; 22.3% ages 38–40; and 12.6% over age 41 (a significant percentage of these births were twins).[5]

Comparing individual IVF clinic's success rates is not always easy because of such inconsistency in methods of reporting. Clinics understandably want their statistics to look good and have found different ways of doing this. Some clinics might include all their IVF patients in their data but will then choose just one particular period of time for analysis. One clinic, for example,[6] gathered data on all the women who began IVF over a period of a few months in mid-2009, and reported that 3 years on, 65–70% of those under 38 years and 40–50% of those between 38 and 43 years, had a baby.

Other clinics might report figures for live births for only those women who have blastocysts (5-day old embryos) to transfer and give a cumulative number over a period of 2 years of attempts.[7] The birth rate when presented like this was 60–80% for women under 38 years of age, and 50–60% for women 38–43 years.

I am often asked: What is the success rate in treating infertility with traditional Chinese medicine (TCM) and how does it compare to in vitro fertilization (IVF)? This is not an easy question to answer. TCM treatment for infertility is a cumulative process; it is not a discrete monthly program, the success of which can be measured per attempt or per cycle. However, now that some IVF clinics report success rates over a period of years rather than per cycle, we can think about making more meaningful comparisons. Controlled clinical trials are not common because of the difficulty in applying control conditions and statistical analysis to Chinese medicine treatment outcomes and there is a paucity of funding. One review, which presents a meta-analysis of the few trials and cohort studies that have been published, found that Chinese herbal medicine improves pregnancy rates twofold within a 4-month period compared with fertility drug treatment or IVF.[8]

Considering all the above, I find that more and more, the treatment options offered to couples coming to my clinic with infertility problems embrace both what Chinese medicine and ART can offer. These two medical models make interesting stable mates and so we shall spend some time examining the different paradigms at work.

THE ART CLINIC

First, we shall examine just what exactly happens in an ART clinic, starting from the most simple to the most complex procedures. Some clinics offer procedures such as ovulation induction, which do not involve manipulation of the eggs and sperm to achieve fertilization without sex, and these are discussed elsewhere (see Ch. 5).

Box 9.1 summarizes the different techniques offered in the reproductive medicine clinic.

Artificial insemination (AI)

Before a couple attempts IVF, some reproductive medicine clinics will suggest less intrusive techniques such as ovulation tracking or ovulation induction accompanied by artificial insemination at the appropriate time. If ovulation is absent or irregular, then there are a number of different drug regimens that can be attempted (discussed in Ch. 5). If the sperm picture is not good, but not hopeless, then washing and sorting the sperm and

---

Box 9.1   Summary of techniques employed in an ART clinic

- AI (artificial insemination) also known as AID (artificial insemination by donor), AIH (artificial insemination by husband) or IUI (intrauterine insemination)
  + Controlled ovarian stimulation
- IVF (in vitro fertilization)
  ± Microsperm injection or ICSI (intracytoplasmic sperm injection)
  ± PGD or preimplantation genetic diagnosis

---

injecting the best of the bunch into the uterus close to the fallopian tubes at the time an egg is being released increases the chance of conception. Cycles of intrauterine insemination may or may not involve manipulation of the woman's hormones with drugs similar to those used in an IVF cycle (but in smaller doses) depending on the clinic and the woman's menstrual cycle history. Progress of follicle development is monitored with blood tests and ultrasounds to predict the day of ovulation. Pregnancy rates with these techniques are lower than with IVF and many patients will progress to IVF if they do not conceive after 3 or 4 rounds of AI.

In vitro fertilization (IVF)

IVF remains the most common protocol offered in an ART clinic.

The way most IVF programs proceed nowadays is explained below (summarized in Box 9.2).

Ovary stimulation

There are a few variations on the IVF theme. They are grouped into long or short cycles (summarized in Box 9.3). Except in the case of the 'natural' cycle, drugs are used to achieve what is a called a controlled hyper-stimulation of the ovaries.

Box 9.2   Steps in an IVF cycle

- The ovaries are hyper-stimulated with drugs to produce a number of ripe eggs
- These are collected by a needle inserted through the vaginal wall
- The eggs are placed in a Petri dish in a special medium and mixed with a sperm sample
- Embryologists monitor (or aid) the fertilization of the eggs and the development of any embryos over the next 3–5 days
- At 3 or 5 days, an embryo will be returned to the uterus
- Any remaining embryos will be frozen

Box 9.3   Different types of drug regimens used in IVF

- Long downregulated (agonist) cycle (± ICSI)
- Short (antagonist) cycle (± ICSI)
- Short (agonist) cycle (± ICSI)
- Natural cycle (± ICSI)

Choice of cycle type and drugs depends on the age of the woman and what she has already tried with or without success, or on the individual preference of the IVF doctor, or sometimes on what drugs are currently available or the subject of recent studies.

The long downregulated cycle has been the most popular method for stimulating multiple egg growth in the majority of IVF clinics for the past few decades. In some clinics, this is still the case, however the short downregulated cycle is now becoming a more common and popular regimen since drugs are taken for fewer days.

LONG DOWNREGULATED (AGONIST) CYCLE (± ICSI)

To persuade the ovaries to produce multiple eggs, the menstrual cycle must be manipulated. In the menstrual cycle, prior to IVF being performed, the woman is given 'downregulating' drugs. These are gonadotrophin-releasing hormone (GnRH) agonists (called Lucrin/Lupron (Luprorelin) injection or Synarel (Nafarelin) nasal spray), which prevent the pituitary gland from producing hormones and thus interfering with the programed effects of the stimulatory drugs. (See Box 9.4 for other drug names.)

The agonist drugs cause a flare of FSH and LH as they stimulate, then inhibit the pituitary gland.

Once a period comes, and a blood test shows that the natural hormone levels are at baseline, drugs to stimulate the follicles in the ovaries can be given. These follicle-stimulating hormone (FSH) preparations (Gonal-F or Puregon or Follistim) are given by injection.

You may remember from Chapter 2 that in a normal menstrual cycle, anywhere between 1 and 30 follicles (depending on age), known as recruits, will begin to develop under the influence of FSH. However, only one (occasionally two) of these developing follicles will become dominant and release an egg in response to the FSH that a woman produces naturally.

In an IVF cycle, administration of daily injections of FSH will keep the level of this hormone constant and high, and thus encourage more of the recruits to grow and develop into large follicles containing mature eggs that can be collected surgically.

No amount of administered FSH will stimulate more follicles than are available to be recruited however. Progress is monitored by blood tests to check the levels of estrogen produced by the growing follicles and by ultrasound to measure the size of these follicles. The duration of FSH administration is also important. The normal length of the follicular phase generally needs to be made available to the growing follicles, although occasionally eggs will ripen more or less rapidly. Ideally, it is approximately 10–14 days after the stimulating drugs are started that the follicles will be large enough and the eggs mature enough to be harvested.

SHORT (ANTAGONIST) CYCLE (± ICSI)

The short cycle is so called because it involves less drug use over fewer days. Thus, the drugs used to prevent the release of eggs from ripened follicles are introduced midway into the stimulation phase, rather than some time before it. Following the same principles as described above for the long downregulated cycle, multiple eggs are stimulated to develop by daily injections of FSH and after approximately 6 days of stimulation, the antagonist drug will be added to ensure that none of these follicles release their eggs.

Like the agonists, the GnRH antagonists are also used to stop the hypothalamus stimulating the pituitary to produce FSH and LH but they do it without first causing the flare of LH, meaning they can be used for a much shorter period of time.

The shorter time of drug administration and the need for fewer injections has meant that this type of IVF cycle has increased in popularity in most clinics. Long-acting FSH preparations, called Elonva (*corifollitropin alfa*) are the next step in markedly reducing numbers of injections.

SHORT (AGONIST) CYCLE (± ICSI)

This variation of the long 'downregulating' protocol is sometimes called a flare cycle. It is less commonly used than the above described cycles.

In the flare cycle, the GnRH agonist is administered from the start of the period (and the FSH begins the next day), and is continued up until the eggs are mature, to suppress ovulation. This is enough time to get past the initial LH surge that agonist causes. The supposed benefit of such an approach is that the agonist will also cause a surge of FSH from the pituitary, which augments the administered dosage of FSH, thereby synergizing the growth of ovarian follicles. But the LH surge at the beginning is not thought to be so good for older women (who might already have elevated LH), possibly spoiling optimal development of ovarian follicles.

The short cycles (antagonist or agonist) offer the opportunity to test the natural levels of the FSH produced by the pituitary before proceeding. Some clinics like to assess ovarian responsiveness with a blood test taken on the 1st day of the cycle. A low FSH (<10 IU/L) indicates that the ovarian reserve is adequate and that the follicles will likely be responsive to the drugs.

A high FSH level indicates poor ovarian response, in which case the patient may be recommended to wait for another month.

'NATURAL' CYCLE WITH NO SUPPRESSION

Sometimes, there are clinical situations where it is advantageous to use no drugs. Of course because few eggs are collected the advantage usually conferred by IVF (that of more chance of creating a good embryo because of more eggs) is lost. This approach may be chosen when there has been repeated failure to respond to the usual drug regimens or the patient has some intolerance to the drugs, particularly the suppressing drugs. In a 'natural' cycle, young women are given no drugs, while older women may be given FSH injections but no suppressing drugs will be employed. Careful tracking is needed and when the lead follicle is nearing maturity, the trigger injection is given and egg collection is scheduled for 34 h later (rather than the usual 36 h for regular IVF, just to be sure to catch the egg before it ovulates). This approach, although rare, is sometimes considered with premature menopause patients who have naturally high levels of circulating FSH.

Box 9.4   Some brand names of IVF medications

FSH – stimulates follicles to grow
- Gonal-F, Puregon, Follistim, Bravelle, Menopur, Repronex, Elonva – injections

GnRH Agonist – blocks pituitary from producing FSH or LH, after initial flare of these hormones
- Lupron, Lucrin, Buserelin – injections
- Synarel – nasal spray

GnRH Antagonist – blocks pituitary from producing FSH or LH
- Orgalutron, Cetrotide, Cetrorelix, Ganirelix – injections

hCG – trigger to prepare oocytes for collection
- Pregnyl, Ovidrel, Profasi, Novarel – injections

Progesterone – for luteal support after embryo transfer
- Progesterone – injection, pessaries
- Prometrium, Cyclogest – pessaries
- Prometrium, Utrogestan – capsules
- Crinone, Prochieve – gel

hCG for luteal support after embryo transfer
- Pregnyl – injection

Egg collection, oocyte pick-up (OPU)

Once ultrasounds indicate that there is a cohort of follicles all approaching an ideal 20 mm in size, a trigger injection of human chorionic gonadotrophin, hCG, which in these circumstances acts like the luteinizing hormone (LH) that provokes ovulation, is given to mature the eggs and prepare the follicles to release them. (Occasionally if there has been a history of ovarian hyperstimulation syndrome (see below), then a dose of an agonist such as Synarel will be used to supply the LH surge. But before they escape (close to 36 h after the trigger), a needle guided by the surgeon's hand will penetrate each follicle and gently extract it via the vagina. This is called oocyte pick-up or retrieval. In an ideal case, there will be plenty of eggs collected (5–10, sometimes more). The number varies and depends on some known factors such as age, and on some as yet unknown factors. The sperm (freshly donated in a private room often furnished with whisky and glossy 2D sex goddesses) are washed and sorted. Eggs meet sperm in a specially formulated medium in a Petri dish and (what's left of) nature takes its course – or not.

Once an egg is successfully penetrated by a sperm, an extraordinary and complex series of events takes place. The chromosomes of the egg and the chromosomes of the sperm line up, and if the fit is good a new potential life begins.

However, sometimes this stage needs a little bit of help from the embryologist.

Intracytoplasmic sperm injection

Intracytoplasmic sperm injection (ICSI) may be performed as part of either the long or the short protocols. This technique involves the injection of a sperm directly into the cytoplasm of a harvested egg using a very fine needle. ICSI is usually performed where the sperm are unable to fertilize the egg under their own steam, e.g., if the sperm count is very low, or the sperm are not very motile, or are affected by antibodies. It is a technique that can sometimes be used to help men whose semen contains no sperm, because of a congenital or infective blockage or after vasectomy (the sperm may be collected from further up the reproductive tract). Before ICSI, at best 5% of infertile men could be treated; with it, the potential for infertile men to father children has increased many fold. With ICSI, any man who produces sperm, even if the sperm are never ejaculated, or if the sperm-making cells in the testes are defective, or even if the sperm die before they get anywhere, can potentially become a father. The method has been so successful that some IVF clinics do not even bother with normal fertilization, but simply inject sperm into the egg, hoping for higher fertilization rates.

Some additional fine tuning can be added to the ICSI procedure. This includes choosing a sperm from those that bind to a substance called hyaluron (referred to as PICSI), since only mature and structurally sound sperm will bind to this substance. Some clinics are using very high magnification of sperm (7000 instead of 400 times), particularly when there is a finding of high DNA fragmentation, to improve choice of the best sperm for ICSI. This is sometimes referred to as MICSI.

It is now accepted (by many IVF doctors) that with the advent of ICSI, male infertility should be no impediment at all to conception. Some andrologists (and Chinese medicine practitioners and naturopaths), however, feel that the health and vitality of the sperm is something that can and should be addressed rather than circumnavigated. While most of the focus has been on the age and quality of the egg, there is also evidence that the age and quality of the sperm influences not only fertility but also the integrity of the embryo (see Ch. 7).

Once fertilization occurs successfully and an embryo forms, it will be incubated in carefully controlled conditions and if after 3–5 days the embryo is still alive and dividing, it is ready to be transferred back to the womb where it belongs.

Preimplantation genetic diagnosis

In the case of known inherited genetic disorders in the couple or their family, one last procedure remains before the embryo is transferred.

Some cells are removed from the embryo and are analyzed for chromosomal disorders. This technique, called preimplantation genetic diagnosis (PGD) can diagnose hundreds of different genetic disorders. Only those embryos that pass the screening will be available for transfer or freezing. PGD, which can now analyze all the chromosomes of an embryonic cell, is sometimes advised for older women who are at higher risk of having chromosomal abnormalities in their embryos or women who have had previous chromosomal abnormality in a pregnancy or repeated implantation failure or repeated pregnancy losses.

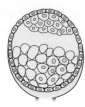

Figure 9.1 Day 3 and Day 5 embryos.

Embryo transfer

A fine plastic catheter that has been loaded with the chosen embryo/s, is passed through the cervix into the uterus. The deposited embryo is held snuggly by the front and back walls of the uterus. It cannot fall out.

Embryos will sometimes be transferred at 3 days of age, particularly if there are not so many of them. But in the case where there are several embryos to choose from, allowing them to grow longer permits the embryologist to see which embryos are the fittest (Fig. 9.1).

At the Morula stage, when the embryo is between 8–64 cells, it is not always easy to identify embryos with appropriate development potential. Approximately 40% of the embryos that look good on Day 3 will fail to progress to Day 5.

Embryos are able to develop to Day 3 using the maternal genomic drive. The embryo's genome (which is made up of both maternal and paternal genetic material) is not activated until after 3 days and if there is a chromosome problem in the embryo, then its development may slow down or stop at this point. Also, if the embryo lacks the necessary ability to make energy, it will have difficulty continuing to divide and create new cells.

At 5 days, the embryo is called a blastocyst and has a greater chance of survival after transfer than do younger embryos. Usually, one blastocyst is transferred through the cervix to the uterus (called blastocyst transfer or BT); any more and the risk of multiple pregnancy is too great. Some IVF clinics will try to increase their pregnancy statistics by transferring larger numbers, but doing so can seriously compromise the health of resulting pregnancies and babies if there are multiple conceptions.

Frozen embryo or cryoblastocyst transfer

When a number of oocytes are collected and successfully fertilized as part of a stimulated IVF cycle, the number of embryos produced may be well in excess of what can be transferred at the time. Those embryos not transferred back to the uterus can be frozen for future use when they will be defrosted a few hours before a carefully timed transfer to an early luteal phase uterus. In a frozen embryo transfer cycle there may be some drug manipulation of the woman's hormonal status, as in an IVF cycle, but less so. Estrogen may be prescribed to ensure the uterine lining thickens and, after the transfer, progesterone is given. But often there is a 'natural' cycle transfer, wherein no drugs are given but ovulation is tracked to correctly time the transfer. Some clinics find they get a higher pregnancy rate with fresh embryo transfers but studies have also found that pregnancies from frozen embryos have reduced miscarriage and complication rates,[9] and that frozen embryo cycles are better for endometriosis patients.[10]

Implantation

The success of the next stage, implantation, depends on the environment inside the uterus, the uterine lining and most importantly, on the embryo itself. If the embryo is strong and has its genetic programing up and running well, it will very likely succeed in implanting and continue to develop. As you may remember from Chapter 8, a majority of embryos do not have what it takes to go the long haul from egg and sperm chromosome line up to a fully viable pregnancy, because there is plenty of opportunity for chromosomal blunders in this completely new genetic blueprint. Current ART knowledge does not allow for predicting the genetic viability of a particular embryo by its appearance or the vigorousness of its cell division, so after transfer it becomes a nerve-wracking case of wait-and-see with fingers crossed.

Despite the fact there may be several of them, the corpus lutei, which are needed to provide progesterone for the next stage do not function. The use of the downregulating drugs prevents the production of LH which is needed to stimulate the corpus luteum. That plus the fact that when the eggs are aspirated from the follicles at OPU some of the cells which are needed to form the corpus luteum are also removed which means that the corpus lutei, will need some additional help from an external source of progesterone. Thus progesterone injections, pessaries or gel may be given at this stage, or two or three injections of hCG (which has a structure very similar to LH) may be given to boost corpus luteum function.

Ovarian hyperstimulation syndrome

Ovarian hyperstimulation syndrome (OHSS) is an iatrogenic complication of IVF, the pathogenesis of which is poorly understood. It occurs in the days following the injection of hCG given to trigger final egg maturation and preparation for collection and is exacerbated by further hCG injections given in the luteal phase or by pregnancy. Mild hyperstimulation occurs in up to 25% of IVF patients and moderate to severe in up to 5%.

The main symptoms are ovarian enlargement, ascites (caused by leakage of fluid from follicles, increased capillary permeability or rupture of follicles), and hypovolemia (decreased blood volume that can increase risk of thrombosis). In severe cases, the blood flow to the kidneys is reduced and urine output falls dramatically or ceases altogether. In very severe cases, there is leakage of fluid into the chest cavity, giving rise to shortness of breath.

Enlargement of the ovaries can cause abdominal pain, nausea, and vomiting. Increased intra-abdominal pressure due to extra fluid accumulating in the abdominal space causes distenion, discomfort and pain. Blood from ruptured cysts, protein-rich fluid, and inflammatory mediators can all cause peritoneal irritation contributing to abdominal pain. If the pain is very acute it may indicate ovarian torsion, rupture of cysts, or hemorrhage.

There are some warning signs that might occur during the medication phase of the IVF cycle (especially in women of young age, those with low body weight, or with polycystic ovarian syndrome, or those who have had previous episodes of hyperstimulation).

- A large number, i.e., 15–30, of intermediate sized follicles (10–14 mm)

- High estrogen levels; some women experience OHSS at E2 levels of 2000–5000 pg/mL but levels can rise to 40 000 pg/mL in extreme cases

- Early symptoms (e.g., abdominal bloating and discomfort, mild nausea, weight gain, edema, lethargy and diarrhea prior to OPU).

If OHSS is pronounced, then the embryo transfer will be delayed for a future date and any embryos will be frozen awaiting that future opportunity.

Some clinics will use a different trigger if there is a clear risk of OHSS. Lucrin or Lupron can be used instead of hCG to provide a surge of LH which prepares the oocytes for collection in women on short antagonist IVF cycles. Since the surge is short lived, hyperstimulation is less likely. Extra luteal support in the form of estrogen and progesterone will be added in these cases.

REFERENCES

1.   Australian Bureau of Statistics. *Catalogue no. 3301.0.* Sydney: ABS; 2007.
2.   Vajta G, Rienzi L, Cobo A, et al. Embryo culture: can we perform better than nature? *Reproductive BioMedicine Online* 2010;**20**(4):453–69.

3.   Herbert DL, Lucke JC, Dobson AJ. Birth outcomes after spontaneous or assisted conception among infertile Australian women aged 28 to 36 years: a prospective, population-based study. *Fertil Steril* 2012;**97**(3):630–8.

4.   Australian Institute of Health and Welfare. *Assisted reproductive technology in Australia and New Zealand* 2009 http://www.aihw.gov.au/publication-detail/?id=10737420465&tab=2.

5.   Society for Assisted Reproductive Technology. *IVF success rate reports.* http://www.sart.org/.

6.   Genea. *IVF success rates* 2012. http://www.genea.com.au/How-we-can-help/Our-Success/IVF-Success-Rates/Genea-IVF-Success-Rates.

7.   IVF Australia. *IVF Australia success rates* 2012 http://www.ivf.com.au/ivf-success-rates.aspx.

8.   Ried K, Stuart K. Efficacy of traditional Chinese herbal medicine in the management of female infertility: A systematic review. *Complement Ther Med* 2011;**19**(6):319–31.

9.   Kalra S, Ratcliffe SJ, Milman L, et al. Perinatal morbidity after in vitro fertilization is lower with frozen embryo transfer. *Fertil Steril* 2011;**95**(2):548–53.

10. Mohamed AM, Chouliaras S, Jones CJ, et al. Live birth rate in fresh and frozen embryo transfer cycles in women with endometriosis. *Eur J Obstet Gynecol Reprod Biol* 2011;**156**(2):177–80.

Assisted reproduction technology and traditional Chinese medicine

10

Chapter Contents

INFERTILITY PATIENTS AND THEIR TREATMENT NEEDS

Where does a couple looking for fertility treatment start?

Many patients will make their first appointment in the TCM (traditional Chinese medicine) clinic, based on their philosophical preferences and recommendations made by friends or the family doctor. Some patients will be wondering which is the correct approach for them. Is ART (assisted reproduction technology) or TCM better – For different types of patients? – For different types of infertility? – For different stages of infertility treatment? The answer is Yes on all counts and the advice given by the primary practitioner needs to be thoroughly informed (see Box 10.1).

The sort of treatments appropriate for patients who fall into the first four categories in Box 10.1 are those that we have discussed in the previous chapters. Patients who have had bad reactions to the drugs prescribed in ART clinics may need some rehabilitation, both physiologic in correcting the menstrual cycle, and emotional. Where there is Kidney weakness (which is the case for most functional infertility), Chong and Ren vessel function is vulnerable to disruption. What happens during an IVF cycle causes massive disruption to the natural function of the Chong and Ren vessels.

Where Kidney deficiency in the woman undergoing IVF is significant (this is the woman who is older, or who ovulates irregularly and poorly, who may have been trying to become pregnant for a long time), high doses of follicle stimulating drugs will be required to get a minimal response. Such high doses or repeated use can jeopardize what was already fragile ovary function, sometimes catastrophically. In the worst case scenario, menstrual cycles do not recover and a (peri)-menopausal pattern sets in.

For women in this category (men's Kidney energy is not challenged directly by IVF), the aim of treatment is to restore Kidney Yin and Yang function in a regular cyclical fashion. Applying the principles outlined in Chapter 4 is the correct approach; however, be prepared for a longer than usual period of Kidney Yin reinforcement. In addition, Liver and Heart Qi stagnation will always need addressing after a failed IVF cycle – in some women more than others.

It is the last group mentioned in Box 10.1, those couples who wish to try everything, who present some unique challenges in the clinic. The combining of Chinese medical therapy with IVF requires careful thought – and like all the ART techniques of the last few decades, some experimentation. This is an area ripe for research – already underway in many countries (see below).

Such a combination throws TCM into a cutting-edge modern medical arena, but the beauty of this oldest of all existing medical systems is that it is universally applicable and unceasingly flexible. Even if the patient is taking drugs that stop the pituitary gland dead in its tracks; is having surgical procedures to remove artificially ripened

---

Box 10.1   Different patients, different needs

Couples[a] who are having difficulty conceiving but are not yet ready to try IVF

Some of these patients become pregnant with the help of TCM, some move onto the ART clinic after a certain time.

Couples who want 'natural medicine'

Some couples who consult a TCM doctor do so because they have a philosophical attachment to the use of natural medicines and a fear of doctors, surgery, and drugs. In some cases, these couples have made a choice not to use ART because they are concerned about the possible risks to the baby. Many of these couples are committed to maintaining their own good health and are often well educated and informed. If their infertility is 'unexplained', then often TCM will uncover a possible cause, and because these patients are generally healthy, compliant and motivated, the results are often good. However, in some of these cases (e.g., tubal blockage or very low sperm count), it is just not in the best interests of the couple to rely on TCM when their only real hope of conception is to try and overcome their objections or fear and embrace sensibly the help modern medicine can offer. Often hearing such advice from a trusted TCM doctor – on the other side of the fence, so to speak – can help to break down fears, and referral to a compassionate specialist in ART is the next step.

Couples for whom IVF has failed or is not appropriate

This group constitutes a large proportion of patients seeking Chinese medicine treatment and includes women who:

- have completed three or more IVF cycles without success (most IVF successes are within the first 3 cycles)
- showed no response or a paradoxical response to the drugs used during IVF
- are over 43 (IVF success is rare in this age group, unless donor eggs are used).

Couples preparing for IVF

Some couples who are planning to use IVF, or to return to IVF after a break, wish to prepare themselves (and their gametes) by using a therapy that enhances their health in the hope of increasing chance of success.

Combining treatments

The last group of couples who seek TCM treatment for infertility are those who wish to try everything, usually all together!

---

[a] The term 'couple' here includes heterosexual and lesbian couples but also applies to single women using sperm donors.

gametes from their glandular homes; or is experiencing intense emotional stress, the doctor of Chinese medicine can still make a diagnosis incorporating all those factors and their effect on the body and mind, and can prescribe treatment which not only focuses on the particular imbalance but may also work with the medical interventions to make their results better and their side-effects less.

Referral to ART clinics is sometimes made too early and sometimes inappropriately. Some couples spend a lot of money and take unnecessary risks using drastic measures, when simple alternative methods could have been just as effective if they had been well enough informed to pursue them. Remember our patient in Chapter 1 with sharp corners? On the other hand, some patients pursue 'natural' therapies for too long, when their main or only chance of success is to use IVF.

We can put couples having difficulty falling pregnant into a number of different groups, according to their age and the cause of the infertility. Out of this, some generalizations and recommendations can be made (see Box 10.2).

Box 10.2　Choosing the right treatment

Major impediment to fertility – ART

Certain disorders leave open only one choice. For blocked tubes or very low (or absent) sperm counts, IVF is the best choice.

Minor impediment – young woman – TCM or other medicines

Minor impediment – older woman – ART or combination of ART/TCM

Relatively minor impediments to fertility (e.g., slightly low sperm counts, irregular ovulation, mild endometriosis and vague hormonal imbalances) tend to delay pregnancy rather than prevent it outright. Such factors can be treated with the less-invasive therapies first, e.g., nutritional regimens, TCM or clomifene.

Older women in this group might increase their chances of falling pregnant by using TCM, e.g., as preparation for or during ART procedures.

Combination of minor or undiagnosed factors – long-term infertility – TCM or ART

If a couple has been trying for a long time to have a child but there are no major pathologic factors in either party, it might be the combination of a number of minor factors all operating together that is preventing pregnancy. Statistical analysis tells us that two minor factors in combination can reduce fertility so dramatically that it can take on average 7 years to get pregnant; three minor factors in combination increase this disturbing figure to 40 years.[1]

The answer in allopathic medicine is not to treat the minor problems but to circumnavigate them and orchestrate the conception in the laboratory (IVF). You may remember from Chapter 1 that allopathic medicine expects that its treatment of major impediments to fertility (with drugs or surgery) will make a useful difference but that its treatment of minor or subtle factors may involve risks which outweigh the benefits.

The opposite applies to TCM: not only do subtle (and functional) problems respond better than major (and structural) abnormalities but also, because Chinese medicine views the body as a whole, a combination of subtle problems can be dealt with all at once. If the combination of factors all occur in one of the partners, e.g., a long irregular menstrual cycle, inadequate levels of luteal phase hormones and mild endometriosis – then chances are they will all be seen as manifestations or complications of the one primary imbalance. In the example above, the TCM doctor might diagnose 'Kidney Yin and Yang deficiency leading to Blood stasis'. One prescription can supplement Kidney Yin and Yang and regulate Blood (although the skilful doctor will emphasize different aspects at different times in the menstrual cycle).

Box 10.2   Choosing the right treatment—cont'd

If the combination of factors occurs in both of the partners, e.g., irregular periods and low sperm count, then both partners will need treatment.

No detectable abnormality – TCM

There is another situation where ART specialists advocate medical procedures to assist conception, and that is when, even though all the investigations show no abnormality no pregnancy is occurring. ART is usually recommended if the couple has failed to become pregnant over a certain length of time, e.g., ≥1 year. It is reasoned that time and chance have had more than enough opportunity to produce a pregnancy but the hurdle (even though it has no label) is clearly too big.[2]

Once again, this rationale does not apply to the TCM perspective. For example, if a woman has a Kidney Yin deficiency at age 29 years, it is more likely than not that she will still have a Kidney Yin deficiency at age 34, unless steps have been taken to address it. So her infertility persists, despite many years of trying to conceive. However, intervention to strengthen the Kidney Yin even after 5 years of attempting to become pregnant is a valid and often effective clinical approach before resorting to ART.

Some older women (38+) with unexplained (other than age-related) infertility may benefit from a combined approach of TCM and IVF in the hope that the lower IVF pregnancy rate of this age group can be lifted a little.

Table 10.1   Summary of treatment options

Cause of infertility	Approach to treatment
Major impediment	ART
Minor impediment	
Young woman	TCM, nutritional or lifestyle program, drugs
Older woman	ART plus TCM
Combination of more than one minor factor	TCM or ART
No abnormality diagnosed	TCM, nutritional or lifestyle program

A summary of these treatment options is given in Table 10.1. If at times there can be a serendipitous marriage between the two medical systems to achieve reasonably rapid and effective results, then we have found a happy solution. Infertility is an area where both Western and Chinese medical systems have strong, effective approaches and both have much to gain by listening to and using the strengths of the other.

COMPARING DIFFERENT INFERTILITY TREATMENTS

ART and TCM have such different approaches, philosophical underpinnings, and methods, that we might question whether they can in fact work together. But examining the context and comparing the approach, techniques and emphasis of these different types of treatment will afford us insights into ways they might best complement each other.

IVF and TCM – different approach

Traditional Chinese medicine is a medical therapeutic treatment and IVF is essentially a technologic strategy. IVF does involve drugs but they are not used in a therapeutic way, they are used to artificially stimulate many follicles

Table 10.2   IVF and TCM – different approach

IVF	TCM
Technological regimen	Therapeutic treatment
Sophisticated and involved	Basic and minimally invasive
Clinical personnel	Clinical personnel
Infertility specialist – drugs and surgery, pathology tests	Infertility specialist
Anesthetists – local or general anesthetics	Herbs and acupuncture
Nurses – injections and blood samples	Diet and lifestyle
Radiologists – ultrasounds	Exercise, Qi Gong
Embryologists – monitor fertilization and embryo development	Some pathology tests

to ripen – a process called controlled ovarian hyperstimulation. IVF does not look at the means to an end, it skips straight to the end. TCM can only work by improving or correcting the means (i.e., the Kidney deficiency, the Liver Qi stagnation, etc.), which hopefully leads to healthier gametes and healthier offspring. Table 10.2 outlines the different methodology and style inherent in these two approaches.

The IVF clinic is sophisticated and uses advanced technology such as ultrasound equipment, blood testing labs, surgical tools, microscopes, and incubators. The Chinese medicine clinic is equipped with herbs and needles, and often only two bits of machinery – scales and a battery operated stimulator for electroacupuncture.

An IVF clinic is staffed with large numbers of people with different roles, reflecting the complexity of the technology.

The TCM clinic is often just one specialist who prescribes and administers different sorts of treatment and recommends relevant lifestyle changes. Sometimes pathology tests are ordered; these won't necessarily change the treatment approach but they may indicate prognosis and progress.

IVF and TCM – different techniques

If we are to compare the philosophy behind the techniques used in these two medical models (see Table 10.3) the key feature is the holistic nature of TCM and the reductionist paradigm of modern medicine. In Western medicine, the mind and body are separated and the body is viewed, analyzed and treated as an entity which can be understood only by reducing it to its component parts. Such a Cartesian viewpoint, where we reduce the body to basic components separated from the whole, is nowhere so clearly shown as in IVF where the sperm and egg are put together outside the body in a dish in the laboratory.

TCM looks at, and treats, the whole body and mind – the patient feels better, fertility is improved but in some cases the treatment process may be too slow to meet the specific needs of the patient.

The risks of IVF are yet to be fully elucidated. The procedure at a few decades old, is relatively new. From the TCM doctor's point of view, it is the emphasis on quantity over quality that is the concern. The Kidney Jing, that hard-to-measure *quality* of inheritance, is ignored by IVF clinics. It may be some time before this risk, if it is real, can be fully assessed because large numbers of IVF babies have not yet tried to reproduce themselves.

Risks inherent in IVF to the mother include ovarian hyperstimulation syndrome and a higher frequency of pregnancy complications. An increased risk of developing non-invasive ovarian tumors has been shown in IVF patients.[3] Other risks to the woman doing IVF include ovarian hyperstimulation syndrome, and side-effects of the drugs including abdominal discomfort, fatigue, and headaches. Chinese medicine treatment, because it has been

Table 10.3   IVF and TCM — different techniques

IVF	TCM
Reductionist	Holistic
New	Time tested
Possible side-effects	Few side-effects
Some risk to mother and baby	No risk to mother or baby demonstrated
Quick acting	Slow acting

tested and filtered through many hundreds of years of close observation has few side-effects or risks. Occasional digestive upset (from herbs) or bruising (from acupuncture) may occur.

Risks to the baby include higher rates of premature delivery, low birth weight, neonatal or later morbidity and birth defects. Such hazards are more pronounced in cases of multiple pregnancies but still apparent in singletons conceived with IVF.[4–7]

It is thought that some of these risks may be due to the infertility itself rather than the ART procedures. From our point of view, if the infertility was related to poor Kidney Jing in the first place, it is not surprising that this may be visited upon the offspring. TCM treatment of Kidney deficiency related infertility only succeeds if the Kidney is bolstered such that conception occurs and proceeds to a viable pregnancy and healthy offspring. Of course the sort of research done on IVF babies has not been done on babies conceived with the help of Chinese medicine, so it is impossible to assess the validity of this assumption.

However, the type of infertility appears not to influence adverse outcomes, i.e., women who were doing IVF because they had blocked tubes or because of male factor infertility showed no difference in adverse perinatal outcomes from other women. This indicates that the increase in adverse outcomes is more likely to be due to the procedures themselves than to the infertility which leads to their use.[8]

There is also evidence that defects in IVF babies are due to imprinting or epigenetic effects, i.e., the process (mediated by DNA methylation and stable chromatin modifications) by which certain genes are switched off or kept active. We know that in those first few days of life, chemical pollutants, dietary components, temperature changes and other external stresses can exert long-lasting effects on development, metabolism, and health, sometimes even persisting in subsequent generations.[9–12] The impact of IVF culture medium and embryo manipulation is necessarily being closely examined in this context.

ART involves the manipulation of early embryos at a time when they may be particularly vulnerable to external disturbances. We know that environmental influences during embryonic and fetal development influence the individual's susceptibility to cardiovascular disease[13] and it appears that IVF children may indeed be at risk of vascular dysfunction similar in magnitude to that in children suffering from type 1 diabetes mellitus.[14] Angiomas appear to be more prevalent among IVF children.[15]

Intracytoplasmic sperm injection (ICSI), in particular, has some biologists worried. If sperm are unable to make it as far as the fallopian tubes to fertilize an egg, presumably they are substandard and are rightly being discriminated against by the heartless but necessary process of natural selection. Further, if the sperm collected in an IVF procedure and placed in a Petri dish with some eggs are still unable to carry out fertilization, their biologic credentials are further in doubt. In Chinese medicine terms, we would describe sperm that lack the necessary to carry out penetration and fertilization of egg cells as reflecting quite serious Kidney Jing deficiency. This is not a good thing to be visited upon the putative new life. Of course, if the Jing is so deficient that it is incompatible with life, then the stages of cleavage and division that should happen after the sperm is injected into the egg will not proceed.

These concerns about lack of Kidney Jing do not apply to the sperm collected from men who have had a vasectomy or have some other mechanical blockage. In this case, there is no reason to think that their essential vitality (or Kidney Jing) is in any way defective, and relying on the methods of ART may be the only hope they have for becoming fathers (or becoming fathers again). Similarly, the effects of infections or exposure to radiation or chemicals that are short term should not have lasting effects on the Kidney Jing.

The artificial insertion of the sperm into the egg cytoplasm can change the way the sperm chromosomes line-up with the egg chromosomes (especially the X chromosome),[16] and there is an increased risk of babies having a sex chromosome disorder if they are conceived after ICSI from a father with a very poor sperm count.[17] There are higher than normal rates of embryopathy after ICSI.[18] And a higher incidence of birth defects compared with IVF babies conceived without ICSI.[19] Overall, absolute numbers of babies born with birth defects in babies conceived using ART are small; less than 10%. Many of the birth defects are minor and can be corrected.

Other risks associated with ART concern the pregnancy itself. A retrospective study found significant increases in odds ratio for gestational hypertension, placenta previa, need for cesarean section, and pre-term birth in IVF (singleton) pregnancies.[20] ICSI appears to be related to a higher incidence of pre-term births and low birth weight babies.[21]

IVF is quick acting – a cycle is over in 4–6 weeks. However, not every IVF patient is pregnant in that time. Some IVF clinics have observed that if someone is going to get pregnant with IVF, they will most likely do so within 3 stimulated cycles.

On the other hand, improving the general health of the would-be parents and especially their gametes, can be quite a lengthy process, in particular the oocytes. It takes up to 9 months to nourish a follicle and its egg through all its stages of development from a nascent preantral stage. Sperm develop over a 3-month period and appear to respond quite rapidly to some treatment – some studies saw improvements after just 5 weeks of acupuncture treatment (see Ch. 7).

Typically, a treatment cycle with TCM that aims at improving the environment of the ovary and the eggs, might span 4–6 months or more, compared with the 4–6 weeks of a single IVF treatment cycle. TCM also aims to improve female fertility in other ways – specifically improving ovary function, regulating the menstrual cycle and balancing hormones. In this case, results can be seen more quickly, often around 3 months. In the case of relaxing the fine muscles of the fallopian tubes, the effect can be more immediate.

In summary, where TCM treatment of infertility is holistic, time tested and generally slow acting with few side-effects and little risk, IVF is specialized, relatively new and quick to get results but not without possible (though small) risk to mother and baby.

However, the results IVF achieves ensure that it is a technique which is here to stay. Most of the common criticisms made by patients about IVF (it is invasive, impersonal, experimental, and expensive) are compensated for by the fact that it provides results for a good number of the couples who use it. The price of any powerful and rapid medical protocol is the inherent risk involved (as we saw in Ch. 1).

IVF and TCM – different emphasis

The scope and emphasis of the two different sorts of treatments differ markedly. Table 10.4 summarizes this comparison.

No matter how each patient presents, the IVF protocol is pretty much the same. There will be minor variations in doses of ovary-stimulating drugs, and there will occasionally be variations on timing of administration. But use of different drugs is often dictated by what is new or available, rather than the specific needs of an individual patient. The expertise of the fertility specialist comes therefore not so much in changing the prescription or timing for the dose of one of the drugs but from the technical surgical skill required when removing tiny egg cells from the ovary and transferring fragile embryos back to the uterus. And it is the expertise of scientists and embryologists who work in laboratories developing ways of managing eggs, sperm and embryos when they are outside of the body that has brought with it increased success rates and new techniques.

Table 10.4   IVF and TCM – different emphasis

IVF	TCM
Quantity of eggs	Quality of eggs
ICSI	Number, shape and vitality of sperm
Thickness of endometrium	Quality of endometrium
Few protocol variations	Endless treatment variations

It is generally understood that IVF is essentially a numbers game – it increases the odds of success by increasing the numbers of eggs produced in a given month. This technique does not aim to affect the *quality* of the egg; rather it aims to increase the *quantity* of eggs, in the hope that in a large number, at least one will have what it takes.

The thickness of the lining of the uterus is the other factor measured by the radiographer. If it is inadequate, there is not much that the fertility specialist can do about it. If it is too thin (<6 mm), the transfer of any embryos may need to be postponed to a subsequent cycle in the hope that the endometrium might be adequate for a frozen embryo transfer.

The general health of the couple, in the absence of major pathology, is of minor concern. Whether the male partner has enough motile sperm is even becoming less important now in the days of ICSI. Sperm parameters will be measured but abnormalities are not treated (except for antioxidants in the case of DNA fragmentation) – they are circumnavigated with ICSI.

In contrast, Chinese medicine considers the overall health of the person (with special emphasis on Kidney Qi) who is making the gametes, based on the supposition that this will translate into healthier gametes. We know that the greatest determinant of a viable pregnancy is a viable embryo, which in turn depends largely on the fusion of healthy and compatible gametes. Unlike IVF, TCM treatment is not a numbers game. Treatment with Chinese medicine on its own does not usually increase the number of eggs ovulated. But it can influence some aspects of egg quality. This will be discussed below in detail when we look at TCM treatment for women preparing to do IVF.

In the clinic, we also use acupuncture to enhance release of the egg into and its journey down the fallopian tubes. In addition, TCM treatment aims to improve the fallopian tube environment and the endometrium thickness and quality. Chinese medicine can also influence the quality and vitality of the sperm.

The correct application of Chinese medicine in the treatment of infertility (as we saw in Ch. 4) is complex and demanding of its practitioners. Unlike the IVF treatment regimen, TCM has an endless number of variations – as numerous as the patients themselves. The skill of the TCM infertility specialist is in the correct diagnosis of subtle patterns of dysfunction, the correct prescription of herbs and their doses, the correct timing of the medicine, and the technical skill involved in applying acupuncture if that is part of the treatment program.

IN THE CLINIC – COMBINING TCM AND ART

Reputable texts of Chinese medicine can describe, with some authority, the presentation and treatment of different diseases and conditions based on some hundreds of years of observation and analysis by many generations of doctors working in clinics in China, refining and testing their protocols.

When it comes to treating patients using ART, none of us, here or in China, have more than a few years' experience, and while what we have to offer the ART patient is no doubt valid and useful, we are not yet at the stage where textbooks stating 'clinical truths' can be published.

Hence, we will broach some ideas based on TCM principles but acted upon a new clinical (and pathologic, in the broad sense of the word) condition, namely, the patient with 'controlled ovarian hyperstimulation'. However, we are not going to try and 'cure' this condition obviously, but we may try to enhance the 'pathologic process' and at the same time, contain it and protect the Zheng Qi of the patient. This is indeed new territory for a TCM doctor, and a different way of thinking.

Not only is this new treatment territory we find ourselves in, but also it may be a new clinical setting. Integrative medicine is one of the new frontiers many doctors are exploring and the combination of TCM and IVF is one of the stages it is being played out on increasingly. Driven by the demands of IVF patients, more IVF clinics are interested in working with acupuncturists and in some cases, are employing them.

The impetus for IVF patients to seek out acupuncture has its origins in some research published in 2002 that indicated that there was a small but significant increase in pregnancy rates if IVF patients had acupuncture on a certain day of their IVF treatment. The infertility chat rooms on the internet were soon full of this news. Since then, there has been more research, the results of which confirm this finding in some cases, or refute it in others. Hence, what claims can be made for acupuncture and TCM, what information is true and useful for IVF patients and indeed the place of acupuncture in the treatment of IVF patients in general, must be carefully assessed. It is contingent on all Chinese medicine practitioners to maintain vigilant and professional integrity in the face of demands from a particularly vulnerable and desperate section of the community.

TCM and IVF – points of influence

Before we talk in more detail about diagnosing and treating the IVF patient, let us recap the stages of an IVF treatment cycle and identify the points at which TCM may have a contribution to make. We have looked at the conceptual, philosophical, and practical differences between TCM and IVF. It is in fact these very differences that give the two methods the potential to skillfully complement or enhance each other's strengths. The contributions of TCM and IVF influence fertility at different times at different levels and in different ways.

Figure 10.1 shows the points of influence of the two medical systems and Box 10.3 describes more fully the relative usefulness of the IVF and TCM at different stages of the path toward a viable pregnancy. Seen this way, it appears there may be a convenient dovetailing of the complementary contributions of TCM and IVF.

Diagnosis of the IVF patient

Diagnosis of the IVF patient begins and continues the way all our patients are diagnosed. That is with a collection of signs and symptoms much as we described in Chapter 4. If your patient has already undergone one or more IVF cycles, then information from this will add to your repertoire of diagnostic tools. It is not

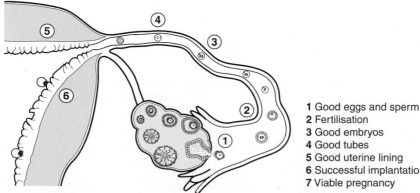

1 Good eggs and sperm
2 Fertilisation
3 Good embryos
4 Good tubes
5 Good uterine lining
6 Successful implantation
7 Viable pregnancy

Figure 10.1 The different points where IVF and TCM influence fertility.

Box 10.3   The different points where IVF and TCM influence fertility

Good eggs and good sperm – TCM is useful

This stage, the first one, is the most important stage of all. TCM doctors talk about the vitality and quality of the gametes in terms of Kidney Jing. Strong Kidney Jing makes for strong, healthy gametes. The way the eggs develop and the development and behavior of the sperm depend on Kidney Yin and Yang. These terms and what they mean in terms of treatment or intervention were all described in detail in Chapters 2 and 4. Chinese medicine can exert far-reaching influence on fertility at this point. We will discuss egg quality and TCM further below.

Improving sperm quality is a relatively accessible goal. Good nutrition with vitamin and antioxidant supplementation, avoidance of toxic chemicals and appropriate lifestyle changes already go a long way to helping sperm counts and motility. Acupuncture is effective in improving motility and morphology. If the couple is young, then using Chinese medicine over a period of time (up to 1 year) can usually help even very compromised sperm (see Ch. 7).

Fertilization – IVF is useful

Getting the sperm and the eggs together is what IVF techniques are all about – this is the second stage in Figure 10.1. In cases where there is a blockage in the tubes, or the sperm are unable to reach the egg under their own steam, IVF creates a solution. If sperm are unable to fertilize the egg, then ICSI is employed to create an embryo.

Good embryos – TCM is useful, but may also need IVF

The third stage is the early development of the embryo. This is a function of the quality of the sperm and egg, how they fuse and the compatibility of their genetic material. As such, both TCM, to improve quality of gametes, and IVF, to help the two get together, can contribute.

Good tubes – IVF circumnavigates (TCM has limited usefulness)

Good tubes are necessary for natural conception but not for IVF. Treatment by Chinese medicine aims to improve the elasticity, the secretions and the internal environment of the fallopian tubes, but for absolute obstructions, microsurgery is required or IVF can be employed to bypass the tubes altogether. Acupuncture is thought to be useful in facilitating movement in the tubes and preventing spasm of the fine muscles in the walls of the tubes.

Good uterine lining – TCM is useful

Studies during IVF procedures have shown that pre-ovulatory endometrium thickness and ultrasound appearance is predictive of embryo implantation rates. Less than 9 mm sagittal thickness and triple line appearance is associated with a reduction in live birth rate per embryo transfer. Women with poor endometrium development have a history of (thus far) unexplained IVF failure or early recurrent miscarriage. And for each millimeter decrease in endometrial thickness, there is a 12% relative increase in the risk of an adverse perinatal outcome.[22]

With Chinese medicine, we aim to increase the thickness and the quality of the lining of the uterus by building the Blood, Yin and Yang and promoting corpus luteal function in producing high levels of progesterone and increasing blood flow to the uterus.[23]

Implantation – TCM is useful

If the embryo is a viable one, and the stage and extent of development of the endometrium is correct, it is expected that implantation will proceed. Little influence can be exerted by ART at this stage, except ensuring that transfer of embryos is made at the right time and with the right instruments. Chinese herbs and acupuncture can influence blood flow and reduce contractions of the uterus. Studies have shown that

> ### Box 10.3 The different points where IVF and TCM influence fertility—cont'd
>
> acupuncture applied at the time of embryo transfer in an IVF procedure may improve implantation and pregnancy rates (we shall discuss this further below).
>
> **Viable pregnancy**
>
> If all the steps leading up to this stage have been successful, then in most cases the pregnancy will survive to produce a healthy baby. Chinese medicine is sometimes used in the early stages of pregnancy if there is any sign that the mother's body is weakening and a miscarriage threatens. At the later stages, Chinese medicine is used if the baby's growth is not optimal, and even later again, acupuncture will be employed if the baby is overdue or labor proves difficult.

uncommon for patients coming to a TCM clinic requesting treatment for infertility to have a history of unsuccessful IVF cycles.

IVF history – a new diagnostic factor

Some of the pertinent questions you will ask the patient who has a history of IVF attempts are listed in Box 10.4.

> ### Box 10.4 Questions we ask about IVF history
>
> - How many stimulated IVF cycles?
> - How many mature eggs collected? (Dose of FSH required?)
> - How many fertilized? (with ICSI?)
> - How many embryos viable on Day 3 and on Day 5?
> - How many transfers of 'fresh' embryos overall?
> - How many frozen embryos transferred overall?
> - How many pregnancies, biochemical or viable?

HOW MANY STIMULATED IVF CYCLES?

The number of cycles already attempted not only gives you some idea of how fertile or not this couple is, but also allows an assessment of Kidney Jing stores. If a woman has completed a large number of cycles (≥5), especially if these have been over a short period of time, then it is likely her reserves will be depleted. Further evidence for this will be gleaned by the answers to the questions below.

HOW MANY MATURE EGGS COLLECTED? (DOSE OF FSH REQUIRED?)

A good response to the FSH drugs and plenty of ripe follicles with plenty of eggs collected indicates good Kidney Jing. Few eggs or high doses of FSH drugs imply depleted Kidney Jing (i.e., the pool of follicles available for recruitment is small). If a patient has done a number of IVF cycles it is useful to note how the response to the FSH drugs changes over time. If there is a trend to reduced numbers of eggs with repeated cycles, or a trend to higher FSH doses, then the depletion of Kidney Jing is being accelerated by the IVF process itself (or by aging). However, if egg numbers remain reasonably steady with repeated cycles and the dose of FSH administered does not rise, then ovarian reserve and resilience is good and the reason for the infertility is likely something other than poor egg quality or low Kidney Jing.

HOW MANY EGGS FERTILIZED? (WITH ICSI?)

This information gives us an indication of the maturity or quality of the eggs, as well as of the sperm function. If the eggs collected are immature, then some factor important to their development is lacking, likely the Kidney Yin or Jing.

If ICSI is required, then it usually indicates that sperm function is poor, although it should be noted that some clinics do ICSI routinely, whether there is a male factor or not.

HOW MANY EMBRYOS VIABLE ON DAY 3 AND ON DAY 5?

How the embryos develop tells us a lot about the energy of the eggs. As we discussed in Chapter 4, it is the egg cells that must provide the capacity to make the energy to drive the first few days of embryo cell division. If the egg is defective or has inadequate vitality, then the embryos will not develop past Day 3. This is an indication of low Kidney Jing or Yin or Yang. Or, since the genome of the embryo, made up of both mother's and father's chromosomes, must control growth after Day 3, sperm defects may also manifest at this stage.

HOW MANY TRANSFERS OF EMBRYOS IN TOTAL?

If a significant number of embryos (especially if they are blastocysts) has been transferred without a viable pregnancy eventuating, it is possible that there may be an issue with implantation. In this case, we turn our attention to the endometrium and look closely at any issues (such as immune factors) that might impact there – Blood or Yin deficiency, Blood stagnation or internal Heat can all contribute.

HOW MANY PREGNANCIES (BIOCHEMICAL OR VIABLE) AND MISCARRIAGES?

This information likewise tells about the success of implantation. Frequent early stage miscarriage indicates the possibility of immune factors rejecting the embryo, or some other failure of implantation or placentation. Once again, we need to look closely at Blood stasis or internal Heat, but also at Kidney Yang deficiency.

IVF history and TCM diagnosis

Let us now revisit our diagnostic categories relating to causes of infertility and include the information we get from the patient who has completed one or more IVF cycles.

Each of the diagnoses in Box 10.5 is characterized by symptoms and signs that we became familiar with in Chapter 4. For patients who have undergone IVF treatment, we can expand those characteristics. Women of different constitutions will react differently to different aspects of the IVF process. Symptoms or signs manifesting during, or related to the IVF cycle. As discussed in Chapter 4, it is important to realize that these categories are slightly contrived in the sense that they seldom occur in isolation. Real life means that they more often appear in crossover and mixed patterns. However, starting with discrete patterns like this, and describing some predictable responses to IVF treatments within the context of these patterns, gives us the manageable base from which we then create our diagnoses with the flexibility that clinical situations require.

Box 10.5   **Female functional infertility diagnoses**

- Insufficient Kidney Jing
- Insufficient Kidney Yin
- Insufficient Kidney Yang
- Heart Qi stagnation
- Liver Qi stagnation
- Blood stagnation
- Phlegm-Damp accumulation

INSUFFICIENT KIDNEY JING

SIGNS OF INSUFFICIENT KIDNEY JING

- Underdeveloped sexual characteristics
- Late puberty, irregular cycles, amenorrhea
- Constitutional weakness
- BBT shows no pattern
- Low AMH
- Ovaries not responsive to FSH drugs, estrogen levels slow to rise
- Poor egg quality, few embryos
- Long recovery time for ovaries after IVF.

Women who are constitutionally Kidney Jing deficient tend to be frail and in more marked or obvious cases will have small hips and breasts and possibly small underactive ovaries. This woman likely started menstruating quite late and may have an irregular cycle. Her BBT charts may not show clear development of Kidney Yin to Kidney Yang in the luteal phase. Women in this category are born with low ovarian reserve. This may be related to genetic factors or factors operating during her mother's pregnancy or in early infancy or childhood.

When such a woman is given FSH drugs, the blood tests will not show rapidly rising estrogen levels, indicating a poor response from the ovaries. In these cases, the FSH drugs may need to be continued longer than usual. If eggs are harvested, there are usually low numbers and egg quality is not optimal.

(*Note* Kidney Jing deficiency that is not constitutional but due to damage and depletion is also a common cause of infertility and poor response to IVF drugs, however the constitutional signs described above may not present in this case).

INSUFFICIENT KIDNEY YIN

SIGNS OF INSUFFICIENT KIDNEY YIN

- Long or short menstrual cycles
- Scanty fertile mucus
- Scanty period flow
- Restless and anxious
- BBT long or short follicular phase
- High FSH, low AMH
- Poor response to IVF drugs, low estrogen levels
- Thin endometrium
- Poor egg quality, few embryos
- Long recovery time for ovaries after drug stimulation.

This is the most common diagnosis seen in infertility clinics in the West. Women in their late 30s and early 40s who are peri-menopausal often fall into this category. Their menstrual cycles may have subtly shortened if the Yin deficiency has given rise to some internal Heat, and this may also be manifesting in nervous system symptoms, such as disturbed sleep and anxiety.

If the Yin deficiency is accompanied by, or has led to, Blood deficiency, the menstrual cycles may be longer than 28 days and the flow may become scanty. Scanty and dark flow can also be a result of internal Heat arising from Yin deficiency.

When Yin and Blood are lacking, the endometrium will not develop well and ultrasounds will show a thin lining (<10 mm at time of egg collection).

As in the previous category, the administration of FSH drugs may need to be extended and doses may need to be increased if the ovaries are not responding. These women do not produce large numbers of eggs and those they do produce are not always of good quality. Side-effects such as flushing or anxiety or irritability are possible. Hyperstimulation is unlikely in this category.

After an unsuccessful IVF cycle, the ovaries may take some time to recover as Yin and Blood stores are gradually replenished and the Chong vessel refills.

Some women with immune factors contributing to infertility may fall into this category.

INSUFFICIENT KIDNEY YANG

SIGNS OF INSUFFICIENT KIDNEY YANG

- Short menstrual cycle, luteal phase defect
- Low libido, motivation
- Lethargy, slow metabolism
- Low back pain with period
- Menstrual flow, with tissue fragments
- BBT low or short luteal phase
- Low progesterone in mid-luteal phase
- Slow embryo growth in vitro, fewer blastocysts
- Fatigue and/or depression during IVF
- Biochemical pregnancies or early miscarriages.

You may have diagnosed this patient with a Kidney Yang deficiency before she embarked on IVF, if her BBT charts had indicated a short luteal phase. Women with Yang deficiency tend to be lethargic, and this can be exacerbated markedly by drugs used during the IVF cycle. Depression or low mood may accompany the fatigue. While egg numbers may be adequate, often these do not make embryos that make it to blastocyst stage. Embryos may be transferred on Day 3 but implantation or sustained growth of the embryo may fail in these cases, resulting in a negative HCG test or a biochemical pregnancy (very low HCG). Women with untreated Kidney Yang deficiency who do conceive, are less able to support early stage pregnancy and may need more progesterone supplementation (or Kidney Yang herbs).

HEART QI STAGNATION

SIGNS OF HEART QI STAGNATION

- Irregular or no ovulation
- Recent or historical emotional factors
- Pituitary/hypothalamus dysfunction
- Anxiety, insomnia, palpitations
- BBT unstable, especially follicular phase
- Early miscarriage
- Emotional lability during IVF, low resilience
- Few IVF cycles.

Some forms of amenorrhea fall into this category (as seen in Ch. 5) but Heart Qi stagnation does not always disturb the menstrual cycle. The most common symptom confirming this diagnosis will be anxiety, insomnia, or palpitations. Women with instability of the Shen find doing IVF very emotionally taxing, and hence do not often cope with more than 1 or 2 cycles.

If there is no Kidney factor, then numbers of eggs and embryos are expected to be adequate. These women gain enormous benefit from acupuncture support during the IVF cycle, although there will still inevitably be some emotional cost. Where pregnancy does occur, this group of women will be strongly advised to continue acupuncture for the 1st trimester, to ensure the Shen is stable, the Bao and Luo mai are secured and the uterus stays closed.

LIVER QI STAGNATION

SIGNS OF LIVER QI STAGNATION

- Irregular periods
- Ovulation pain, delayed ovulation
- Premenstrual syndrome
- Fallopian tube constriction
- Prone to frustration and irritability
- BBT unstable, especially luteal phase
- Abdominal pain and swelling during IVF
- Emotional volatility, headaches during IVF.

Liver Qi stagnation is not such a common cause of infertility on its own, and where it is, it is a pattern that is easily rectified with Chinese medicine. However, the impatient manner that women with Liver Qi stagnation exhibit often takes them to the IVF clinic prematurely. In the absence of any other pathology, egg and embryo quality is not of concern.

They tend to suffer side-effects such as headaches, abdomen discomfort and bloating, and irritability. There is a slightly increased risk of ovarian hyperstimulation syndrome with these patients, especially if they have been diagnosed with PCOS. Acupuncture during the IVF cycle is useful for these patients to reduce stress and ease side-effects.

BLOOD STAGNATION

SIGNS OF BLOOD STAGNATION

- Chong vessel not filled and emptied smoothly
- Endometrium uneven, clotty period flow, spotting
- Heart function (and circulation) compromised
- Polyps, fibroids, tumors, endometriosis
- Blocked tubes, ovarian cysts, pituitary tumors
- Pain
- Immune factors – implantation/placentation failure
- Poor egg quality, few embryos.

Blood stagnation is a reasonably common pattern seen in the IVF clinics. In fact, IVF was initially designed for patients with blocked tubes (which is one form Blood stagnation can take). Most other forms of substantial Blood stagnation, such as endometriosis, polyps, cysts, and large fibroids will be dealt with surgically before IVF is attempted. More subtle Blood stagnation in the form of immune or clotting factors will be treated with blood thinning medications and Chinese herbs. Blood stagnation, as we saw in Chapter 5, and shall see below, appears to have deleterious effects on egg quality.

PHLEGM-DAMP

SIGNS OF PHLEGM-DAMP

- Cysts, including polycystic ovarian syndrome
- Blocked tubes, pituitary tumor
- Vaginal discharge, no fertile mucus
- Overweight
- Periods may be irregular, with thick or mucusy flow
- Persistent weight gain after IVF
- Bloating and abdomen discomfort during IVF
- Large numbers of follicles during IVF (may be immature).

Women with Phlegm-Damp can have a difficult time with IVF, becoming lethargic and easily putting on weight, which is hard to move after the IVF cycle, whether they have conceived or not. These patients feel quite uncomfortable during IVF and acupuncture is useful for relief.

Patients diagnosed with PCOS often fall into this category and they are at increased risk of ovarian hyperstimulation syndrome. Large numbers of eggs may be retrieved but in these circumstances, they are not generally of good quality.

In summary, most of these categories of infertility benefit from TCM treatment prior to attending the IVF clinic, and some benefit greatly from treatment during the IVF cycle. Treatment of the IVF patient before and during the cycle is discussed in Chapter 11.

REFERENCES

1. Jansen R. *Getting pregnant*. Sydney: Allen and Unwin; 2003, 391.

2. Jansen R. *Getting pregnant*. Sydney: Allen and Unwin; 2003, 389.

3. van Leeuwen FE, Klip H, Mooij TM, et al. Risk of borderline and invasive ovarian tumors after ovarian stimulation for in vitro fertilization in a large Dutch cohort. *Hum Reprod* 2011;**26**(12):3456–65.

4. Finnström O, Källén B, Lindam A, et al. Maternal and child outcome after in vitro fertilization – a review of 25 years of population-based data from Sweden. *Acta Obstet Gynecol Scand* 2011;**90**:494–500.

5. Klemetti R, Gissler M, Sevón T, et al. Children born after assisted fertilization have an increased rate of major congenital anomalies. *Fertil Steril* 2005;**84**(5):1300–7.

6. Olson CK, Keppler-Noreuil KM, Romitti PA, et al. In vitro fertilization is associated with an increase in major birth defects. *Fertil Steril* 2005;**84**(5):1308–15.

7. Reefhuis J, Honein MA, Schieve LA, et al. and the National Birth Defects Prevention Study. Assisted reproductive technology and major structural birth defects in the United States. *Hum Reprod* 2009;**24**(2):360–6.

8. Chung K, Coutifaris C, Chalian R, et al. Factors influencing adverse perinatal outcomes in pregnancies achieved through use of in vitro fertilization. *Fertil Steril* 2006;**86**(6):1634–41.

9. Feil R, Fraga MF. Epigenetics and the environment: emerging patterns and implications. *Nat Rev Genet* 2012;**13**:97–109.

10. Maher ER. Imprinting and assisted reproductive technology. *Hum Mol Genet* 2005;**14**:133–8.

11. Maher ER, Brueton LA, Bowdin SC. Beckwith-Wiedemann syndrome and assisted reproduction technology (ART). *J Med Genet* 2003;**40**:62–4.

12. Ludwig M, Katalinic A, Gross S. Increased prevalence of imprinting defects in patients with Angelman syndrome born to subfertile couples. *J Med Genet* 2005;**42**:289–91.

13. Barker DJ. The origins of the developmental origins theory. *J Intern Med* 2007;**261**:412–7.

14. Scherrer U, Rimoldi SF, Rexhaj E, et al. Systemic and pulmonary vascular dysfunction in children conceived by assisted reproductive technologies. *Circulation* 2012;**125**:1890–6.

15. Viot G, Epelboin S, Olivennes F. Is there an increased risk of congenital malformations after ART? Results from a prospective French long-term survey of a cohort of 15162 children. *Hum Reprod* 2010;**25**(Suppl 1):i53–5.

16. Terada Y, Luetjens CM, Sutovsky P, et al. Atypical decondensation of the sperm nucleus, delayed replication of the male genome, and sex chromosome positioning following intracytoplasmic human sperm injection (ICSI) into golden hamster eggs: does ICSI itself introduce chromosomal anomalies?. *Fertil Steril* 2000;**74**(3):454–60.

17. Jansen R. *Getting pregnant*. Sydney: Allen and Unwin; 2003, 149.

18. Lathi RB, Milki AA. Rate of aneuploidy in miscarriages following in vitro fertilization and intracytoplasmic sperm injection. *Fertil Steril* 2004;**81**:1270–2.

19. Davies MJ, Moore VM, Willson KJ, et al. Reproductive technologies and the risk of birth defects. *N Engl J Med* 2012;**366**:1803–13.

20. Poikkeus P, Gissler M, Unkila-Kallio L, et al. Obstetric and neonatal outcome after single embryo transfer. *Hum Reprod* 2007;**22**:1073–9.

21. Aytoz A, Camus M, Tournaye H, et al. Outcome of pregnancies after intracytoplasmic sperm injection and the effect of sperm origin and quality on this outcome. *Fertil Steril* 1998;**70**:500–5.

22. Chung K, Coutifaris C, Chalian R, et al. Factors influencing adverse perinatal outcomes in pregnancies achieved through use of in vitro fertilization. *Fertil Steril* 2006;**86**(6):1634–41.

23. Stener-Victorin E, Waldenstrom U, Andersson SA, et al. Reduction of blood flow impedance in the uterine arteries of infertile women with electro-acupuncture. *Hum Reprod* 1996;**11**:1314–7.

Traditional Chinese medicine treatment of the IVF patient

11

Chapter Contents

USING TCM IN PREPARATION FOR AN IVF CYCLE

Once a full TCM diagnosis of the cause of infertility or other conditions is made, we follow the protocols outlined in detail in Chapter 4.

In an ideal situation, 6–9 months of ovary 'make over' is advisable. This allows time to remove factors that might be toxic to ovary and uterine health, like internal Heat or Damp, stagnant Blood (such as is found in endometriosis, PCOS, pelvic inflammatory disease, etc.), and includes identifying and avoiding workplace and domestic pollutants and lifestyle changes such as optimizing good diet and minimizing certain dietary 'indiscretions'. It is also an appropriate period of time over which Kidney Jing can be replenished with herbs and the function of Kidney Yin and Yang can be improved with tonics for the Yin, Yang, Qi and blood. This will not increase the number of eggs in the ovaries but well nourished eggs in a balanced hormonal environment can be more responsive to stimulation by FSH from the pituitary or the pharmacist's EpiPen. However, it is rare that a patient who has reached the point of considering IVF, or doing further IVF, will be in a position to spend 9 months doing this sort of preparation. Often, anything is better than nothing, and I try to persuade patients to consider at least 3 months of preparation before starting IVF (again).

Some women who are not infertile but are doing IVF due to male factor infertility will choose to use TCM treatment to prepare their body for optimal outcomes. A diagnosis is done in the usual way, considering the constitution and any symptoms. But additionally, we are mindful of increasing ovarian resilience and response by boosting Kidney function, and will also be mindful of clearing any signs of stagnation in the uterus. It is usually the case that a shorter preparation time is necessary for these women, unless there are significant general health issues.

Our approach to treatment of women with infertility will be according to the four categories of infertility we have previously described (Kidney deficiency, Liver/Heart Qi stagnation, Blood stagnation, Phlegm-Damp obstruction). We shall discuss each of these categories and describe a simplified approach to treatment with herbs that can be undertaken in the weeks or months leading up to IVF.

Kidney deficiency (and egg quality)

A large number of the women seeking help for infertility from the Chinese medicine clinic and the IVF clinic fall into a Kidney deficient category. These are often women in their late 30s and early 40s, or those who are depleted by overwork. If they have already attempted some IVF cycles they will often have heard from their specialist that their egg quality is not so good.

Egg quality is something mentioned in hallowed terms in IVF clinics because it is somewhat unfathomable and seemingly beyond the influence of the IVF specialists or scientists. Some ovaries age more quickly than others and unfortunately, neither acupuncture nor Chinese herbs (nor much else) can increase the number of eggs left in the ovary or change the integrity of the chromosomes. Nobody, not even the most skilled doctor, can improve the genetic quality of an 'old' egg because its genetic material was created decades earlier, when the woman was an embryo herself, and it has been subject to the relentless cellular wear and tear of decades. However, there is more to an egg than just its DNA and it is in consideration of its other components that we hope to apply some influence.

The environment that eggs occupy during their lengthy maturation process inside the follicles of the ovary has an impact on what shape they are in before meeting a sperm (with or without an IVF embryologist in attendance). They need a good blood supply, sufficient oxygen, adequate amounts of the right nutrients, the right hormone signals and the capacity to supply enough energy to the embryo.

This has important implications, particularly for eggs that are coming from slightly older ovaries (or where AMH levels are low or FSH levels are elevated) and possibly for eggs coming from women with PCOS or endometriosis.

The question is, can Chinese medicine be used to rejuvenate some oocyte characteristics by improving delivery of oxygen and nutrition to the developing egg and enhancing capacity to make energy (ATP), thus increasing the chances of making viable embryos? There is evidence to say that it can.

Research has shown that eggs that come from follicles with optimal blood supply and oxygen content have higher fertilization rates and developmental potential leading to improved IVF outcomes.[1]

The blood supply to the follicles in older ovaries is reduced at the later stages of their development, meaning that these eggs do not receive optimal oxygen or nutrition,[2] which may be a contributing factor to the poor quality of older eggs. Unlike chromosomal integrity, this *is* something we can influence.

Acupuncture has been shown to promote the growth of new blood vessels (angiogenesis)[3] and to specifically increase blood flow to the ovaries.[4]

In summary, we could say that the use of certain acupuncture point combinations, stimulated with a gentle electrical pulse can promote blood supply, and delivery of nutrition and oxygen to the follicles and therefore hope to improve their potential to fertilize and create embryos. Another way we may be able to improve egg quality is by improving the egg's capacity to make energy so that it can impart this enhanced capacity onto an embryo after fertilization. The organelles in the cytoplasm of the oocyte, called the mitochondria, have been identified as possible markers for egg and embryo quality. These powerhouses of the cell, which are donated from the egg to the embryo, are responsible for providing energy for cell division and metabolism in a process called aerobic respiration.

Those oocytes that consume more oxygen before fertilization (i.e., have more active aerobic respiration), are the ones which form better quality embryos.[5]

The early pre-implantation embryo occupies a low oxygen environment (the fallopian tube or the Petri dish in the IVF lab) and relies on anaerobic as well as aerobic respiration. By the time the embryo reaches the uterus (Day 5 or 6), it needs not only good numbers of mitochondria but optimal mitochondrial function and ATP production via aerobic respiration to succeed in implanting.[6]

It is at this level that Chinese medicine hopes to exert some beneficial influence by ensuring the number and activity of the mitochondria in the ripening eggs is optimal. We know that eggs with more energy (ATP) have a better chance of making viable embryos and that the rate of division and successful implantation of embryos has more to do with how much energy they have than with maternal age. However, the mitochondria of older eggs are not so good at producing ATP[7] and the eggs of poor responders to IVF drugs have three times less mitochondria than those of good responders.[8]

Similarly, it is known that older follicles have fewer antioxidant defenses against cellular damage caused by aerobic respiration and oxidative stress,[9] and that this too is related to poorer IVF outcomes.[10]

The ART embryologists have been experimenting with adding younger mitochondria to the eggs from older women to see if this helps to make better embryos. The Chinese herbalist uses Kidney Yang herbs to do the something similar. These are the herbs that we saw added to fertility formulas in the late stages of the follicular phase (Phase 3) (see Ch. 4).

Interestingly, researchers have shown that it is precisely these particular herbs (used in fertility clinics in China for many centuries!) that markedly enhance mitochondrial activity and ATP production in laboratory studies on mice, while other herb categories such as Qi or Yin tonics have little effect on mitochondrial ATP production. These same herbs were shown to enhance antioxidant defenses at the cellular level.[11]

What the ancients knew from trial and error scientists are now proving in labs. We must bear in mind however, that for the doctor of TCM, the clinical experience of thousands of years of Chinese herbalists treating infertility carries more weight than the lab findings examining mouse tissues. That is not to say it isn't satisfying when a new science can verify an old one.

Thus, we might surmise that the Kidney Yang herbs that are taken in the days leading up to ovulation, when the egg is maturing, can boost mitochondrial function, which then gives a newly formed embryo an advantage by dint of increased energy making capacity to aid development and successful implantation.

The herbs in Box 11.1 were found to increase ATP output in mice tissues. They are listed in descending order of effectiveness.

Box 11.1   Herbs shown to increase ATP production in laboratory studies

Suo Yang

Tu Si Zi

Rou Cong Rong

Bu Gu Zhi

Du Zhong

Gu Sui Bu

Xian Mao

Ba Ji Tian

Jiu Cai Zi

Yin Yang Huo

Xu Duan

Thus, when we are choosing which Yang herbs to add to our formulas in the days before ovulation, we might consider not only the characteristics we examined in Chapter 4 when constructing our formulas but also the potency they have shown in laboratory tests.

Back to the clinic and to our patient who is concerned with egg quality, we must recognize that we have a condition, Kidney deficiency, that is not one that responds quickly to treatment – it takes time, rest, regular routines, reduced stress, adequate sleep, good nutrition and the sorts of treatments a doctor of Chinese medicine can provide.

However, time is usually the one thing these women often don't have. They are anxious to get to the IVF clinic, or back to the IVF clinic, hounded by the ticking of the biological clock and the sound of their IVF specialists voice saying, 'You shouldn't have left it so long!' But the sad irony is that for these women, IVF or repeated IVF, only drains the Kidney further.

WHAT TO DO? …

In the case of a woman who is older or who has responded poorly in previous IVF cycles and now wishes to add a TCM approach, we focus especially on ovarian function and egg quality. This is done in exactly the way we described previously, by focusing on strongly reinforcing Kidney Jing, Yin and Blood. Ideally, this is done over a period of 6 months or more but even if only 3 months of strong Kidney Jing and Yin nourishment can be maintained alongside important lifestyle changes, then some changes will be achieved and hopefully responsiveness and resilience of the ovary will be sufficiently improved.

If your patient is actively trying to conceive, then use the treatment principles outlined in Chapter 4 for Kidney Jing and/or Yin deficiency. However, your patient may now be planning or waiting to do IVF and may no longer be trying so actively to conceive naturally. You and she may prefer an approach that is a little simpler than the complex 4-Phase one. In this case, you can combine the ideas inherent in both Phases 2 and 4 to create a formula which can be taken all month.

A comprehensive formula which combines both Gui Shao Di Huang Tang with Kidney Jing and Yang tonics is appropriate for across the board use in Phases 2, 3, and 4.

Herbal formula — Such a formula can be modified to take into account Yin-deficient Heat with the addition of Zhi Mu and Huang Bai. If the Spleen is weak you may need to increase the amount of Sha Ren and reduce the amount of Shu Di.

Gui Shao Di Huang Tang (Angelica Peonia Rehmannia decoction) modified

Shu Di	12 g	Radix Rehmanniae Glutinosae Conquitae
Shan Yao	9 g	Radix Dioscorea Oppositae
Shan Zhu Yu	9 g	Fructus Corni Officinalis
Fu Ling	9 g	Sclerotium Poriae Cocos
Mu Dan Pi	9 g	Cortex Moutan Radicis
Ze Xie	6 g	Rhizoma Alismatis
Dang Gui	9 g	Radix Angelicae Sinensis
Bai Shao	9 g	Radix Paeoniae Lactiflorae
Dan Shen	9 g	Radix Salviae Miltiorrhizae
Sha Ren	6 g	Fructus seu Semen Amomi
Tu Si Zi	9 g	Semen Cuscatae
Bu Gu Zhi	9 g	Fructus Psoraleae
Xiang Fu	6 g	Rhizoma Cyperi Rotundi
He Huan Pi	9 g	Cortex Albizziae Julibrissin
Suo Yang	6 g	Herba Cynomorii Songarici
Lu Jiao Pian	6 g	Cornu Cervi Parvum
Zi Shi Ying	6 g	Fluoritum

This expanded version of Gui Shao Di Huang Tang prepares a woman for IVF by reinforcing the Kidney Yin, Yang, and Jing, and calming the mind.

This formula can be taken for 3 or more months, with a break during the period if required. As we saw in Chapter 4, the main action of Gui Shao Di Huang tang is to reinforce Kidney Yin and the Blood. Here, we add herbs that support Kidney Yang as well, and herbs to calm the mind and keep the Qi and blood moving smoothly, so that it is applicable at all times of the cycle. Should your patient conceive during this preparation time, then switch formulas to one focusing on miscarriage prevention (see below).

During the menstrual period, a formula based on Tao Hong Si Wu Tang (see Ch. 4) could be taken.

Acupuncture treatment used to prepare for IVF will take into account patient circumstances, constitutional factors and the time of the cycle. (Follow the principles outlined in Ch. 4, and refer to Tables 4.1–4.7.)

Heart and Liver Qi stagnation (and sleep and stress)

As mentioned above, it is women with Heart and Liver Qi stagnation who benefit greatly from treatment during the IVF cycle, however preparatory treatment to regulate the cycle and calm the nervous system will also pay dividends. Sometimes in a big way, these patients are quite likely to respond quickly to acupuncture and may conceive before the (next) IVF cycle.

Treatment protocols following the 4 Phases are those found in Chapter 4. If, however, a simpler approach is required, then combining an expanded version of Gui Shao Di Huang Tang with elements of Xiao Yao San or Gan Mai Da Zao Tang could be taken all month to prepare your patient and her ovaries for IVF.

Herbal formula — The formula of choice is:

Gui Shao Di Huang Tang (Angelica Peonia Rehmannia decoction) with Xiao Yao San (Bupleurum and Tangkuei powder) and Gan Mai Da Zao Tang (Licorice, Wheat, and Jujube Decoction) modified

Shu Di	9 g	Radix Rehmanniae Glutinosae Conquitae
Shan Yao	9 g	Radix Dioscorea Oppositae
Shan Zhu Yu	9 g	Fructus Corni Officinalis
Dang Gui	9 g	Radix Angelicae Sinensis
Bai Shao	9 g	Radix Paeoniae Lactiflorae
Dan Shen	9 g	Radix Salviae Miltiorrhizae
Fu Ling	9 g	Sclerotium Poriae Cocos
Mu Dan Pi	9 g	Cortex Moutan Radicis
Ze Xie	9 g	Rhizoma Alismatis
Sha Ren	3 g	Fructus seu Semen Amomi
Tu Si Zi	9 g	Semen Cuscatae
Bu Gu Zhi	6 g	Fructus Psoraleae
Xiang Fu	6 g	Rhizoma Cyperi Rotundi
He Huan Pi	9 g	Cortex Albizziae Julibrissin
Chai Hu	9 g	Radix Bupleuri
Fu Xiao Mai	6 g	Semen Tritici Aestivi Levis
Da Zao	6 pieces	Fructus Zizyphi Jujuba
Gan Cao	6 g	'Radix Glycyrrhizae Uralensis

Using this sort of formula to prepare for IVF will provide support for the Kidney Yin and Yang and Blood at the same time adding a little more focus on regulation of the Heart and Liver Qi. The actions of Gui Shao Di Huang Tang and Xiao Yao San we have discussed before. The sweetness of Da Zao, Gan Cao and Fu Xiao Mai (Gan

Mai Da Zao Tang) soothe the mind and relieve melancholy and sadness, commonly experienced by patients who have given up the possibility of conceiving naturally.

Should your patient conceive during this preparation time, then switch the formula to one focusing on early pregnancy support (see below).

During the menstrual period, a formula based on Tao Hong Si Wu Tang (see Ch. 4) could be taken. For acupuncture protocols, please refer to Tables 4.1–4.7 for general prescriptions, alongside modifications for Liver and Heart stagnation, Table 4.8.

Reducing stress

Apart from regulating the menstrual cycle and helping your patient's mood, there is good reason to regulate the Liver Qi and reduce stress hormone levels before IVF. We know that stress can have a negative impact on IUI[12] and IVF outcomes,[13] and that women who have taken active measures to reduce their stress have had better results with IVF than those who don't, especially if they are doing their second or more cycles.[14–16] Women who do not feel depressed before starting IVF treatment conceive twice as often as women who are depressed before treatment,[17,18] so ensuring healthy and unobstructed Liver Qi can have significant implications for a future IVF cycle.

Some researchers suspect that stress may impact specific factors in the endometrium as well as its general effects on hormones. It is not so easy to directly examine endometrial implantation sites in women trying to conceive, but studies on animal models have revealed a negative impact of stress on uterine receptivity and number of implantation sites.[19] Stress, and its affect on fertility in general is discussed in Chapter 12.

The formula above addresses many of the aspects of infertility related to stress, but in more severe cases, the dose of He Huan Pi can be increased.

Improving sleep

Sleep quality and quantity (see also Ch. 12) should be a focus of our attention in the patient with an unstable Shen planning to do IVF, particularly if she suffers from insomnia. People with chronic insomnia tend to have higher levels of some cytokines, notably interleukin-6 and tumor necrosis factor.[20] These immune factors can impact implantation of the embryo and placental development. Some researchers have proposed that a suboptimal cytokine environment can contribute to miscarriage.[21] Certain cytokines can lead to clotting of the placental vessels in cases of early or late pregnancy loss, or interference of angiogenesis in cases of occult pregnancy loss.

The formula above can be further modified with Shen calming agents such as Mu Li and Suan Zao Ren, in the case of insomnia.

Blood stagnation

Treatment in the 3 cycles before IVF can be very useful in going some way to resolving blood stagnation, which might affect oocyte or endometrium quality. Most Blood stagnation pathologies affect the endometrium, whether they be ones that require surgery such as large submucosal fibroids or polyps, or ones not always so amenable to surgery such as adenomyosis, endometritis or diffuse endometriosis. Some forms of Blood stagnation appear to affect the egg quality as well as the endometrium quality, and this is also amenable to treatment. For example there is some evidence to show that Chinese herbs improve egg quality in patients with endometriosis by reducing inflammatory markers in the follicular fluid.[22]

Treatment protocols are those described in Chapter 4 with a large emphasis on clearing stagnation during Phase 1, during the menstrual flow. In this way, we hope to alter the endometrium and the way it forms in the hope that this will reduce risk of implantation failure. This sort of treatment aims to minimize the effect of immune and clotting factors which can jeopardize implantation and placenta formation.

Improving the hormonal and immune milieu of the ovaries of these patients with endometriosis with acupuncture or Chinese herbs in the months before doing IVF could have benefits similar to treatment of older ovaries, i.e., an improvement in the egg quality.

The progress of your treatment may be effectively monitored by menstrual symptoms such as pain or the nature of the menstrual flow.

A simplified approach using herbs in preparation for IVF would be the use of a Phase 1 type of formula such as that below, during the period, and at other times of the cycle if natural conception is not being attempted. Where your patient is still attempting to conceive, use the formula below (Tao Hong Si Wu tang modified) during the period followed by the next formula (Gui Shao Di Huang tang plus Tao Hong Si Wu tang modified) for the rest of the cycle to prepare the ovaries for the IVF drugs.

Herbal formula — The formula of choice is:

Tao Hong Si Wu tang (Persica Carthamus Four Substances decoction) modified

Dang Gui	9 g	Radix Angelicae Sinensis
Chi Shao	9 g	Radix Paeoniae Rubra
Chuan Xiong	6 g	Radix Ligustici Wallichii
Tao Ren	9 g	Semen Persicae
Hong Hua	9 g	Flos Carthami Tinctorii
Gui Zhi	3 g	Ramulus Cinnamomi Cassiae
Dan Shen	9 g	Radix Salviae Miltiorrhizae
Shan Zha	6 g	Fructus Crataegi
Pu Huang	9 g	Pollen Typhae
Wu Ling Zhi	9 g	Excrementum Trogopterori
Yan Hu Suo	12 g	Rhizoma Corydalis Yanhusuo
Xiang Fu	9 g	Rhizoma Cyperi Rotundi
Xu Duan	9 g	Radix Dipsaci
Chuan Niu Xi	6 g	Radix Cyathulae

This formula which expands the reach of Tao Hong Si Wu tang (described in Ch. 4) is single pointed in its application to clearing Blood stasis and can be taken in the weeks leading up to an IVF cycle in patients who show clear signs of stasis, such as menstrual clots or abdomen pain. If the stasis is material and substantial in the form of endometriosis or fibroids then the relevant sections in Chapter 5 or Chapter 8 should be consulted.

Gui Shao Di Huang tang (Angelica Peonia Rehmannia decoction) and Tao Hong Si Wu tang (Persica Carthamus Four Substances decoction) modified

Shu Di	9 g	Rehmanniae Glutinosae Conquitae
Shan Yao	9 g	Dioscorea Oppositae
Shan Zhu Yu	9 g	Fructus Corni Officinalis
Dang Gui	9 g	Radix Angelicae Sinensis
Bai Shao	9 g	Radix Paeoniae Lactiflorae
Dan Shen	9 g	Radix Salviae Miltiorrhizae
Mu Dan Pi	9 g	Cortex Moutan Radicis
Fu Ling	9 g	Sclerotium Poriae Cocos

Ze Xie	9 g	Rhizoma Alismatis
Sha Ren	3 g	Fructus seu Semen Amomi
Tu Si Zi	9 g	Semen Cuscatae
Bu Gu Zhi	6 g	Fructus Psoraleae
Xiang Fu	6 g	Rhizoma Cyperi Rotundi
He Huan Pi	9 g	Cortex Albizziae Julibrissin
Tao Ren	9 g	Semen Persicae
Hong Hua	9 g	Flos Carthami Tinctorii
Pu Huang	9 g	Pollen Typhae
Wu Ling Zhi	9 g	Excrementum Trogopterori

This formula is an expanded version of Gui Shao Di Huang Tang combined with Tao Hong Si Wu tang (both described in Ch. 4) and other herbs to clear stagnation. The patient preparing for IVF can take this throughout the cycle to reinforce the Kidneys and clear stasis but should she conceive it should be discontinued and a formula to support early pregnancy given (see below).

In the case of endometriosis, formulas described in Chapter 5 should be taken in preparation for IVF (and natural conception avoided). Fibroids should also be addressed before doing IVF if they are large or multiple and affecting the endometrium; these treatments are covered in the Blood stagnation sections of Chapters 4 and 8.

For acupuncture protocols please refer to Tables 4.1–4.7 for general prescriptions, alongside modifications for Blood stasis, Table 4.9.

Phlegm-Damp (and weight loss)

Blockages caused by Phlegm-Damp should be addressed before IVF. Although mucus secretions in the fallopian tubes will be circumnavigated by the IVF process, the presence of Phlegm-Damp in the Uterus does not create a desirable environment for the transferred embryo.

Herbal formula — The formula of choice is:

Gui Shao Di Huang Tang (Angelica Peonia Rehmannia decoction) plus Jian Gu Tang (Strengthen and Consolidate decoction) modified

Nu Zhen Zi	9 g	Fructus Ligustri Lucidi
Han Lian Cao	9 g	Herba Ecliptae Prostratae
Shan Yao	9 g	Dioscorea Oppositae
Shan Zhu Yu	9 g	Fructus Corni Officinalis
Ji Xue Teng	9 g	Radix et Caulis Jixueteng
Bai Shao	9 g	Radix Paeoniae Lactiflorae
Dan Shen	9 g	Radix Salviae Miltiorrhizae
Mu Dan Pi	9 g	Cortex Moutan Radicis
Fu Ling	15 g	Sclerotium Poriae Cocos
Ze Xie	9 g	Rhizoma Alismatis
Sha Ren	6 g	Fructus seu Semen Amomi
Yi Yi Ren	15 g	Semen Coicis Lachryma-jobi
Dang Shen	9 g	Radix Codonopsis Pilulosae
Bai Zhu	9 g	Rhizoma Atractylodis Macrocephalae

Tu Si Zi	9 g	Semen Cuscatae
Ba Ji Tian	9 g	Radix Morindae Officinalis
Yin Yang Huo	9 g	Herba Epimedii
Zao Jiao Ci	6 g	Spina Gleditsiae Sinensis
Dan Nan Xing	6 g	Rhizoma Arisaematis

This simplified approach, which can be used at any time of the menstrual cycle in the weeks before the IVF cycle begins, uses a modified Gui Shao Di Huang tang and combines it with a formula such as Jian Gu Tang (both described in Ch. 4), to strengthen the Kidneys and the Spleen and remove Phlegm-Damp.

Should your patient conceive during this preparation time, then switch formulas to one focusing on early pregnancy support (see below).

During the menstrual period, a formula based on Tao Hong Si Wu tang could be taken (see Ch. 4).

For acupuncture protocols, see Tables 4.1–4.7 for general prescriptions, alongside modifications for Phlegm-Damp accumulation, Table 4.10.

Losing weight

In the case of overweight patients, including patients with PCOS, acupuncture and herbs that aim to clear Damp can be extremely useful. We know that loss of weight and reduction in insulin resistance will improve ovarian function and egg quality. IVF success rates are higher in women with normal range BMIs. Acupuncture and herbs can be used to promote lipolysis, reduce appetite and increase metabolism generally. Weekly acupuncture sessions serve not only to boost Spleen and Stomach function to improve metabolism, but provide a regular checking in point where diet and exercise schedules are monitored and weight is measured. Patients with Phlegm-Damp accumulation can be difficult to motivate so persistence and encouragement is needed. But it is good to remind them that it is the initial mobilizing of Damp that is the crucial step in improving ovarian function. Once the first 10% of body weight is lost, or even 5 kg, ovary function will start to improve and the patient will be more motivated to continue with the treatment and the relevant lifestyle changes. (For more discussion on this topic, see Chs 5 and 12).

Note that it is not only women who need to pay attention to weight. It appears that obesity affects sperm negatively and this is discussed further in Chapters 7 and 12.

At the same time as helping weight loss, Chinese medicine can contribute to an improved environment in which eggs are maturing. Acupuncture using Spleen and Stomach points, which promote clearing of Damp, has been shown to reduce the elevated levels of testosterone and luteinizing hormone in women with PCOS both of which are thought to have a negative impact on egg quality.[23] Some IVF specialists use Metformin or Glucophage 'off-label' to achieve something similar.

Like improving Kidney function, clearing Phlegm-Damp is not a quick process. However, patients in this category are often younger and have more time to prepare for IVF; 3–6 months is ideal. (See Chs 4 and 5 for more discussion of treatments for Phlegm-Damp Infertility.)

Preparation for IVF for men

It is worthwhile treating male factor infertility even if the couple plan to do IVF with ICSI. If the sperm vitality improves, ICSI may not be necessary. If it improves enough, IVF may not be necessary! (For the treatment of male factor infertility, see Ch. 7.)

Herbal formula — The formula below for reinforcing Kidney Yin, Yang and Jing and nourishing and invigorating Blood and Qi is applicable to any Kidney deficiency male factor infertility and should be taken for

TCM TREATMENT OF THE IVF PATIENT

some weeks or months before the IVF cycle. It can be taken in small doses by partners of women doing IVF who have no male factor but who would like to maximize sperm quality.

Bu Shen Yi Jing fang (Supplement the Kidneys Benefit the Jing formula) modified

Tu Si Zi	9 g	*Semen Cuscatae*
Fu Pen Zi	12 g	*Fructus Rubi Chingii*
Nu Zhen Zi	9 g	*Fructus Ligustri Lucidi*
Gou Qi Zi	9 g	*Fructus Lycii Chinensis*
He Shou Wu	12 g	*Radix Polygoni Multiflori*
Sheng Di	9 g	*Radix Rehmanniae Glutinosae*
Shan Zhu Yu	9 g	*Fructus Corni Officinalis*
Dang Shen	9 g	*Radix Codonopsis Pilulosae*
Dan Shen	9 g	*Radix Salviae Miltiorrhizae*
Hong Hua	6 g	*Flos Carthami Tinctorii*
Huang Qi	12 g	*Radix Astragali*
Yin Yang Huo	9 g	*Herba Epimedii*

Bu Shen Yi Jing fang was discussed in Chapter 7.

If there are signs of Heat then replace Huang Qi and Yin Yang Huo with Huang Bai (*Phellodendri Cortex*) 9 g and Zhi Mu (*Anemarrhenae Rhizoma*) 9 g.

Acupuncture is applicable to male factor infertility and is recommended in the weeks before doing IVF for the same reasons that herbs are recommended, i.e., to maximize the chances of success and the possibility of not requiring ICSI. If the partner of a woman who will be doing IVF has a normal semen analysis but wishes to maximize chances of a good outcome, it is quite reasonable to offer acupuncture treatment based on his constitution and symptoms (if any), combined with points that have been shown in research to improve microcirculation in the testes.[24] This is particularly useful if the patient is over 35 and/or has any signs or symptoms of Blood stagnation or Kidney deficiency.

Treatment will be continued for a course of 10 or 12 treatments, or weekly until the sperm donation on the day of OPU. (For further discussion of appropriate treatment where there is male factor infertility, see Ch 7.)

Acupuncture points — Choose from the following (and see Table 11.1):

SP-6	Sanyinjiao
Ren-4	Guanyuan
K-6	Zhaohai
ST-36	Zusanli
ST-29	Guilai
K-3	Taixi
BL-23	Shenshu
BL-52	Zhishi
DU-4	Mingmen
ST-30	Qichong
LIV-5	Ligou
LIV-8	Ququan
SP-10	Xuehai
PC-6	Neiguan
BL-32	Ciliao
BL-33	Zhongliao

369

CO-4	Hegu
CO-11	Quchi
LIV-3	Taichong
GB-41	Zu linqi
GB-27	Wushu

Table 11.1   Acupuncture points suggested for use with male patients in preparation for IVF

Treatment goal	Acupuncture points
To reinforce Kidney Jing, Yin and Yang[a]	Ren-4, K-6, K-3, BL-23, BL-52, DU-4
To resolve Blood or Qi stagnation[b]	ST-30, LIV-5, 8, SP-10, PC-6, BL-32, 33
To clear Damp Heat[b]	CO-4, CO-11, GB-41, GB-27, LIV-8.
To regulate Liver Qi, relieve stress[b]	LIV-3 CO-4
To reinforce Spleen/Stomach Qi[a]	Ren-6, SP-6, ST-36
To calm shen, relieve insomnia[a]	HT-7, PC-6, DU-20
To increase blood flow in the testicles[c]	ST-29, SP-6

[a]Use even method.
[b]Use reducing method.
[c]Use electroacupuncture (10 Hz) joining SP-6 to ST-29 on the same side for 5–20 min.

Box 11.2   Summary of influences on sperm quality, follicular microenvironment and egg quality in preparation for IVF

- Increase blood supply (oxygen and nutrients) to the testicles with acupuncture
- Increase blood supply (oxygen and nutrients) to the follicles with acupuncture
- Improve ovarian function by regulating hormone levels (e.g., LH, testosterone, insulin) with acupuncture
- Reduce stress hormones associated with reduced IVF success with acupuncture
- Increase oocyte mitochondrial ATP output with certain Chinese herbs
- Enhance follicle antioxidant defenses with certain Chinese herbs
- Improve follicle environment by reducing inflammatory cytokines with certain Chinese herbs.

In summary, there are many ways we can use TCM to help couples prepare for IVF, both in terms of useful lifestyle and physiologic changes such as diet and weight loss, and improvements to sleep and stress levels and so on but also, specifically in terms of maximizing egg and sperm quality. Box 11.2 summarizes some of the useful ways (based on early research findings) we can possibly help couples in the months before they embark on IVF.

TREATMENT DURING THE IVF CYCLE

When treating the IVF patient in the TCM clinic, we do exactly what we always do as Chinese medicine doctors, and analyze precisely what we see in front of us from a TCM perspective and administer treatment according to our diagnosis and according to what we have learnt about the treatment of infertility from experts over the centuries of TCM history. Some of what we learned (see Ch. 4) about specifically timed treatments for female functional infertility will still apply in the context of an IVF cycle, however we will need to make some adjustments for altered physiologic conditions and symptoms arising as a result of IVF drugs. This is a new frontier for Chinese medicine doctors, both in the West and also for those in China. We do not yet have the wealth of experience of generations of experts working with IVF patients to guide or inform our approach to treatment. What I present here is a brief summary of programs we have been developing in specialist support clinics set up in Australia for IVF patients. These clinics have seen several thousand patients at the time of writing, with the result that a lot of data has been collected. This sort of information, along with the clinical experience and trials being run by our and other centers will, over time, inform and refine treatment that is appropriate and most advantageous for the patient preparing for, and undertaking IVF. But in terms of TCM, clinical experience is still in its early days, and until such time as more experience and data is available, all the treatment suggestions made below must be seen as just that – considered suggestions.

Chinese medical treatment of internal disorders including infertility, relies on herbal medicine; while this approach may well be comfortable from the Chinese medicine doctor's point of view, it can be worrying from the IVF specialist's point of view. There is a concern that there may be unexpected or unfavorable interactions with the IVF drugs. This is a valid concern, since no studies have been done that I am aware of which examine the interaction of Chinese herbs with IVF drugs. Uncontrolled interference with medications can cloud the clinical picture.

If fruit juices like apple, orange, or grapefruit can interact with drug metabolizing enzymes and drug uptake transporters[25] then we must assume that herbs may do something similar (although IVF patients are not told to avoid fruit juice, yet!).

Anecdotally, there are Chinese medicine practitioners and IVF specialists in this country who are quite happy to combine the two medicines and apparently with no untoward effect, in fact possibly the opposite. However, these practitioners are in the minority, and at the support clinics we do not prescribe herbs during the drug phase of the IVF cycle (up until egg collection). Until drug interaction studies have been done, most Chinese herbalists should take the cautious approach of advising their patients to stop taking Chinese herbs for a 5–7 day washout period before they begin taking their IVF drugs (the half-life of most aqueous herbal compounds is measured in hours rather than days or weeks, so this timeframe is more than adequate). This applies especially in the case of the agonist and antagonist downregulating drugs. These drugs prevent the pituitary gland producing hormones to stimulate the ovaries, and prescribing herbs that promote reproductive function (Kidney tonics) at the same time is counterintuitive, at least theoretically. Our clinical observations (and those of thousands of gynecologists in China before us) indicate that Kidney Yin herbs have the capacity to promote ovarian activity and increase their estrogen output, e.g., many patients report more regular menstrual cycles, stronger menstrual flow and specifically, increased secretions of cervical mucus when they take these herbs. However, we don't know the mechanism by which these herbs are achieving this. We can say however, that the use of Kidney tonic herbs to promote ovarian function at the same time as the administration of FSH is at least theoretically, a clinically congruent action.

Additionally, we need to be aware of overall drug load on the liver's detoxification systems. Women who are getting side-effects like nausea, headaches, rashes or fatigue may be showing signs of an overloaded liver. Adding more substances to the mix may risk exacerbation of these symptoms or worse.

Having made this point loud and clear, I now wish to add that there are circumstances where the addition of Chinese herbs to an IVF cycle appears to be useful and also acceptable. If an IVF patient has completed two or more stimulated cycles, with poor response to the IVF drugs and no or very few embryos produced, then patients and their specialists may well be looking for something else to try. This is often where the Chinese herbalist can step in, with the encouragement of the patient and the blessing of the IVF specialist (or at least a 'we have nothing to lose' viewpoint). We hope that treating Kidney deficiency may increase the responsiveness of the ovaries to the drugs (given enough time), and that treating Blood or Qi stagnation may increase implantation rates.

Since downregulating and FSH drugs are given by injection (or by nasal spray), interference of uptake and absorption by herbs taken orally may not be a critical issue, however separate timing of administration of IVF drugs and herbs by 4h is recommended to reduce possible interactions. Response to the herbs and the drugs should be monitored regularly and doses of herbs reduced if the patient is getting side-effects such as nausea, dizziness, or headaches.

For cycles involving the transfer of frozen embryos, there is no contraindication to the taking of Chinese herbs. Similarly, in artificial insemination cycles where downregulating drugs are not being used, there is no contraindication to the use of Chinese herbs. The use of Chinese herbs with ovulation inducing drugs such as clomifene has been well documented and researched in China and is strongly recommended.

We mustn't forget however, that preparation with Chinese medicine treatment for ovary health and gamete vitality is best done well before IVF is started (3–9 months). While that opportunity does not always exist, it is important that patients and IVF specialists realize that it is the contribution that can be made before the IVF cycle that is the real place of Chinese medicine.

Of course it goes without saying that concerns about drug interactions do not apply to acupuncture, which can and should continue to be applied according to standard TCM diagnostic and treatment procedures (combined with research-based protocols where appropriate) during the IVF cycle. The use of Kidney channel points with their possible stimulatory action on the pituitary or the ovary during a downregulated phase, is unlikely to adversely impact a pituitary gland that has been switched off pharmaceutically.

The practitioner must have a good understanding of the IVF process and will take into account all clinical symptoms or side-effects arising as a result of the IVF drugs into his/her diagnosis.

4-Phase TCM treatment during the IVF cycle

Treatments according to the 4 Phases we described in Chapter 4 can be modified for use during the IVF cycle. In Chapter 4, when we applied the 4-Phase treatments we maintained a close awareness of the natural physiology of the menstrual cycle and applied treatments that followed these. However, in the case of the IVF patient, we must now be aware of the physiology of the drug manipulated ovary. Rather than enhancing the natural processes of the menstrual cycle as we did in Chapter 4, we must now track and support what are essentially pathologic states as some of the pituitary and hypothalamus activity is shut down and the ovaries are artificially hyper-stimulated.

Suggestions made here for herbal prescriptions to be taken during the IVF cycle (for those patients who have a history of poor response to IVF drugs, as discussed above) follow the requirements of each of the 4 Phases of the menstrual cycle, manipulated as it is. However, in comparison with the complex and many layered approach to treatment of infertility the doctor of TCM takes as primary practitioner, here we take a simpler role as a support practitioner to the IVF specialist.

We need to be clear about what it is exactly that we are supporting in this physiologically artificial and manipulated situation. Essentially, we are assisting the patient emotionally and her ovaries physiologically. Our aims are to:

• support the ovaries (the Kidneys) to promote optimal response to the FSH drugs

• reduce stress and anxiety and bolster the patient's resilience

• manage side-effects of the drugs.

Assisting the ovaries as they are induced by non-physiologic doses of FSH to ripen multiple eggs means in TCM terms supporting the Kidneys; this is usually achieved with the use of herbal medicine. This sort of treatment will most often be requested by the 'poor responder', as we discussed above. The ovaries of women with depleted Kidney Qi, or those who have done a lot of IVF cycles, tend to respond poorly to stimulation by IVF drugs.

IVF patients who do not need this support (the 'good responders' who produce adequate numbers of eggs and younger women) may request Chinese medicine treatment during their IVF cycle to deal with stress, anxiety and side-effects. This is best achieved with acupuncture and administration of herbal medicine is not indicated in these cases.

The guiding prescriptions offered as support for IVF patients who are not good responders and have a history of failed IVF cycles address the immediate situation (namely, ripening of ovarian follicles) as much as the patient with her original infertility diagnosis. Hence, compared with the guiding formulas described in Chapter 4, there are fewer modifications required relating to the original cause of fertility.

Here, we will describe the 4 Phases of the menstrual cycle modified to take into account the effects of the drugs used in an IVF cycle. For women on a long downregulated IVF cycle, drugs will be administered before we actually get to Phase 1 (the menstrual phase) and these GnRH agonist drugs tend to delay the period. At this point, what is required is regulation of Qi and Blood to encourage menstrual flow and to prevent stagnation. Acupuncture to regulate the movement of Qi and Blood is particularly helpful at this time. Additionally, we want to support the Kidneys and their Jing, as they prepare for the demands on them once the stimulating drugs commence. Except in the circumstances described above, herbs are not usually prescribed during this downregulating phase and if your patient has been taking herbs in the preparation phase for IVF, then she will usually be advised to discontinue them before she starts the GnRH agonist.

Once the period arrives, we shall arrange our treatment according to the 4 Phases as described below.

Phase 1 (menstrual period) Day 1–3

DRUGS: FSH ± GNRH AGONIST

You will recall that the main aim of Phase 1 treatment is to encourage an efficient removal and remodeling of the endometrial layers such that the uterine environment is conducive for implantation of an embryo that might arrive later in the cycle.

Acupuncture points — Acupuncture is usefully applied in this phase to promote movement of Qi and Blood – choose from the points below and see Table 11.2:

CO-4	Hegu
SP-6	Sanyinjiao
SP-10	Xuehai
SP-8	Diji
Ren-6	Qihai
Tituo xue	
KI-14	Siman
BL-25	Dachangshu
BL-30	Baihuangshu
BL-32	Ciliao
Shiqizhui	
BL-31–34	Baliao
PC-5	Jianshi

Herbal formula — In the case of Blood stagnation (clotty or painful periods, or history of endometriosis, etc.), the use of Blood moving herbs should be considered.

Tao Hong Si Wu tang (Persica Carthamus Four Substances decoction) modified (for use during IVF cycle in restricted circumstances – Phase 1)

Dang Gui	12g	Radix Angelicae Sinensis
Bai Shao	9g	Radix Paeoniae Lactiflorae

Chuan Xiong	6 g	Radix Ligustici Wallichii
Tao Ren	6 g	Semen Persicae
Hong Hua	9 g	Flos Carthami Tinctorii
Yi Mu Cao	9 g	Herba Leonuri Heterophylli
Xiang Fu	12 g	Rhizoma Cyperi Rotundi
Ji Xue Teng	12 g	Radix et Caulis Jixueteng
Shan Zha	6 g	Fructus Crataegi
Dan Shen	12 g	Radix Salviae Miltiorrhizae
Chuan Niu Xi	6 g	Radix Cyathulae

Tao Hong Si Wu Tang is the ideal basis for a formula applied during the period at the start of an IVF cycle because it has a gentle but firm action on the movement of blood and at the same time builds up Blood, i.e., it helps replace blood at same time it is being lost through menstruation. It is augmented with herbs such as Yi Mu Cao and Chuan Niu Xi to encourage a thorough shedding of the lining and Dan Shen and Shan Zha to facilitate this movement. The addition of Qi regulators such as Xiang Fu, promotes the action of Qi leading the Blood and ameliorates cramping of the uterus.

In the case of Blood stagnation (clotty or painful periods, or history of endometriosis, etc.), the use of stronger blood moving herbs (Yan Hu Suo, Wu Ling Zhi, Pu Huang) should be considered. FSH drugs are commenced during this phase, usually on Day 2. Support of follicle stimulation, with herbs or acupuncture, will begin in the next phase however.

Phase 2 (follicle development) Day 4 to approx. Day 11

DRUGS: FSH ± GNRH AGONIST OR ANTAGONIST

FSH drugs stimulate the ovaries to ripen a number of eggs from the available cohort of recruits. Because the agonist drug (or the antagonist drug introduced on about Day 6 of stimulation) will stop the pituitary

Table 11.2   Acupuncture points[a] suggested for use during an IVF cycle: menstrual phase

Treatment goal	Acupuncture points
To open the uterus and encourage downward movement and a smooth and thorough discharge of the menstrual flow	CO-4 with SP-6
To moderate this action and hold the Qi	Ren-6
To treat all aspects of the Blood, both its movement and its supplementation and control heavy bleeding if there is Heat	SP-10
To remove obstructions to Blood flow	SP-8
To move Blood in the Chong channel	KI-14
To regulate the Qi in the uterus and moderate the descending action of SP-6	Tituo
To regulate Qi in the lower Jiao	BL-25 and BL-30
To regulate Qi specifically in the Uterus	BL-32, Shiqizhui
To regulate Qi, particularly if there is pain in the sacrum	Baliao (BL-31–34)
To make Blood flow smoothly, relieve pain, calm the mind	PC-5

[a]Use reducing method on leg and trunk points and even method needling on wrist points.

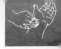

from responding to the rising levels of estrogen and triggering ovulation, many follicles continue to develop unhindered.

The process of folliculogenesis, as you will remember from Chapter 2, relies on Kidney Yin and Blood and draws on Kidney Jing stores. During an IVF cycle, the growth of more follicles than usual means there will be a larger draw on these resources than in a natural cycle and hence, greater Kidney support may be required. The rise in Yin and Blood and the effect of the FSH drugs (and the herbs if they are used) will be measured in the rise of estrogen and in the growth of the follicles seen on ultrasound. This will happen more rapidly for some patients than for others. In an ideal case this phase of follicle stimulation will last approximately 7 or 8 days, during which time several follicles ripen steadily at about the same rate to reach 13 or 14 mm, and at the same time, the uterine lining gradually thickens. It is common to feel the Kidney pulse fill out during this and the next phase as the follicles grow. If there are side-effects from the drugs and the process of hyperstimulating the ovaries, it may also be felt on the Liver pulse (which may become tight and wiry) and Spleen pulse (which may become weak).

In some cases, the ultrasounds may show that after several days of FSH injections, the follicles are not growing as expected or that there are few of them. The IVF specialist will usually increase the dose of FSH in this case, and the projected date for egg collection might be delayed. On the other hand, sometimes follicles develop more rapidly than expected and are ready for collection after only a few days of stimulation. Neither the slow nor the rapid growing follicles represent an ideal situation and it is preferable that follicles ripen in a time frame similar to a natural cycle (i.e., over about 2 weeks).

• Acupuncture

Acupuncture at this point supports the Kidneys and the Blood and regulates the function of the Ren and Chong vessels (such as it is). Maintaining Chong vessel function as much as possible and promoting unfettered movement of Liver Qi in the abdomen, may help the regular and ordered growth of the recruited follicles so that they grow at a similar rate. This increases the possibility of collecting more eggs at the correct stage of maturity on the day of egg collection.

Moving the Liver and Heart Qi helps relieve stress and calm the emotions and since we know that women who feel more stressed during IVF procedures (measured by raised heart beat and high systolic blood pressure) have significantly lower implantation rates it is important to continue treatment at this time.[26] Some side-effects such as headaches may be apparent, however the physiological pressure and abdomen discomfort caused by enlarged ovaries does not usually come into play until late in this phase or in the next.

It is useful to incorporate some of the research based protocols (described below) which increase blood flow to the ovaries and uterus. This will aid in getting maximal delivery of nutrients, oxygen and drugs to the follicles as they are developing, and in promoting the development of lining of the uterus as the Blood in the Chong channel increases.

In the case that estrogen levels are slow to rise and follicles are slow to grow then increasing blood flow to the ovaries with acupuncture may facilitate drug delivery to stimulate follicle growth. Likewise, in the case that the endometrium is thin, using acupuncture points which improve blood flow to the uterus may be helpful.

Acupuncture points — Choose from the list below (and see Table 11.3):

Ren-7	Yinjiao
KI-5	Shuiquan
KI-8	Jiaoxin
KI-13	Qixue
KI-3	Taixi
KI-6	Zhaohai
SP-6	Sanyinjiao

ST-36	Zusanli
Ren-4	Guanyuan
BL-23	Shenshu
ST-27	Daju
BL-28	Pangguanshu
BL-57	Chengshan
SP-4	Gongsun
PC-6	Neiguan
ST-30	Qichong
ST-28	Shuidao
ST-29	Guilai
SP-9	Yinlingquan
SP-6	Sanyinjiao
SP-10	Xuehai
Zigong	
LIV-3	Taichong
LIV-5	Ligou
LIV-8	Ququan
Yin Tang	
HT-7	Shenmen
HT-4	Lingdao
Ren-14	Juque
CO-4	Hegu
GB-20	Fengchi
DU-20	Baihui

Herbal formula — If a considered decision has been made to prescribe herbs during an IVF cycle for a patient with previous poor response, then those that reinforce Kidney Jing, Yin and Blood will be required.

Table 11.3 Acupuncture points[a] suggested for use during an IVF cycle: stimulation phase

Treatment goal	Acupuncture points
To regulate Ren and Chong vessels	Ren-7, KI-5, KI-8, KI-13
To encourage Blood production (build endometrium)	ST-36, LIV-3, BL-17, BL-20, SP-10
To support Kidney Yin and Jing	KI-3, KI-5, KI-6, SP-6, BL-23, Ren-4, ST-27
To increase Blood flow to the uterus[b]	BL-28, BL-23, SP-6, BL-57, SP-4, PC-6, ST-30
To increase Blood flow to the ovaries[b]	ST-28, ST-29, SP-6, SP-9
To regulate Qi around the ovaries	ST-28, ST-29, Zigong, LIV-5, LIV-8
To stabilize Shen	Yin Tang, HT-7, HT-4, Ren-14
To treat headaches, depression, irritability	CO-4, LIV-3, YT, GB-20, DU-20

[a]Use even method needling. Acupuncture applied twice a week (or more) is recommended during this phase.
[b]Use electroacupuncture (10 Hz) linking abdomen or lower back points to Spleen points on the lower leg.

Gui Shao Di Huang tang (Angelica Peonia Rehmannia decoction) modified

Shu Di	12 g	Radix Rehmanniae Glutinosae Conquitae
Shan Zhu Yu	9 g	Fructus Corni Officinalis
Shan Yao	9 g	Radix Dioscorea Oppositae
Dang Gui	9 g	Radix Angelicae Sinensis
Bai Shao	9 g	Radix Paeoniae Lactiflorae
Dan Shen	9 g	Radix Salviae Miltiorrhizae
Ji Xue Teng	9 g	Radix et Caulis Jixueteng
Mu Dan Pi	9 g	Cortex Moutan Radicis
Fu Ling	9 g	Sclerotium Poriae Cocos
Ze Xie	6 g	Rhizoma Alismatis
Sha Ren	6 g	Fructus seu Semen Amomi
Tu Si Zi	9 g	Semen Cuscatae
Bu Gu Zhi	6 g	Fructus Psoraleae
Xiang Fu	9 g	Rhizoma Cyperi Rotundi
Wu Yao	3 g	Radix Linderae Strychnifoliae
Yin Yang Huo	6 g	Herba Epimedii
Lu Jiao Pian	6 g	Cornu Cervi Parvum
Zi Shi Ying	6 g	Fluoritum
He Huan Pi	12 g	Cortex Albizziae Julibrissin
Suan Zao Ren	9 g	Semen Ziziphi Spinosae

We use this expanded version of Gui Shao Di Huang tang (described in Ch. 4) to support Kidney Jing, Yin, and Yang to promote follicle growth. As well as encouraging follicle development we want to protect the Kidneys from being drained by the artificial stimulation by external FSH.

The Blood tonic herbs nourish and promote circulation of blood to promote endometrial growth, and Qi regulating herbs prevent Qi stagnation occurring as the ovaries swell.

Herbs that calm the mind are added in recognition of the emotional stress associated with infertility in general and doing IVF in particular. Previously, we used mind calming herbs in Phase 2 formulas (see Ch. 4) for another reason. In a natural conception cycle, a stable Shen is important to ensure Bao vessel function and follicle growth. In the case of the IVF patient, this is no longer so relevant since the FSH stimulation of the follicles comes from an injection rather than from the pituitary gland, hence this aspect of Bao vessel function is supplanted. Some Kidney Yang herbs are added in recognition of the fact that a 'poor responder' likely has deficiencies of Kidney Yin and Yang, and that the eggs will be (hopefully) steadily maturing under the influence of the FSH drugs (reaching the more Yang phase of their development).

Phase 3 (approx. Day 11–14, follicle maturation, trigger injection + egg collection)

DRUGS: FSH + GNRH AGONIST OR ANTAGONIST + HCG TRIGGER

By Phase 3, the phase in which ovulation occurs in a natural menstrual cycle, physiological events take an even larger departure from normal. The ovaries are by now in quite an unnatural state. The FSH drugs continue to stimulate the ovaries and the follicles will reach their maximal size in this phase, however they are inhibited from releasing eggs by the action of the agonist or antagonist drugs. Once the eggs reach the appropriate size (around 20 mm), the trigger injection will be given. This finalizes the last stages of maturation and loosens the eggs from their follicle housing so they can be flushed out. In a natural cycle Phase 3 spans the days leading up to ovulation and the events immediately afterwards. In the IVF cycle Phase 3 continues only up until the day of egg collection.

This is a more intense time of the IVF cycle as the moment for egg collection approaches. Ultrasounds and blood tests are often done more frequently at this juncture so as to determine the best time for collection. Stress and anxiety relating to the results of these tests and the number and size of the follicles often builds at this time. The crucial nature of the timing of the hCG trigger injection (administered exactly 36h before the egg collection) adds to the anxiety for some.

• Acupuncture

Acupuncture is very useful at this point to address side-effects that may be worrying the patient. Most commonly, these are related to Liver Qi stagnation. There are several reasons that the Liver may be strained or overworked. First, there is the profound disruption to a natural physiologic cycle that is overseen by the Liver. By this stage of the IVF cycle, the ovaries may be swelling in the abdomen and obstructing Liver Qi and there will be unusually large amounts of estrogen taxing the liver's enzymes in addition to metabolism of the IVF drugs. Headaches, abdomen distension and pain, irritability and nausea are indications that the Liver Qi needs treatment.

Insomnia and anxiety are signs that the Heart Qi and the Shen need attention.

Dizziness is a less common symptom but may indicate Liver wind. Research-based acupuncture protocols which increase blood flow to reproductive organs can be continued in this phase.

It is in Phase 3 that warning signs of excessive hyperstimulation may appear (high blood estrogen levels or large numbers of follicles on ultrasound or severe abdomen distension), and the practitioner should be aware of these and take timely action. Treatment will be largely symptomatic at this stage, based primarily on regulating Liver Qi in the abdomen. (We discuss treatment of ovarian hyperstimulation syndrome below). The points chosen in the days before egg collection will be similar to those Phase 3 points described in Chapter 4. However, while the integrity and activity of the fallopian tubes were of prime concern there, in this case they are irrelevant.

Acupuncture points — Choose from the points below (and see Table 11.4):

Ren-4	Guanyuan
KI-6	Zhaohai
KI-13	Qixue
K-14	Siman
SP-13	Fushe
KI-5	Shuiquan
KI-8	Jiaoxin
Zigong	
SP-6	Sanyinjiao
KI-4	Dazhong
Ren-6	Qihai
ST-28	Shuidao
ST-29	Guilai
SP-6	Sanyinjiao
LIV-5	Ligou
LIV-8	Ququan
GB-34	Yanglingquan
Ren-12	Zhongwan
Ren-9	Shuifen
PC-4	Ximen
PC-6	Neiguan
HE-5	Tongli
HE-7	Shenmen
Yintang	

Table 11.4   Acupuncture points[a] suggested for use during an IVF cycle: trigger injection and egg collection phase

Treatment goal	Acupuncture points
To support Kidneys and promote growth of the follicles/eggs (days before trigger injection)	Ren-4, KI-6, KI-13, K-14
To boost Kidney Yang and promote final maturation of follicles/eggs (day of trigger injection)	KI-5, KI-8, Zigong, SP-6
To enhance Kidney function and stabilize emotions	KI-4
To regulate Qi, relieve abdomen distension (lower), promote circulation to ovaries	Ren-6, ST-28, ST-29, SP-6, LIV-5, SP-13, Ah Shi points
To regulate Qi, relieve abdomen distension (upper)	GB-34, Ren-12, LIV-5, LIV-8, REN-9
To regulate Liver Qi, relieve irritability, depression or headaches	LIV-3, CO-4
To calm Liver wind, relieve dizziness	LIV-8, CO-11
To clear Heat, relieve rashes	SP-10, CO-11
To regulate the Heart Qi, calm the mind, relieve insomnia	PC-4, 5 or 6, HE-5, 7, Yintang

[a]Use local and leg points with reducing method and even method with wrist points. The choice of abdomen or back points can be guided by sensations or pain.

Herbal formula — Just as the information from the blood tests and ultrasounds lets the IVF specialist know when to administer the trigger injection, this information will also let you know when you need to change the formula (in the case that you and the IVF doctor have made a decision to include herbs). It is when the follicles are measuring around 12–14 mm (i.e., they are approx 3–4 days from maturity) that you should prescribe a formula that continues to support Kidney Yin but will now contain more Kidney Yang tonic herbs in higher doses than before. This is to provide a final boost to the energy making capacity of the eggs before they are harvested.

In some women, as the ovaries swell with multiple follicles, abdominal discomfort increases as does distension. Thus the Phase 3 formulas will contain more herbs that regulate Qi to alleviate distension. Promoting Liver Qi movement also enables your patient to deal with stress.

Blood moving herbs with blood thinning qualities, such as those found in Phase 3 formulas in Chapter 4, are not included in this formula because of the impending surgical procedure. For the same reason, the patient will be advised to stop the formula altogether before the trigger injection, i.e., approx. 48 h before the egg collection procedure. Thus, this formula is for short use only, 2–3 days. Because we are not relying on correct functioning of the Bao Vessel for ovulation, we do not need to emphasize herbs to stabilize the Shen in the same way we did when we prescribed treatment in Phase 3 of a natural cycle. Similarly, we do not need to be concerned with the free movement of the fallopian tubes or the production of cervical mucus.

Bu Shen Cu Pai Luan is a Phase 3 formula used to support Kidney Yin and boost Kidney Yang while regulating the Qi to prepare for ovulation.

Bu Shen Cu Pai Luan Tang (Reinforce Kidney and Ovulation formula) modified

Bai Shao	9 g	*Radix Paeoniae Lactiflorae*
Nu Zhen Zi	9 g	*Fructus Ligustri Lucidi*
Shan Yao	9 g	*Dioscorea Oppositae*
Shan Zhu Yu	9 g	*Fructus Corni Officinalis*

Tu Si Zi	12 g	Semen Cuscatae
Bu Gu Zhi	6 g	Fructus Psoraleae
Rou Cong Rong	9 g	Herba Cistanches
Suo Yang	6 g	Herba Cynomorii Songarici
He Huan Pi	9 g	Cortex Albizziae Julibrissin
Xiang Fu Cu	12 g	Rhizoma Cyperi Rotundi
Qing Pi	3 g	Pericarpium Citri Reticulatae Viride
Ju He	3 g	Semen Citri Reticulatae
Li Zhe He	3 g	Semen Litchi
Wu Yao	3 g	Radix Linderae Strychnifoliae

This variation of Bu Shen Cu Pai Luan (described in Ch. 4) incorporates the Kidney Yang tonics that boost ATP production which we discussed above, and we hope will confer an enhanced energy making capacity to the eggs and hence to the embryo. These are combined with a strong Qi regulating element (the last five herbs listed, above), to emphasize circulation of Qi around the ovaries as they enlarge with a number of swollen follicles.

Phase 3 ends with egg collection. The patient is usually advised to rest for the rest of the day, because of the invasiveness of the procedure (with or without general anesthetic) and the possible physical trauma, but to consider returning for acupuncture in the days following.

THE MALE PARTNER'S ROLE

The spotlight has been on the ovaries and follicles, but it is at this moment that the sperm need to play their part.

As far as the male partner is concerned, we know that improving sperm motility and morphology can takes several weeks but, even in the short term, sperm vitality can be influenced. Electroacupuncture (and in some cases moxa) applied to the lower abdomen just before sperm donation, may help not only 'performance' and 'stage fright' but also galvanize the sperm for their task in the Petri dish.

Acupuncture points — Choose from the points below (and see Table 11.5):

K-3	Taixi
K-6	Zhaohai
LU-7	Lieque
Ren-4	Guanyuan
Ren-6	Qihai
DU-20	Baihui
ST-29	Guilai
SP-6	Sanyinjiao
SP-10	Xuehai
LIV-5	Ligou
LIV-8	Ququan
PC-6	Neiguan
Yin Tang	
LIV-3	Taichong
CO-4	Hegu
GB-41	Zu linqi
TH-5	Weiguan

Table 11.5   Acupuncture points[a] suggested for use during an IVF cycle: male partner on day of sperm donation

Treatment goal	Acupuncture points
Reinforce K Qi	Ren-4[b] K-3, K-6, LU-7
Fortify Yang	Ren-4 and 6 with moxa (if there is Cold), DU-20
Reinforce and regulate Qi and Blood supply	ST-29[c], SP-6, SP-10, LIV-5, 8, PC-6
Reduce anxiety	YT, LIV-3, CO-4 (20 min only)
Clear Damp in Lower Jiao, if necessary	GB-41, TH-5

[a]Use local and leg points with mild reducing method and even method with wrist points.
[b]Use deep but gentle needling with deqi traveling downwards.
[c]5 or 10 min of electroacupuncture (10 Hz) joining ST-29 to SP-6 on the same side.

Phase 4a (Day 14–Day 16/19, from egg collection to embryo transfer)

DRUGS: PROGESTERONE SUPPORT (PESSARIES, INJECTIONS, GEL) OR HCG INJECTIONS

Phase 4 in a natural cycle begins a few days after ovulation. For treatment of the IVF patient, we have divided Phase 4 into two parts, the first part spanning the days immediately after egg collection up until the embryo transfer (this may be anywhere between 2 and 5 days, during which time the embryo is in the incubator); and the second part from the day after the transfer of the embryo and up to the pregnancy test or the period.

ACUPUNCTURE – AFTER EGG COLLECTION

Acupuncture administered in the 2–3 days after egg collection aims at restoring normal Qi and blood flow in the channels through the reproductive organs, settling any tissue trauma, reducing effects of internal bleeding, reducing swelling of the ovaries and promoting circulation in the lining of the uterus. We do this by clearing Blood stasis, re-establishing Chong and Ren function, regulating Liver Qi and supporting Kidney function, especially Kidney Yang. By so doing, we aim to create favorable implantation conditions.

Additionally, help with managing stress is usually required. This is a nerve-racking time as your patient waits to hear whether her eggs have fertilized, and then whether the embryo(s) are developing. IVF clinics will usually report the total number of embryos on the day after fertilization and then will leave them undisturbed until the 3rd day, in incubator conditions that mimic as closely as possible the environment of the fallopian tube. If a reasonable number of embryos have survived at this point, the embryologist will suggest leaving them for another 2 days until they reach blastocyst stage.

Acupuncture points — Choose from the points below (and see Table 11.6):

Ren-7	Yinjiao
Ren-3	Zhongji
K-14	Siman
PC-6	Neiguan
SP-4	Gongsun
LIV-5	Ligou
LIV-4	Zhongfeng
GB-34	Yanglingquan
GB-27	Wushu

Ah Shi points on the abdomen

SP-10	Xuehai
SP-8	Diji
ST-29	Guilai
ST-30	Qichong
BL-57	Chengshan
BL-32	Ciliao
Ren-4	Guanyuan
Ren-6	Qihai
K-13	Qixue
K-6	Zhaohai
K-3	Taixi
BL-23	Shenshu
HT-7	Shenmen
Yin Tang	
DU-20	Baihui

Herbal formula — Now that the eggs are collected and the downregulating drugs are no longer required, drug–herb interactions are of less concern, and IVF patients can feel comfortable with taking herbs if they so wish, whether or not they have taken them at other times of their IVF cycle. There is no known or theoretical contraindication to using Chinese herbs at the same time as the exogenous progesterone (or hCG) that is administered at this phase.

Herbs to prepare the uterus for implantation are now prescribed. We combine some of the principles of treatment from Phase 3 with Phase 4 treatment principles.

This formula can be commenced after egg collection on the same day and will be continued for 6 or 7 days until the time the embryo implants – in other words, until a day or two after the transfer of a blastocyst, or 3–4 days after the transfer of a Day 3 embryo. Our treatment is focused on removing any stasis resulting from internal bleeding after the surgical removal of the eggs, and preparing the endometrium which may have been adversely affected by the drugs and hormone levels of the stimulation phase. Stability of the Shen and the Bao vessel is important in Phase 4a and 4b to keep the uterus closed.

Table 11.6 Acupuncture points[a] suggested for use during an IVF cycle: Phase 4a, after egg collection

Treatment goal	Acupuncture points
To regulate Qi and Blood in the Ren and Chong channels	Ren-7, Ren-3, K-14, PC-6, SP-4
To regulate Liver Qi, reduce swelling, alleviate pain	LIV-5, LIV-4, GB-34, GB-27 or Ah Shi points on the abdomen
To regulate Blood, clear Blood stasis, promote circulation to the endometrium	SP-10, SP-8, ST-29, ST-30, BL-57, BL-32
To boost Kidney Yang	Ren-4, Ren-6, K-13, K-6, K-3, BL-23
To calm the Shen	HT-7, YT, DU-20

[a]Use local and leg points with mild reducing method and even method with wrist and head points.

We modify the same formula Bu Shen Cu Pai Luan, with herbs to regulate the Blood as well as the Qi.

Bu Shen Cu Pai Luan (Reinforce Kidney Ovulation formula) modified

Dang Gui	9 g	Radix Angelicae Sinensis
Chi Shao	6 g	Radix Paeoniae Rubra
Bai Shao	6 g	Radix Paeoniae Lactiflorae
Hong Hua	3 g	Flos Carthami Tinctorii
Ji Xue Teng	9 g	Radix et Caulis Jixueteng
San Qi	3 g	Radix Pseudoginseng
Shan Yao	6 g	Dioscorea Oppositae
Shu Di	6 g	Rehmanniae Glutinosae Conquitae
Nu Zhen Zi	6 g	Fructus Ligustri Lucidi
Mu Dan Pi	6 g	Cortex Moutan Radicis
Fu Ling	6 g	Sclerotium Poriae Cocos
Tu Si Zi	12 g	Semen Cuscatae
Xu Duan	12 g	Radix Dipsaci
Zi Shi Ying	6 g	Fluoritum
He Huan Pi	9 g	Cortex Albizziae Julibrissin
Xiang Fu	9 g	Rhizoma Cyperi Rotundi

Bu Shen Cu Pai Luan (described in Ch. 4) is modified here with herbs which clear Blood stasis and maintain Shen stability. Support Kidney Yin and Yang, clear blood stasis, calm the mind.

To the original Bu Shen Cu Pai Luan, we add Ji Xue Teng to gently encourage Blood circulation in the endometrium, which alongside the Kidney Yin and Yang support we hope will create an optimal environment conducive to implantation. San Qi is added to address any internal bleeding from the egg collection procedure.

Zi Shi Ying and He Huan Pi are added to calm the Shen.

ACUPUNCTURE – THE DAY OF EMBRYO TRANSFER

Acupuncture is often performed on the day of embryo transfer. If the embryo transferred is a blastocyst, it is anticipated that implantation will happen within the following day or 2. If the embryo was transferred at 3 days, then implantation will occur in the following few days. Implantation is a complex event. Subtle changes in immune factors, up or downregulation of implantation factors, blood supply, hormone levels and so on, can all influence the delicate interaction of uterus and embryo. Equally, subtle external influences may exert an effect on implantation – like laughing, or being hypnotized, or having acupuncture. Such influences increase the endorphin level, or decrease the cortisol level or change certain cytokines levels or any number of other subtle biochemical or physiological changes about which we still know very little. Acupuncture points are chosen for their ability to support Kidneys and regulate local Qi and Blood flow with the aim of creating favorable implantation conditions. It may well be the fact that some of these points will reduce factors that hinder implantation, such as uterine contractions or autoimmune or clotting factors but at this stage, the mechanism of acupuncture's action at the time of implantation has not been elucidated. We will discuss the clinical trials that look at the effect of acupuncture or other interventions on the day of embryo transfer below. Most of these clinical trials have applied acupuncture both before and after the transfer on the same day. The trials that applied acupuncture stimulation only after the transfer, or on the day before the transfer, claim to achieve similar results. Thus, the acupuncture schedule you choose may be dictated by factors such as time and convenience, as much as clinical trial results. Most of the trials used the same acupuncture prescription with little or no variation (see below).

Table 11.7   Acupuncture points[a] suggested for use during an IVF cycle: Phase 4a, at embryo transfer

Treatment goal	Acupuncture points
To regulate Liver Qi, reduce uterine cramping	LIV-3, GB-34, CO-4
To regulate Blood, clear stasis, promote circulation to the endometrium	SP-10, SP-8, ST-29
To promote production of Blood and Qi	ST-36, SP-6
To boost Kidney Yang	Ren-4, Ren-6, K-6, K-3
To regulate the activity of the Chong and Ren vessels	Ren-7
To calm the Shen	HT-7, PC-6, YT, DU-20

[a]Use local and leg points with mild reducing method and even method with wrist points. Abdomen points are used only in the treatments before the embryo transfer.

Acupuncture points — Choose from the points below (and see Table 11.7):

LIV-3	Taichong
GB-34	Yanglingquan
CO-4	Hegu
SP-10	Xuehai
SP-8	Diji
ST-29	Guilai
ST-36	Zusanli
SP-6	Sanyinjiao
Ren-4	Guanyuan
Ren-6	Qihai
K-6	Zhaohai
K-3	Taixi
Ren-7	Yinjiao
HT-7	Shenmen
PC-6	Neiguan
Yin Tang	
DU-20	Baihui

Phase 4b (from day after embryo transfer until pregnancy test or period, implantation)

DRUGS: PROGESTERONE PESSARIES, INJECTIONS OR GEL OR HCG INJECTIONS

Implantation and development of the early placenta occurs in this phase. We support this process with treatment that reinforces Kidney, Spleen, and the Blood. Some IVF patients describe this waiting period as the most difficult time of the whole cycle. Now that there is no longer attention from the nurses, doctors, and radiographers, the support of the acupuncturist plays an important role.

Table 11.8   Acupuncture points[a] suggested for use during an IVF cycle: Phase 4b, between embryo transfer and pregnancy test

Treatment goal	Acupuncture points
To boost Kidney Yang	K-6, K-5
To regulate Liver Qi, reduce uterine cramping	GB-34, LIV-3, LIV-4, LIV-5, LIV-9, LIV-11
To regulate Blood in the Liver, Kidney and Ren channels and address Liver Blood deficiency	LIV-8, LIV-3, KI-5
To invigorate the Spleen and Stomach and promote production of Blood and Qi	ST-36, BL-17, BL-20, BL-21
To calm the Shen, safeguard the Bao Luo vessel	YT, DU-20, Ren-15, HE-5, HE-7, K-9
To relieve stress and regulate Liver Qi in the upper body	LIV-5, PC-6, PC-7, PC-5

[a]Use local and leg points with mild reducing method and even method with wrist points. Avoid abdomen and lower back points.

Acupuncture points — Choose from the points below (and see Table 11.8):

Yin tang	
DU-20	Baihui
Ren-15	Jiuwei
HE-5	Tongli
HE-7	Shenmen
GB-34	Yanglingquan
LIV-3	Taichong
LIV-4	Zhongfeng
LIV-5	Ligou
LIV-9	Yinbiao
LIV-11	Yinlian
LIV-8	Ququan
KI-5	Shuiquan
ST-36	Zusanlin
BL-17	Geshu
BL-20	Pishu
K-9	Zhubin
K-6	Zhaohai
KI-5	Shuiquan
PC-6	Neiguan
PC-7	Daling
PC-5	Jianshi

Herbal formula — From this point, we focus on nourishing Kidney Yin and Yang, with the aim of supporting the secretory function of the endometrium and the implantation of the embryo. Kidney Yang herbs have been observed to increase progesterone levels and may be useful in supporting the action of hCG injections, which are given to promote corpus luteum function at this stage or supplementing any exogenous progesterone. Adequate progesterone levels are important to maintain endometrium function and support early pregnancy. There is no danger in having too much progesterone. Nourishing Blood supports nutrition to the endometrium, as does the use of Spleen Qi tonics. Herbs which regulate Qi in the abdomen ameliorate the cramping symptoms that the supplemental progesterone can cause.

You Gui Wan (Restore the Right Kidney pill) plus Yu Lin Zhu (Fertility Pearls) modified

Bai Zhu	12 g	Rhizoma Atractylodis Macrocephalae
Fu Ling	9 g	Sclerotium Poriae Cocos
Dang Gui	9 g	Radix Angelicae Sinensis
Bai Shao	9 g	Radix Paeoniae Lactiflorae
Shu Di	9 g	Radix Rehmanniae Glutinosae Conquitae
Shan Zhu Yu	9 g	Fructus Corni Officinalis
Shan Yao	9 g	Dioscorea Oppositae
Tu Si Zi	12 g	Semen Cuscatae
Xu Duan	12 g	Radix Dipsaci
Du Zhong	6 g	Cortex Eucommiae Ulmoidis
Ba Ji Tian	9 g	Radix Morindae Officinalis
Xiang Fu	9 g	Rhizoma Cyperi Rotundi
Gan Cao	3 g	Radix Glycyrrhizae Uralensis

Yu Lin Zhu and You Gui Wan are formulas we discussed in Chapter 4. This combination reinforces Kidney Yin and warms Kidney Yang, nourishes Blood, supports Spleen and regulates Qi.

If there are immune factors which may be implicated in impaired implantation, then consider adding Huang Qi in a large dose (20 g). For clotting factors, we might consider Dan Shen in a small dose, however most patients diagnosed with clotting factors will be taking low molecular weight heparin, and the addition of extra blood thinning agents will not be necessary.

CASE HISTORY – MELISSA

Melissa (36) had been trying to have a baby for 5 years, with no luck. Her infertility was a mystery. All investigations of herself and her husband showed no discernible abnormality. She visited an ART specialist who recommended an IUI procedure. This procedure involves stimulation of the ovaries by injected FSH preparations and, when the ultrasound and blood tests indicate that ovulation is imminent, a selected and scrubbed-up sample of sperm is injected into the uterus near the entrance of the fallopian tubes.

Melissa underwent this procedure four times. She did achieve one pregnancy, but sadly it was followed by a miscarriage. One thing that was discovered during these procedures was that her ovaries were quite unresponsive to the drugs and were slow to produce eggs. In fact, one of her ovaries, the right one, showed no response at all in three out of the four procedures. From ultrasound investigations during other (drug-free) cycles, it seemed that the ovary was quite dormant.

She decided to see what TCM could offer. She told me her cycle was regular at 28 or 29 days. Her BBT (basal body temperature) charts showed ovulation at day 14, which was followed by an adequate to low luteal phase. Premenstrually, she became moody and had sore breasts. Periods were normal and trouble-free. At midcycle she saw stretchy fertile mucus for 3 days. She was healthy and cheerful despite the tortuous path her infertility had led her. The pulse was normal and her tongue was red on the edges and the tip.

We had few clues here, but the lack of ovarian response during the IUI cycles indicated some Kidney deficiency. One other interesting clue emerged when she started using urine ovulation kits and found that her levels of LH were too low to be detected. In a TCM framework, this might indicate that it is the influence of Kidney Yang that is failing. Her BBT charts gave some hint of this too.

She took herbs based on the standard protocol outlined in Chapter 4, but after 3 months when she was not pregnant, we discussed the possibility of her doing IVF. There was so little symptomatology for me to assess the progress of any TCM treatment, her Kidney deficiency manifested only at the level of the ovary itself, and without constant blood tests and ultrasounds, it was difficult to monitor change. By doing IVF we would discover more about her ovary responses to the drugs (which are administered for longer than in an IUI cycle) and more about the eggs themselves and their ability to fertilize. She agreed to try IVF; the results were illuminating, if depressing.

She underwent 2 IVF cycles in which few eggs were collected (three from the left ovary only each time), but when these eggs were fertilized, the embryos that formed were very fragmented and failed to divide. Recovery from these cycles was long. Melissa suffered severe Shen disturbance, manifesting as insomnia, anxiety, dizziness, and fatigue. After each IVF cycle, it took 3 more cycles to return to a regular 28-day cycle.

However, armed with the information gleaned from the behavior of the eggs and the embryos during IVF, I had another way to approach treatment. Before and during Melissa's procedure, we would now strongly reinforce the Kidney Jing to try and influence the nature of the eggs themselves and their ability to respond to hormonal stimulation. This was achieved by taking the following formula of herbs, which strengthen Kidney Jing, Yang and Yin. Some cooling herbs were added to counteract the Heat in the Yang tonics.

Zi He Che*	3 g	Placenta Hominis
Lu Jiao Pian	6 g	Cornu Cervi Parvum
Dong Chong Xia Cao	3 g	Cordyceps Chinensis
Tu Si Zi	12 g	Semen Cuscatae
Suo Yang	6 g	Herba Cynomorii Songarici
Rou Cong Rong	9 g	Herba Cistanches
Shu Di	9 g	Radix Rehmanniae Glutinosae Conquitae
Dang Gui	9 g	Radix Angelicae Sinensis
Shan Zhu Yu	9 g	Fructus Corni Officinalis
Shan Yao	9 g	Radix Dioscorea Oppositae
Zhi Mu	12 g	Radix Amenarrhena
Huang Lian	3 g	Rhizoma Coptidis
Xiang Fu	9 g	Rhizoma Cyperi Rotundi
Dan Shen	9 g	Radix Salviae Miltiorrhizae

Melissa took these herbs for 2 weeks and then embarked on another IUI protocol. To everybody's surprise, her ovaries – including the dormant right one – responded enthusiastically to the FSH drugs. The response was so good that she produced far too many eggs to do an insemination as the risk of multiple pregnancy was too high. So the insemination was cancelled and the eggs collected, as in an IVF cycle. Out of eight eggs, four fertilized with no fragmentation and three developed into blastocysts that were of a good enough quality to freeze. Sadly, none of those blastocysts went the distance to a viable pregnancy. Melissa underwent IVF again, taking herbs at the same time, and again produced embryos which developed well and did not fragment, but did not implant. A fifth and final IVF program combined with the Jing tonic herbs finally brought with it the long sought-after pregnancy. Melissa had an uneventful pregnancy and gave birth to a large healthy baby girl.

*Zi He Che is a restricted substance in some countries.

CASE HISTORY – DAVID

David (30), a businessman, wanted desperately to be a dad but for unknown reasons, his sperm did not have what it takes. His count was low, motility was low and there were too few sperm of normal morphology. His wife was healthy and had a normal cycle. In the 5 years they had been trying to have a baby, they had tried preconception programs, taking many vitamins and eating organic food, and had undergone 2 IVF cycles. A number of blastocysts were obtained after ICSI was performed to bring about fertilization. Pregnancy, however, eluded them.

David was fit and healthy, with good libido and sexual function. His pulse was full and tight and his tongue was quite red.

He was prescribed herbs to reinforce Kidney Yin and Yang, clear Heat and regulate Blood.

Shu Di	9 g	Radix Rehmanniae Glutinosae Conquitae
Sheng Di	12 g	Radix Rehmanniae Glutinosae
Nu Zhen Zi	9 g	Fructus Ligustri Lucidi
Gou Qi Zi	9 g	Fructus Lycii Chinensis
Dang Gui	9 g	Radix Angelicae Sinensis
Bai Shao	9 g	Radix Paeoniae Lactiflorae
He Shou Wu	9 g	Radix Polygoni Multiflori
Bai Zhu	6 g	Rhizoma Atractylodes Macrocephalae
Huang qi	9 g	Radix Astragali
Dan Shen	9 g	Radix Salviae Miltiorrhizae
Tao Ren	6 g	Semen Persicae
Tu Si Zi	15 g	Semen Cuscatae
Fu Pen Zi	9 g	Fructus Rubi Chingii
Ba Ji Tian	9 g	Radix Morindae Officinalis
Xiang Fu	6 g	Rhizoma Cyperi Rotundi
Huang Lian	3 g	Rhizoma Coptidis
Gan Cao	3 g	Radix Glycyrrhizae

He took this formula for 4 months and then he and his wife tried another IVF cycle. When it came time for the ICSI procedure, the embryologists discovered that the sperm were able to successfully fertilize a good number of eggs unaided. The vitality of the sperm had improved sufficiently to fertilize an egg in a dish but not enough to achieve a conception naturally.

The script was changed to incorporate more Yang tonics when David reported that the pressure to perform was starting to affect sexual function. In addition, herbs to clear Damp-Heat were added because the most recent sperm analysis showed some debris in the semen. Additions:

Xu Duan	9 g	Radix Dipsaci
Lu Rong	6 g	Cornu Cervi Parvum
Xian Mao	6 g	Rhizoma Curculiginis Orchioidis
Long Dan Cao	9 g	Radix Gentianae Scabrae
Huang Qin	6 g	Radix Scutellariae

He tolerated these well and sexual function improved.

A fourth IVF was attempted, in which his sperm performed even more impressively and fertilized even more eggs spontaneously; however, no pregnancy eventuated. This story ends with an application for adoption. The toll of infertility and failed IVF attempts was exacting too great a price on this couples' relationship.

CASE HISTORY – FREYA

Freya (40) had been trying to conceive since she was 37. There was no reason for her infertility or for the fact that the four stimulated IVF cycles she'd undergone hadn't worked either. During each cycle, she produced a good number of eggs, all of which fertilized and most of which reached the blastocyst stage. With two embryos transferred each cycle, she had plenty left for freezing. However, several transfers of the frozen embryos (two or three embryos each time) had failed also. Freya decided to add TCM to her regimen.

She reported that her cycles were regular at 29 days. She knew when she ovulated, because she saw plenty of good-quality fertile mucus and felt ovarian discomfort. Her BBT charts indicated ovulation around Day 15 or 16; her luteal phase was high and steady. The follicular phase showed some instability, with several peaks. Before her period, she became irritable and bloated; her period was pretty much pain-free but the flow was scanty and dull red. She suffered from insomnia, headaches on waking, and sore eyes. She presented as a bright, chatty and anxious woman. Her Liver pulse was choppy and her Heart pulse had a knotted quality. The Kidney pulses were thready. The tongue had pale sides and a purplish hue.

In TCM terms, she was Liver and Heart Blood deficient with signs of stagnation. My guess was that the Bao Mai (from the Heart) and Bao Luo (from the Kidneys) were affected, which meant inadequate nourishment of the Uterus. This may have been the reason why the embryos were not implanting.

For 2 cycles, she took herbs to replenish the Liver and Heart Blood and increase its circulation. In addition, she took herbs to strengthen Kidney function.

Shu Di	9g	*Radix Rehmanniae Glutinosae Conquitae*
Dang Gui	9g	*Radix Angelicae Sinensis*
Bai Shao	9g	*Radix Paeoniae Lactiflorae*
Gou Qi Zi	15g	*Fructus Lycii Chinensis*
Long Yan Rou	9g	*Arillus Euphoriae Longanae*
Shan Zhu Yu	9g	*Fructus Corni Officinalis*
Chuan Xiong	6g	*Radix Ligustici Wallichii*
Dan Shen	9g	*Radix Salviae Miltiorrhizae*
Yu Jin	9g	*Tuber Curcumae*
Suan Zao Ren	15g	*Semen Ziziphi Spinosae*
Xiang Fu	9g	*Rhizoma Cyperi Rotundi*

Acupuncture points: Ren-7, Ren-3, ST-30, KI-14, KI-3, LIV-3, PC-6, SP-6

After midcycle, we varied this formula by removing Chuan Xiong and Yu Jin, reducing Dan Shen to 6g and including Tu Si Zi 9g and Zi Shi Ying 9g.

Acupuncture points: KI-14, KI-6, LIV-3, PC-7

After 2 months of taking these herbs, Freya reported that she saw more fresh red blood with her period, she was sleeping better, her spirits were better, and she was feeling more optimistic. Heart and Liver pulses improved and her tongue was not quite so pale. However, she had still not conceived and decided to try another FET cycle. In preparation, she took herbs during the period and, so she could say she'd tried everything, she had a surgical dilatation and curettage (D&C) as well.

Chuan Xiong	6g	*Radix Ligustici Wallichii*
Dan Shen	9g	*Radix Salviae Miltiorrhizae*
Yu Jin	9g	*Tuber Curcumae*
Yi Mu Cao	9g	*Herba Leonuri Heterophylli*
Wu Ling Zhi	9g	*Excrementum Trogopterori*
Shan Zha	9g	*Fructus Crataegi*
Dang Gui	12g	*Radix Angelicae Sinensis*
He Shou Wu	12g	*Radix Polygoni Multifori*

Acupuncture points: SP-10, SP-6, Ren-6, LIV-8, PC-6

After the period, she took herbs to nourish Blood and Yin and calm the Shen:

Shu Di	9g	*Radix Rehmanniae Glutinosae Conquitae*
Shan Yao	9g	*Radix Dioscorea Oppositae*
Shan Zhu Yu	9g	*Fructus Corni Officinalis*
Dang Gui	9g	*Radix Angelicae Sinensis*
Bai Shao	9g	*Radix Paeoniae Lactiflorae*
Chuan Xiong	6g	*Radix Ligustici Wallichii*
Yu Jin	6g	*Tuber Curcumae*
Suan Zao Ren	9g	*Semen Ziziphi Spinosae*
Bai Zi Ren	9g	*Semen Biotae Orientalis*
Mu Li	9g	*Concha Ostrea*
Huang Lian	3g	*Rhizoma Coptidis*

Acupuncture points: Ren-4, KI-6, HE-7, PC-6, SP-6, Yin Tang

From midcycle and just before the transfer of three embryos she took:

Shu Di	9 g	Radix Rehmanniae Glutinosae Conquitae
Bai Shao	9 g	Radix Paeoniae Lactiflorae
Dan Shen	6 g	Radix Salviae Miltiorrhizae
Mu Li	9 g	Concha Ostrea
Suan Zao Ren	12 g	Semen Ziziphi Spinosae
Tu Si Zi	9 g	Semen Cuscatae
Xu Duan	9 g	Radix Dipsaci
Fu Pen Zi	9 g	Fructus Rubi Chingii
Rou Cong Rong	6 g	Herba Cistanches
Xiang Fu	6 g	Rhizoma Cyperi Rotundi

She had her last acupuncture treatment on the morning of the transfer:

Yin Tang, PC-6, LIV-3, SP-6, Ren-4, KI-14

At 10 days later, she received a positive pregnancy test – with the highest progesterone readings the clinic had ever seen. She continued with herbs to secure the pregnancy.

Sang Ji Sheng	15 g	Ramulus Sangjisheng
Tu Si Zi	15 g	Semen Cuscatae
Xu Duan	9 g	Radix Dipsaci
Du Zhong	9 g	Cortex Eucommiae Ulmoidis
Nu Zhen Zi	9 g	Fructus Ligustri Lucidi
Han Lian Cao	12 g	Herba Ecliptae Prostratae
Bai Shao	9 g	Radix Paeoniae Lactiflorae
MuLi	9 g	Concha Ostrea
Huang Qin	9 g	Radix Scutellariae
Suan Zao Ren	12 g	Semen Ziziphi Spinosae

The pregnancy was somewhat problematic, with intermittent bleeding throughout, but baby Sam was born on time and healthy.

*Zi He Che is a restricted substance in some countries.

OVARIAN HYPER-STIMULATION SYNDROME

The main symptoms of ovarian hyper-stimulation syndrome (OHSS) usually manifest in Phase 4, although warning signs can occur as early as Phase 2 during stimulation of the follicles. Such a disturbance of water metabolism is more likely to occur in patients with Kidney deficiency, and secondarily in those with Spleen (and Lung) deficiency and stagnation of Qi and Blood.

Kidneys, Spleen, and Lungs are responsible for fluid movement in the upper, middle and lower Jiao, respectively.

Moderate or severe OHSS itself is an acute and excess condition and our first priority is to mobilize fluids then to support Kidney, Spleen (and Lungs). Qi and Blood stagnation may also need to be addressed. Herbal treatment focuses on regulating water metabolism in the body by using diuretic herbs and promoting Kidney Yang and Spleen Qi.

Herbal formula — The Phase 4b formula (You Gui wan plus Yu Lin Zhu modified) can be further modified to correct water metabolism with the addition of:

Huang Qi	20–30 g	Radix Astragali
Zhu Ling	15 g	Polyporus
Ze Xie	15 g	Rhizoma Alismatis

and increasing Fu Ling (*Poria*) to 15 g.

If there is marked stasis, and embryo transfer has been postponed for another time,

Dan Shen (*Radix Salviae Miltiorrhizae*) 15–20 g, can be added.

Acupuncture points — Choose from the points below (and see Table 11.9):

Ren-9	Shuifen
Ren-5	Shimen
ST-28	Shuidao
K-5	Shuiquan
SP-9	Yinlingquan
BL-22	Sanjiaoshu
BL-28	Pangguanshu
SJ-10	Tianjing
LIV-4	Zhongfeng
CO-6	Pianli
K-14	Siman
BL-32	Ciliao
GB-26	Daimai
GB-27	Wushu
GB-28	Weidao
Ren-17	Shanzhong
LU-7	Lieque
LU-1	Zhongfu

Table 11.9   Acupuncture points[a] suggested for use during an IVF cycle: Phase 4, OHSS

Treatment goal	Acupuncture points
To regulate water passages and alleviate pain and distension of abdomen	Ren-9, Ren-5, ST-28, K-5, SP-9
To promote removal of fluids via the bladder	BL-22, BL-28
To descend rebellion, alleviate shortness of breath, ascites	SJ-10, LIV-4, CO-6, Ren-17
To resolve accumulations and swelling via the Dai Channel	GB-26, GB-27, GB-28
To regulate Qi and Blood, clear stasis	K-14, BL-32
To regulate water passages and descend Lung Qi	LU-7, LU-1
To regulate water passages and benefit Kidney	K-7

Treatment should be applied twice a week or in more severe cases every 2nd day or daily.
[a]Use points with reducing method. Needle abdomen points very shallowly.

THE POSITIVE PREGNANCY TEST

A pregnancy achieved after a period of (female) subfertility needs careful nurturing in the first few weeks. This patient's risk of miscarriage is raised compared to women with no history of fertility difficulties.

Acupuncture once a week is recommended. The idea behind our treatments at this stage is to support the Kidney Qi and to stabilize the Bao vessel and Bao channel so that the uterus remains closed.

Some research has indicated that just the act of monitoring early pregnancy seems to help reduce miscarriage rates in women with a history of pregnancy loss,[27] and many IVF clinics offer similar services now, with weekly blood tests and/or ultrasounds. The rising hCG in the blood tests or the growing fetus on the ultrasound provides confirmation that helps to settle the Shen and stabilize the Bao Mai.

In the acupuncture clinic, we can offer something similar in the way of reassurance of a healthy pulse picture (a strong gliding quality on the Kidney position is ideal, although it is not every viable pregnancy that shows this in the early days). But we can do something more. Using herbs and acupuncture points to support Kidney and Spleen Qi will support endometrial function and nourishment of the developing fetus. By using herbs and points which calm the Shen, we shall be ensuring the Bao Mai is stable and the uterus remains closed.

Acupuncture points — Choose from the points below (and see Table 11.10):

Yin Tang
DU-20   Baihui
PC-6   Neiguan
K-9   Zhubin
K-6   Zhaohai
ST-36   Zusanli
HT-7   Shenmen
LIV-3   Taichong
GB-34   Yanglingquan
K-4   Dazhong

Herbal formula — There is some evidence from clinical trials to show that using Chinese herbs to support the Kidneys and the Spleen in the early part of pregnancy, reduces miscarriage rates after IVF cycles.[28]

The formula used in this research 'Gu tai tang' or Protect Fetus decoction has many different versions, but fundamentally they all aim to support Kidney and Spleen Qi while nourishing the blood and quieting the fetus.

Table 11.10   Acupuncture points[a] suggested for use in the early stage of pregnancy after an IVF cycle

Treatment goal	Acupuncture points
To stabilize Shen	YT, DU-20, PC-6, HT-7, K-4, K-9
To support Kidney Qi	K-6
To support Spleen Qi	ST-36
To alleviate residual abdominal discomfort or ovarian swelling	LIV-5, GB-34

[a]Use points with even method. Avoid abdomen and lower back points.

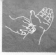

Herbal formula for use after a positive pregnancy test in an IVF cycle; Yishen Gutai Tang (Nourish Kidney and Protect Fetus) modified. Reinforce Kidney and Spleen Qi, nourish Blood and quiet the fetus.

Yishen Gutai Tang (Nourish Kidney and Protect Fetus decoction) modified

Tu Si Zi	20 g	Semen Cuscatae
Du Zhong	15 g	Cortex Eucommiae Ulmoidis
Xu Duan	15 g	Radix Dipsaci
Sang Ji Sheng	15 g	Ramulus Sangjisheng
Bai Zhu	15 g	Rhizoma Atractylodis Macrocephalae
Huang Qin	9 g	Radix Scutellariae Baicalensis
Gou Qi Zi	12 g	Fructus Lycii Chinensis
Dang Shen	12 g	Radix Codonopsis Pilulosae
Bai Zhu	12 g	Rhizoma Atractylodis Macrocephalae
Da Zao	3 pieces	Fructus Zizyphi Jujuba
Sha Ren	3 g	Fructus seu Semen Amomi
He Shou Wu	12 g	Radix Polygoni Multiflori

If there is any bleeding, add:

E Jiao	15 g	Gelatinum Asini
Zhu Ma Gen	9 g	Radix Boehmeriae

For Morning sickness, see Chapter 4.

THE NEGATIVE PREGNANCY TEST

If the IVF cycle has not succeeded, then the treatment priorities are to re-establish Chong and Ren channel function, clear stagnation of Qi and Blood, reinforce Spleen and Kidney function and to treat Lungs and Heart for grief and sadness. The menstrual cycle immediately after an IVF cycle will sometimes be longer than usual, as the ovaries may take some time to recover.

Weekly acupuncture treatment is useful at this time and should be continued until at least one good menstrual cycle has been achieved. Then the patient may start preparing for another IVF cycle using the suggestions for herb and acupuncture prescriptions made earlier.

If she is not planning on repeating IVF so soon, or she plans to try and conceive naturally, then a 3-month program can be constructed using the protocols outlined in Chapter 4, or above.

Acupuncture points — Choose from the points below (and see Table 11.11):

SP-6	Sanyinjiao
SP-4	Gongsun
PC-6	Neiguan
LU-3	Tian Fu
LIV-5	Ligou
K-6	Zhaohai
SP-10	Xuehai
K-3	Taixi
Ren-3	Zhongji

Ren-7	Lingdao
HT-7	Shenmen
HT-4	Lingdao
Yin Tang	
Ren-6	Qihai
ST-28	Shuidao

This concludes our discussion on the use of Chinese medicine for the patient doing IVF, before, during and after her cycle (Table 11.12). As I stated at the outset, it will be some decades of careful observation in the clinic and informed and considered clinical experimentation before we can become expert in this sort of treatment. However I am, as are my colleagues, thrilled to be part of this exciting era of exploring the frontiers of reproductive medicine and the place that Chinese medicine can play in it. Some intrepid clinicians and researchers have already made wonderful contributions to this area and it is only just the beginning! This is what we shall discuss next.

RESEARCH ON ACUPUNCTURE AND IVF

Many IVF patients heard about the possible benefits of combining acupuncture with their IVF cycle after results of a small trial were published in 2002. This was followed by a spate of repeat trials from 2006 onwards. More than 20 trials, of varying quality, which look at the effect of acupuncture on the day of embryo transfer have been published in peer reviewed journals. While many of these have shown a positive effect on pregnancy rates when acupuncture is used, a number of other trials have shown no effect.

The abstracts of the many studies to-date that investigate the effect of acupuncture done at the time of embryo transfer, can be found online.[29,30]

Despite the fact that the jury is still out on whether acupuncture performed in this way is actually increasing pregnancy rates, many IVF patients are seeking out acupuncture as an adjunctive treatment. And, despite lack of consistent evidence of increased pregnancy rates, there is no doubt that IVF patients generally appreciate the increased well-being they experience as a result of the acupuncture. This has been shown in clinical studies to have the effect of reducing the stress and distress experienced during the cycle and increasing resilience and ability to cope with repeated IVF cycles if they are necessary.[31–34]

Table 11.11   Acupuncture points[a] suggested for use following a negative pregnancy test after an IVF cycle

Treatment goal	Acupuncture points
To re-establish Chong channel function	SP-4, PC-6
To regulate Chong and Ren channels	Ren-3, Ren-7
To alleviate grief and sadness, benefit sleep	LU-3, HT-7, HT-4, YT
If bleeding after IVF cycle persists for longer than usual	SP-10, K-3
To relieve abdominal bloating or discomfort	Ren-6, ST-28, LIV-5, SP-6
To strengthen the Kidney Qi	Ren-4, K-6

[a]Use points with even method.

Table 11.12 Summary of herbal formulas suggested for use by IVF patients

Summary of formulas used in preparation for IVF

Clinical presentation	Time of administration	Principle of treatment	Guiding formula (see also Appendix 4)	Plus	Minus
Poor egg quality or over 35 years or previous failed IVF cycles.	3–6 months Taken throughout the cycle or Phase 2, 3, or 4.	Supplement Kidney Yin, Yang, and Jing, calm the mind	Gui Shao Di Huang tang	Dan Shen Sha Ren Tu Si Zi Bu Gu Zhi Xiang Fu He Huan Pi Suo Yang Lu Jiao Pian Zi Shi Ying	
Stress or distress, irregular cycles, PCOS, menstrual symptoms.	1–3 months Taken throughout the cycle or Phase 2, 3, or 4.	Supplement Kidney Yin and Yang, and regulate Liver and Heart Qi	Gui Shao Di Huang Tang with Xiao Yao San and Gan Mai Da Zao Tang	Sha Ren Tu Si Zi Bu Gu Zhi Xiang Fu He Huan Pi Dan Shen	Sheng Jiang Bo He Bai Zhu
Pain or masses, menstrual symptoms.	1–6 months Taken during Phase 1, or whole cycle for 1–2 cycles if not trying to conceive.	Clear Blood stasis	Tao Hong Si Wu tang	Chi Shao Gui Zhi Dan Shen Shan Zha Pu Huang Wu Ling Zhi Yan Hu Suo Xiang Fu Xu Duan Chuan Niu Xi	Shu Di Bai Shao

Table 11.12 Summary of herbal formulas suggested for use by IVF patients—cont'd

Clinical presentation	Time of administration	Principle of treatment	Guiding formula (see also Appendix 4)	Plus	Minus
Pain or masses, menstrual symptoms.	3–6 months Taken during whole cycle. If conception occurs stop the formula.	Supplement Kidneys. Clear Blood stasis	Gui Shao Di Huang tang and Tao Hong Si Wu tang	Pu Huang Wu Ling Zhi Sha Ren Tu Si Zi Bu Gu Zhi Xiang Fu He Huan Pi Mu Dan Pi	Chuan Xiong
Excess weight (PCOS)	3–6 months Taken throughout the cycle or Phase 2, 3, or 4. If conception occurs stop the formula.	Supplement Kidneys. Clear Phlegm-Damp	Gui Shao Di Huang Tang plus Jian Gu Tang	Zao Jiao Ci Dan Nan Xing Sha Ren Ji Xue Teng Dan Shen Nu Zhen Zi Han Lian Cao	Shu Di Dang Gui

Male partner preparation for IVF

Poor semen analysis or older man (over 35 years)	3–6 months	Supplement the Kidneys, nourish Qi and Blood	Bu Shen Yi Jing fang	Sheng Di Hong Hua *With Heat* Huang Bai Zhi Mu	Rou Cong Rong Ba Ji Tian Suo Yang Lu Jiao Pien Bai Shao Mu Dan Pi

Summary of formulas used during IVF (after 2 or more failed cycles)

IVF cycle (poor responder only) Menstrual period Drugs: FSH ± GnRH agonist	Phase 1 Day 1–3	Regulate Blood and Qi, replenish Blood	Tao Hong Si Wu tang	Yi Mu Cao Xiang Fu Ji Xue Teng Shan Zha Dan Shen Chuan Niu Xi	Shu Di

Continued

Table 11.12 Summary of herbal formulas suggested for use by IVF patients—cont'd

Clinical presentation	Time of administration	Principle of treatment	Guiding formula (see also Appendix 4)	Plus	Minus
IVF cycle (poor responder only) Follicle development Drugs: FSH ± GnRH agonist or antagonist	Phase 2 Day 4 to approx. Day 11	Supplement Kidney Yin, Yang and Jing, Blood and calm the mind	Gui Shao Di Huang tang	Dan Shen Ji Xue Teng Sha Ren Tu Si Zi Bu Gu Zhi Xiang Fu Wu Yao Yin Yang Huo Lu Jiao Pian Zi Shi Ying Suan Zao Ren He Huan Pi Suan Zao Ren	
IVF cycle (poor responder only) Follicle maturation, egg collection Drugs: FSH + GnRH agonist or antagonist + hCG trigger	Phase 3 Day 11–14 approx. From follicle size 12 mm to 12 h before trigger injection.	Supplement Kidney Yin, boost Kidney Yang, regulate Qi and Blood	Bu Shen Cu Pai Luan	Wu Yao Shan Zhu Yu Bu Gu Zhi He Huan Pi Xiang Fu Cu Qing Pi Rou Cong Rong Suo Yang He Huan Pi Xiang Fu Cu Qing Pi Li Zhe He Ju He	Dang Gui Shu Di Chi Shao Dan Pi Fu Ling Xu Duan Wu Ling Zhi Hong Hua

Table 11.12 Summary of herbal formulas suggested for use by IVF patients—cont'd

Clinical presentation	Time of administration	Principle of treatment	Guiding formula (see also Appendix 4)	Plus	Minus
IVF cycle Preparing for embryo transfer. Drugs: Progesterone support (pessaries, injections; gel) or hCG injections	Phase 4a Day 14–day 16/19 approx. Between egg collection and embryo transfer	Supplement Kidney Yin, boost Kidney Yang, clear Blood stasis, calm the mind	Bu Shen Cu Pai Luan	Zi Shi Ying He Huan Pi Xiang Fu Ji Xue Teng San Qi	Wu Ling Zhi
IVF cycle Implantation of embryo Drugs: Progesterone support (pessaries, injections; gel) or hCG injections	Phase 4b Day 16/19–day 28 approx. From embryo transfer until pregnancy test	Supplement Kidney Yin, warm Kidney Yang, nourish Blood, support Spleen, regulate Qi	You Gui wan plus Yu Lin Zhu	Xiang Fu Xu Duan	Lu Jiao Pian Dang Shen Chuan Xiong

Ovarian hyperstimulation syndrome

Clinical presentation	Time of administration	Principle of treatment	Guiding formula (see also Appendix 4)	Plus	Minus
IVF cycle High estrogen, abdomen distension, dizziness, etc.	Phase 4 or from trigger injection	Supplement Kidneys, support Spleen, regulate Qi and promote diuresis	You Gui wan plus Yu Lin Zhu	Huang Qi Zhu Ling Ze Xie Fu Ling (extra) Xiang Fu Xu Duan (Dan Shen)	Lu Jiao Pian Dang Shen Chuan Xiong

Pregnancy support

Clinical presentation	Time of administration	Principle of treatment	Guiding formula (see also Appendix 4)	Plus	Minus
Early pregnancy	Until week 10 or 12	Supplement Kidneys, warm the womb, settle the fetus, support the Spleen.	Yishen Gutai Tang	E Jiao Zhu Ma Gen if spotting	

Additionally, it has been shown that acupuncture increases blood flow to the uterine lining and (in rats) to the ovaries. This theoretically could mean increased drug delivery and nutrition to these areas. Many clinics that offer acupuncture treatment to IVF patients combine the points that increase blood flow to ovaries and the uterus during the stimulation phase of the cycle when the woman is using the FSH drugs, and then points used in the above mentioned trials at the time of embryo transfer.

Effects on implantation and pregnancy rate

It is thought that the acupuncture points applied on the day of embryo transfer may confer some advantage to the process of implantation.

The original investigators said that they chose acupuncture points that 'relax the uterus according to the principles of TCM' and that 'because acupuncture influences the autonomic nervous system, such treatment should optimize endometrial receptivity.' They state that the points they chose 'stimulate Taiying meridians (Spleen) and Yangming meridians (Stomach, Colon) to result in better blood perfusion and more energy in the uterus' and that stimulation of other points, aimed to 'sedate the patient and stabilize the endocrine system.'

A number of subsequent reviews have postulated that the effect of acupuncture given at the time of transfer might be to reduce contractions in the uterus, change the immune milieu, increase blood flow or to relax the patient and reduce cortisol. It has been noted that pregnancy and implantation rates are negatively impacted by uterine contractions at the time of transfer.[35] One study on rats found that acupuncture reduced uterine contractions.[36]

One group thought that acupuncture might reduce endometrial motility and uterine contractions and therefore facilitate implantation of the embryo but when they tested this theory with ultrasound, they found little difference in the movement of the uterus at transfer between acupuncture and non-acupuncture groups.[37]

Another clinic[33] has shown that acupuncture (whether by pricking the points or penetrating the points) reduces levels of the stress hormone cortisol, and also reduces the vascularity of the endometrium. They wondered if just having the patients lie down and relax before their embryo transfer might have the same result but found that it didn't and that the acupuncture was the active intervention.

We don't yet know exactly what effect cortisol level has on implantation, although stress has definitely been shown to be associated with lower fertility[38] and lower implantation rates.[26]

Another study looked at the effect of repeated electroacupuncture treatments (using points which have been shown to increase blood flow to the uterus) before and during the drug phase of an IVF phase, on the serum cortisol and prolactin levels. They found that cortisol and prolactin levels were higher (cortisol still in normal physiologic range, but prolactin higher than normal physiologic range) in the acupuncture group than the control group for the week prior to embryo transfer, although the difference was not sustained after EPU.[39]

Endorphin levels, or other stress markers like adrenalin, sympathetic nervous system activity or heart rate have not to-date been measured in trials looking at the effect of acupuncture on implantation.

Acupuncture points used on the day of embryo transfer (ET)

Nearly all researchers using acupuncture (or electrical stimulation on acupuncture points) at the time of ET have used (for the treatment group) the original points used in the trial in 2002.[40] Results have varied (in terms of pregnancy rates), despite use of the same points. The acupuncture protocol was varied in some trials.[41–43] Box 11.3 summarizes the points used in these trials.

Another small study looked at the effect of hypnosis and another at the effect of laughter on IVF patients having embryo transfer. In both cases, the 'treatment' groups showed a higher pregnancy rate than the control group, indicating that stress reduction might have a beneficial effect on implantation.[44,45]

Box 11.3   Acupuncture points used in clinical trials investigating the effect of acupuncture at time of embryo transfer

Points used before embryo transfer

PC-6, SP-8, LIV-3, DU-20, ST-29

Ear points: shenmen, zhigong (uterus), neifenmi (endocrine), naodian (sympathetic or brain)

(variations/additions: Zigong, SP-10, Ren-6).

Points used after embryo transfer

ST-36, SP-6, CO-4, SP-10

Ear points: shenmen, zhigong (uterus) neifenmi (endocrine)

(variations/additions: Ren-4, Ren-6, ST-29, PC-6, SP-8, K-3, BL-23, Ear points: pizhixia).

Effects on endometrium

We do not yet fully understand the effects of increased or decreased blood flow to the uterus or its lining on implantation. Electroacupuncture performed on certain points appeared to increase blood flow to the uterus of women taking downregulating drugs of the type used in IVF cycles in a small clinical trial, although these women were not actively doing IVF[46] and the endometrium itself was not examined in this study.

One group,[33] found that acupuncture (using the Paulus pre-transfer points, manual stimulation only) performed just before embryo transfer during an IVF cycle, reduced vascularity or endometrium volume. Less vascularity of the endometrium may promote a more hypoxic environment and since the mammalian embryo develops in a low-oxygen environment (especially during its first 5 days when it is normally traveling down the fallopian tube to the uterus), this may confer an advantage. This local hypoxia promotes angiogenesis (growth of new blood vessels) in anticipation of the demands of the growing embryo for oxygen and nutrients.[47,48]

Interestingly, acupuncture has also been shown to promote angiogenesis (in rat brains, using EA on DU-26).[49]

It may be an interesting combination of acupuncture-induced reduction of endometrial vascularity and hypoxia, combined with an increased stimulus to angiogenesis from both the acupuncture and the hypoxia that benefits implantation. If some types of acupuncture treatment do indeed promote a hypoxic environment that is advantageous to implantation and early embryo development, TCM doctors would be advised to avoid applying those acupuncture treatments which have been shown to increase blood flow to the uterus (see Box 11.4, below) at the time of embryo transfer, or the days following. In fact, these points were included in those treatments applied during the drug stimulation phase of the IVF cycle when the uterine lining is thickening. Most acupuncturists would be reluctant to apply electroacupuncture to the lower back, abdomen or Spleen points at the time of implantation in any case.

Additionally, we should be wary at this time of using herbs that have been shown to increase blood flow to the uterus.[50]

CONCLUSION

A number of advances have occurred in ART in the last 2 decades, much of it driven by the innovative work of embryologists who are working on developing the best conditions in which embryos form and thrive in vitro. What happens in the ovary before they get their hands on the egg and once the embryo is returned to the womb

Box 11.4   Acupuncture points shown in clinical trials to affect blood flow to uterus

BL-28, 23

High frequency (100 Hz) pulses of 0.5 ms duration

BL-57, SP-6

Low frequency (2 Hz) pulses of 0.5 ms duration

(Women taking GnRH agonists, showed reduction of uterine artery impedance.[46])

LIV-3, SP-6, ST-28, Zigong, Ren-6, Ren-4

Low frequency (10 Hz) for 30 min

(Women taking FSH and GnRH antagonist drugs, showed reduction of uterine artery impedance.[51])

PC-6, SP-8, LIV-3, DU-20, ST-29

(One treatment, before embryo transfer, no electro-stimulation, showed reduced vascularity of endometrium.[33])

ST-28 and SP-6

Points in abdominal and the hindlimb muscles of rats, corresponding to above points.

(Low-frequency 2 Hz EA at 3 and 6 mA elicited significant increases in ovarian blood flow.[4])

---

is more of a mystery. Ovary function, the follicular milieu and the quality of the egg are mostly things viewed by ART specialists as being hard wired in a woman's genetic script and therefore out of reach. Similarly, the receptive or not so receptive, uterine environment is described as the hidden frontier by these specialists; they cannot see what happens after they put the embryo back and they cannot experiment ethically with women who have new embryo/s on board.

But it is precisely these inaccessible areas that we hope to work with. The strength of Chinese medicine is its ability to foster subtle balance – and doctors of Chinese medicine are used to working with the hidden and the subtle.

As long as we continue to focus intently on the balance of the Kidney Yin and the Yang, the Qi and the Blood, clearing Heat, Cold, Stasis or Damp, as needed, then we can improve the follicular and the uterine environment.

It may well be the case that some of our Kidney Yang herbs increase DHEA production or enhance oocyte mitochondrial function, or that the Kidney Yin herbs reduce oxidative damage inside the follicle. Or indeed, that acupuncture reduces the levels of inflammatory markers, increases nutrition and oxygen to the follicle and helps to create the correct balance of immune factors required for the survival of the fledgling embryo and its early development. While this is interesting to us, it does not fundamentally change the TCM diagnosis we make, or the treatment we apply.

Many TCM practitioners who work in integrated settings are attempting to achieve a balance between a traditional approach based on history, empirical knowledge and comprehension of Chinese medicine theory with the findings from clinical trials conducted on IVF patients. Ideally, we root our diagnosis and treatment in TCM principles while using research findings to augment the effectiveness of what we do where appropriate.

It is a challenging and stimulating arena requiring careful, inquiring reflective practice and data collection, and well thought out clinical trials, so that in some decades to come, we will have a substantial body of knowledge and discovery that will inform future doctors of Chinese medicine who treat IVF patients.

1. Bhal PS, Pugh ND, Gregory L, et al. Perifollicular vascularity as a potential variable affecting outcome in stimulated IUI treatment cycles. *Hum Reprod* 2001;**16**:1682–9.

2. Van Blerkom J, Antczak M, Schrader R. The developmental potential of the human oocyte is related to the dissolved oxygen content of follicular fluid: association with vascular endothelial growth factor levels and perifollicular blood flow characteristics. *Hum Reprod* 1997;**12**:1047–55.

3. Du Y, Shi L, Li J, et al. Angiogenesis and improved cerebral blood flow in the ischemic boundary area were detected after electroacupuncture treatment to rats with ischemic stroke. *Neurol Res* 2011;**33**(1):101–7.

4. Stener-Victorin E, Kobayashi R, Kurosawa M. Ovarian blood flow responses to electro-acupuncture stimulation at different frequencies and intensities in anaesthetized rats. *Auton Neurosci* 2003;**108**:50–6.

5. Tejera A, Herrero J. de los Santos MJ. Oxygen consumption is a quality marker for human oocyte competence conditioned by ovarian stimulation regimens. *Fertil Steril* 2011;**96**(3):618–23.

6. Lonergan T, Bavister B, Brenner C. Mitochondria in stem cells. *Mitochondrion* 2007;**7**(5):289–96.

7. Dumollard R, Duchen M, Carroll J. The role of mitochondrial function in the oocyte and embryo. *Curr Top Dev Biol* 2007;**77**:21–49.

8. May-Panloup P, Chrétien MF, Jacques C, et al. Low oocyte mitochondrial DNA content in ovarian insufficiency. *Hum Reprod* 2005;**20**:593–7.

9. Tarin JJ, Gomez-Piquer V, Pertusa JF, et al. Association of female aging with decreased parthenogenetic activation, raised MPF, and MAPKs activities and reduced levels of glutathione S-transferases activity and thiols in mouse oocytes. *Mol Reprod Dev* 2004;**69**:402–10.

10. Wiener-Megnazi Z, Vardi L, Lissak A, et al. Oxidative stress indices in follicular fluid as measured by the thermochemiluminescence assay correlate with outcome parameters in in vitro fertilization. *Fertil Steril* 2004;**82**(Suppl 3):1171–6.

11. Ko KM, Leon TY, Mak DHF, et al. A characteristic pharmacological action of 'Yang-invigorating' Chinese tonifying herbs: Enhancement of myocardial ATP-generation capacity. *Phytomedicine* 2006;**13**:636–42.

12. Demyttenaere K, Nijs P, Steeno O, et al. Anxiety and conception rates in donor insemination. *J Psychosom Obstet Gynaecol* 1988;**8**:175–81.

13. Ebbesen S, Zachariae R, Mehlsen MY, et al. Stressful life events are associated with a poor in-vitro fertilization (IVF) outcome: a prospective study. *Hum Reprod* 2009;**24**(9):2173–82.

14. De Liz TM, Strauss B. Differential efficacy of group and individual/couple psychotherapy with infertile patients. *Hum Reprod* 2005;**20**:1324–32.

15. Klonoff-Cohen H, Natarajan L. The concerns during assisted reproductive technologies (CART) scale and pregnancy outcomes. *Fertil Steril* 2004;**81**(4):982–8.

16. Domar A, Rooney KL, Wiegand B. Impact of a group mind/body intervention on pregnancy rates in IVF patients. *Fertil Steril* 2011;**95**(7):2269–73.

17. Thiering P, Beaurepaire J, Jones M, et al. Mood state as a predictor of treatment outcome after in vitro fertilization/embryo transfer technology (IVF/ET). *J Psychosom Res* 1993;**37**(5):481–91.

18. Demyttenaere K, Bonte L, Gheldof M, et al. Coping style and depression level influence outcome in in vitro fertilization. *Fertil Steril* 1998;**69**(6):1026–33.

19. Kondoh E, Okamoto T, Higuchi T, et al. Stress affects uterine receptivity through an ovarian-independent pathway. *Hum Reprod* 2009;**24**:945–53.

20. Rogers NL, Szuba MP, Staab JP, et al. Neuroimmunologic aspects of sleep and sleep loss. *Semin Clin Neuropsychiatry* 2001;**6**(4):295–307.

21. King K, Smith S, Chapman M, et al. Detailed analysis of peripheral blood natural killer (NK) cells in women with recurrent miscarriage. *Hum Reprod* 2010;**25**(1):52–8.

22. Lian F, Li X, Sun Z. Effect of Quyu Jiedu Granule on Microenvironment of Ova in Patients with Endometriosis. *Chin J Integr Med* 2009;**15**(1):42–6.

23. Stener-Victorin E, Jedel E, Janson PO, et al. Low-frequency electroacupuncture and physical exercise decrease high muscle sympathetic nerve activity in polycystic ovary syndrome. *Am J Physiol Regul Integr Comp Physiol* 2009;**297**(2):R387–95.

24. Cakmak YO, Akpinar IN, Ekinci G, et al. Point- and frequency-specific response of the testicular artery to abdominal electroacupuncture in humans. *Fertil Steril* 2008;**90**:1732–8.

25. Farkas D, Greenblatt DJ. Influence of fruit juices on drug disposition: discrepancies between in vitro and clinical studies. *Expert Opin Drug Metab Toxicol* 2008;**4**(4):381–93.

26.   Gallinelli A, Roncaglia R, Matteo ML, et al. Immunological changes and stress are associated with different implantation rates in patients undergoing in vitro fertilization-embryo transfer. *Fertil Steril* 2001;**76**(1):85–91.

27.   Liddell HS, Pattison NS, Zanderigo A. Recurrent miscarriage – outcome after supportive care in early pregnancy. *Aust N Z J Obstet Gynaecol* 1991;**31**(4):320–2.

28.   Ying Liu, Jing-zhi Wu. Effect of gutai decoction on the abortion rate of in vitro fertilization and embryo transfer. *Chin J Integr Med* 2006;**12**(3):189–93.

29.   Acupuncture IVF. *Support Clinic*. Research and reviews htt p://www.acupunctureivf.com.au/pages/research_by_cat.php?research_type_id=1.

30.   Acupuncture IVF. *Support Clinic*. Research and reviews htt p://www.acupunctureivf.com.au/pages/research_by_cat.php?research_type_id=8.

31.   Domar AD, Meshay I, Kelliher J, et al. The impact of acupuncture on in vitro fertilization outcome. *Fertil Steril* 2009;**91**(3):723–6.

32.   De Lacey S, Smith C, Paterson C. Building resilience: An exploration of women's perceptions of the use of acupuncture as an adjunct to IVF. *BMC Complement Altern Med* 2009;**9**:50.

33.   So EW, Ng EH, Wong YY, et al. A randomized double blind comparison of real and placebo acupuncture in IVF treatment. *Hum Reprod* 2009;**24**(2):341–8.

34.   Balk J, Catov J, Horn B, et al. The relationship between perceived stress, acupuncture, and pregnancy rates among IVF patients: a pilot study. *Complement Ther Clin Pract* 2010;**16**(3):154–7.

35.   Fanchin R, Righini C, de Ziegler D, et al. Effects of vaginal progesterone administration on uterine contractility at the time of embryo transfer. *Fertil Steril* 2001;**75**:1136–40.

36.   Kim J, Shin KH, Na CS. Effect of acupuncture treatment on uterine motility and cyclooxygenase-2 expression in pregnant rats. *Acupunct Electrother Res* 1991;**16**:1–5.

37.   Paulus W, Zhang M, Strehler E, et al. Motility of the endometrium after acupuncture treatment. *Fertil Steril* 2003;**80**(Suppl 3):131.

38.   Buck Louis GM, Lum KJ, Sundaram R, et al. Stress reduces conception probabilities across the fertile window: evidence in support of relaxation. *Fertil Steril* 2011;**95**(7):2184–9.

39.   Magarelli PC, Cridennda DK, Cohen M. Changes in serum cortisol and prolactin associated with acupuncture during controlled ovarian hyperstimulation in women undergoing in vitro fertilization-embryo transfer treatment. *Fertil Steril* 2009;**92**(6):1870–9.

40.   Paulus WE, Zhang M, Strehler E, et al. Influence of acupuncture on the pregnancy rate in patients who undergo assisted reproduction therapy. *Fertil Steril* 2002;**77**(4):721–4.

41.   Dieterle S, Ying G, Hatzmann W, et al. Effect of acupuncture on the outcome of in vitro fertilization and intracytoplasmic sperm injection: a randomized, prospective, controlled clinical study. *Fertil Steril* 2006;**85**:1347–51.

42.   Moy I, Milad MP, Barnes R, et al. Randomized controlled trial: effects of acupuncture on pregnancy rates in women undergoing in vitro fertilization. *Fertil Steril* 2011;**95**:583–7.

43.   Zhang R, Feng XJ, Guan Q, et al. Increase of success rate for women undergoing embryo transfer by transcutaneous electrical acupoint stimulation: a prospective randomized placebo-controlled study. *Fertil Steril* 2011;**96**(4):912–6.

44.   Levitas E, Parmet A, Lunenfeld E, et al. Impact of hypnosis during embryo transfer on the outcome of in vitro fertilization–embryo transfer: a case-control study. *Fertil Steril* 2006;**85**:1404.

45.   Friedler S, Glasser S, Azani L, et al. The effect of medical clowning on pregnancy rates after in vitro fertilization and embryo transfer. *Fertil Steril* 2011;**95**(6):2127.

46.   Stener-Victorin E, Waldenstrom U, Andersson SA, et al. Reduction of blood flow impedance in the uterine arteries of infertile women with electro-acupuncture. *Hum Reprod* 1996;**11**:1314–7.

47.   Genbacev O, Joslin R, Damsky CH, et al. Hypoxia alters early gestation human cytotrophoblast differentiation/invasion in vitro and models the placental defects that occur in preeclampsia. *J Clin Invest* 1996;**97**(2):540–50.

48.   Breier G. Angiogenesis in embryonic development – a review. *Troph Res* 2000;**14**:11–5.

49.   Du Y, Shi L, Li J, et al. Angiogenesis and improved cerebral blood flow in the ischemic boundary area were detected after electroacupuncture treatment to rats with ischemic stroke. *Neurol Res* 2011;**33**(1):101–7.

50.   Wing T, Sedlmeier E. Measuring the effectiveness of Chinese Herbal Medicine in improving female fertility. *J Chin Med* 2006;**80**:22.

51.   Ho M, Huang LC, Chang YY, et al. Electroacupuncture reduces uterine artery blood flow impedance in infertile women. *Taiwan J Obstet Gynecol* 2009;**48**(2):148–51.

SECTION 4

Lifestyle and Fertility

Diet and lifestyle

12

Chapter Contents

INTRODUCTION

In this chapter, we will consider the effect of diet and lifestyle on fertility. Here we combine Chinese medicine advice which has evolved over many hundreds of years with that which medical research has uncovered in just the last few years. The infertility patients who consult a Chinese medicine doctor are often well educated and may have a lot of questions. In the interests of trying to cover all the relevant areas related to infertility and preparing to conceive, I have included information in this chapter that is not part of traditional Chinese medicine, but should help the clinical specialist be as informed as possible.

There is a dizzying amount of information and misinformation handed out to prospective parents: what they should eat – what they shouldn't eat – which pills they should swallow – which they should not – what activities they should do – and not do. Attempts to follow all of this advice is enough to make any couple trying to conceive tense and miserable! However, being sensible and responsible about one's diet and lifestyle not only safeguards health but can pay large dividends in gamete and embryo quality. Additionally, it is now recognized that mother's nutritional status at the time of conception can have significant implications on the health of the future baby and the adult it will grow into.[1]

Jing

Jing is considered to be very precious; it is the life spring sourced in our deepest origins, a substance or energy inherited from our parents. In that sense, it is a finite bundle which must be conserved because it is not so easy to replenish it once spent. Healthy Kidney Jing is vitally important for fertility.

Previous generations of Chinese people were very aware of conserving their energy reserves. They were taught early in life to pace themselves, to move gently through life, not rush at it all at once, as we tend to do in the West. For Chinese people a long life is a desired goal and something they actively foster. This means they must look after their Jing and use it sensibly like a steady drip feed, which gets topped up on a regular basis. In so many parts of modern Western culture we adopt the philosophy of 'live hard and die young,' rather than thinking and planning, while we are still in our 20s, to be well and healthy in our 80s or 90s. Observing patients in the clinic of a well-known, elderly and wise Chinese doctor in New York in the 1980s, I had the opportunity to see these differing approaches to life. Every day, New Yorkers, driven by ambition and circumstance, would come to the clinic complaining of myriad different disorders. They were often young people who were working 70 or 80h a week just to keep their feet on the bottom rung of the Big Apple ladder. The old Chinese doctor would look at their faces carefully, take their pulses and say 'can't you rest a little more?' Usually, he was met with squawks of protest or looks of blank incomprehension. Slowing down or resting was just not part of the script for success. But if such a lifestyle persists, then the price is paid – in Jing and Yin currency.

It is the balanced path through life which helps to conserve Jing. Life doesn't have to be quiet externally if our internal environment is quiet, i.e. if the mind can remain stable and still, but for most of us this is difficult when living in the midst of so much stimulation and stress. Likewise, rushing all the time doesn't just make us stressed, it exhausts us. And if we keep going on an empty tank, the Jing is consumed.

Jing can also be depleted in a more sudden and dramatic way if there is a major crisis, e.g., recovery from an accident or serious illness draws deeply on life reserves. People in terrifying and dangerous situations like war and famine may also need to drain Jing supplies rapidly just to survive.

There are many ways that Jing is used up in the normal course of living and this is, of course, the nature of life. Jing is intimately related to reproductive processes and one of the more obvious expenditures of Jing is the semen and sperm spent with every ejaculation. The Chinese were strong believers in conserving the Jing by practicing semen conservation techniques, i.e. having sex without ejaculation. However, this book is about achieving pregnancy, so further discussion of semen conservation techniques will have to be sought elsewhere. In a man with poor Jing and low Kidney energy, however, it is always wise to limit sexual activity (including masturbation) and focus on spending Jing reserves only at the fertile time of his partner.

The sexual secretions of women are not considered to be so depleting to the Jing as is the loss of semen. Since these secretions do not contain gametes, they do not have such a direct connection to the Jing. Rather, they reflect Kidney Yin reserves; these too can be drained somewhat by excessive sexual activity. However, every menstrual cycle in which an ovulation occurs requires contribution from the Jing. It is when no more Jing contributions can be made (i.e., there are no more viable eggs) that menstrual cycles cease and menopause has arrived. Thus, women spend their Jing too in the normal processes of the menstrual cycle during the reproductive years. Celibacy in a woman cannot preserve Jing in the same way it can for a man. Stopping ovulation altogether, as happens, e.g., in women taking the oral contraceptive pill, may preserve some aspects of Jing, although it does so at a price.

The production of a whole new baby human during pregnancy draws heavily on the Qi, Blood and Jing resources of the mother. Anything which damages the DNA in the chromosomes (such as X-rays and mutagenic chemicals) is said to be damaging to the Jing. Some of the epigenetic effects of assisted reproduction technology (see Ch. 10) could also be of concern as far as Jing is concerned.

There are some ways Jing can be nourished, although clearly even the most careful lifestyle and nourishing diet cannot replace the Jing that must necessarily be spent in living. Some Taoist and Qi Gong practices can protect and nurture the Jing; similarly, there are Ayurvedic and Buddhist practices that aim to do the same.

Jing and food

Food substances which are designed by nature to nourish offspring can enhance many different levels of energy, including the Jing. Substances, e.g. royal jelly, which is produced by bees to nourish their larvae, offer this type of nourishment.

Eggs of birds, such as chickens or ducks, are one of nature's most complete protein food packages and represent a type of Jing themselves, containing as they do the gametes of the female of the species. Similarly, fish eggs or roe are a form of Jing themselves and provide useful food if we wish to nourish our own Jing. Caviar may be precious not just because it is so rare and expensive but also because it is such a marvelous Jing tonic.

Seeds and nuts contain not only fertilized germ cells but also supplies for the immediate nutritional requirements of the potential new plant; hence, they are useful sources of Jing nourishment. In fact eating a handful of walnuts a day for 3 months has been shown to improve all sperm parameters. Pollen, which is made up of plant germ cells, is also a form of Jing and therefore a potentially useful supplement for Jing deficiency.

Some animal organs and tissues nourish the Jing. For example, bone marrow (especially that from pig spine) can be used to make a particularly good Jing-strengthening soup. Brains fall into a similar category to bone marrow. Animal organs such as kidneys also provide the sort of nourishment which can support the Jing. Oysters, with their aphrodisiac reputation, bolster Jing by delivering essential minerals like zinc to the sperm-manufacturing cells.

Other plant products which nourish Jing are seaweeds and algae. These plants provide trace elements which are necessary for many processes in the body, including the production of the gametes and the hormones which control their development.

Additional foods reported to have a special effect on the Jing are: artichoke leaf, nettles, oats, and raw milk.[2]

Yin

Yin cannot exist or be described except with reference to Yang, its opposite force. The Yin energy of the body is the internal, quiescent, restorative, and moistening force to balance Yang's more outward, active, stimulating, and warming force. When we try and make parallels with our understanding of physiology from the Western point of view, it is sometimes said that Yin reflects anabolic activities (synthesizing and storing) and Yang reflects catabolic (energy-producing) activities. Or that Yin reflects the function of the parasympathetic nervous system that controls internal homeostasis, whereas Yang reflects the activity of the sympathetic nervous system that controls our responses to stimuli.

Yin is essentially an internal and quiet energy. An overly stimulating and rushed lifestyle damages it by not allowing time for rest and regeneration. It is such a lifestyle which turns up our slow drip feed of Jing, draining it more rapidly than is healthy and at the same time creating an imbalance between Yin and Yang by indulging in more Yang active times than Yin 'resting' times. Such a lifestyle depletes both Jing and Yin, which spells doom for fertility. Those fortunate people born with plentiful and strong Jing energy may sustain quite some Yin deficiency without the Jing being depleted but eventually a frantic life catches up with everyone – lucky are those for whom it doesn't happen until old age, when fertility is no longer an issue! Yin deficiency in the absence of Jing deficiency can still compromise fertility. Restoring damaged Yin energy, although not quite so difficult as dealing with deficient Jing, is still not an easy clinical task. Yin-deficient women, especially older ones (speaking from the ovary's perspective) find getting and staying pregnant a challenge. Their juices are dried up, i.e., they have little fertile mucus to carry the sperm safely into the uterus, and the lining of the uterus can be thin. The development of the egg too is compromised if the Yin is inadequate. And men are not immune from the damaging effects of the Yin-hungry lifestyle; internal Heat which develops as a result of Yin deficiency can have very dire repercussions for the development and maturation of sperm.

Yin can be nourished and rebuilt by attention to inner calm. Meditation, Tai Chi, and regular walks in serene natural environments recharge Yin. Modifying those habits or behavior patterns which increase mental stimulation excessively and heat or dry the body will also help Yin. For example, trying to fit too much into one day and skimping on sleep and meal times undermines the Yin and should be avoided or limited in those with a tendency to be Yin-deficient or in those wishing to preserve their Yin.

Modern work places may be hazardous for the Yin. Long hours in front of computer screens, or around other electrical machinery such as photocopiers, drains and dries the body, as does the stale air in the air conditioning of large sealed office blocks. Antidotes to such influences need to be sought out on a regular basis in areas of naturally high negative ions such as rainforests, river banks, and the ocean.

Toxic fumes associated with some trades and professions (e.g. manufacturers of glues, paints and solvents, photographers who develop their own photos in darkrooms, cleaners and dry cleaners) appear to have a damaging effect on the Jing and Yin. Under these conditions, the developing eggs or sperm become less able to create viable embryos (see Environmental pollutants, below, and Ch. 8).

Severe or recurrent febrile illnesses or the loss of large quantities of blood can deplete and damage Yin.

Yin and food

Attention to lifestyle habits and avoiding stimulating drinks and foods has more impact on conserving or recovering the Yin than does making specific additions to the diet. In general, diets composed of foods which are rich in nutrients and not overly stimulating are those which nourish the Yin. A diet of fruits and vegetables and adequate protein (especially tofu, fish, and milk) is one which fortifies the Yin. On the other hand, drinking too much coffee and eating very spicy food can consume Yin. Some texts recommend the following specific foods: barley and millet; string beans; asparagus; all dark-colored beans; dark fruits like blackberry, mulberry, and blueberry; seaweeds; and animal products, including fish eggs, dairy produce, duck, and pork.[3]

One word about soy before recommending it as a good addition to the diet of Yin-deficient men with poor sperm counts – it has been found that men who eat even moderate quantities of soy-based foods regularly produce a third less sperm per milliliter than men who consume no soy-based foods.[4] One cup of soy milk or one serving of tofu, tempeh, or soy burgers every other day provides enough isoflavone content to affect the sperm. It is thought that the phytoestrogens may interfere with hormonal signals that govern sperm production.

Including soy-based foods in the diet won't affect most men, but if there is also obesity (fat also produces estrogens) and if a man's sperm count is low, or even low-to-normal, soy foods could tip the estrogen/testosterone balance in the wrong direction and reduce sperm count further.

Ensuring that the body is well hydrated is also important. Yin-deficient people are often thirsty and dry. Drinking a lot, however, will not necessarily hydrate the tissues if the fluid passes straight through the body and is excreted (see Fluid intake, below).

Yin can be damaged by chronic dieting (to the point where the body is malnourished) and by the use of recreational drugs.

Yang

Yang deficiency often develops out of a Yin deficiency, but can also be provoked by certain environments, behavior, and diet. Living and working in icy climates or even damp cold ones can damage the Yang. The external Cold can enter the body, through specific channels or organs and inhibit or weaken the inner Fire of Yang. If the Yang of the body (and therefore its Wei Qi or natural defences) is weakened, Cold can enter even more easily. For example, in the first days of a woman's period, her body is slightly Yang deficient (because she is losing body heat with the blood loss) and is more vulnerable to direct attack of Cold to the Uterus because the Chong channel is open. It is for this reason that Chinese women (and Asian women in general) are advised not to swim in cold water during their periods. If the Cold restricts or inhibits the rapid and easy flow of the blood it can 'stagnate', setting the stage for many gynecological problems later, including infertility.

When Kidney Yang is damaged, so is fertility in both men and women. Libido will be poor in both sexes, and in women, the function of the corpus luteum and the processes of implantation of a newly fertilized embryo into the uterine lining will be compromised. Kidney Yang deficiency in men can lead to impotence and/or low sperm counts and motility.

A Yang-deficient body is one without enough driving or warming energy, so that metabolism and mental processes become sluggish. The body and limbs easily feel cold and lethargic, and motivation and assertiveness diminish. As much as Yin needs rest and a quiet mind to regenerate itself, Yang needs movement and stimulation to feed it. Providing there is a good Yin base, and activity and stimulation are appropriate for the circumstances, Yang will benefit from activity and physical exercise. When the Yang is already weak and motivation is very low, the first few steps are difficult. In cases like this, the use of strong Yang tonics (like deerhorn and ginseng capsules) and the appropriate diet will help to motivate a Yang-deficient person into initiating the appropriate changes in their life. This may be as simple as beginning a gentle exercise program, or it may be as challenging as being assertive in an unfavorable work situation.

Yang and food

Yang benefits from a diet that is warming. This means eating foods which are nutrient or calorie-rich such as protein or carbohydrate and eating foods which have been cooked. It also means avoiding ice-cold drinks and foods like ice cream. Methods of cooking such as long slow baking or simmering will increase the Yang Qi in foods. Cooking foods like fruits can reduce their cooling nature and addition of some spices like ginger, shallots, or cinnamon can increase Yang Qi in foods. Very hot spices like cayenne and chilli certainly add Heat to food and in moderation can be helpful in raising a sluggish metabolism. When very pungent spices are eaten a lot (as they are in some very hot and tropical climates), they can have the opposite effect, i.e. become cooling, because they provoke sweating. Stimulants like coffee are favored by Yang-deficient people because the adrenaline (epinephrine) they provoke creates an impression of internal Heat and activity. However, it is false Yang, and eventually consumes reserves rather than stimulating them.

The organs most commonly affected by Yang deficiency are the Spleen and the Kidney. For the person with weak Yang Qi, a diet of raw and Cold foods can quickly douse the inner Fire, creating problems of Spleen and Kidney Yang deficiency. This will manifest first, as digestive symptoms such as bloating and loose stools. If this situation continues, it can start to mimic a chronic food allergy picture, where many foods become difficult to digest and stamina and mental concentration are affected. Fluid is not metabolized efficiently and edema or puffiness may occur in some parts of the body.

Texts of Chinese dietetics recommend the following additions to the diet: garlic, onion, chicken, lamb, trout, salmon, lobster, shrimp, prawn, mussel, black beans, walnuts, chestnut, pistachio, raspberry, and quinoa.[5]

Qi and Blood

The vitality and actions of the internal organs can be described not only in terms of Jing, Yin, and Yang but also in terms of their Qi and Blood. While Qi is an immaterial substance which we translate as energy, the TCM concept of Blood includes the material substance we can see (the red stuff in our veins) and many aspects of nourishment of the body. Plentiful Blood and Qi makes us more substantial and resilient in both physical and emotional ways.

When the Blood and Qi is adequate and moves well, all the tissues are well nourished and the complexion appears to be a good color. A pale tongue is a sure sign that the Blood reserves are low.

Healthy Qi requires rest, movement and flexibility. Exercise builds Qi and the capacity for producing Qi, providing it is done in an appropriate way. For some people this means aerobic workouts or athletic training. For people at the other end of the spectrum, this means gently stretching the limbs or walking slowly around the block. For most of us, an exercise program somewhere in the middle is appropriate. As the lungs work more, so does the Qi. The nature of work in the city, often sedentary, often stressful, combined with eating too much or in a rush does not help the Qi move smoothly; rather, a regular routine plus a sensible exercise program will help the Qi build and move.

Spleen Qi is important for the absorption and metabolism of food and the production of Blood. Just as important is the patency of the Liver and Heart Qi (see also Stress, below).

Qi and food

A diet of varied fresh and tasty food eaten in an unhurried and regular daily routine will benefit the Spleen Qi and ensure its capacity to transform the nutrients in food into the myriad molecules that are required for all the thousands of biochemical processes which occur every moment in every organ and tissue.

When Qi (especially Spleen Qi) is weak or is obstructed, there will be bloating after eating, and other digestive symptoms. The judicious use of herbs and spices in cooking can be helpful, as can foods which specifically help to maintain circulation of Liver Qi. Drinking warm water with a little lemon or lime juice to add a sour flavor is a useful Liver Qi invigorating start to the day. To support the Spleen Qi, foods should be lightly cooked and balanced in flavor and nature. The diet should include some with sweet, some with bitter, and some with pungent flavors. The sweet flavor is found in root vegetables and grains and these usually form the base of a meal. If eaten in excess, however, they can create stagnation. Bitter leaves like arugula (rocket) or watercress help digestion and pungent foods like onions, garlic, coriander or chives (even small amounts of chilli) also help digestion and Qi movement.

Chinese people sip green teas during meals to facilitate digestion (especially of fats) and the custom of French and Mediterranean people of drinking wine during the meal has now become an international habit. In careful moderation, wine can be a useful tool in regulating Qi and helping digestion. Spirits, likewise, can move the Qi. Because spirits add a lot of Heat to the system, however, they must be taken sparingly.

There are many aspects of the menstrual cycle which depend on plentiful Blood. Liver Blood is an important component of menstruation and is one way we can describe the Blood-storing function of the Uterus in TCM terms. When periods become very scanty, it is said that Liver Blood is deficient. This means the uterine lining is thin and lacks nourishment. Blood deficiency can contribute to poor semen quality.

Blood and food

Diet and the way we digest foods is very important if we are trying to build up the Blood. In Western medicine, a severely Blood-deficient person might be called anemic, and iron would be prescribed so that more hemoglobin could be manufactured. The way TCM doctors see it, is that although iron is very important, equally important are the cofactors and the process itself which makes hemoglobin from iron. Adequate cofactors are ensured by using whole foods as the source of iron and the process of making hemoglobin happens efficiently if the Spleen Qi is strong.

$$Iron \xrightarrow{\text{Cofactors and Spleen Qi}} \text{Hemoglobin in the blood}$$

Foods which build Blood best are meats and poultry, and especially stocks and soups made from bones. Such stocks provide Blood-fortifying bone marrow and also calcium from the bones (if a little vinegar is added to leach it out). Small amounts of meats which have been marinated before cooking, or stewed in casseroles for a long time, will provide rapid nourishment to the Blood. Egg yolk and legumes also help to nourish the Blood, as do grains, green leafy vegetables, beetroots, red wine, and stout. Substances which build the Blood after menstruation are an important component of diet and herbal prescriptions. With this in mind, Chinese and other Asian women commonly eat special soups made with chicken and herbs after the period. For example, post-menstrual soup is made by boiling a whole chicken with a selection of herbs and vegetables. These include carrots, mushrooms, shallots, and sweet potato. Herbs which are often added include Shan Yao (yam), Gou Qi Zi (Lycium berries), Long Yan Rou (Longan fruit), and Sheng Jiang (ginger). The resulting stock makes a nutritious post-menstrual soup – some chicken meat can be added if desired.

Heat in the Blood is a condition which develops from internal imbalance or from external factors like excess consumption of Heating foods. Foods which are obviously heating and stimulating, like chilli, pepper, and coffee, can contribute to Heat in the Blood, as can alcohol, especially spirits. If Heat in the Blood is manifesting in the form of heavy periods or skin rashes, then such foods should be avoided. In general, Heat is not conducive to the development of good-quality sperm or eggs or a thick endometrium.

To allow the Blood to flow freely during the period, sour, astringent foods should be avoided. If consumed in excess, such foods can inhibit or temporarily stop the flow. For example, during the period, vinegar and pickles, some sour fruits like grapefruits and gooseberries and sour yogurt should be limited or avoided. In general, very fatty foods are not advisable because they slow the blood and make it thicker and easier to stagnate.

Phlegm-Damp

When we discussed the various TCM patterns of infertility, we mentioned three categories other than Kidney weakness, these were: Liver and Heart Qi stagnation, Blood stagnation, and Phlegm-Damp accumulation. Of these three, it is Phlegm-Damp accumulation which is most related to diet.

Phlegm-Damp creates an internal environment of congested and stagnant fluids. Excess mucus forms in the gastrointestinal tract and bowel movements become sluggish and unformed. The lungs and other parts of the respiratory tract can also become congested with fluid or mucus. The urine becomes cloudy if the bladder is affected. Obesity, diabetes, and heart disease can develop. In terms of fertility, we are concerned mostly with congested or stagnant fluids blocking the cervix (pathologic vaginal discharges or inflammation), or the tubes (mucus and inflammation), or affecting the ovaries (cysts), or the uterine lining (excess secretions). Damp in men can contribute to impotence, prostatitis, discharges from the penis or thick congealed semen – all of which have an affect on sperm. Phlegm-Damp in both men and women can manifest as fatty deposits around the abdominal organs. If a person has a tendency to Damp or already manifests pathologic manifestations of it, then Damp-clearing herbs will be prescribed. Such therapy must be supported by the appropriate diet.

Phlegm-Damp and food

Poor eating habits or poor digestive function allows accumulation of Phlegm-Damp. A diet which is unlikely to create Damp is one which has few fatty rich foods and includes foods which help to mobilize fluids and break up congestion. Herbal digestives are often taken by Chinese people after a meal to help to avoid Damp accumulating, e.g., hawthorn flakes after eating heavy meats. Where there is already evidence of internal Phlegm-Damp (weight gain), reducing intake of fatty meats, dairy products, sweets (especially chocolate and ice cream), bread, and fried foods is important. Dairy products are one of the main dietary culprits for many Westerners, milk and cheese being such a popular part of the diet in countries like Australia, New Zealand, UK, France, and America. It is well known by nutritionists that adult Caucasians often lose the capacity to digest the components of dairy (specifically lactose) as they mature, and in the case of many Asians, that capacity was not there even in childhood. Some studies relate the inability to digest dairy products (or galactose, a sugar found only in milk) or overconsumption of dairy products, to impaired ovarian function.[6] High levels of galactose appear to be toxic to ovarian germ cells and trials have been done to examine its association with premature ovarian failure.[7]

However, for women who can digest lactose and galactose and who do not have a tendency to Phlegm-Damp, then milk or dairy products can be an important source of protein and calcium.

In a case where infertility is related to Phlegm-Damp in the lower Jiao, a diet based on aromatic rice (and some millet and barley) with the addition of broad beans, chick peas and, especially, adzuki beans, will support the Spleen and drain Damp.[8]

The *Clinical Handbook of Internal Medicine*, Vol. 2, Chapter 26, provides more in depth discussion of diets for different constitutions with appropriate food inclusions or exclusions.[9]

FLUID INTAKE

Drinking enough fluid is an important part of a good diet. Water is the major component of the human body. Every system in the body depends on water. Blood is 83% water; muscles are 75% water; the brain is 74% water, and even bone is 22% water. Water lubricates every joint in the body. Water is used in the digestion and absorption of food and nutrients and the elimination of digestive wastes.

Not everyone, however, is able to make effective use of the fluid they drink. People with Yin deficiency tend to have tissues which are less well hydrated and lubricated. They often feel dry and thirsty and may have dry skin and hair, especially if their condition is complicated with Yin-deficient Heat. But no matter how much they drink, the tissues remain somewhat dehydrated and liquid tends to pass straight through them. From the point of view of the nourishing fluid around the egg in the follicle, the fluid in the fallopian tubes and the fluid levels in the endometrium as it prepares to sustain a fetus, keeping moisture levels up is obviously very important. This is why such emphasis is placed on clearing Heat and reinforcing Yin in the follicular phase of the menstrual cycle. In men, the quality and quantity of the semen which nourishes the sperm is dependent on healthy Yin and moisture levels. TCM doctors use Yin tonic herbs (such as Mai Dong and Tian Dong) to encourage tissues in the body to hold more fluid. A daily fluid intake of eight or more glasses of liquid which does not contain sugar, salt, or caffeine should be advised.

Interestingly, people with Damp constitutions also make poor use of the fluid they imbibe. Unlike the Yin-deficient types who can't hold liquid in their tissues, Damp people hold too much fluid in their tissues, which become boggy and congested. The lack of easy fluid movement in and out of the cells means that as a vehicle for nutritional factors and wastes, it is most inefficient. In the case of constitutional Damp, herbs are given which help to alter the osmotic balance between the intra- and extracellular fluids such that liquid moves out of the tissues and into the bloodstream, from where it can be drained from the body via the kidneys and bladder. Damp people should not drink large quantities of water until this process is happening efficiently.

One last reason why adequate water intake is important, is to keep the blood circulating well. You will know by now that Blood stagnation is a pathology that crops up frequently in infertility and other gynecological disorders. While Blood stagnation is a TCM term which covers a lot of complex pathologic changes in different tissues, it is a process which actually starts at the level of the circulation of blood in the capillary. When the body is dehydrated (even mildly and even before much thirst is registered), the blood becomes thicker and circulation in the far reaches of the tiniest capillaries is retarded. If this situation is repeated over and over, day after day, month after month, then Blood stagnation develops.

PRECONCEPTION DIETS

So what does in fact constitute a healthy diet for those preparing to conceive (who don't need to lose or gain weight), one that will maximize their nutritional status and their fertility? This will vary enormously depending on the country, the culture, urban or rural environs, economic status, and individual constitutions and preferences. In the USA, one large study tried to define some of the parameters of a diet which promoted fertility.[10]

413

The Nurses Health Study followed nearly 20 000 women over several years and correlated pregnancy attempts with diet and lifestyle factors. They recorded higher pregnancy rates when women had what they defined as a 'fertility diet.' Their findings were summarized with this advice:[11]

Choose whole grains and other unrefined carbohydrates rather than highly refined carbohydrates that quickly boost blood sugar and insulin.

Eat more vegetable protein, like beans and nuts, and less animal protein.

Avoid trans-fats, found in many commercial products and fast foods. Use more unsaturated vegetable oils, such as olive oil, and cut back on saturated fat from red meat and other sources.

Get plenty of iron from fruits, vegetables, beans and supplements (not from red meat).

Drink coffee, tea and alcohol in moderation and skip sugared sodas.

Drink a glass of whole milk or eat a dish of full-fat yogurt every day.

Take a multivitamin with folic acid and other B vitamins.

If you are overweight, lose 5 to 10 percent of your body weight. Start a daily exercise plan (if you are already quite lean, don't overdo it).

We could summarize general diet advice even further with the words of esteemed author Michael Pollan, who writes extensively about our modern food production and eating habits.[12] His mantra is *Eat food. Not too much. Mostly plants.*

To this we would add, *Enjoy*! And we would add an artful TCM touch emphasizing balance, taste, flavor, appeal and ease of digestion, alongside an awareness of the season and an individual's constitution.[9]

We know that nutritional status at the time of conception can be critical in determining the health of the baby and future adult (particularly in terms of cardiovascular disease and diabetes),[13–15] hence it is important that women take steps to ensure their diet includes sufficient nutrients. In general, a diet that includes plenty of fresh fruit and vegetables and sufficient protein, will provide the nutrition needed to create a healthy environment for the new embryo. However, it may be wise to add supplements to ensure intake of certain essential vitamins (such as folate) particularly where the diet is not ideal.

NUTRITIONAL SUPPLEMENTS

The British Association for the Promotion of Preconception Care, called Foresight, has for many years dispensed information about diet and lifestyle to prospective parents. They have sponsored research which supports the notion that healthy, well-nourished parents have healthy pregnancies and make healthy babies.[16] Their advice includes a sound, well-balanced, and 'clean' (i.e., no junk food or added chemicals) diet and the optimum intake of many vitamins and minerals, namely: zinc, selenium, manganese, potassium, magnesium, iron, iodine, calcium, chromium, boron, vitamins A, B complex, C, D, E, folic acid, and essential fatty acids.[17]

It has long been recognized that nutrients such as calcium and iron are important for the health of the pregnant woman and her baby. We now know that lack of folic acid can have dire consequences on the early development of the nervous system of the fetus, causing neural tube defects such as spina bifida. As more research is carried out on different nutrients, their role in fetal development will be elucidated. The above-mentioned nurses study found that women who took supplemental vitamins had a better chance of conceiving.[18]

Finding a good prenatal supplement which incorporates essential vitamins and minerals is important and consultation with a local naturopath or nutritionist for guidance may be advisable. A full discussion of the roles and dosage requirements of all these supplemental nutrients is outside the scope of this text, however it is worth noting that there are some nutrients that modern diets seem to be lacking, and which may be the cause of some disturbances in fetal development. Consumption of iodine has dropped in many countries (except those where a lot of seaweed is eaten), to levels that have caused concern for infant brain development. Iodine deficiency in the mothers' diet can lead to miscarriage, premature birth and significant developmental delays in affected children.[19] Hence, it is important that women take a vitamin preparation containing 150 μg iodine daily, in preparation for and during pregnancy and lactation to supplement iodine intake from the diet;[20,21] the total daily intake should be 250 μg.[22] Dietary sources are seafood, dairy and eggs, and some vegetables. In some countries, foods like bread are fortified with iodine to prevent a public health problem. However, the amount of iodine in dietary sources is inadequate for pregnant and breast-feeding women.

Similarly, vitamin D levels are inadequate in a large number of women who are pregnant or preparing to conceive. Very few foods (other than some fatty fish) have significant amounts of vitamin D in them and the primary source, the action of sunshine on the skin, is limited in the lives of many modern women who work inside and seldom see the sun. Vitamin D deficiency adversely affects bone health and brain development of the baby, but also increases risk of heart disease, type 1 diabetes and cancer as the baby grows into an adult.[23]

In summary, women preparing to conceive should take a prenatal multivitamin supplement and should check this for inclusion of adequate folate (500–1000 μg), Vitamin D and iodine. Women are often recommended to add Fish oil and CoQ10 capsules to a preconception vitamin preparation if it is not included.

Many patients who have had a poor response to IVF or who have been diagnosed with poor ovarian reserve are recommended by their specialist to take DHEA (dehydroepiandrosterone). This is a hormone that is produced by the ovaries and the adrenal glands and is an essential prerequisite for ovarian follicular steroidogenesis, specifically follicular testosterone.[24] However, DHEA levels decline with age. Some clinical studies on small numbers of IVF patients classified as poor responders, have shown promising effects of DHEA supplementation (75 mg/day for 6–12 weeks) on outcomes such as number of mature oocytes, embryos, pregnancies, and live births.[25,26]

Other supplements sometimes suggested by clinics to their IVF patients who have not responded well include:

Arginine – supplementation with this amino acid has been examined in several small studies which show conflicting results, arginine supplementation being associated with both better IVF outcomes in earlier trials but worse outcomes in more recent studies.[27–29]

Melatonin (N-acetyl-5-methoxytryptamine) – this hormone is secreted during the night by the pineal gland to regulate a variety of pathways related to circadian rhythms and reproduction. It has been shown in one study to reduce intra-follicular oxidative damage, and increase fertilization and pregnancy rates in IVF poor responders at a dose of 3 mg per night for 5–6 weeks leading up to egg retrieval.[30,31]

Inositol – a naturally occurring carbohydrate that is found in phospholipids which function as cellular mediators of signal transduction in metabolic regulation and growth. One recent trial claimed that using Inositol 4 g/day, and Melatonin 3 mg/day together, improved oocyte quality and pregnancy rates.[32]

Men who are preparing to have a child and who do not have an ideal diet are recommended to take a general vitamin supplement and fish oils. A high intake of omega-3 fats such as those found in fish oils is associated with better sperm morphology.[33]

Men whose sperm have a high degree of DNA fragmentation are recommended to take antioxidants, such as Vitamins C and E.[34]

Drinking Rooibos tea or green tea also benefits men with a high degree of DNA fragmentation.[35]

WEIGHT

Does weight matter? Body weight that varies from a defined norm in either direction can affect fertility. Restriction of calorie intake has an immediate effect on the pituitary hormones acting on the ovary[36] and a loss of even 10%

of body weight below the standard can cause ovulatory problems and reduced fertility. More extreme weight loss (as in anorexia nervosa) can inhibit ovulation altogether. Even in women with regular weight, low body fat can negatively affect ovulation. This is observed in women who train seriously for athletic and sporting events and stop ovulating until such time as their exercise regimen is reduced and their body fat builds up again. If infertility is the result of the body deciding it cannot support the huge caloric requirements of pregnancy and breast-feeding because it does not have enough adipose tissue, the remedy may be as simple as consuming more calories. For some women who have very low appetites or who have difficulty eating enough or digesting larger quantities of food, some work may need to be done to invigorate Spleen Qi. For women who cannot put on weight no matter what they eat, then treatment to build the Yin, cool internal Heat and calm the Shen must accompany a good diet. Both herbal tonics and acupuncture can invigorate the Spleen Qi, supplement the Yin, or clear internal Heat and thus encourage less sympathetic nervous system activity and more weight gain.

We do not have any evidence to indicate that low BMI affects men's fertility in the same way. Very thin men with poor sperm counts will likely be Yin deficient and will need to be treated for this and any internal Heat over some time.

On the other side of the coin, it is well known that overweight women can have difficulty conceiving. This difficulty is sometimes related to polycystic ovary syndrome (PCOS), sufferers of which often experience weight gain. (We have discussed the relationship between polycystic ovaries and the condition called Phlegm-Damp accumulation and impaired fertility in Ch. 5.) With an excess of Damp accumulation (with or without PCOS), ovulation frequency and egg quality may be reduced. The follicular fluid surrounding the eggs of obese women is different to that of moderate weight women and maturation within this environment is detrimental to the eggs.[37,38] It has been shown that overweight women do less well with IVF[39] and suffer more risks during pregnancy.

Researchers who have examined the effect of obesity on placental function in animal models advise women that in order to make a good functioning placenta they should lose weight well before conceiving and not just switch to a good diet once they are pregnant. They describe fat deposit patterns in placentas of the obese rats in their trial, such that the nutrient supply region is just half the size of that of a normal-weight mother, even when both were eating the same healthy diet. As a result, obese mothers gave birth to babies that were 17% smaller than they should have been, risking lifelong consequences.[40]

But it is not only excess weight in women that we must concern us. Although not all reports agree, there is growing evidence that excess weight in men also has a negative effect on ability to reproduce; sperm counts reduce significantly as BMI and abdominal fat increase[41] and men who are overweight are more likely to suffer erectile dysfunction.[42]

When the embryos of overweight men doing IVF are examined at Day 4 or 5 (when paternal genetic influence comes into play) there is evidence of impaired development. Overall studies show there is decreased blastocyst development, and fewer conceptions when the male partner is overweight.[43]

There is certainly enough compelling evidence to persuade both partners in a couple to try and reach a reasonable BMI before trying to conceive or do IVF.

It is not only the increased chance of achieving a healthy pregnancy but the health of the child may also be affected by the weight of the parents.

Mice studies have shown that obese fathers can have offspring (especially daughters) that are prone to obesity and insulin resistance. Obesity can actually change the microRNA of the sperm revealing that a man's diet can affect the epigenome of his sperm, a non-genetic mechanism to inform the next generation of environmental change. Another compelling reason to lose weight before conception.[44]

Losing weight

A Damp condition often causes weight gain or even obesity because the body's metabolism is severely hampered by the congestion of stagnant fluids. Treatment consists of clearing Damp generally, so that metabolism improves and specifically so that ovulation proceeds. The weight loss that follows is usually accompanied by a return of fertility.

It is encouraging for your overweight patients to know that a little bit of weight loss goes a long way to improving fertility. Losing just 5 kg is a manageable target for most and once the Damp starts to mobilize reproductive health quickly responds. Just moving the metabolism a little bit in the direction of burning off fat stores can stimulate ovarian activity, improve egg and sperm quality, and increase fertility.

Chinese herbs are often prescribed to help weight loss. They regulate bowel transit time, reduce fluid retention, encourage efficient metabolism and increase energy levels. Herbs which specifically boost the function of the Spleen in transforming and transporting foods and clearing Damp are a good support to metabolism.

Formulas such as Xiang Sha Liu Jun Zi tang whose function is to Harmonize the Digestion, are a good basis from which to start.

Xiang Sha Liu Jun Zi tang (Six-Gentleman decoction with Aucklandia and Amomum)

Chao Bai Zhu	12 g	Rhizoma Atractylodis Macrocephalae
Fu Ling	12 g	Sclerotium Poriae Cocos
Dang Shen	15 g	Radix Codonopsis Pilulosae
Ban Xia	9 g	Rhizoma Pinelliae
Sha Ren	6 g	Fructus seu Semen Amomi
Chen Pi	6 g	Pericarpium Citri Reticulate
Gan Cao (Zhi)	6 g	Radix Glycyrrhizae Uralensis
Mu Xiang	6 g	Radix Saussureae seu Vladimiriae

For poor sleep add:

Suan Zao Ren	9 g	Semen Ziziphi Spinosae

For poor digestion from overeating or food stagnation add:

Chao Mai Ya	12 g	Fructus Hordei

For fluid retention add:

Ze Xie	9 g	Rhizoma Alismatis

For constipation or sluggish bowels add:

Rou Cong Rong	9 g	Herba Cistanches

There are some further additions that can be made, in the short term, to stimulate digestion and movement in the digestive tract, i.e., remove food stagnation and phlegm.

These include the following seeds and fruits:

• Lai Fu Zi – Radish seed – especially for digestion of carbohydrate

• Shan Zha – Hawthorn berry – especially for digestion of meat

• Bing Lang – Areca seed – to clear food and Phlegm-Damp stagnation in the digestive tract

- Da Fu Pi – Areca peel – to clear food and Phlegm-Damp stagnation in the digestive tract

- Jue Ming Zi – Cassia seeds – for constipation (but only if Spleen Qi is not too weak)

- Bai Jie Zi – Mustard seeds – to help remove Phlegm-Damp stagnation in digestive tract

- Zhi Ke – Citrus peel – to move the Qi and prevent stagnation in the intestines.

(Other citrus peels such as Chen Pi, Qing Pi, Ju Pi and Fo Shou can also be used for this).

Adding herbs such as those below, when cooking a pot of porridge, provides a nourishing meal with the recommended fiber to help control insulin resistance and also helps to clear Phlegm-Damp

Yi Yi Ren	30 g	Semen Coicis Lachryma-Jobi
Shan Zha	15 g	Fructus Crataegi
Yi Mu Cao	30 g	Herba Leonuri Heterophylli
Bai Bian Dou	20 g	Stir baked Dolichos Lablab

Acupuncture for weight loss

Acupuncture can be used effectively to stimulate the action of the Spleen Qi in regulating metabolism and clearing Damp. Many studies have examined the effect of acupuncture on weight loss, generally with positive outcome.[45] Additionally, acupuncture appears to increase insulin sensitivity, which makes weight loss easier in those patients who have insulin resistance.[46]

Using acupuncture points on the ear helps some patients control their appetites by stimulating the auricular branch of the vagal nerve and raising serotonin levels, both of which increase tone in the smooth muscle of the stomach and suppress food cravings.[47]

Other points on the body are used to stimulate the body's metabolism and encourage more efficient breakdown of stored energy (fat, in other words), reduce food cravings, and improve circulation. And there are other points that are used to improve sleep and mood. It is well documented that tired sleep-deprived people do not lose weight so easily, and that depression and anxiety do not encourage good food choices or diet control.[48]

Electroacupuncture applied to points on the abdomen and limbs body can promote lipolytic activity (destruction of fat cells) to reduce fat accumulation.[49]

Choose from the following points (and see Table 12.1):

Ren-3	Zhongji
Ren-6	Qihai
SP-6	Sanyinjiao
SP-9	Yinlingquan
GB-27	Wushu
GB-28	Weidao
GB-41	Zu Linqi
TH-5	Waiguan
ST-28	Shuidao
ST-40	Fenglong
SP-3	Taibai
TH-6	Zhigou
TH-10	Tianjing
LI-11	Quchi

CO-4   Hegu
ST-36   Zusanli
ST-25   Tianshu
DU-20   Baihui
Yin Tang
Ren-9   Shuifen
GB-34   Yanglingquan
LIV-3   Taichong
Ear points; Mouth, Lung, Stomach, Hunger, Shen Men

Acupuncture as a strategy to encourage weight loss and reduce insulin resistance needs to be repeated frequently, preferably 3 times a week. Frequent acupuncture can help reduce the appetite making portion size reduction easier. It also provides regular support both physically and mentally.

Despite these useful clinical strategies, it is important to realize that weight gain and loss are complex issues often tangled up with emotional coping patterns learned in childhood. Treatment to help a patient lose weight is not quite as easy as I have made it sound. This text is not the place to explore the many issues involved in weight loss, gain or obesity but awareness of some of the difficulties coupled with plenty of optimistic encouragement will help you to help your patient stick with treatment. It is worth reiterating that weight loss just needs to **start** – once the Damp is mobilizing, many positive changes will be seen in mood, energy, and ovary and testicle function.

Weight loss diets

The scope and focus of this book does not allow an in depth look at different diets employed for weight loss, besides which it is a complex and for many an emotional minefield fraught with obsessions and unhealthy behavior. We shall briefly look at some general and widely held as sensible dietary plans for weight loss and include a Chinese medicine perspective.

Table 12.1   Acupuncture points[a] used to promote weight loss

Treatment goal	Acupuncture points
To promote Stomach and Spleen function	ST-36, SP-6, Ren-12, Ren-6, Ear point; Stomach
To clear Phlegm-Damp	ST-40, SP-3, SP-9, GB-41, TH-5, GB-27/28
To promote regulate bowel movements	ST-25, TH-6, Ren-6, DU-20
To clear Heat to reduce appetite	ST-44, CO-11, CO-4, Ear point; Hunger
To reduce stress and indigestion	LIV-3, GB-34
To improve sleep and mood	YT, DU-20, Ear point; Shen Men
To regulate metabolism of fluids in the San Jiao	TH-6, TH-10, Ren-9
For food addiction or compulsive eating	Ear point; Mouth, Lung
To treat insulin resistance[b]	ST-28, SP-6, SP-9

[a]Reinforcing or reducing technique is used; electroacupuncture can be applied to abdomen, Ear or Large Intestine or Stomach points 2–10 Hertz, 20 min.
[b]Electroacupuncture to treat insulin resistance uses abdomen points linked to Spleen points on the inner leg.

We spoke briefly about a 'good' diet to promote health and fertility above. Here, we shall refine that basic advice to formulate a diet that not only provides good prenatal nutrition but helps weight loss. Some general pointers apply which can be summarized thus for your overweight patient trying to conceive:

- Choose delicious fresh food, vegetables and fruits in season, mix colors and make flavors interesting with herbs and spices. Enjoy your food. Sit down to eat it, away from the work desk, away from the television.

- Chew slowly, savor each mouthful. When you eat too fast, you don't give the stomach time to tell the brain that it's had enough – so you keep on eating. It takes 20 minutes for brain-signaling hormones to signal the brain that it no longer needs food.

- Be a little bit French in your eating patterns – choose excellent quality food, even if it is a bit more expensive. Just eat less of it. Spoil yourself.

- Have three meals a day, with small healthy snacks in between. Do not skip meals. Have your meals on smaller plates so you reduce your quantities. Only one plate per meal. No second helpings.

- Have protein at least once a day; this can be lean meat, chicken, fish, tofu, eggs, lentils, or legumes.

- Use home-made vegetable soups to replace one meal per day (the evening meal is best); these are nutritious, low calorie and satisfying because they stay in the stomach longer than solid meals.

- Do not have iced water with your meals. Have a few sips of wine (but no more than a few sips) or have a digestive tea like Oolong or Pu Erh if you want to drink with your meals.

- Stop all drinks that contain sugar or artificial sweeteners.

- Stop all processed foods like cakes, biscuits, and white breads.

- Limit carbohydrates – only one or two small slices of bread a day, and very modest servings of rice, noodles, or pasta rather than large ones.

- Cut out fatty and fried foods, although small amounts of good oils (e.g., olive oil, avocado), should be included.

Patients with weight problems will almost always have some degree of Spleen dysfunction. We discussed some ideas about supporting Spleen function in our discussion of Qi and Damp above. When we want to boost the Spleen function of our patients and encourage good metabolism, we need to encourage good eating patterns. Patients with Spleen issues may on the one hand, crave and indulge in inappropriate amounts of starchy and sweet foods, or on the other hand, become obsessed with unhealthy unbalanced diets. We need to steer them down the middle path and encourage a holistic context to healthy eating based on regular routines, choosing the right foods for the right time and season, and their personal constitution combined with enough movement.

The TCM practitioner will help the overweight patient to find the appropriate food choices and design a weight loss diet specific to his or her needs. That is one that is easy to digest and light. Cooked foods (rather than the raw foods commonly recommended), aromatic spices, and fragrant herbs make digestion easy. Frequent intake of small portions of warming foods containing protein and avoidance of sweet foods are conducive to healthy Spleen function. In the case of Phlegm-Damp accumulation that is giving rise to Heat, some more cooling foods might be incorporated, or at least the more heating foods may need to be avoided. We can also encourage the addition of some specific foods which have been shown to inhibit weight gain and promote weight loss. The polyphenols present in green tea, grape seeds, orange, grapefruit, and blueberries can help move the Damp. They have been shown to combat adipogenesis at the molecular level and in some cases, also induce lipolysis or reduce insulin resistance.[50,51] Drinking green tea before doing exercise can support the break down of visceral adipose tissue. An alternative to green tea, oolong tea, has also been found to have good weight loss properties.[52]

For more discussion of specific foods to be included in or excluded from a diet to support Spleen Qi and reduce Damp and Phlegm, see Vol. 2 of the *Clinical Handbook of Internal Medicine*.[9]

For discussion of the role that exercise and sleep play in weight loss, see below.

EXERCISE

In general, exercise is an essential component of maintaining good health. Exercise can greatly enhance fertility as it manages weight, promotes blood flow and hormone balance, and counteracts stress.

As part of a weight loss program, it is essential, especially where there is insulin resistance. Exercise builds muscle tissue and increases skeletal muscle insulin sensitivity. This means that pancreatic production of insulin drops and blood levels are lower. With less insulin in the blood, less sugar is converted to fat.

Where insulin resistance is making weight loss difficult, very short bursts of high intensity training appears to be helpful. The time investment in this sort of training is small and manageable by even the busiest of patients.[53]

Exercise also lowers levels of the stress hormone, cortisol. Not only does this improve mood and allow for better stress management but it also reduces the deposition of visceral fat, which is seen in some women with PCOS.

From the Chinese medicine perspective exercise is an important support for weight loss – not only for the burning up of calories but also for the improved circulation of blood and fluids which helps disperse the Damp. Programs that support PCOS sufferers to lose weight have found that exercise in a group context adds an important psychological component to recovery. Since Damp is an internal environment which can cause sluggishness, low motivation, and depression, this sort of encouragement is important.

However, exercise can be overdone. One study found that women who exercised daily were three times more likely to have fertility problems than women who were not so active.[54]

Another study indicated that vigorous exercise did not give women doing IVF any advantage, rather the opposite. Women who were used to exercising vigorously for more than 4 h a week had a lower rate of pregnancy than those who exercised less. The data showed that, in particular, intense cardiovascular exercise such as running, cycling, and stair climbing was detrimental to IVF outcomes.[55]

The Chinese medicine practitioner is well placed to assess the appropriateness or otherwise of vigorous exercise. Exercise is advised to our patients because it promotes Lung function and moves the Qi and Blood, thus building the capacity of the body to manufacture more Qi and Blood and use fuel efficiently. However, women who do intense cardiovascular exercise for several hours a week, on top of a busy work schedule, may be depleting their Blood and Yin reserves somewhat, even though their Qi may still be healthy. Thus for keen exercisers who are not finding it easy to conceive, the advice is to reduce exercise sessions to three a week (1 h max. each time) and to exercise at moderate levels only. For those women who suffer from fatigue due to very low reserves of Qi, gentle exercise which gathers energy rather than spends it, is more useful. Exercise such as Tai Chi or yoga or gentle walking helps to build internal energy and calm the nervous system rather than working the heart and muscles.

Sperm of men who engage in moderate exercise appear to have better motility than that of sedentary men.[56] However, some sports are thought not to be so good for sperm production and quality. These include sports which overheat the body, such as long distance or grueling athletics, and those which put sustained pressure on the testicles like cycling. On the other hand, anecdotally, swimming or surfing (i.e., chilling the testicles) appears to be good for sperm health.

In summary, some words of advice for your patient about exercise in general and for losing weight:

- You need to move. And make moving enjoyable.

- If you are highly motivated, go to the gym three times a week to do aerobic classes

- *or* walk daily and briskly for 30 min in a pleasant green environment

- *or* engage regularly in some other strenuous activity you enjoy.

- For men, choose swimming rather than cycling or long distance running.

- If you are less enthusiastic about exercise, get a personal trainer who will tailor exercise to your needs and provide the motivation to keep going. Or join a boot camp exercise group which meets several times a week, or set one up with your friends.

- A small time investment of high intensity training helps reduce insulin resistance (a personal trainer is useful for this sort of exercise program).

- For those people for whom this level of activity is not possible or advisable, then gentle movement like Tai Chi or yoga is appropriate. These forms of movement can still help weight loss, albeit more slowly – Tai Chi, e.g., burns as many calories as downhill skiing! And as the Qi recovers, the capacity to metabolize more efficiently increases.

STRESS

No matter how stressful life can be, it is more stressful if there is difficulty in achieving a pregnancy. Why? We all arrive in this world assuming the 'God-given' right to reproduce ourselves. Even if we haven't given it much conscious thought, because it is written in our genes, it is a very strong biologic imperative. At the bottom line, reproducing is our genes' main agenda! And to have that most fundamental of drives put in question or thwarted outright is undermining and distressing at a profound level to so many aspects of ourselves – both conscious and unconscious. If the molecular screaming from the DNA in the tissues is not enough, added to that are all the expectations society has, especially of women, to do their bit in perpetuating the race, the family, and the family name. This pressure is felt very acutely by women in developing nations where a woman's worth is measured in terms of offspring, usually male offspring. Such is still the case in much of China.

In addition, so many of the current generation of women in the West have been brought up on the notion that they can have it all – career, income, wealth, and then children. But society at large didn't get the same message. The circumstances which most women face in the work and public arena strongly disadvantage child-bearing in the ideal fertile years; those between 25 and 35 years of age. The added frustration so many women experience when they discover that getting pregnant when you are 40 isn't just like putting another item on the day's agenda, accelerates stress levels markedly. These are women who have become used to writing their own scripts and then successfully actualizing them, and it is a cruel blow to discover that biology is not always quite so cooperative.

Once a couple embarks on a modern technological treatment program for infertility, a whole new set of stresses arrives. The demands of frequent clinic visits, intrusive procedures, drug side-effects and financial pressures can take their toll on all but the most optimistic of people. For couples who do not achieve pregnancy after many attempts, keeping a positive frame of mind becomes increasingly difficult. The fraught question of when to stop trying must be faced, but when new developments in assisted reproduction technology (ART) are constantly announced, the couple who thought they had tried everything are suddenly thrown back into the arena with the hope of success this time.

How does stress affect fertility? Western specialists will usually say that stress has little or no effect on fertility, except to perhaps reduce the frequency of intercourse if either partner, especially the male, is feeling extremely stressed.[57]

Not everybody agrees. Some specialists at the Harvard Medical School[58] point out that stress has been implicated, along with depression, in ovulation irregularities, and in men attending IVF clinics, emotional stress can be associated with abnormal sperm development.[59]

Depression among infertile women is found to be just as severe as the depression experienced by those with life-threatening diseases such as cancer, heart disease, and AIDS. The cruel irony is that this depression can then contribute further to the infertility.

Studies of women undergoing IVF show that those who exhibit lower levels of measurable physiological stress have a higher chance of success,[60] while those with more stressful lives do less well.[61] Feeling relaxed and unstressed favors natural (non-IVF) conception, according to studies which measure mood states on standard psychometric tests,[62] while raised levels of physiologic stress markers correlate with reduced conception rates.[63]

The positive effect of feeling relaxed on conception rates in these studies was not thought to be due to increased frequency of intercourse.

Doctors of Chinese medicine look at some of the more subtle manifestations or ramifications of stress and recognize the impact of these on fertility. Feeling content and relaxed usually indicates, in our TCM frame of reference, healthy and unobstructed Heart and Liver Qi (among other things). (We have already discussed the impact that Heart Qi stagnation can have on ovulation in Ch. 4.) According to Chinese medicine, the Heart is the emotional center of the body and houses the spirit. When the Qi in the Heart becomes obstructed (the cause is always emotional), the messages which the Heart should send to the ovaries via the Bao vessel do not arrive and eggs are not stimulated to ripen. Mental stress which affects the Heart therefore can frequently upset the rhythm of the menstrual cycle. If the effect of the stress on the Heart is severe, then periods may stop altogether, i.e., there may be no messages from the Heart to the ovaries for a long time. When ovulation is disrupted for a very long time (years), it can be harder to re-establish the Bao vessel function. The emotions that affect the Heart are anxiety and mental anguish. Difficulty in becoming pregnant can certainly cause these sorts of feelings, as can relationship difficulties. Addressing the Heart Qi is recognized as a very important part of TCM infertility treatment.

The Liver Qi is also easily obstructed by stress. The sorts of stress we are talking about here are those day-to-day frustrations which can make us feel irritable, such as finding the milk has gone off after you've poured it into your morning cup of tea; the car breaking down; conflict at work. The Liver Qi which is responsible for overseeing the smooth running of many cycles in our bodies can also be upset if daily routines are not regular. An extreme example of this is the difficulty experienced by flight attendants on international flights in maintaining regular routines, which means their Liver Qi easily becomes obstructed.

The Liver not only has influence over cycles in the body but also over the movement of Qi in the pelvis and chest. Stress-related Liver Qi stagnation can be responsible for tension in the fallopian tubes, preventing the passage of the egg, sperm, or embryo. Liver Qi stagnation can also manifest later in the cycle in the premenstrual week, with breast tenderness and swelling, abdomen bloating and perhaps cramping. While these are clear clinical signs that Liver Qi is obstructed, there doesn't appear to be direct impediment to fertility at this point, unless the Liver Qi stagnation has led to Blood stagnation and the endometrium is therefore not favorable for implantation.

Acupuncture is well known for its ability to reduce the effects of stress and as such, has an important place in treatment of infertility patients, particularly those undergoing IVF. A number of studies have been done which look at the effect of acupuncture on perceived stress levels of women undergoing IVF.[64-68]

Acupuncture, which calms the Shen and promotes smooth movement of Liver Qi will nearly always have a rapid and positive effect on stress levels.

Exercise is a useful strategy for moving the Qi and disengaging the mind. Massage can do the same. A regular rhythm of life is important in mitigating the effects of stress and stagnation of Qi. One of the most effective means to prevent Qi stagnation is meditation, completely emptying the mind of all its chatter and allowing the body and mind to be completely untrammeled. If this can be achieved (and it is by no means as simple as it sounds), then Qi and Blood have no place to become stagnant.

SLEEP

The connection between sleep and fertility is not always self-evident, although getting to bed early with your partner may for some couples have obvious benefits.

It is often not recognized that the quality and quantity of your sleep influences sex hormones, sperm production, ovulation, immune factors, weight gain, mood, stress levels, and longevity, as well as the more obvious stamina. Getting enough good quality sleep is an essential part of preparing for conception for all of these reasons.

From our point of view as TCM practitioners, sleep is of paramount importance in nourishing Blood and building Qi, nurturing Kidney Yin and Kidney Yang. You may remember from our earlier discussions on the preservation of Yin (and Jing), that times when the body and mind are at complete rest are crucial for restoring and recuperating stores of essential energy.

It is increasingly recognized that sleep deprivation is not only very common (it is estimated by the US National Sleep foundation that 70% of us in the developed world don't get enough sleep) but that it can also damage many aspects of health. Studies in the past have indicated that the average adult benefits from 8 or 9 h of sleep every night, but the typical American or Australian city worker may only get 7, and many get considerably less without ever catching up (for some reason Europeans seem to have a healthier attitude to sleep and, in general, are less sleep deprived).

Sleep and sex hormones

Lack of sleep affects ovulation, causing menstrual irregularity and delaying conception. A large proportion (50%) of women who work in notoriously sleep-deprived professions, e.g., flight attendants, nurses, and other night-shift workers experience irregular and erratic periods and in some cases, infertility.[69,70]

In many cases, these women stop having periods altogether. Sleep disrupted by night-shifts at the time of ovulation and conception may also increase the odds of miscarriage. In general, getting <8 h a night sleep is considered a risk factor for 1st trimester miscarriage.[71] In an ideal world, men and women trying to conceive should avoid shift work, or skimping on sleep, or if this is impossible, they should make a concerted effort to catch up on sleep when they can.

Lack of sleep can also cause a slump in sperm production. Testosterone production in men occurs during the night, normally increasing by 20–30% and cutting back on sleep drastically reduces testosterone levels.[72] This may be one of the reasons for the observed decline in male fertility in modern times.

One of the main functions of sleep in TCM physiology is to allow the Liver Blood to gather and build. This is important for normal Liver Qi movement and in maintaining sufficient Heart Blood. Lack of sleep and insufficient Liver and Heart Blood resources create a vicious cycle where maintaining sleep becomes more and more difficult. When Heart Blood is deficient, the Shen becomes unsettled and deep sleep is illusive. This creates the stage for Bao Mai dysfunction, menstrual irregularities, and risk of miscarriage. Additionally, chronic lack of sleep draws on Kidney reserves, depleting Kidney Yin, Yang and Jing and compromising potential fertility.

Conversely, levels of sex hormones have a profound effect on sleep patterns, especially in women, which in turn has an effect on neuroendocrine functioning. Since the same part of the brain that regulates sleep–wake hormones also stimulates daily pulses of reproductive hormones for men and women, some feedback between these systems is likely. Women who suffer from premenstrual symptoms have been shown to get less of the deep slow brain wave stages of sleep than asymptomatic women.[73] Here we see the connections between Liver Qi stagnation, Liver Blood deficiency and sleep.

Sleep and metabolism

Sleep scientists at the University of Chicago have found that those who suffer from an accumulated sleep debt may develop serious ongoing health problems. Sleep deprivation causes alterations in metabolic and endocrine function that show all the hallmarks of aging. The odds of becoming obese and developing metabolic syndrome (including diabetes, heart disease, high blood pressure) are nearly doubled in men and women who sleep <6 h, compared with those who sleep between 7 and 8 h/night.[74–77]

Being overweight or obese has significant deleterious effects on fertility in men and women (as we saw above). Weight loss is an important part of improving fertility but it is hard to lose weight if sleep is inadequate. In fact, weight loss programs are 50% less effective if they are not accompanied by adequate sleep. Less sleep results in increased hunger but lower resting metabolic rate; a sure recipe for weight gain, not weight loss. Lack of sleep also raises levels of ghrelin. This hormone not only reduces energy expenditure but promotes the retention of fat.[78]

Over and over, overweight, overworked women, or overweight mothers of young families have demonstrated that being chronically tired (failing Spleen Qi) can make you fat, and now the clinical research confirms it!

So important is the role of sleep in weight loss that the Stanford Sleep Medicine Center in California has suggested that sleep needs to be included in weight loss packages that have traditionally focused on just diet and exercise. Skipping sleep does not just consume Kidney energy, it risks damaging the Spleen.

We spend Qi all day, every day, some of us more than others. The only way to replenish this essential resource is to take in fuel, keep breathing, and to rest. We are all familiar with the role of the Spleen in maintaining good metabolism, the efficient movement, absorption and use of nutrients, and removal of waste products. When the Spleen Qi weakens and any of these steps are compromised, then fat deposits occur, boggy congested tissue starts to appear and weight is gained. Alongside eating the right foods in the right quantity, and breathing, sleep is essential to safeguard optimal Spleen function.

Sleep and stress

Anxiety levels increase incrementally, the longer sleep loss continues. Sleep restriction affects biologic mechanisms involved in the stress response. The two major neurobiologic transmitters of the stress response (cortisol regulation and sympathovagal balance) show significant changes after just a few days of sleep restriction.[79] However, emotional and physiologic stress caused by lack of sleep is reversible once sleep loss is recovered.[80]

Levels of stress hormones are higher and thyroid hormones are also disrupted when sleep is cut short. Mental sharpness and the ability to concentrate effectively and remember, have been shown to be affected by inadequate sleep.

Lack of sleep and the resulting compromised stores of Liver Blood creates the conditions for Heart Blood deficiency and a disturbed Shen and mental agitation, and also Liver Qi stagnation and enhanced stress reactions. Lack of Blood and Qi feeding the brain will also contribute to memory problems.

Sleep and the immune system

The complex and intimate interactions between sleep and the immune system have been the focus of study for several years. The equally complex and intimate interactions of immune factors and fertility are also currently the object of intense research.

We know that certain immune factors (cytokines) regulate sleep and in turn are altered by sleep and sleep deprivation. People with chronic insomnia tend to have higher levels of some cytokines, notably interleukin-6 and tumor necrosis factor.[81] These immune factors can impact on certain parts of the reproductive system, particularly implantation of the embryo and placental development. Some researchers have proposed that a suboptimal cytokine environment can contribute to miscarriage.[82]

Certain cytokines can lead to clotting of the placental vessels in cases of early or late pregnancy loss, or interference of angiogenesis in cases of occult pregnancy loss. Disturbed sleep also increases inflammatory processes in the body.[83] Thus, regulating the immune system, particularly in its autoimmune aspects, is another reason for encouraging sufficient and sound sleep.

Ensuring smooth movement of Blood and Qi and adequate Kidney Yin levels will help prevent the scenarios we often see in autoimmune conditions, i.e., Heat and inflammation from Yin deficiency and Blood stasis from insufficient Blood or poor Qi movement.

Although not so related to reproductive issues directly, other immune issues, i.e., inadequate defenses against infection, are seen more often in sleep-deprived people. Here we see a consequence of reduced Wei Qi from compromised Kidney Yang function.

A good night's sleep

What, then, does sufficient and sound sleep actually mean?

It means allowing the body to build resources like the Blood, the Qi, the Yin and the Yang, all of which fit into our picture of optimal fertility in the many different ways we have outlined above. This takes a lot of hours of maintaining a deeply quiescent state of the mind and body.

It may be the case that those hours before midnight, which our grandmothers always told us were the most important, are the time that the Kidney Yang in particular is recuperated. Certainly, it is in those first few hours of sleep when we experience slow brain wave sleep, the deepest type of sleep, that growth hormone is secreted, and the first stage of learning and memory is carried out as newly acquired information is sent from the hippocampus to the cortex. The early morning hours of sleep seem to be the time when the mind gets its rejuvenation and when the second stage of learning is carried out as memory is solidified in the cortex during the replays of REM (rapid eye movement) sleep.[84]

With the clarifying and steadying action on the mind which early morning dream sleep (REM) brings, the deep levels of Yin have the chance to recuperate too. In summary, it is the early bedtime and the early morning hours of sleep that are important for regenerating Kidney Yin and Yang.

Attention to sleep is especially important after the age of 30, when both capacity for deep sleep and the production of growth hormone start to decline quite rapidly,[85] paralleling the decline in Kidney Yin and Yang which begins at this time.

In summary, sleep is clearly important for many reasons: preserving the Spleen Qi and Liver Blood, regulating the Heart Qi, and regenerating Kidney Yin and Yang. For couples trying to get pregnant, long and deep sleep is very important even if it no longer comes quite so easily once they are past their mid-30s. Acupuncture and herbal remedies are quite effective at helping to achieve healthy sleep patterns as we all know. (For representative herbal formulae and acupuncture point prescriptions for various types of sleep disturbance, refer to the *Clinical Handbook of Internal Medicine*, Vol. 1.)[86]

OUR DAILY DRUGS

Could those constant habits of imbibing, inhaling, or swallowing our daily props be affecting fertility? It seems that coffee, alcohol, cigarettes, and marijuana are not such a good idea for someone who is having difficulty falling pregnant. Sure we all know of people who smoke like chimneys, drink like fish, and down cups of coffee like Italians or Brazilians, and who still manage to have broods of children – but that's not the point. The point is that if fertility is compromised for some reason, then all the factors which reduce it further must be addressed.

Caffeine

A large study carried out by the Yale Medical School found that the risk of infertility (which they defined as not being able to conceive after 12 months) was 55% higher for women drinking just 1 cup of coffee per day; 100% higher for women drinking 1.5–3 cups per day; and 176% higher for >3 cups per day,[87] and this was backed up 5 years later by a study in Europe, which found that high caffeine intake in women slowed rates of conception.[88] The effect of caffeine on the fertility of men has not been examined to the same extent but one study did find a delay in conception related to caffeine intake though the dose was not significant.[89] Additionally, there is evidence that coffee drinking in men and women increases miscarriage rates and that caffeine intake during pregnancy has a negative influence on fetal growth.[90,91]

Most studies indicate that it is the consumption of ≥300 mg of caffeine daily that can lead to fertility problems. It is estimated that >20% of Australians and Americans drink more than 350 mg/day. So, coffee drinkers having difficulty falling pregnant may well be advised to reduce their intake significantly, switch to low-caffeine varieties of tea, or to find alternatives for their morning and afternoon cuppas.

Alcohol

Many couples are told that they should stop drinking alcohol altogether in preparation for conception. But the evidence for such prohibition is not clear cut. Exploring the literature on the effect of alcohol on fertility, it would appear that alcohol has little effect on fertility in some countries and a dramatic effect in others. For example, the Italians are quite sure that alcohol intake has no negative effect on their ability to fall pregnant.[92] Similarly, other large studies carried out in a number of countries in Europe have been able to demonstrate no relationship between moderate alcohol intake of men and women and ability to get pregnant,[93] although heavier consumption (defined as >8 drinks a week) did have a negative effect.

A study in Denmark[94] showed that women who drank moderately (2 glasses a week to 2 glasses a day) conceived more quickly than those who didn't drink at all. However, before advising all prospective parents to raid their cellars, it should be noted that these results do not mean that consuming alcohol is better for fertility than not drinking alcohol at all. Non-drinkers differ from moderate drinkers in many other aspects; for instance, they may have a weaker constitution or other health problems that can influence fertility, directly or indirectly. In addition, alcohol drinkers may have a higher frequency of sexual intercourse.

Women do metabolize alcohol much less efficiently than men and there is certainly evidence to suggest that alcohol can increase incidence of some gynecological and other disorders which might contribute to infertility. Alcohol consumption is associated with altered estrogen and progesterone levels as well as menstrual irregularities and increased incidence of endometriosis, abnormalities in the ovaries, impaired implantation and blastocyst development and the early onset of menopause.[95]

Some studies have found evidence that moderate drinking by women (5–10 drinks per week) is linked to lower fertility and increased miscarriage.[96] And others have found a definite relationship between even modest alcohol consumption in women (<5 drinks/week) and delay in conception.[97,98]

Alcohol consumption by men in many of these studies seemed to have little effect on fertility of the couple. However, very heavy drinking on the part of the male partner significantly negatively impacts the time it takes for a couple to conceive.[99] Excessive alcohol consumption can induce testicular atrophy, impotence, reduced libido, and cause a deterioration in sperm count.[100]

It therefore seems that evidence can be found to support either camp on this issue, but most professionals working in the field of fertility will advise against too much alcohol consumption on the part of either partner for both general health reasons and consideration of health of the gametes. Completely restricting all alcohol intake in couples (with no history of, or reasons for infertility) planning to become pregnant is not justified.

There is however some good evidence to suggest that couples should abstain from alcohol in the lead up to starting an IVF cycle. Consumption of as few as four alcoholic drinks per week (either partner) is associated with a decrease in IVF live birth rate.[101] Other researchers have found that alcohol consumption by the woman in the month before IVF meant reduced numbers of eggs collected and by the male partner meant reduced live birth rates.[102] The European Society of Human Reproduction and Embryology has issued guidelines for ART specialists, saying that: 'Fertility treatment should not be provided to women whose alcohol consumption is more than moderate levels, and to those unwilling or unable to reduce their consumption.'[103]

427

From a TCM point of view, excessive or chronic use of alcohol can increase internal Heat or Damp-Heat. Thus, a patient with a tendency to a Hot or Damp-Heat constitution (especially the larger or ruddy type), who is trying to conceive will be advised to limit alcohol severely. On the other hand, colder or Qi-deficient patients trying to conceive may positively benefit from small amounts of red wine taken with food. The doctor of Chinese medicine should be able to give discerning and educated advice to individual patients about the consumption of alcohol.

Once pregnancy is confirmed, then all or nearly all alcohol consumption by the mother should be avoided for the duration of the pregnancy and breast-feeding. Alcohol has been shown to have effects on the child both before and after birth.

Nicotine

The effect of smoking has been examined by many researchers and the general consensus here is the same. Most studies have shown negative effects of smoking on reproduction, and in couples where either partner smokes, it takes longer for them to conceive.[104]

Female smokers also experience the menopause earlier than usual. Additionally, smoking has been strongly associated with tubal factor infertility, and it has been linked to increased rates of miscarriage. The effects of smoking are also felt at the level of the uterine lining, affecting its receptivity to the embryo.[105]

Smoking has also been shown to have a deleterious effect on sperm counts. On average, smoker's sperm counts are nearly 20% lower than non-smokers. And when smokers stop smoking, their sperm counts were seen to rise between 50% and 800%, indicating that toxic chemicals in the tobacco have a very deleterious effect on sperm production but that these effects can be reversed.[106]

Marijuana

Women trying to conceive are generally advised to avoid marijuana. This is on the strength of animal studies which showed that THC (the active ingredient in marijuana) is toxic to the developing egg and at certain levels, could delay ovulation markedly.[107]

There is also ample evidence demonstrating a damaging effect by THC on sperm production and function. Sperm production and motility have been shown to be drastically reduced in heavy marijuana smokers and new research indicates that the THC might also interfere with the binding of the sperm to an egg and its ability to fertilize it.[108]

Junk food

A junk food diet is one which is high in fat and sugar and low in nutrients. Fat and sugar are not actually drugs, however many of us are addicted to them.

A diet high in fat, especially trans-fat, such as that found in many processed and take away foods, is associated with lower sperm counts, whereas higher intake of omega-3 fats (in fish and some vegetable oils) improves sperm quality.[32]

Men who eat a lot of processed foods (and meat) have poorer sperm quality (in particular motility) than men who eat more fresh foods and fish.[109] Men who drink 1.2 litres (a quart) or more of cola daily have sperm counts almost 30% lower than men who drink no cola.[110] This finding could be related to the caffeine or the sugar content of such a high consumption of cola. The excessive amount of sugar would certainly contribute to insulin resistance and excess weight (which we saw above had a negative impact on fertility).

Assessing the effect of junk food on egg quality is more difficult than it is for sperm, however the diet that appeared to promote fertility in the Nurses study quoted above was based on whole foods and avoided junk foods.[9,10]

Eating more whole foods appears to have a good effect on reducing C Reactive protein (CRP) levels which are correlated with fertility in women.[111]

Other drugs

Anti-inflammatory drugs

There is some evidence that taking non-steroidal anti-inflammatory drugs (NSAIDs) for arthritic or painful conditions may interfere with the chemical signals which allow release of the egg at ovulation time, producing a well-characterized syndrome known as LUFS or luteinized unruptured follicle syndrome. This phenomenon was noticed in women taking either the standard class of NSAIDs[112] or the new generation of anti-inflammatory drugs, called COX-2 inhibitors (trade names Celebrex and Vioxx). Stopping the medication reversed the effect, and ovulation was no longer delayed.[113,114] In animal studies, even aspirin could inhibit ovulation.[115]

Antidepressants

We know there are negative effects on pregnancy outcome and fetal health when women take antidepressants, however less is known about their effect on fertility.

Taking SSRIs (selective serotonin reuptake inhibitors) during pregnancy is associated with increased risk of miscarriage,[116] and twice as many pre-term births and delayed head growth[117] (although it should be noted that untreated depression is also associated with slower fetal growth). Some SSRIs (fluoxetine or paroxetine) are suspected of increasing the risk of cardiovascular malformations in the fetus[118] and others of disrupting sleep patterns of the fetus in utero.[119] Research is continuing to assess the impact of manipulating serotonin levels with SSRI drugs in utero on the fetal brain growth and other organs. In the meantime, the fact that acupuncture has proved effective at treating depression during pregnancy gives women an alternative.[120]

Should we advise women to stop SSRI medication while trying to conceive? Probably not until such time as there is evidence that they impair fertility more than depression does. However, addressing the causes of the depression will be a main aim of the TCM practitioner as part of the treatment to enhance fertility and prepare for a healthy pregnancy. One small study has indicated that acupuncture is as effective as the conventional pharmaceutical approaches in treating major depression.[121]

SSRIs in some reports have shown an adverse effect on sperm count (which was reversible once the medication was stopped) and impairment of sexual function.[122–124]

ENVIRONMENTAL POLLUTANTS

Many years ago, the Pregnancy and Lifestyle Study (PALS) carried out in Australia looked at the effects of toxic chemicals in the environment on the fertility and miscarriage rates of some thousands of couples. The results[125] revealed that lifestyle, life circumstances, and environment had a major impact on fertility and miscarriage rates. Unfortunately, exposure to environmental pollutants has increased markedly over the ensuing years since this study and it is difficult for most couples to avoid the chemicals that are in our air, water, food, houses, and workplaces. We don't yet know all the ramifications for reproductive health but many pesticides and plastics have been shown to have hormone disrupting abilities.

We mentioned the effects of such endocrine disruptors on sperm manufacture in Chapter 7. But it is not just the sperm that are vulnerable. Mammalian females are born with a finite number of primordial follicles, the majority of which remain in a quiescent state for many years. Because they cannot be regenerated, these 'resting' oocytes are particularly vulnerable to damage by synthetic chemical compounds which trigger abnormal rates of atresia with disastrous effects on female fertility as oocyte quality is compromised and ovarian reserve is depleted.[126–128]

This has already been shown to be the case with some known toxic chemicals such as those in cigarette smoke, which are associated with early menopause.

There is some suggestion that exposure of baby girls to pesticides in utero can increase the risk of PCOS.[129]

Air pollution in general is correlated with reduced fertility. When many thousands of women attending an IVF clinic were assessed for exposure to local air pollution (at home and at the IVF clinic), there was a clear and disturbing link between higher exposure, particularly to nitrogen dioxide and fine air-borne particulate matter, reduced numbers of pregnancies and live births.[130]

Once a woman is pregnant, even relatively low ambient air pollution exposure can affect birth weight.[131] (To read more about the effect of environmental toxins on miscarriage rates, please see Chs 7 and 8.)

Some chemicals commonly used in the workplace and the home affect the fertility of both men and women.[132] For example, commonly encountered fumes such as dry cleaning liquid, petrol, ammonia, and nail polish remover can interfere with fertility in susceptible people. Hand cleansing gels (containing triclosan) used in hospitals and more generally, are also under scrutiny by the Food and Drug Administration in the USA, in this regard.

Likewise many chemicals used in industry and agriculture are now the subject of scrutiny. These include polychlorinated biphenyls (PCBs) used in solvents, paints, and many industrial products; phthalates used in plastics and nail polish; dioxins found in pesticides; polybrominated diphenyl ethers (PBDEs) used as flame retardants in polyurethane foam, electronics, carpets and textiles; bisphenol A (BPA) found in hard clear plastics, food and drink cans and cartons, water pipes, dentistry sealants, and thermal cash register receipts; perfluorinated compounds (PFCs) used for grease resistant coatings; 4-vinylcyclohexene diepoxide (VCD), a by-product of the manufacture of many products including rubber tires and insecticides; trichloroethylene (TCE) a solvent and degreaser; alkylphenol ethoxylates (APEs) surfactants in laundry detergents, stain removers, and all-purpose cleaners and glycol ethers; organic solvents used in many household cleaning products – and there are many others. Some of these chemicals are now banned but are nevertheless extremely persistent in the environment and in living organisms.

Polychlorinated biphenyls (PCBs)

This family of chemicals, which includes DDT, concentrates through the food chain, accumulates in fat tissue, and comprises the bulk of organochlorine residues in human tissues. They can be detected in follicular fluid of infertile women doing IVF.[133] Human reproductive toxicity of PCBs has been examined in studies of fishing communities, fish eaters and the general population.[134,135] The level of PCBs (and phthalates) are higher in the semen of infertile men than that of men with normal fertility. The highest concentrations were found in fish eaters.[136] More Y chromosome bearing sperm are manufactured in men who are exposed to higher levels of PCBs, and sperm motility overall is reduced.[137,138]

Polybrominated diphenyl ethers (PBDEs)

We are exposed to PBDEs which can leach out into the environment and accumulate in human fat cells mostly through food and house dust. These chemicals are endocrine disruptors which have a damaging effect on male reproductive hormones and fertility.[139,140] Additionally, PBDE levels are associated with increased odds of subclinical hyperthyroidism in pregnant women (and therefore increased risks of adverse pregnancy outcomes)[141] and can compromise fetal health resulting in low birth weight babies.[142]

Phthalates

The general population is exposed to phthalates through consumer products, as well as diet and medical treatments. Phthalates are thought to have damaging effects on fertility, particularly on sperm.[143]

Bisphenol A (BPA)

BPA is another ubiquitous chemical in the industrial world, which has the potential to interfere with biological processes because its structure resembles estrogen. More than 90% of the US population have detectable levels of urinary BPA.

Research has shown that BPA disrupts normal development of oocytes and increases DNA fragmentation in sperm.[144,145]

Women with higher serum or urinary levels of BPA not only have poorer quality oocytes, but also reduced fertilization rates and higher implantation failure rates in IVF cycles.[146,147]

It is not only in fertility stakes that this common environmental pollutant causes damage. BPA also appears to affect in utero development, particularly of baby girls. Those girls who are exposed in utero show impaired behavioral and emotional regulation when they are toddlers.[148]

Perfluorinated compounds (PFCs)

Grease-resistant products are often coated with this compound, including stick-resistant cookware, dental floss, and carpets. Exposure to PFCs risks lower conception rates, i.e., it takes longer to become pregnant.[149]

4-vinylcyclohexene diepoxide (VCD)

VCD is a metabolite of a product released during the manufacture of rubber tires, flame retardants, insecticides, plasticizers, and antioxidants. It is well known as an ovarian toxicant and has been shown to quickly destroy oocytes in animal studies.[150]

Trichloroethylene (TCE)

TCE is used as a solvent and degreaser. Mechanics and others who work with engines are frequently exposed to this chemical and the seminal fluid of mechanics contains discernible levels of TCE.[151] Others are exposed to TCE through contaminated drinking water; seepage of this compound into groundwater has raised health concerns in many locations.

Exposure of mice to TCE affects the ability of sperm to fertilize eggs, even at levels that have no discernible effect on the testes or the count or motility of the sperm. Similarly, maturing oocytes are susceptible to even very short in vivo exposures to TCE which reduces their ability to be fertilized and form embryos.[152]

Alkylphenol ethoxylates (APEs)

APEs are commonly used in cleaning products like laundry powder and cleaning products used in the kitchen. The breakdown products of these detergents are found throughout the natural environment now, especially in the waterways, where they are wreaking havoc with the reproductive systems of some aquatic organisms such as turtles, fish, and frogs. APEs are also found in house dust and food[153,154] and have been shown to have damaging effects on the reproductive system in laboratory studies.[155]

Some countries have taken steps to ban these chemicals.

Glycol ethers

Glycol ethers are a large group of organic solvents used in industry and the home as glass cleaners, carpet cleaners, floor cleaners and oven cleaners. They are absorbed as volatile fumes from the air by the skin as well as inhalation.

Animal studies have reported testicular damage, reduced fertility, early embryonic death, birth defects, and delayed development from inhalation and oral exposure to the glycol ethers.[156] Occupational exposure to glycol ethers has also been shown to result in reproductive and developmental impacts in humans. Studies of exposed male workers show that glycol ethers can reduce sperm counts and pregnant women exposed to glycol ethers in their work environments are significantly more likely to have children with birth defects such as neural tube defects and cleft lip.[157,158]

Heavy metals

Exposure to heavy metals has also been implicated in reproductive disorders and fetal mal-development. Mercury – which is present in fish at the top of the feeding chain (e.g. tuna or shark), in some industrial chemicals used in printing processes and in leaking dental amalgams – is antagonistic to zinc, a mineral thought to be very important in many body functions, including gamete manufacture. Some populations with high blood mercury levels are less fertile than those with lower levels.[159]

Lead, which is found in all city dust, contaminated soil and water, and in painted finishes in older houses (pre-1960), can affect sperm manufacture and can cause miscarriages. High blood levels of lead in men are associated with delayed conception.[160] Lead also interferes with the metabolism of iron, an important mineral in reproductive health.

Cadmium is another heavy metal which, when present at high blood levels in women, has been associated with pregnancy loss and delayed conception.[160] It is used in the manufacturing process of plastics, ceramics, metals, rubber, pesticides, some refined foods, and cigarettes. Air-borne particles of Cadmium (e.g., from cigarette smoke) can travel over long distances and may be accumulated in animals, fish, and plants. Like mercury, it is antagonistic to zinc.

Electromagnetic fields

Cell phones (mobile phones)

There is growing evidence in both animals and humans that chronic exposures to cell phone radiation, far below existing standards, can impair sperm function and count. There is a concern that the mobile phone kept in the trouser pocket may lead to significant exposure of the testicles. One human study found a 59% decline in sperm count in men who used cell phones for ≥4h/day as compared with those who did not use cell phones.[161] This and other studies have described deleterious effects on sperm viability, motility, and morphology related to mobile phone use.[162,163]

While keeping in mind that there may be other lifestyle factors which accompany a lot of mobile phone use, it is probably a good idea to recommend that men do not keep their phone in their jeans pocket.

To date, no studies have examined the effect of mobile phone radiation on egg quality, however it has been noted that thyroid function in rats is reduced after exposure to such radiation after only 30min a day for 4 weeks. If the same effect is seen in future studies in humans, then women will be well advised to limit mobile phone use, since optimal thyroid function is important for fertility and during pregnancy.[164]

Other animal studies have linked exposure to cell phone radio frequencies during pregnancy with increased levels of ADHD in offspring. These studies have not as yet been done in humans, but a warning to limit excessive use of mobiles while trying to conceive and when pregnant is one that some doctors give.[165]

Laptops

Laptops employing Wi-Fi appear to affect sperms' motility and damage the DNA.[166] The effect is compounded if the laptop is in fact kept on the lap! Scrotal temperature increases significantly after just 1h of use like this and it is well established that heating the testicles reduces sperm manufacture.[167]

The question is then: 'Is it possible to avoid air pollution, PCBs, BPAs. PFCs, APEs, PBDEs, etc., heavy metal contamination and electromagnetic fields, without leaving the planet or becoming completely neurotic?' When we start to look closely at what is in our environment today it is hard to avoid the conclusion that what we are exposed to and what we are consuming may not be very good for our gametes.

Of course, the fact is we cannot avoid all these chemicals and EMFs and Chinese medicine does not have a magic formula to protect from the exposure we face to these on a daily basis. The fact is also that the majority of people living in urban and rural environments do manage to have children and healthy ones at that.

Nevertheless, for couples having difficulty conceiving (especially if it is 'unexplained') and for couples who want to maximize their health and that of their offspring, then limiting exposure where possible to chemicals and EMFs is a good idea.

Eating a diet based on organic produce will limit exposure to pesticides. Organic in this context means food which has been grown or raised without exposure to artificial fertilizers, pesticides, antibiotics, or hormones. While Western-trained specialists generally attach little importance to eating organic food, specialists in IVF clinics are aware of just how important it is that embryos are not exposed to toxic chemicals of any sort, at any level. Much of the dramatic improvement in IVF success rates is due to steady improvement of the quality of items and reagents used in the laboratory procedures. Thus, the water used to make the culture medium is now purified to a very great degree, so that not even miniscule amounts of chemicals contaminate it and dishes and other items that hold embryos are made of special plastics, which do not leak any contaminants. Purification of the air of general volatile organic contaminants in IVF surgeries and laboratories protects embryos further, and to this end, anyone handling or working with eggs and embryos does not wear perfumed skin or hair products. Laboratories in several locations have found higher embryo survival rates and fewer miscarriages when the air is purified.[168,169]

Therefore, the advice given to couples trying to conceive and those newly pregnant to avoid pesticides and other chemicals and fumes, appears to have a sound basis in terms of safeguarding the well-being of the embryo.

In addition to trying to load the diet with plenty of fresh fruits and vegetables of organic origin, protein sources also need to be carefully chosen. Finding certified organic sources of meat and poultry will reduce exposure to contaminants and hormones and is advisable for everyone, but especially for those couples who have difficulty concciving.

Fish is an extremely important food source, however in order to reduce consumption of PCBs and phthalates, large fish near the top of the aquatic food chain should be avoided. Deep sea, short-lived fish such as salmon, cod, herring, perch, and mackerel should be eaten, while fish from lakes or rivers, which can be high in pollutants, should be avoided unless they come from a known pristine environment. Wild sources of fish are preferable to farmed sources in terms of nutrients and pollutants. It is important to find good sources of fish, both when trying to conceive and also once pregnant. The omega-3s that come from regular dietary fish intake prevent the development of a pro-inflammatory state (related to an excess of omega-6) that contributes to a number of complications including preterm birth, hypertension and postpartum depression. In addition, fetal deficiency of omega-3 fats may place infants at risk for allergic disease and suboptimum neuropsychiatric development.[170]

To limit exposure to BPA, it is best not to heat or microwave food in plastic containers or to cover it with plastic wrap. In general, avoidance of foods packaged in plastic or cans is a good idea and storing foods and liquids in glass is preferable to plastic.

To avoid PFCs, it is advisable to be wary of non-stick cookware, however before the dental floss is discarded, it is worth noting that there may be benefits to flossing that outweigh any increase in exposure to PFCs from floss. Researchers have found in retrospective studies that women with gum disease take longer to conceive than women without. Gum disease however does not prevent conception outright and may be associated with other lifestyle factors that reduce fertility.[171]

To avoid the chemicals found in commercial cleaning products, sourcing non-toxic ones or making your own is advisable. Recipes using vinegar, baking or washing sodas, natural soaps, lemon, or cornstarch can be found easily on the internet, and many companies now sell such products.

Many preconception programs recommend avoidance of gadgets that emit electromagnetic radiation as much as possible, and suggest removal of all such devices (phones, TVs, clock radios, computers, electric blankets, etc.) from the bedroom. Electromagnetic radiation can disturb sleep patterns, so this is probably a good idea.

Using the laptop in battery mode reduces radiation compared with when it is plugged into the mains, and it should never be used on a lap which has testicles! Mobile phones are best kept away from testicles too, until we have a more definitive understanding of how EMFs affect sperm.

Let us now reduce all this information into bite sized, digestible pieces for your patient:

- Don't smoke (anything).

- Sleep 7 or 8 h a night.

- Exercise regularly but not too much. Make it fun.

- Eat organic foods where possible and enjoy a good wholesome tasty diet.

- Take a preconception vitamin formula.

- Drink plenty of fluids – but not of the alcoholic or caffeinated variety.

- Have plenty of sex but not at the cost of adequate sleep.

- Avoid fumes where ever possible.

- Don't worry too much or get stressed about trying to follow all of the above advice.

REFERENCES

1. Barker DJ, Eriksson JG, Forsén T, et al. Fetal origins of adult disease: Strength of effects and biological basis. *Int J Epidemiol* 2002;**31**:1235–9.

2. Leggett D. *Recipes for self healing*. Totnes: Meridian Press; 1999, 96, 139.

3. Leggett D. *Recipes for self healing*. Totnes: Meridian Press; 1999, 108.

4. Chavarro JE, Toth TL, Sadio SM, et al. Soy food and isoflavone intake in relation to semen quality parameters among men from an infertility clinic. *Hum Reprod* 2008;**23**(11):2584–90.

5. Leggett D. *Recipes for self healing*. Totnes: Meridian Press; 1999, 103.

6. Cramer DW, Xu H, Sahi T. Adult hypolactasia, milk consumption and age-specific fertility. *Am J Epidemiol* 1994;**139**(3):282–9.

7. Bandyopadhyay SJ, Chakrabarti S, Banerjee S, et al. Galactose toxicity in the rat as a model for premature ovarian failure: an experimental approach readdressed. *Hum Reprod* 2003;**18**(10):2031–8.

8. Leggett D. *Recipes for self healing*. Totnes: Meridian Press; 1999, 120.

9. Maclean W, Lyttleton J. Stomach and spleen. *Clinical handbook of internal medicine*. **Vol. 2**: Sydney: University of Western Sydney; 2002, Ch. 26:862.

10. Chavarro JE, Rich-Edwards JW, Rosner BA, et al. Diet and lifestyle in the prevention of ovulatory disorder infertility. *Obstet Gynecol* 2007;**110**:1050–8.

11. Chavarro JE. *The fertility diet*. London: McGraw-Hill; 2007.

12. Pollan M. *In defense of food: An eater's manifesto*. London: Penguin Books; 2008.

13. Barker DJ. Developmental origins of adult health and disease. *J Epidemiol Comm Health* 2004;**58**:114–5.

14. Le Clair C, Abbi T, Sandhu H, et al. Impact of maternal undernutrition on diabetes and cardiovascular disease risk in adult offspring. *Can J Physiol Pharmacol* 2009;**87**(3):161–79.

15. Tappia PS, Gabriel CA. Role of nutrition in the development of the fetal cardiovascular system. *Exp Rev Cardiovasc Ther* 2006;**4**(2):211–25.

16. Roberts J. The foresight program. *J Austr Coll Nutr Environ Med* 1995;**14**(2):16.

17. Naish F, Roberts J. *The natural way to better babies*. Sydney: Random House; 1996, 57.

18. Chavarro JE, Rich-Edwards JW, Rosner BA, et al. Use of multivitamins, intake of B vitamins, and risk of ovulatory fertility. *Fertil Steril* 2008;**89**:668–76.

19. Renner R. Dietary iodine: why are so many mothers not getting enough?. *Environ Health Perspect* 2010;**118**(10):A438–42.

20. The Public Health Committee of the American Thyroid Association. Iodine supplementation for pregnancy and lactation–United States and Canada: recommendations of the American Thyroid Association. *Thyroid* 2006;**16**(10):949–51.

21. NHMRC Public Statement. *Iodine supplementation for pregnant and breastfeeding women*. January 2010www.nhmrc .gov.au/_files_nhmrc/publications/attachments/new45_statement.pdf.

22. World Health Organization Secretariat. World Health Organization technical consultation on the prevention and control of iodine deficiency. *Public Health Nutrition* 2007;**10**:1606–11.

23. Kaludjerovic J, Vieth R. Relationship between vitamin D during perinatal development and health. *J Midwifery Womens Health* 2010;**55**(6):550–60.

24. Haning RV, Hackett RJ, Flood CA, et al. Plasma dehydroepiandrosterone sulfate serves as a prehormone for 48% of follicular fluid testosterone during treatment with menotropins. *J Clin Endocrinol Metab* 1993;**76**:1301–7.

25. Barad D, Gleicher N. Effect of dehydroepiandrosterone on oocyte and embryo yields, embryo grade and cell number in IVF. *Hum Reprod* 2006;**21**(11):2845–9.

26. Wiser A, Gonen O, Ghetler Y, et al. Addition of dehydroepiandrosterone (DHEA) for poor-responder patients before and during IVF treatment improves the pregnancy rate: A randomized prospective study. *Hum Reprod* 2010;**25**(10):2496–500.

27. Bódis J, Várnagy A, Sulyok E, et al. Negative association of l-arginine methylation products with oocyte numbers. *Hum Reprod* 2010;**25**(12):3095–100.

28. Battaglia C, Regnani G, Marsella T, et al. Adjuvant l-arginine treatment in controlled ovarian hyperstimulation: a double-blind, randomized study. *Hum Reprod* 2002;**17**(3):659–65.

29. Battaglia C, Salvatori M, Maxia N, et al. Adjuvant L-arginine treatment for in-vitro fertilization in poor responder patients. *Hum Reprod* 1999;**14**(7):1690–7.

30. Tamura H, Takasaki A, Taketani T, et al. The role of melatonin as an antioxidant in the Follicle. *J Ovarian Res* 2012;**5**:5.

31. Tamura H, Takasaki A, Miwa I, et al. Oxidative stress impairs oocyte quality and melatonin protects oocytes from free radical damage and improves fertilization rate. *J Pineal Res* 2008;**44**(3):280–7.

32. Unfer V, Raffone E, Rizzo P, et al. Effect of a supplementation with myo-inositol plus melatonin on oocyte quality in women who failed to conceive in previous in vitro fertilization cycles for poor oocyte quality: a prospective, longitudinal, cohort study. *Gynecol Endocrinol* 2011;**27**(11):857–61.

33. Attaman J, Toth T, Furtado J, et al. Dietary fat and semen quality among men attending a fertility clinic. *Hum Reprod* 2012;**27**(5):1466–74.

34. Greco E, Iacobelli M, Rienzi L, et al. Reduction of the incidence of sperm DNA fragmentation by oral antioxidant treatment. *J Androl* 2005;**26**(3):349–53.

35. Awoniyi DO, Aboua YG, Marnewick J, et al. Protective effects of rooibos (Aspalathus linearis), green tea (Camellia sinensis) and commercial supplements on testicular tissue of oxidative stress-induced rats. *Phytother Res* 2012;**26**(8):1231–9.

36. Loucks AB, Heath EM. Dietary restriction reduces luteinizing hormone (LH) pulse frequency during waking hours and increases LH pulse amplitude during sleep in young menstruating women. *J Clin Endocrinol Metab* 1994;**78**(4):910–5.

37. Norman RJ, Robker R, Xing Y, et al. Eshre abstracts O-188. Components of follicular fluid from obese women induce adverse metabolic defects in cumulus-oocyte complexes. *Hum Reprod* 2011;**26**(Suppl 1):1–353.

38. Robker RL, Akison LK, Bennett BD, et al. Obese women exhibit differences in ovarian metabolites, hormones, and gene expression compared with moderate-weight women. *J Clin Endocrinol Metab* 2009;**94**(5):1533–40.

39. Luke B, Brown MB, Missmer SA, et al. The effect of increasing obesity on the response to and outcome of assisted reproductive technology: a national study. *Fertil Steril* 2011;**96**:820–5.

40. Strakovsky RS, Yuan-Xiang PA. Decrease in DKK1, a WNT inhibitor, contributes to placental lipid accumulation in an obesity-prone rat model. *Biol Reprod* 2012;**86**(3):81.

41. Paasch U, Grunewald S, Kratzsch J, et al. Obesity and age affect male fertility potential. *Fertil Steril* 2010;**94**(7):2898–901.

42. Esposito K, Giugliano F, Di Palo C, et al. Effect of lifestyle changes on erectile dysfunction in obese men. *JAMA* 2004;**291**(24):2978–84.

43. Bakos HW, Henshaw RC, Mitchell M, et al. Paternal body mass index is associated with decreased blastocyst development and reduced live birth rates following assisted reproductive technology. *Fertil Steril* 2011;**95**(5):1700–4.

44. Ohlsson Teague EMC, Fullston T, Palmer NO,. Sperm microRNAs are differentially expressed in obese fathers – novel candidate paternal dietary signals to offspring. Oral presentation at the 14th World Congress on Human Reproduction. Melbourne: 2011; 30 Nov–3 Dec.

45. Rerksuppaphol L. Acupuncture: A novel remedial contrivance for obesity. *J Med Health Sci (Thai)* 2010;**17**:1.

46. Liang F, Koya D. Acupuncture: is it effective for treatment of insulin resistance?. *Diab Obes Metab* 2010;**12**:555–69.

47. Shen EY, Hsieh CL, Chang YH, et al. Observation of sympathomimetic effect of ear acupuncture stimulation for body weight reduction. *Am J Chin Med* 2009;**37**(6):1023–30.

48. Cabioglu MT, Ergene N, Tan U. Electroacupuncture treatment of obesity with psychological symptoms. *Int J Neurosci* 2007;**117**:579–90.

49. Zhang H, Peng Y, Liu Z, et al. Effects of acupuncture therapy on abdominal fat and hepatic fat content in obese children: a magnetic resonance imaging and proton magnetic resonance spectroscopy study. *J Alt Comp Med* 2011;**17**(5):413–20.

50. Moghe SS, Juma S, Imrhan V, et al. Effect of blueberry polyphenols on 3T3-F442A preadipocyte differentiation. *J Med Food* 2012;**15**(5):448–52.

51. Seymour EM, Tanone II , Urcuyo-Llanes DE, et al. Blueberry intake alters skeletal muscle and adipose tissue peroxisome proliferator-activated receptor activity and reduces insulin resistance in obese rats. *J Med Food* 2011;**14**(12):1511–8.

52. He RR, Chen L, Lin BH, et al. Beneficial effects of oolong tea consumption on diet-induced overweight and obese subjects. *Chin J Integr Med* 2009;**15**(1):34–41.

53. Little JP, Gillen JB, Percival ME, et al. Low-volume high-intensity interval training reduces hyperglycemia and increases muscle mitochondrial capacity in patients with type 2 diabetes. *J Appl Physiol* 2011;**111**(6):1554–60.

54. Gudmundsdottir SL, Flanders WD, Augestad LB. Physical activity and fertility in women. *Hum Reprod* 2009;**24**(12):3196–204.

55. Morris SN, Missmer SA, Cramer DW, et al. Effects of lifetime exercise on the outcome of in vitro fertilization. *Obstet Gynecol* 2006;**108**(4):938–45.

56. Murakami M, et al. Leisure-time exercise behavior influences semen parameters in men attending an infertility clinic. *Fertil Steril* 2011;**96**(3):S71.

57. Jansen R. *Getting pregnant*. Sydney: Allen and Unwin; 1997, 10.

58. Barbieri RL, Domar AD, Loughlin KR. *6 Steps to increased fertility*. New York: Simon and Schuster; 2000.

59. Clarke RN, Klock SC, Geoghegan A, et al. Relationship between psychological stress and semen quality among in-vitro fertilization patients. *Hum Reprod* 1999;**14**(3):753–8.

60. Facchinetti F, Matteo ML, Artini GP, et al. An increased vulnerability to stress is associated with a poor outcome of in vitro fertilization-embryo transfer treatment. *Fertil Steril* 1997;**67**(2):309–14.

61. Ebbesen SM, Zachariae R, Mehlsen MY, et al. Stressful life events are associated with a poor in-vitro fertilization (IVF) outcome: a prospective study. *Hum Reprod* 2009;**24**(9):2173–82.

62. Sanders KA, Bruce NW. A prospective study of psychosocial stress and fertility in women. *Hum Reprod* 1997;**12**(10):2324–9.

63. Louis GM, Lum KJ, Sundaram R, et al. Stress reduces conception probabilities across the fertile window: evidence in support of relaxation. *Fertil Steril* 2011;**95**(7):2184–9.

64. Balk J, Catov J, Horn B, et al. The relationship between perceived stress, acupuncture, and pregnancy rates among IVF patients: A pilot study. *Comp Ther Clin Pract* 2010;**16**(3):154–7.

65. So EW, Ng EH, Wong YY, et al. A randomized double blind comparison of real and placebo acupuncture in IVF treatment. *Hum Reprod* 2009;**24**(2):341–8.

66. De Lacey S, Smith C, Paterson C. Building resilience: An exploration of women's perceptions of the use of acupuncture as an adjunct to IVF. *BMC Complement Alt Med* 2009;**9**:50.

67. Domar AD, Meshay I, Kelliher J, et al. The impact of acupuncture on in vitro fertilization outcome. *Fertil Steril* 2009;**91**(3):723–6.

68. Hinks J, Coulson C. An assessment of the demand and importance of acupuncture to patients of a fertility clinic during investigations and treatment. *Hum Fertil* 2010;**13**(S1):3–21.

69. Lawson CC, Whelan EA, Lividoti Hibert EN, et al. Rotating shift work and menstrual cycle characteristics. *Epidemiology* 2011;**22**:305–12.

70. Nurminen T. Shift work and reproductive health. *Scand J Work Environ Health* 1998;**24**(Suppl 3):28–34.

71. Samaraweera Y, Abeysena C. Maternal sleep deprivation, sedentary lifestyle and cooking smoke: Risk factors for miscarriage: A case control study. *Aust N Z J Obst and Gyn* 2010;**50**:352–7.

72. Leproult R, Van Cauter E. Effect of 1 week of sleep restriction on testosterone levels in young healthy men. *JAMA* 2011;**305**(21):2173–4.

73. Lee KA, Shaver JF, Giblin EC, et al. Sleep patterns related to menstrual cycle phase and premenstrual affective symptoms. *Sleep* 1990;**13**(5):403–9.

74. Spiegal K, Leproult R, Van Cauter E. Impact of sleep debt on metabolic and endocrine function. *Lancet* 1999;**354**(9188):1435–9.

75. Hublin C, Partinen M, Koskenvuo M, et al. Sleep and mortality: a population-based 22-year follow-up study. *Sleep* 2007;**30**(10):1245–53.

76. Buxton OM, Cain SW, O'Connor SP, et al. Adverse metabolic consequences in humans of prolonged sleep restriction combined with circadian disruption. *Sci Transl Med* 2012;**4**(129):129–43.

77. Van Cauter E, Leproult R, Plat L. Age-related changes in slow wave sleep and REM sleep and relationship with growth hormone and cortisol levels in healthy men. *J Am Med Assoc* 2000;**284**(7):861–8.

78. Nedeltcheva AV, Kessler L, Imperial J, et al. Exposure to recurrent sleep restriction in the setting of high caloric intake and physical inactivity results in increased insulin resistance and reduced glucose tolerance. *J Clin Endocrinol Metab* 2009;**94**(9):3242–50.

79. Huang W, Kutner N, Bliwise DL. A systematic review of the effects of acupuncture in treating insomnia. *Sleep Med Rev* 2009;**13**:73–104.

80. Wu H, Zhao Z, Stone WS, et al. Effects of sleep restriction periods on serum cortisol levels in healthy men. *Brain Res Bull* 2008;**77**(5):241–5.

81. Rogers NL, Szuba MP, Staab JP, et al. Neuroimmunologic aspects of sleep and sleep loss. *Semin Clin Neuropsychiatry* 2001;**6**(4):295–307.

82. King K, Smith S, Chapman M, et al. Detailed analysis of peripheral blood natural killer (NK) cells in women with recurrent miscarriage. *Hum Reprod* 2010;**25**(1):52–8.

83. Vgontzas AN, Zoumakis E, Bixler EO, et al. Adverse effects of modest sleep restriction on sleepiness, performance, and inflammatory cytokines. *J Clin Endocrinol Metab* 2004;**89**:2119–26.

84. Stickgold R, Hobson JA, Fosse R, et al. Sleep, learning, and dreams: off-line memory reprocessing. *Science* 2001;**294**(5544):1052–7.

85. Van Cauter E, Plat L. Physiology of growth hormone secretion during sleep. *J Pediatr* 1996;**128**(5 Pt 2):S32–7.

86. Maclean W, Lyttleton J. *Clinical handbook of internal medicine.* Sydney: University of Western Sydney; 2000, 826.

87. Dulgosz L, Brachs MB. Coffee reduces fertility. *Epidemiol Rev* 1992;**14**:83.

88. Bolumar F, Olsen J, Rebagliato M, et al. Caffeine intake and delayed conception: a European multicenter study on infertility and subfecundity. European Study Group on Infertility and Subfecundity. *Am J Epidemiol* 1997;**145**(4):324–34.

89. Curtis KM, Savitz DA, Arbuckle TE. Effects of cigarette smoking, caffeine consumption, and alcohol intake on fecundability. *Am J Epidemiol* 1997;**146**(1):32–41.

90. Infante-Rivard C, Fernandez A, Gauthier R, et al. Fetal loss associated with caffeine intake before and during pregnancy. *J Am Med Assoc* 1993;**270**(24):2940–3.

91. Ford JH, MacCormack L, Hiller J. Pregnancy and lifestyle study. *Mut Res* 1994;**313**:153–64.

92. Parazzini F, Chatenoud L, Di Cintio E, et al. Alcohol consumption is not related to fertility in Italian women. *BMJ* 1999;**318**(7180):397.

93. Olsen J, Bolumar F, Boldsen J, et al. Does moderate alcohol intake reduce fecundability? A European multicenter study on infertility and subfecundity. European Study Group on Infertility and Subfecundity. *Alcohol Clin Exp Res* 1997;**21**(2):206–12.

94. Juhl M, Nyboe Andersen A-M, Grønbæk M, et al. Moderate alcohol consumption and waiting time to pregnancy. *Hum Reprod* 2001;**2001**(16):2705–9.

95. Gill J. The effects of moderate alcohol consumption on female hormone levels and reproductive function. *Alcohol* 2000;**35**:417–23.

96. Bradley KA, Badrinath S, Bush K, et al. Medical risks for women who drink alcohol. *J Gen Int Med* 1998;**13**(9):627–39.

97. Jensen TK, Hjollund NH, Henriksen TB, et al. Does moderate alcohol consumption affect fertility? Follow up study among couples planning first pregnancy. *BMJ* 1998;**317**(7157):505–10.

98. Grodstein F, Goldman MB, Cramer DW. Infertility in women and moderate alcohol use. *Am J Public Health* 1994;**84**(9):1429–32.

99. Hassan MA, Killick SR. Negative lifestyle is associated with a significant reduction in fecundity. *Fertil Steril* 2004;**81**(2):384–92.

100. Muthusami KR, Chinnaswamy P. Effect of chronic alcoholism on male fertility hormones and semen quality. *Fertil Steril* 2005;**84**:919–24.

101.   Rossi BV, Berry KF, Hornstein MD, et al. Effect of alcohol consumption on in vitro fertilization. *Obstet Gynecol* 2011;**117**(1):136–42.

102.   Klonoff-Cohen H, Lam-Kruglick P, Gonzalez C. Effects of maternal and paternal alcohol consumption on the success rates of in vitro fertilization and gamete intrafallopian transfer. *Fertil Steril* 2003;**79**:330–9.

103.   Dondorp W, de Wert G, Pennings G, et al. ESHRE Task Force on Ethics and Law. Lifestyle-related factors and access to medically assisted reproduction. *Hum Reprod* 2010;**25**(3):578–83.

104.   Hassan MA, Killick SR. Negative lifestyle is associated with a significant reduction in fecundity. *Fertil Steril* 2004;**81**(2):384–92.

105.   Soares SR, et al. Cigarette smoking affects uterine receptiveness. *Hum Reprod* 2007;**22**(2):543–7.

106.   Vine M. The effect of smoking on sperm counts. *Fertil Steril* 1994;**6**(1):35–43.

107.   Smith CG. Marijuana and the reproductive cycle. *Science News* 1983;**123**(13):March 26.

108.   Schuel H, Chang MC, Burkman LJ, et al. Cannabinoid receptors in sperm. In: Nahas G, Sutin KM, Harvey D, editors. *Marihuana and medicine*. New Jersey: Humana Press; 1999. p. 335–45.

109.   Gaskins AJ, Colaci D, Mendiola J, et al. Dietary patterns and semen quality in young men. *Fertil Steril* 2011;**96**(3):S8.

110.   Jensen TK, Swan SH, Skakkebæk NE, et al. Caffeine intake and semen quality in a population of 2,554 young Danish men. *Am J Epidemiol* 2010;**171**(8):883–91.

111.   Gaskins AJ, Mumford S, Rovner AJ, et al. Whole grains are associated with concentrations of high sensitivity c-reactive protein among premenopausal women. *J Nutr* 2010;**140**(9):1669–76.

112.   Smith G, Roberts R, Hall C, et al. Reversible ovulatory failure associated with the development of luteinized unruptured follicles in women with inflammatory arthritis taking non-steroidal anti-inflammatory drugs. *Br J Rheumatol* 1996;**35**(5):458–62.

113.   Norman RJ. Reproductive consequences of COX-2 inhibition. *Lancet* 2001;**358**(290):1287–8.

114.   Pall M, Fridén BE, Brännström M. Induction of delayed follicular rupture in the human by the selective COX-2 inhibitor rofecoxib: a randomized double-blind study. *Hum Reprod* 2001;**16**:1323–8.

115.   Zanagnolo V, Dharmarajan AM, Endo K, et al. Effects of acetylsalicylic acid (aspirin) and naproxen sodium (naproxen) on ovulation, prostaglandin, and progesterone production in the rabbit. *Fertil Steril* 1996;**65**(5):1036–43.

116.   Nakhai-Pour HR, Broy P, Bérard A. Use of antidepressants during pregnancy and the risk of spontaneous abortion. *Can Med Assoc J* 2010;**182**(10):1031–7.

117.   El Marroun H, Jaddoe VW, Hudziak JJ, et al. Maternal use of selective serotonin reuptake inhibitors, fetal growth, and risk of adverse birth outcomes. *Arch Gen Psychiatry* 2012;**69**(7):706–14.

118.   Malm H, Artama M, Gissler M, et al. Selective serotonin reuptake inhibitors and risk for major congenital anomalies. *Obstet Gynecol* 2011;**118**:111–20.

119.   Mulder EJ, Ververs FF, de Heus R, et al. Selective serotonin reuptake inhibitors affect neurobehavioral development in the human fetus. *Neuropsychopharmacology* 2011;**36**:1961–71.

120.   Manber R, Schnyer RN, Lyell D, et al. Acupuncture for depression during pregnancy: a randomized controlled trial. *Obstet Gynecol* 2010;**115**(3):511–20.

121.   Allen JJB, et al. The efficacy of acupuncture in the treatment of major depression in women. *Psychol Sci* 1998;**9**(5):397.

122.   Tanrikut C, Schlegel PN. Antidepressant-associated changes in semen parameters. *Urology* 2007;**69**(1):185.e5–7.

123.   Safarinejad MR. Sperm DNA damage and semen quality impairment after treatment with selective serotonin reuptake inhibitors detected using semen analysis and sperm chromatin structure assay. *J Urol* 2008;**180**(5):2124–8.

124.   Relwani R, Berger D, Santoro N, et al. Semen parameters are unrelated to BMI but vary with SSRI use and prior urological surgery. *Reprod Sci* 2011;**18**(4):391–7.

125.   Ford JH, MacCormack L, Hiller J. Pregnancy and lifestyle study. *Mut Res* 1994;**313**:153–64.

126.   Hoyer PB, Sipes IG. Assessment of follicle destruction in chemical-induced ovarian toxicity. *Annu Rev Pharmacol Toxicol* 1996;**36**:307–31.

127.   Sobinoff A, Pye V, Nixon B, et al. Adding insult to injury: effects of xenobiotic-induced preantral ovotoxicity on ovarian development and oocyte fusibility. *Toxicol Sci* 2010;**118**(2):653–66.

128.   Sobinoff AP, Mahony M, Nixon B, et al. Understanding the villain: DMBA-induced preantral ovotoxicity involves selective follicular destruction and primordial follicle activation through PI3K/Akt and mTOR signaling. *Toxicol Sci* 2011;**123**(2):563–75.

129.   Wohlfahrt-Veje C, Andersen HR, Schmidt IM, et al. Early breast development in girls after prenatal exposure to non-persistent pesticides. *Int J Androl* 2012;**35**(3):273–82.

130.   Legro RS, Sauer MV, Mottla GL, et al. Effect of air quality on assisted human reproduction. *Hum Reprod* 2010;**25**(5):1317–24.

131. Brauer M, Lencar C, Tamburic L, et al. A cohort study of traffic-related air pollution impacts on birth outcomes. *Environ Health Perspect* 2008;**116**:680–6.

132. Huel G, Mergler D, Bowler R. Spontaneous abortion after chemical exposure. *Br J Ind Med* 1990;**47**:400–4.

133. Drbohlav P, Jirsová S, Masata J, et al. Relationship between the levels of toxic polychlorinated biphenyls in blood and follicular fluid of sterile women. *Ceska Gynekol* 2005;**70**(5):377–83.

134. Toft G, Hagmar L, Giwercman A, et al. Epidemiological evidence on reproductive effects of persistent organochlorines in humans. *Reprod Toxicol* 2004;**19**:526.

135. Longnecker MP, Korrick SA, Moysich KB. Human health effects of polychlorinated biphenyls. In: Schecter A, Gasiewicz TA, editors. *Dioxins and health.* 2nd edn Hoboken, NJ: John Wilcy; 2003. p. 679–728.

136. Rozati R, Reddy PP, Reddanna P, et al. Role of environmental estrogens in the deterioration of male factor fertility. *Fertil Steril* 2002;**78**(6):1187–94.

137. Tiido T, Rignell-Hydbom A, Jönsson B, et al. Exposure to persistent organochlorine pollutants associates with human sperm Y: X chromosome ratio. *Hum Reprod* 2005;**20**(7):1903–9.

138. Toft G, Jönsson BAG, Lindh CH, et al. Semen quality and exposure to persistent organochlorine pollutants. *Epidemiology* 2006;**17**(4):450–8.

139. Meeker JD, Stapleton HM. House dust concentrations of organophosphate flame retardants in relation to hormone levels and semen quality parameters. *Environ Health Perspect* 2010;**118**:318–23.

140. Akutsu K, Takatori S, Nozawa S, et al. Polybrominated diphenyl ethers in human serum and sperm quality. *Bull Environ Contam Toxicol* 2008;**80**:345–50.

141. Chevrier J, Harley KG, Bradman A, et al. Polybrominated diphenyl ether (PBDE) flame retardants and thyroid hormone during pregnancy. *Environ Health Perspect* 2010;**118**:1444–9.

142. Chao HR, Wang SL, Lee WJ, et al. Levels of polybrominated diphenyl ethers (PBDEs) in breast milk from central Taiwan and their relation to infant birth outcome and maternal menstruation effects. *Environ Int* 2007;**33**:239–45.

143. Hauser R, Meeker JD, Duty S, et al. Altered semen quality in relation to urinary concentrations of phthalate monoester and oxidative metabolites. *Epidemiology* 2006;**17**:682–91.

144. Machtinger R, Hauser C, Combelles C, et al. The impact of bisphenol A (BPA) on human oocyte meiotic maturation. *Fertil Steril* 2011;**96**(3):S7.

145. Wu DH, Leung Y-K, Thomas MA, et al. Bisphenol A (BPA) confers direct genotoxicity to sperm with increased sperm DNA fragmentation. *Fertil Steril* 2011;**96**(3):S5.

146. Ehrlich S, Williams PL, Missmer SA, et al. Urinary bisphenol A and implantation failure among women undergoing in vitro fertilization. *Fertil Steril* 2011;**96**(3):S6.

147. Fujimoto VY, Kim D, vom Saal FS, et al. Serum unconjugated bisphenol A concentrations in women may adversely influence oocyte quality during in vitro fertilization. *Fertil Steril* 2011;**95**(5):1816–9.

148. Braun J, Kalkbrenner AE, Calafat AM, et al. Impact of early-life bisphenol a exposure on behavior and executive function in children. *Pediatrics* 2011;**128**:873–82.

149. Fei C, McLaughlin JK, Lipworth L, Olsen J. Maternal levels of perfluorinated chemicals and subfecundity. *Hum Reprod* 2009;**24**(5):1200–5.

150. Hoyer PB, Devine PJ, Hu X, et al. Ovarian toxicity of 4-vinylcyclohexene diepoxide: a mechanistic model. *Toxicol Pathol* 2001;**29**(1):91–9.

151. Forkert PG, Lash L, Tardif R, et al. Identification of trichloroethylene and its metabolites in human seminal fluid of workers exposed to trichloroethylene. *Drug Metab Dispos* 2003;**31**(3):306–11.

152. DuTeaux SB, Berger T, Hess RA, et al. Male reproductive toxicity of trichloroethylene: sperm protein oxidation and decreased fertilizing ability. *Biol Reprod* 2004;**70**(5):1518–26.

153. Guenther K, Heinke V, Thiele B, et al. Endocrine disrupting nonylphenols are ubiquitous in food. *Environ Sci Technol* 2002;**36**:1676–80.

154. Calafat A, Kuklenyik Z, Reidy JA, et al. Urinary concentrations of bisphenol A and 4-nonylphenol in a human reference population. *Environ Health Perspect* 2005;**113**:391–5.

155. Hossaini A. In utero reproductive study in rats exposed to nonylphenol. *Reprod Toxicol* 2001;**15**(5):537–43.

156. U.S. EPA Glycol Ethers Hazard Summary. U.S. EPA, Air Toxics Division, January 2000, www.epa.gov/ttn/atw/hlthef/glycolet.html

157. Lamb JC, Gulati DK, Hommel LM, et al. Ethylene glycol monobutyl ether. *Environ Health Perspect Suppl* 1997;**105**(Suppl 1).

158. Hardin BD, Goad PT, Burg JR. Developmental toxicity of diethylene glycol monomethyl ether (diEGME). *Fundam Appl Toxicol* 1986;**6**:430–9.

159. Choy CM, Lam CW, Cheung LT, et al. Infertility, blood mercury concentrations and dietary seafood consumption: a case-control study. *BJOG* 2002;**109**(10):1121–5.

160. Bock R, McGrath J. NIH study links high levels of cadmium and lead in blood to pregnancy delay. US Dept Health and Human Services, NIH News, Feb. 8, 2012.

161. Agarwal A, Deepinder F, Sharma RK, et al. Effect of cell phone usage on semen analysis in men attending infertility clinic: an observational study. *Fertil Steril* 2008;**89**(1):124–8.

162. De Iuliis GN, Newey RJ, King BV, et al. Mobile phone radiation induces reactive oxygen species production and DNA damage in human spermatozoa in vitro. *PLoS One* 2009;**4**(7):e6446.

163. Falzone N, Huyser C, Becker P, et al. The effect of pulsed 900-MHz GSM mobile phone radiation on the acrosome reaction, head morphometry and zona binding of human spermatozoa. *Int J Androl* 2011;**34**(1):20–6.

164. Koyu A, Cesur G, Ozguner F, et al. Effects of 900 MHz electromagnetic field on TSH and thyroid hormones in rats. *Toxicol Lett* 2005;**157**(3):257–62.

165. Aldad TS, Gan G, Gao XB, et al. Fetal radiofrequency radiation exposure from 800–1900 Mhz-rated cellular telephones affects neurodevelopment and behavior in mice. *Sci Rep* 2012;**2**:312.

166. Avendaño C, Mata A, Sarmiento S, et al. Use of laptop computers connected to internet through Wi-Fi decreases human sperm motility and increases sperm DNA. *fragmentation Fertil Steril* 2012;**97**(1):39–45.

167. Sheynkin Y, Welliver R, Winer A, et al. Protection from scrotal hyperthermia in laptop computer users. *Fertil Steril* 2011;**95**(2):647–51.

168. Matson P. *Access National Newsletter*. Sydney: Access Infertility Network; 2000.

169. Talwar P. *Manual of assisted reproductive technologies and clinical embryology*. New Delhi: JP Medical; 2012.

170. Mozurkewich E, Berman DR, Chilimigras J. Role of omega-3 fatty acids in maternal, fetal, infant and child wellbeing. *Expert Rev of Obstet Gynecol* 2010;**5**(1):125–38.

171. Hart R, Doherty DA, Newnham IA, et al. Periodontal disease – a further potentially modifiable risk factor limiting conception – a case for a pre-pregnancy dental check-up?. *Hum Reprod* 2011;**26**(Suppl 1):1–353.

Herbs – Pinyin, Chinese, and Latin characters

Ai Ye	艾叶	*Folium Artemisiae*
Ba Ji Tian	巴戟天	*Radix Morindae Officinalis*
Bai Jiang Cao	败酱草	*Herba cum Radice Patriniae*
Bai Mao Gen	白茅根	*Rhizoma Imperatae Cylindricae*
Bai Shao	白芍	*Radix Paeoniae Lactiflorae*
Bai Xian Pi	白藓皮	*Cortex Dictamni Dasycarpi*
Bai Zhi	白芷	*Radix Angelicae*
Bai Zhu	白术	*Rhizoma Atractylodis Macrocephalae*
Bai Zi Ren	柏子仁	*Semen Biotae Orientalis*
Ban Xia	半夏	*Rhizoma Pinelliae*
Bi Xie	萆解	*Rhizoma Dioscorea*
Bian Xu	扁蓄	*Herba Polygone Avicularis*
Bing Lang	槟榔	*Semen Arecae Catchu*
Bo He	薄荷	*Herba Menthae*
Bu Gu Zhi	补骨脂	*Fructus Psoraleae*
Cang Zhu	苍术	*Rhizoma Atractylodes*
Chai Hu	柴胡	*Radix Bupleuri*
Che Qian Zi	车前子	*Semen Plantaginis*
Chen Pi	陈皮	*Pericarpium Citri Reticulate*
Chi Shao	赤芍	*Radix Paeoniae Rubra*
Chuan Bei Mu	川贝母	*Bulbus Fritillariae Cirrhosae*
Chuan Jiao	川椒	*Fructus Zanthoxyli Bungeani*
Chuan Lian Zi	川楝子	*Fructus Meliae Toosendan*

Chuan Niu Xi	川牛膝	*Radix Cyathulae*
Chuan Xiong	川芎	*Radix Ligustici Wallichii*
Da Huang (jiu)	大黄（酒）	*Rhizoma Rhei (wine fried)*
Da Zao	大枣	*Fructus Zizyphi Jujuba*
Dan Nan Xing	胆南星	*Rhizoma Arisaematis (with pig's bile)*
Dan Shen	丹参	*Radix Salviae Miltiorrhizae*
Dan Zhu Ye	淡竹叶	*Herba Lophatheri Gracilis*
Dang Gui	当归	*Radix Angelicae Sinensis*
Dang Shen	党参	*Radix Codonopsis Pilulosae*
Di Gu Pi	地骨皮	*Cortex Lycii Chinensis*
Di Long	地龙	*Lumbricus*
Di Yu	地榆	*Radix Sanguisorbae Officinalis*
Dong Chong Xia Cao	冬虫夏草	*Cordyceps Chinensis*
Du Huo	独活	*Radix Angelicae Pubescentis*
Du Zhong	杜仲	*Cortex Eucommiae Ulmoidis*
E Jiao	阿胶	*Gelatinum Asini*
E Zhu	莪术	*Rhizoma Curcumae Zedoariae*
Fang Feng	防风	*Radix Ledebouriellae Sesloidis*
Fo Shou	佛手	*Fructus Citri Sarcodactylis*
Fu Ling	茯苓	*Sclerotium Poriae Cocos*
Fu Pen Zi	覆盆子	*Fructus Rubi Chingii*
Fu Shen	茯神	*Sclerotium Poriae Cocos Pararadicis*
Fu Xiao Mai	浮小麦	*Semen Tritici Aestivi Levis*
(Zhi) Fu Zi	（制）附子	*Radix Aconiti Charmichaeli Praeparata*
Gan Cao (zhi)	甘草（炙）	*Radix Glycyrrhizae Uralensis*
Gan Jiang	干姜	*Rhizoma Zingiberis Officinalis*
Gan Qi	干漆	*Lacca Sinica Exsiccata*
Gou Qi Zi	枸杞子	*Fructus Lycii Chinensis*
Gou Teng	钩藤	*Ramulus Uncariae Cum Uncis*
Gui Zhi	桂枝	*Ramulus Cinnamomi Cassiae*

Hai Piao Xiao	海螵蛸	*Os Sepiae seu Sepiellae*
Han Lian Cao	旱莲草	*Herba Ecliptae Prostratae*
He Huan Pi	合欢皮	*Cortex Albizziae Julibrissin*
He Shou Wu	何首乌	*Radix Polygoni Multiflori*
Hong Hua	红花	*Flos Carthami Tinctorii*
Hong Teng	红藤	*Caulis Sargentodoxae*
Hou Po	厚朴	*Cortex Magnoliae Officinalis*
Hua Shi	滑石	*Talcum*
Huai Niu Xi	淮牛膝	*Radix Achyranthis Bidentate*
Huang Bai	黄柏	*Cortex Phellodendri*
Huang Jing	黄精	*Rhizoma Polygonati*
Huang Lian	黄连	*Rhizoma Coptidis*
Huang Qi	黄芪	*Radix Astragali*
Huang Qin	黄芩	*Radix Scutellariae Baicalensis*
Huo Ma Ren	火麻仁	*Semen Cannabis Sativae*
Huo Xiang	藿香	*Herba Agastaches seu Pogostei*
Ji Nei Jin	鸡内金	*Endithelium Corneum Gigeraiae Galli*
Ji Xue Teng	鸡血藤	*Radix et Caulis Jixueteng*
Jiang Huang	姜黄	*Rhizoma Curcumae*
Jie Geng	桔梗	*Radix Platycodi Grandiflori*
Jin Ying Zi	金樱子	*Fructus Rosae Laevigatae*
Jing Jie	荆芥	*Herba seu Flos Shizonepetae Tenuifoliae*
Ju He	橘核	*Semen Citri Reticulatae*
Ju Hua	菊花	*Flos Crysanthemi Morifolii*
Ku Shen	苦参	*Radix Sophorae Flavescentis*
Lian Qiao	连翘	*Fructus Forsythiae Suspensae*
Lian Zi Xin	莲子心	*Plumula Nelumbinis Nuciferae*
Long Dan Cao	龙胆草	*Radix Gentianae Scabrae*
Long Gu	龙骨	*Os Draconis*
Long Yan Rou	龙眼肉	*Arillus Euphoriae Longanae*

Lu Gen	芦根	Rhizoma Phragmites Communis
Lu Jiao Pian	鹿角片	Cornu Cervi Parvum (extract of boiling)
Lu Lu Tong	路路通	Fructus Liquidambaris Taiwaniae
Lu Rong	鹿茸	Cornu Cervi Parvum
Ma Huang	麻黄	Herba Ephedrae
Mai Dong	麦冬	Tuber Ophiopogonis
Mai Ya	麦芽	Fructus Hordei
Mang Xiao	芒硝	Mirabilitum
Meng Chong	虻虫	Tabanus Bivittatus
Mo Yao	没药	Myrrha
Mu Dan Pi	牡丹皮	Cortex Moutan Radicis
(Sheng) Mu Li	（生）牡蛎	Concha Ostreae
Mu Tong	木通	Caulis Mutong
Mu Xiang	木香	Radix Saussureae
Nu Zhen Zi	女贞子	Fructus Ligustri Lucidi
Pao Jiang	炮姜	Rhizoma Zingiberis Officinalis
Pi Pa Ye	枇杷叶	Folium Eriobotryae
Pu Gong Ying	蒲公英	Herba Taraxaci Mongolici
Pu Huang	蒲黄	Pollen Typhae
Qi Cao	蛴螬	Holotrichia Vermiculus
Qian Cao Gen	茜草根	Radix Rubiae Cordifoliae
Qian Nian Jian	千年健	Rhizoma Homalomenae Occultae
Qian Shi	芡实	Semen Euryales Ferox
Qing Pi	青皮	Pericarpium Citri Reticulatae Viride
Quan Xie	全蝎	Buthus Martensi
Ren Shen	人参	Radix Ginseng
Rou Cong Rong	肉苁蓉	Herba Cistanches
Rou Gui	肉桂	Cortex Cinnamomi Cassiae
Ru Xiang	乳香	Gummi Olibanum
San Leng	三棱	Rhizoma Sparganii

Pinyin	Chinese	Latin
San Qi	三七	Radix Pseudoginseng
Sang Ji Sheng	桑寄生	Ramulus Sangjisheng
Sang Piao Xiao	桑螵蛸	Ootheca Mantidis
Sha Ren	砂仁	Fructus seu Semen Amomi
Shan Yao	山药	Radix Dioscorea Oppositae
Shan Zha	山楂	Fructus Crataegi
Shan Zhu Yu (Shan Yu Rou)	山茱萸（山萸肉）	Fructus Corni Officinalis
She Chuang Zi	蛇床子	Frucuts Cnidii Monnieri
Shen Qu	神曲	Massa Fermenta
Sheng Di (Huang)	生地（黄）	Radix Rehmanniae Glutinosae
Sheng Jiang	生姜	Rhizoma Zingiberis Officinalis Recens
Sheng Ma	升麻	Rhizoma Cimicifugae
Shi Chang Pu	石菖蒲	Rhizoma Acori Graminei
Shi Gao	石膏	Gypsum
Shu Di (Huang)	熟地（黄）	Radix Rehmanniae Glutinosae Conquitae
Shui Zhi	水蛭	Hirudo seu Whitmaiae
Si Gua Luo	丝瓜络	Vascularis Luffae, Fasciculus
Su Mu	苏木	Lignum Sappan
Su Ye	苏叶	Folium Perillae Frutescentis
Suan Zao Ren	酸枣仁	Semen Ziziphi Spinosae
Suo Yang	锁阳	Herba Cynomorii Songarici
Tai Zi Shen	太子参	Radix Pseudostellariae Heteropyllae
Tao Ren	桃仁	Semen Persicae
Tian Dong	天冬	Tuber Asparagi
Tou Gu Cao	透骨草	Herba Impatiens Balsamina
Tu (Di) Bie Chong	土（地）	Eupolyphagae seu Opisthoplatiae
Tu Si Zi	菟丝子	Semen Cuscatae
Wang Bu Liu Xing	王不留行	Semen Vaccariae
Wu Gong	蜈蚣	Scolopendra Subspinipes
Wu Jia Pi	五加皮	Cortex Acanthopanacis

Wu Ling Zhi	五灵脂	*Excrementum Trogopterori*
Wu Mei	乌梅	*Fructus Pruni Mume*
Wu Wei Zi	五味子	*Fructus Schizandrae Chinensis*
Wu Yao	乌药	*Radix Linderae Strychnifoliae*
Wu Zei Gu	乌贼骨	*Os Sepia seu Sepiellae*
Wu Zhu Yu	吴茱萸	*Fructus Evodiae Rutaecarpae*
Xian Mao	仙茅	*Rhizoma Curculiginis Orchioidis*
Xiang Fu	香附	*Rhizoma Cyperi Rotundi*
Xiao Hui Xiang	小茴香	*Fructus Foeniculi Vulgaris*
Xing Ren	杏仁	*Semen Pruni Armeniacae*
Xu Duan	续断	*Radix Dipsaci*
Xuan Shen	玄参	*Radix Scrophulariae*
Xue Jie	血竭	*Sanguis Draconis*
Yan Hu Suo	延胡索	*Rhizoma Corydalis Yanhusuo*
Ye Jiao Teng	夜交藤	*Caulis Polygoni Multiflori*
Yi Mu Cao	益母草	*Herba Leonuri Heterophylli*
Yi Yi Ren	薏苡仁	*Semen Coicis Lachryma-jobi*
Yi Zhi Ren	益智仁	*Fructus Alpiniae Oxyphyllae*
Yin Yang Huo	淫羊藿	*Herba Epimedii*
Yu Jin	郁金	*Tuber Curcumae*
(Zhi) Yuan Zhi	(炙) 远志	*Radix Polygalae Tenuifoliae*
Zao Jiao Ci	皂角刺	*Fructus Gleditsiae Sinensis*
Ze Lan	泽兰	*Herba Lycopi Lucidi*
Ze Xie	泽泻	*Rhizoma Alismatis*
Zhe Bei Mu	浙贝母	*Bulbus Fritillariae Thunbergii*
Zhi Ke	枳壳	*Fructus Citri seu Ponciri*
Zhi Mu	知母	*Radix Anemarrhena*
Zhi Nan Xing	制南腥	*Rhizoma Arisaematis*
Zhi Zi	栀子	*Fructus Gardeniae Jasminoidis*
Zi Bei Chi	紫贝齿	*Mauritiae Concha*

Zi He Che	紫河车	*Placenta Hominis*
Zi Hua Di Ding	紫花地丁	*Herba Viola cum Radice*
Zi Shi Ying	紫石英	*Fluoritum*
Zhu Ma Gen	苎麻根	*Radix Boehmeria Nivea*
Zhu Ru	竹茹	*Caulis Bambusae in Tueniis*

Herbs which move the Blood

Herbs which can move the Blood are graded into categories according to their actions and relative strength.

HERBS WHICH REGULATE BLOOD MILDLY

These herbs invigorate and encourage circulation of blood in the blood vessels, especially microcirculation in the capillaries. This is achieved by reducing coagulation and accumulation of platelets.

Dang Gui

Ji Xue Teng

Chuan Xiong

Yan Hu Suo

Wang Bu Liu Xing

Lu Lu Tong

HERBS WHICH REGULATE BLOOD AND REMOVE STAGNATION

The next category of herbs encourages circulation, especially in areas where blood circulation has become very sluggish and there is pooling of stagnant blood. Their action is a little stronger than those above, which just encourage efficient circulation, and they will be employed when we see evidence of stasis of Blood, e.g., purple coloration on the skin or tongue, pointed pain (in the abdomen in this case), dark color or clots in the menstrual flow.

Dan Shen

Yi Mu Cao

Tao Ren

Hong Hua

Chuan Niu Xi

Ze Lan

Su Mu

Yu Jin

Wu Ling Zhi

Ru Xiang

Mo Yao

HERBS AND SUBSTANCES WHICH BREAK UP BLOOD AND REMOVE STAGNATION

This category includes herbs and substances which can actually dissolve masses. These are employed when we know (from palpation or from investigative surgery) that there are masses like cysts, fibroids, polyps, endometriosis or breast lumps or tumors. This category includes a number of animal products and these are particularly strong in their Blood-breaking action (and anti-blood-clotting action) and thus have to be used with great caution and in small doses.

Tao Ren

E. Zhu

San Leng

Shui Zhi

Meng Chong

Tu (Di) Bie Chong

Herbs to beware of during pregnancy

HERBS CONTRAINDICATED DURING PREGNANCY

Ba Dou	*Fructus Crotonis*
Ban Mao	*Mylabris*
Chan Su	*Secretio Bufonis*
Che Qian Zi	*Semen Plantaginis*
Chuan Niu Xi	*Radix Cyanthulae*
Da Ji	*Radix Euphorbiae seu Knoxie*
Di Bie Chong	*Eupolyphagea seu Opisthoplatiae*
E Wei	*Asafoetida*
E Zhu	*Rhizoma Curcumae Zedoariae*
Fu Zi	*Radix Aconiti*
Gan Sui	*Radix Euphorbiae Kansui*
Guan Zhong	*Rhizoma Guanzhong*
Hai Long	*Hailong*
Hai Ma	*Hippocampus*
Hong Hua	*Flos Carthami Tinctorii*
Liu Huang	*Sulphur*
Ma Chi Xian	*Herba Portulacae Oleracae*
Ma Qian Zi	*Semen Strychnotis*
Mang Ziao	*Mirabilitum*
Meng Chong	*Tabenus Bivittatus*
Mo Yao	*Myrrha*
Niu Huang	*Calculus Bovis*
Qian Nian Zi	*Semen Pharbitidis*
Qing Fen	*Calomelas*
Qu Mai	*Herba Dianthi*
Ru Xiang	*Gummi Olibanum*
San Leng	*Rhizoma Sparganii*
Shang Lu	*Radix Phytolaccae*
She Gan	*Rhizoma Belamacandae*
She Xiang	*Secretio Moschus Moschiferi*
Shui Zhi	*Hirudo seu Whitmanae*
Tao Ren	*Semen Persicae*
Tian Hua Fen	*Radix Trichosanthis*
Wu Gong	*Scolopendra Subspinipes*
Xiong Huang	*Realgar*
Yan Hu Suo	*Rhizoma Corydalis Yanhusuo*
Yi Mu Cao	*Herba Leonuri Heterophylli*

Yu Ji Hua	*Flos et Fructus Rosae*
Yuan Hua	*Flos Daphnes Genkwa*
Zao Jiao	*Fructus Gleditsae Sinensis*
Zhang Nao	*Camphora*
Zuan Ming Fen	*Natrii Sulphas Exsiccatus*

HERBS TO BE USED WITH CAUTION DURING PREGNANCY

Bai Fu Zi	*Rhizoma Typhonii Gigantei*
Bing Pian	*Borneol*
Chang Shan	*Radix Dichorae Febrifugae*
Chuan Jiao	*Fructus Zanthoxyli Bungeani*
Da Huang	*Rhizoma Rhei*
Dai Zhe Shi	*Haematitum*
Dong Kui Zi	*Semen Abutiloni seu Malvae*
Fan Xie Ye	*Folium Sennae*
Gan Jiang	*Rhizoma Zingiberis Officinalis*
Hou Po	*Cortex Magnoliae Officinalis*
Hua Shi	*Talcum*
Huai Niu Xi	*Radix Achyranthis Bidentatae*
Lou Lu	*Radix Rhapontici seu Echinops*
Lu Hui	*Herba Aloes*
Lu Lu Tong	*Fructus Liquidambaris Taiwanianae*
Mu Tong	*Caulis Mutong*
Pu Huang	*Pollen Typhae*
Rou Gui	*Cortex Cinnamomi Cassiae*
San Qi	*Radix Pseudoginseng*
Su He Xiang	*Styrax Liquidis*
Su Mu	*Lignum Sappan*
Tian Nan Xing	*Rhizoma Arisaematis*
Tong Cao	*Medulla Tetrapanacis Papyriferi*
Wang Bui Liu Xing	*Semen Vaccariae Segetalis*
Xue Jie	*Sanguis Draconis*
Yi Yi Ren	*Semen Coicis Lachryma-jobi*
Yu Jin	*Radix Curcumae*
Yu Li Ren	*Semen Pruni*
Ze Lan	*Herba Lycopi Lucidi*
Zhi Ke	*Fructus Citri seu Ponciri*
Zhi Shi	*Fructus Citri seu Ponciri Immaturis*

REFERENCE

Maclean W. *Clinical handbook of Chinese herbs: desk reference*. Sydney: Pangolin Press; 2011.

Summary of herbal formulas and their uses in this book

AI FU NUAN GONG WAN (ARTEMESIA – CYPERUS WARMING THE UTERUS PILL)

Ai Ye	9 g	Folium Artemesia
Wu Zhu Yu	6 g	Fructus Evodiae Rutaecarpae
Rou Gui	6 g	Cortex Cinnamomi Cassiae
Xiang Fu	9 g	Rhizoma Cyperi Rotundi
Dang Gui	9 g	Radix Angelicae Sinensis
Chuan Xiong	6 g	Radix Ligustici Wallichii
Bai Shao	6 g	Radix Paeoniae Lactiflorae
Huang Qi	6 g	Radix Astragali
Sheng Di	9 g	Radix Rehmanniae Glutinosae
Xu Duan	6 g	Radix Dipsaci

Traditionally used to warm Yang to increase fertility, it is mostly superseded now by formulas which boost Kidney Yang in ways that have been found to increase progesterone production more successfully.

BA ZHEN TANG (EIGHT PRECIOUS DECOCTION)

Shu Di	15 g	Radix Rehmanniae Glutinosae Conquitae
Dang Gui	9 g	Radix Angelicae Sinensis
Bai Shao	9 g	Radix Paeoniae Lactiflorae
Chuan Xiong	6 g	Radix Ligustici Wallichii
Dang Shen	12 g	Radix Codonopsis Pilulosae
Bai Zhu	9 g	Rhizoma Atractylodis Macrocephalae
Fu Ling	9 g	Sclerotium Poriae Cocos
Gan Cao (Zhi)	3 g	Radix Glycyrrhizae Uralensis

Used to aid recovery after miscarriage.

BA ZHEN TANG (EIGHT PRECIOUS DECOCTION)

Dang Gui	9 g	Radix Angelicae Sinensis
Bai Shao	9 g	Radix Paeoniae Lactiflorae
Chuan Xiong	6 g	Radix Ligustici Wallichii
Shu Di	9 g	Radix Rehmanniae Glutinosae Conquitae
Dang Shen	12 g	Radix Codonopsis Pilulosae
Bai Zhu	9 g	Rhizoma Atractylodis Macrocephalae
Fu Ling	12 g	Sclerotium Poriae Cocos
Gan Cao (Zhi)	3 g	Radix Glycyrrhizae Uralensis

This version with slightly different doses treats recurrent miscarriage related to Blood deficiency.

452

BA ZHEN TANG (EIGHT PRECIOUS DECOCTION) MODIFIED

Dang Gui	9 g	Radix Angelicae Sinensis
Shu Di	9 g	Rehmanniae Glutinosae Conquitae
Bai Shao	9 g	Radix Paeoniae Lactiflorae
Chuan Xiong	6 g	Radix Ligustici Wallichii
Dang Shen	12 g	Radix Codonopsis Pilulosae
Dan Shen	9 g	Radix Salviae Miltiorrhizae
Bai Zi Ren	9 g	Semen Biotae Orientalis
Bai Zhu	9 g	Rhizoma Atractylodis Macrocephalae
Fu Ling	9 g	Sclerotium Poriae Cocos
Tu Si Zi	12 g	Semen Cuscatae
Sang Ji Sheng	12 g	Ramulus Sangjisheng
Xiang Fu	9 g	Rhizoma Cyperi Rotundi
Gan Cao (Zhi)	3 g	Radix Glycyrrhizae Uralensis

Used in treatment of Blood deficiency amenorrhea.

BAI ZI REN WAN (BIOTA PILL) MODIFIED

Bai Zi Ren	9 g	Semen Biotae Orientalis
Dan Shen	9 g	Radix Salviae Miltiorrhizae
Chuan Niu Xi	9 g	Radix Cyathulae
Bai Shao	9 g	Radix Paeoniae Lactiflorae
Ze Lan	9 g	Herba Lycopi Lucidi
Xu Duan	9 g	Radix Dipsaci

Added to treatments for Yin deficiency amenorrhea to clear Heat affecting the Heart.

BAI ZI REN WAN (BIOTA PILL) MODIFIED

Bai Zi Ren	9 g	Semen Biotae Orientalis
Dan Shen	9 g	Radix Salviae Miltiorrhizae
Xu Duan	9 g	Radix Dipsaci
Shu Di	9 g	Rehmanniae Glutinosae Conquitae
Chuan Niu Xi	9 g	Radix Cyathulae
Ze Lan	9 g	Herba Lycopi Lucidi
Yu Jin	9 g	Tuber Curcumae
He Huan Pi	9 g	Cortex Albizziae Julibrissin
Yuan Zhi	6 g	Radix Polygalae Tenuifoliae
Fu Ling	9 g	Sclerotium Poriae Cocos

Used for amenorrhea due to Heart Qi stagnation.

BAO YIN JIAN (PROTECTING YIN DECOCTION)

Sheng Di	20 g	Radix Rehmanniae Glutinosae
Shan Yao	12 g	Dioscorea Oppositae

Bai Shao	9g	Radix Paeoniae Lactiflorae
Huang Qin	9g	Radix Scutellariae Baicalensis
Huang Bai	9g	Cortex Phellodendri
Xu Duan	9g	Radix Dipsaci
Gan Cao (Zhi)	3g	Radix Glycyrrhizae Uralensis

Used for threatened miscarriage due to Heat in the Blood.

BAO YIN JIAN (PROTECTING YIN DECOCTION) MODIFIED

Sheng Di	9g	Radix Rehmanniae Glutinosae
Xuan Shen	9g	Radix Scrophulariae
Shan Yao	12g	Radix Dioscorea Oppositae
Bai Shao	9g	Radix Paeoniae Lactiflorae
Huang Qin	6g	Radix Scutellariae Baicalensis
Huang Bai	6g	Cortex Phellodendri
Di Gu Pi	9g	Cortex Lycii Chinensis
Nu Zhen Zi	9g	Fructus Ligustri Lucidi
Han Lian Cao	9g	Herba Ecliptae Prostratae
Suan Zao Ren	15g	Semen Ziziphi Spinosae
Gan Cao (Zhi)	3g	Radix Glycyrrhizae Uralensis

Used for recurrent miscarriage caused by Heat in the Blood.

BI XIE FEN QING YIN (DIOSCOREA SEPARATING THE CLEAR DECOCTION)

Bi Xie	12g	Rhizoma Dioscorea
Yi Zhi Ren	9g	Fructus Alpiniae Oxyphyllae
Wu Yao	9g	Radix Linderae Strychnifoliae
Shi Chang Pu	9g	Rhizoma Acori Graminei

Used for male infertility caused by Damp-Heat.

BU SHEN CU PAI LUAN TANG (REINFORCE KIDNEY AND OVULATION FORMULA)

Dang Gui	9g	Radix Angelicae Sinensis
Chi Shao	9g	Radix Paeoniae Rubra
Bai Shao	9g	Radix Paeoniae Lactiflorae
Shan Yao	9g	Dioscorea Oppositae
Shu Di	12g	Radix Rehmanniae Glutinosae Conquitae
Nu Zhen Zi	9g	Fructus Ligustri Lucidi
Mu Dan Pi	9g	Cortex Moutan Radicis
Fu Ling	12g	Sclerotium Poriae Cocos
Xu Duan	9g	Radix Dipsaci
Tu Si Zi	9g	Semen Cuscatae
Wu Ling Zhi	9g	Excrementum Trogopterori
Hong Hua	6g	Flos Carthami Tinctorii

Used to promote ovulation when a patient has Kidney weakness.

BU SHEN CU PAI LUAN TANG (REINFORCE KIDNEY AND OVULATION FORMULA) MODIFIED

Bai Shao	9 g	Radix Paeoniae Lactiflorae
Nu Zhen Zi	9 g	Fructus Ligustri Lucidi
Shan Yao	9 g	Dioscorea Oppositae
Shan Zhu Yu	9 g	Fructus Corni Officinalis
Tu Si Zi	12 g	Semen Cuscatae
Bu Gu Zhi	6 g	Fructus Psoraleae
Rou Cong Rong	9 g	Herba Cistanches
Suo Yang	6 g	Herba Cynomorii Songarici
He Huan Pi	9 g	Cortex Albizziae Julibrissin
Xiang Fu (Cu)	12 g	Rhizoma Cyperi Rotundi
Qing Pi	3 g	Pericarpium Citri Reticulatae Viride
Ju He	3 g	Semen Citri Reticulatae
Li Zhe He	3 g	Semen Litchi
Wu Yao	3 g	Radix Linderae Strychnifoliae

Used during an IVF cycle in Phase 3 in certain restricted circumstances.

BU SHEN CU PAI LUAN (REINFORCE KIDNEY OVULATION FORMULA) MODIFIED

Dang Gui	9 g	Radix Angelicae Sinensis
Chi Shao	6 g	Radix Paeoniae Rubra
Bai Shao	6 g	Radix Paeoniae Lactiflorae
Hong Hua	3 g	Flos Carthami Tinctorii
Ji Xue Teng	9 g	Radix et Caulis Jixueteng
San Qi	3 g	Radix Pseudoginseng
Shan Yao	6 g	Dioscorea Oppositae
Shu Di	6 g	Rehmanniae Glutinosae Conquitae
Nu Zhen Zi	6 g	Fructus Ligustri Lucidi
Mu Dan Pi	6 g	Cortex Moutan Radicis
Fu Ling	6 g	Sclerotium Poriae Cocos
Tu Si Zi	12 g	Semen Cuscatae
Xu Duan	12 g	Radix Dipsaci
Zi Shi Ying	6 g	Fluoritum
He Huan Pi	9 g	Cortex Albizziae Julibrissin
Xiang Fu	9 g	Rhizoma Cyperi Rotundi

For use during an IVF cycle in Phase 4a (there are fewer restrictions on use of herbs in Phase 4 of an IVF cycle).

BU SHEN GU CHONG TANG (REINFORCE THE KIDNEYS AND CONSOLIDATE THE CHONG VESSEL DECOCTION) MODIFIED

Xu Duan	9 g	Radix Dipsaci
Ba Ji Tian	9 g	Radix Morindae Officinalis
Du Zhong	9 g	Cortex Eucommiae Ulmoidis
Tu Si Zi	9 g	Semen Cuscatae
Dang Gui	9 g	Radix Angelicae Sinensis

Shu Di	9 g	Radix Rehmanniae Glutinosae Conquitae
Gou Qi Zi	12 g	Fructus Lycii Chinensis
Dang Shen	12 g	Radix Codonopsis Pilulosae
Bai Zhu	12 g	Rhizoma Atractylodis Macrocephalae
Da Zao	5 pieces	Fructus Zizyphi Jujuba
Sha Ren	3 g	Fructus seu Semen Amomi

Used after ovulation in patients suffering recurrent miscarriage due to Kidney deficiency.

BU SHEN YI JING FANG (SUPPLEMENT THE KIDNEYS AND BENEFIT THE JING FORMULA)

He Shou Wu	15 g	Radix Polygoni Multiflori
Shu Di	15 g	Radix Rehmanniae Glutinosae Conquitae
Gou Qi Zi	15 g	Fructus Lycii Chinensis
Shan Yao	15 g	Radix Dioscorea Oppositae
Shan Zhu Yu	15 g	Fructus Corni Officinalis
Tu Si Zi	15 g	Semen Cuscatae
Fu Pen Zi	15 g	Fructus Rubi Chingii
Nu Zhen Zi	15 g	Fructus Ligustri Lucidi
Bai Shao	15 g	Radix Paeoniae Lactiflorae
Mu Dan Pi	15 g	Cortex Moutan Radicis
Dang Shen	15 g	Radix Codonopsis Pilulosae
Huang Qi	15 g	Radix Astragali
Yin Yang Huo	15 g	Herba Epimedii
Rou Cong Rong	15 g	Herba Cistanches
Ba Ji Tian	12 g	Radix Morindae Officinalis
Suo Yang	12 g	Herba Cynomorii Songarici
Dan Shen	12 g	Radix Salviae Miltiorrhizae
Lu Jiao Pian	12 g	Cornu Cervi Parvum

Used in the treatment of male infertility related to Kidney deficiency.

BU SHEN YI JING FANG (SUPPLEMENT THE KIDNEYS BENEFIT THE JING FORMULA) MODIFIED

Tu Si Zi	9 g	Semen Cuscatae
Fu Pen Zi	12 g	Fructus Rubi Chingii
Nu Zhen Zi	9 g	Fructus Ligustri Lucidi
Gou Qi Zi	9 g	Fructus Lycii Chinensis
He Shou Wu	12 g	Radix Polygoni Multiflori
Sheng Di	9 g	Radix Rehmanniae Glutinosae
Shan Zhu Yu	9 g	Fructus Corni Officinalis
Dang Shen	9 g	Radix Codonopsis Pilulosae
Dan Shen	9 g	Radix Salviae Miltiorrhizae
Hong Hua	6 g	Flos Carthami Tinctorii
Huang Qi	12 g	Radix Astragali
Yin Yang Huo	9 g	Herba Epimedii

For use by male partner in preparation for IVF.

BU ZHONG YI QI TANG (REINFORCE THE CENTER AND BENEFIT THE QI DECOCTION)

Huang Qi	30 g	Radix Astragali
Dang Shen	15 g	Radix Codonopsis Pilulosae
Bai Zhu	9 g	Rhizoma Atractylodis Macrocephalae
Dang Gui	9 g	Radix Angelicae Sinensis
Chen Pi	6 g	Pericarpium Citri Reticulate
Sheng Ma	6 g	Rhizoma Cimicifugae
Chai Hu	6 g	Radix Bupleuri
Gan Cao (Zhi)	3 g	Radix Glycyrrhizae Uralensis

Used in cases of threatened miscarriage due to Qi deficiency.

BU ZHONG YI QI TANG (REINFORCE THE CENTER AND BENEFIT THE QI DECOCTION) MODIFIED

Huang Qi	15 g	Radix Astragali
Dang Shen	12 g	Radix Codonopsis Pilulosae
Bai Zhu	9 g	Rhizoma Atractylodis Macrocephalae
Dang Gui	9 g	Radix Angelicae Sinensis
Chen Pi	6 g	Pericarpium Citri Reticulate
Sheng Ma	6 g	Rhizoma Cimicifugae
Chai Hu	6 g	Radix Bupleuri
Gan Cao (Zhi)	3 g	Radix Glycyrrhizae Uralensis
Wu Zei Gu	9 g	Os Sepia seu Sepiellae

Used in cases of recurrent miscarriage due to Qi deficiency.

CANG FU DAO TAN WAN (ATRACTYLODES CYPERUS PHLEGM PILL)

Cang Zhu	Rhizoma Atractylodes
Xiang Fu	Rhizoma Cyperi Rotundi
Ban Xia	Rhizoma Pinelliae
Fu Ling	Sclerotium Poriae Cocos
Chen Pi	Pericarpium Citri Reticulate
Dan Nan Xing	Rhizoma Arisaematis
Zhi Ke	Fructus Citri seu Ponciri
Gan Cao (Zhi)	Radix Glycyrrhizae Uralensis
Sheng Jiang	Rhizoma Zingiberis Officinalis Recens
Shen Qu	Massa Fermenta

Patent medicine used in the treatment of PCOS or Phlegm-Damp amenorrhea, or blockage of fallopian tubes by Phlegm-Damp.

CANG FU DAO TAN TANG (ATRACTYLODES CYPERUS PHLEGM DECOCTION) MODIFIED

Cang Zhu	15 g	Rhizoma Atractylodes
Xiang Fu	9 g	Rhizoma Cyperi Rotundi
Ban Xia	9 g	Rhizoma Pinelliae

Fu Ling	15g	Sclerotium Poriae Cocos
Chen Pi	6g	Pericarpium Citri Reticulate
Dan Nan Xing	6g	Rhizoma Arisaematis
Zhi Ke	6g	Fructus Citri seu Ponciri
Gan Cao (Zhi)	3g	Radix Glycyrrhizae Uralensis
Sheng Jiang	3 slices	Rhizoma Zingiberis Officinalis Recens
Shen Qu	6g	Massa Fermenta
Chuan Xiong	6g	Radix Ligustici Wallichii
Chuan Niu Xi	9g	Radix Cyathulae
San Leng	6g	Rhizoma Sparganii
E Zhu	6g	Rhizoma Curcumae Zedoariae
Ze Lan	6g	Herba Lycopi Lucidi

This modification of the above patent medicine treats PCOS and amenorrhea caused by Phlegm-Damp and Blood stagnation.

CANG FU DAO TAN TANG (ATRACTYLODES AND CYPERUS GUIDE OUT PHLEGM DECOCTION) MODIFIED

Cang Zhu	12g	Rhizoma Atractylodis
Fu Ling	15g	Sclerotium Poriae Cocos
Ban Xia	9g	Rhizoma Pinelliae
Sha Ren	6g	Fructus seu Semen Amomi
Fo Shou	3g	Fructus Citri Sarcodactylis
Chen Pi	9g	Pericarpium Citri Reticulate
Dan Nan Xing	6g	Rhizoma Arisaematis
Zhe Bei Mu	6g	Fritillariae Thunbergii Bulbus
Zao Jiao Ci	9g	Spina Gleditsiae Sinensis
Shan Yao	9g	Radix Dioscorea Oppositae
Shu Di	6g	Radix Rehmanniae Glutinosae Conquitae
Bu Gu Zhi	9g	Fructus Psoraleae
Yin Yang Huo	9g	Herba Epimedii
Ji Xue Teng	12g	Radix et Caulis Jixueteng
Zhi Zi	3g	Fructus Gardeniae Jasminoidis

For use with overweight PCOS patients with few or no periods.

CHAI HU TONG LIU YING (BUPLEURUM FREE LODGED PHLEGM FORMULA)

Chai Hu	12g	Radix Bupleuri
Dang Gui	9g	Radix Angelicae Sinensis
Chi Shao	9g	Radix Paeoniae Rubra
Yu Jin	9g	Tuber Curcumae
Su Mu	6g	Lignum Sappan
Si Gua Luo	9g	Vascularis Luffae, Fasciculus
Ju He	3g	Semen Citri Reticulatae

Used to resolve Qi stagnation which is contributing to constriction of the fallopian tubes.

CU PAI LUAN TANG (OVULATION DECOCTION)

Dang Gui	9 g	*Radix Angelicae Sinensis*
Chi Shao	9 g	*Radix Paeoniae Rubra*
Chuan Xiong	6 g	*Radix Ligustici Wallichii*
Hong Hua	6 g	*Flos Carthami Tinctorii*
Dan Shen	9 g	*Radix Salviae Miltiorrhizae*
Ze Lan	9 g	*Herba Lycopi Lucidi*
Ji Xue Teng	15 g	*Radix et Caulis Jixueteng*

Used to promote ovulation in women not suffering any Kidney deficiency.

DA HUANG BIE CHONG WAN (RHEUM EUPOLYPHAGA PILL)

Da Huang	*Rhizoma Rhei*
Tu Bie Chong	*Eupolyphagae seu Opisthoplatiae*
Tao Ren	*Semen Persicae*
Gan Qi	*Lacca Sinica Exsiccata*
Qi Cao	*Holotrichia Vermiculus*
Shui Zhi	*Hirudo seu Whitmaiae*
Meng Chong	*Tabanus Bivittatus*
Huang Qin	*Radix Scutellariae Baicalensis*
Xing Ren	*Semen Pruni Armeniacae*
Sheng Di	*Rehmanniae Glutinosae*
Bai Shao	*Radix Paeoniae Lactiflorae*
Gan Cao (Zhi)	*Radix Glycyrrhizae Uralensis*

This patent medicine is given to remove severe Blood stasis in pelvic inflammatory disease.

DAN ZHI XIAO YAO SAN (MOUTAN GARDENIA FREE AND EASY POWDER)

Chai Hu	9 g	*Radix Bupleuri*
Bai Shao	12 g	*Radix Paeoniae Lactiflorae*
Dang Gui	9 g	*Radix Angelicae Sinensis*
Bai Zhu	9 g	*Rhizoma Atractylodis Macrocephalae*
Fu Ling	15 g	*Sclerotium Poriae Cocos*
Sheng Jiang	3 slices	*Radix Rehmanniae Glutinosae*
Bo He	3 g	*Herba Menthae*
Gan Cao (Zhi)	6 g	*Radix Glycyrrhizae Uralensis*
Mu Dan Pi	9 g	*Cortex Moutan Radicis*
Zhi Zi	6 g	*Fructus Gardenia Jasminoidis*

Used during the luteal phase in the treatment of Liver-Fire.

DAN ZHI XIAO YAO SAN (MOUTAN GARDENIA FREE AND EASY POWDER) MODIFIED

Dang Gui	9 g	*Radix Angelicae Sinensis*
Bai Shao	12 g	*Radix Paeoniae Lactiflorae*

Fu Ling	12g	Sclerotium Poriae Cocos
Bai Zhu	9g	Rhizoma Atractylodis Macrocephalae
Chai Hu	9g	Radix Bupleuri
Mu Dan Pi	9g	Cortex Moutan Radicis
Zhi Zi	6g	Fructus Gardeniae Jasminoidis
Gan Cao (Zhi)	6g	Radix Glycyrrhizae Uralensis
Shan Zhu Yu	9g	Fructus Corni Officinalis
Bo He	3g	Herba Menthae
Sheng Jiang	3g	Rhizoma Zingiberis Officinalis Recens

Used in the treatment of Liver Qi stagnation amenorrhea.

DANG GUI SHAO YAO SAN (ANGELICA PEONIA POWDER) MODIFIED

Dang Gui	9g	Radix Angelicae Sinensis
Bai Shao	15g	Radix Paeoniae Lactiflorae
Fu Ling	9g	Sclerotium Poriae Cocos
Bai Zhu	9g	Rhizoma Atractylodis Macrocephalae
Ze Xie	9g	Rhizoma Alismatis
Dan Shen	6g	Radix Salviae Miltiorrhizae
Gan Cao (Zhi)	3g	Radix Glycyrrhizae Uralensis

Used in the case of threatened miscarriage due to Blood deficiency.

FANG FENG TONG SHENG SAN (LEDEBOURIELLA PILLS WITH MAGICAL EFFECT)

Fang Feng	9g	Radix Ledebouriellae Sesloidis
Jing Jie	9g	Herba seu Flos Shizonepetae Tenuifoliae
Ma Huang	6g	Herba Ephedra
Jie Geng	9g	Radix Platycodi Grandiflori
Bo He	6g	Herba Menthae
Lian Qiao	9g	Fructus Forsythiae Suspensae
Huang Qin	6g	Radix Scutellariae Baicalensis
Zhi Zi	6g	Fructus Gardeniae Jasminoidis
Da Huang (jiu)	6g	Rhizoma Rhei (wine fried)
Shi Gao	9g	Gypsum
Mang Xiao	6g	Mirabilitum
Hua Shi	9g	Talcum
Dang Gui	9g	Radix Angelicae Sinensis
Chuan Xiong	6g	Radix Ligustici Wallichii
Bai Zhu	9g	Rhizoma Atractylodis Macrocephalae
Bai Shao	9g	Radix Paeoniae Lactiflorae
Gan Cao (Zhi)	6g	Radix Glycyrrhizae Uralensis
Sheng Jiang	6g	Rhizoma Zingiberis Officinalis Recens

Used in the treatment of PCOS and amenorrhea caused by Liver Qi stagnation and Phlegm-Damp accumulation.

FU FANG DANG GUI ZHI SHI YE (ANGELICA COMPOUND INJECTION FLUID)

Dang Gui	15 g	Radix Angelicae Sinensis
Hong Hua	9 g	Flos Carthami Tinctorii
Chuan Xiong	9 g	Radix Ligustici Wallichii

An injection of these herbs is used to flush fallopian tubes in an attempt to remove blockages; they may also be administered per rectum.

FU FENG HONG TENG BAI JIANG SAN (SARGENTODOXAE PATRINIAE COMPOUND POWDER)

Dang Gui	9 g	Radix Angelicae Sinensis
Chi Shao	9 g	Radix Paeoniae Rubra
Bai Shao	9 g	Radix Paeoniae Lactiflorae
Hong Teng	15 g	Caulis Sargentodoxae
Bai Jiang Cao	15 g	Herba cum Radice Patriniae
Mu Xiang	6 g	Radix Saussureae seu Vladimiriae
Yan Hu Suo	9 g	Rhizoma Corydalis Yanhusuo
Chai Hu	6 g	Radix Bupleuri
Chen Pi	6 g	Pericarpium Citri Reticulate
Sang Ji Sheng	12 g	Ramulus Sangjisheng
Shan Zha	12 g	Fructus Crataegi
Yi Yi Ren	15 g	Semen Coicis Lachryma-jobi

A formula to be used per rectum in the treatment of pelvic inflammatory disease and fallopian tube blockage.

FU FANG HONG TENG JIAN (SARGENTODOXAE COMPOUND DECOCTION) MODIFIED

Hong Teng	30 g	Caulis Sargentodoxae
Bai Jiang Cao	30 g	Herba cum Radice Patriniae
Pu Gong Yin	15 g	Herba Taraxaci Mongolici
Zi Hua Di Ding	15 g	Herba Viola cum Radice
Ru Xiang	6 g	Gummi Olibanum
Mo Yao	6 g	Myrrha
Mu Xiang	6 g	Radix Saussureae seu Vladimiriae
Dang Gui	9 g	Radix Angelicae Sinensis
Chi Shao	9 g	Radix Paeoniae Rubra
Wu Ling Zhi	9 g	Excrementum Trogopterori
Yi Yi Ren	30 g	Semen Coicis Lachryma-jobi

Another version of this formula can be used per rectum for fallopian tube blockage related to strong Damp-Heat.

GAN MAI DA ZAO TANG (GLYCYRRHIZAE TRITICI ZIZIPHI DECOCTION)

Gan Cao (Zhi)	9 g	Radix Glycyrrhizae Uralensis
Fu Xiao Mai	9 g	Semen Tritici Aestivi Levis
Da Zao	6 g	Fructus Ziziphi Jujubae

Added to Gui Shao Di Huang Tang in the follicular phase if the Shen is disturbed.

GE XIA ZHU YU TANG (ELIMINATING STASIS BELOW THE DIAPHRAGM DECOCTION) MODIFIED

Dang Gui	9 g	Radix Angelicae Sinensis
Chuan Xiong	6 g	Radix Ligustici Wallichii
Tao Ren	9 g	Semen Persicae
Hong Hua	9 g	Flos Carthami Tinctorii
Wu Ling Zhi	9 g	Excrementum Trogopterori
Wu Yao	6 g	Radix Linderae Strychnifoliae
Yan Hu Suo	6 g	Rhizoma Corydalis Yanhusuo
Chi Shao	6 g	Radix Paeoniae Rubra
Mu Dan Pi	6 g	Cortex Moutan Radicis
Chuan Niu Xi	9 g	Radix Cyathulae
Xiang Fu	9 g	Rhizoma Cyperi Rotundi
Zhi Ke	6 g	Fructus Citri seu Ponciri
Zhi Zi	9 g	Fructus Gardeniae Jasminoidis
Hong Teng	9 g	Caulis Sargentodoxae
Gan Cao (Zhi)	3 g	Radix Glycyrrhizae Uralensis

Used to resolve retained pregnancy products after miscarriage or birth which might lead to infection and blocked tubes.

GE XIA ZHU YU TANG (ELIMINATING STASIS BELOW THE DIAPHRAGM DECOCTION) PLUS DAN ZHI XIAO YAO SAN (MOUTAN GARDENIA FREE AND EASY POWDER)

Dang Gui	9 g	Radix Angelicae Sinensis
Chuan Xiong	9 g	Radix Ligustici Wallichii
Tao Ren	9 g	Semen Persicae
Hong Hua	9 g	Flos Carthami Tinctorii
Wu Ling Zhi	9 g	Excrementum Trogopterori
Wu Yao	9 g	Radix Linderae Strychnifoliae
Yan Hu Suo	6 g	Rhizoma Corydalis Yanhusuo
Zhi Zi	6 g	Fructus Gardeniae Jasminoidis
Chi Shao	9 g	Radix Paeoniae Rubra
Mu Dan Pi	9 g	Cortex Moutan Radicis
Xiang Fu	6 g	Rhizoma Cyperi Rotundi
Zhi Ke	6 g	Fructus Citri seu Ponciri
Fu Ling	12 g	Sclerotium Poriae Cocos
Bo He	3 g	Herba Menthae
Gan Cao (Zhi)	3 g	Radix Glycyrrhizae Uralensis

Used to treat blocked tubes caused by Blood stagnation and Heat.

GE XIA ZHU YU TANG (ELIMINATING STASIS FROM BELOW THE DIAPHRAGM DECOCTION) PLUS BU SHEN QU YU FANG (SUPPLEMENT KIDNEY AND DISPEL BLOOD STASIS FORMULA) MODIFIED

Yin Yang Huo	9 g	Herba Epimedii
Xu Duan	9 g	Radix Dipsaci
Tu Si Zi	9 g	Semen Cuscatae

Gou Qi Zi	9 g	Fructus Lycii Chinensis
Huang Qi	9 g	Radix Astragali
Dang Gui	9 g	Radix Angelicae Sinensis
Ze Lan	12 g	Herba lycopi
Dan Shen	9 g	Radix Salviae Miltiorrhizae
San Qi	6 g	Radix Pseudoginseng
Yan Hu Suo	9 g	Rhizoma Corydalis Yanhusuo
Wu Ling Zhi	9 g	Excrementum Trogopterori
Niu Xi	9 g	Radix achyranthis bidentatae
Rou Gui	3 g	Cortex cinnamomi
Tao Ren	6 g	Semen Persicae
Hong Hua	6 g	Flos Carthami Tinctorii
Xiang Fu	9 g	Rhizoma Cyperi Rotundi
(Cu) San Leng	9 g	Rhizoma Sparganii
E Zhu	6 g	Rhizoma Curcumae Zedoariae

Used to treat endometriosis in women with a weak constitution at times when they are not trying to conceive.

GUI SHAO DI HUANG TANG (ANGELICA PEONIA REHMANNIA DECOCTION)

Shu Di	12 g	Radix Rehmanniae Glutinosae Conquitae
Shan Yao	9 g	Radix Dioscorea Oppositae
Shan Zhu Yu	9 g	Fructus Corni Officinalis
Fu Ling	6 g	Sclerotium Poriae Cocos
Mu Dan Pi	6 g	Cortex Moutan Radicis
Ze Xie	6 g	Rhizoma Alismatis
Dang Gui	9 g	Radix Angelicae Sinensis
Bai Shao	9 g	Radix Paeoniae Lactiflorae

This formula is given after the period to build Blood and Kidney Yin. It is also used as a base for many variations used in the post-menstrual phase. It can serve as a guiding formula in the treatment of Yin deficiency amenorrhea.

GUI SHAO DI HUANG TANG (ANGELICA PEONIA REHMANNIA DECOCTION) MODIFIED

Dang Gui	9 g	Radix Angelicae Sinensis
Bai Shao	9 g	Radix Paeoniae Lactiflorae
Shu Di	9 g	Radix Rehmanniae Glutinosae Conquitae
Shan Yao	9 g	Radix Dioscorea Oppositae
Shan Zhu Yu	9 g	Fructus Corni Officinalis
Mu Li	9 g	Concha Ostreae
Yin Yang Huo	9 g	Herba Epimedii
Lu Jiao Pian	9 g	Cornu Cervi Parvum
Zi He Che	6 g	Placenta Hominis
Ren Shen	6 g	Radix Ginseng

Used to treat amenorrhea related to Kidney Jing deficiency. Zi He Che is a restricted substance and is often replaced with other Jing tonics.

GUI SHAO DI HUANG TANG (ANGELICA PEONIA REHMANNIA DECOCTION) MODIFIED

Dang Gui	9 g	Radix Angelicae Sinensis
Bai Shao	9 g	Radix Paeoniae Lactiflorae
Shu Di	9 g	Radix Rehmanniae Glutinosae Conquitae
Shan Zhu Yu	9 g	Fructus Corni Officinalis
Shan Yao	9 g	Radix Dioscorea Oppositae
Fu Ling	15 g	Sclerotium Poriae Cocos
Mu Dan Pi	9 g	Cortex Moutan Radicis
Ze Xie	15 g	Rhizoma Alismatis
Tu Si Zi	9 g	Semen Cuscatae
Du Zhong	6 g	Cortex Eucommiae Ulmoidis
Sha Ren	6 g	Fructus seu Semen Amomi

Used in the treatment of amenorrhea due to Kidney Yin and Yang deficiency with Phlegm-Damp (to be taken with patent remedies).

GUI SHAO DI HUANG TANG (ANGELICA PEONIA REHMANNIA DECOCTION) MODIFIED

Shu Di	9 g	Radix Rehmanniae Glutinosae Conquitae
Shan Yao	9 g	Radix Dioscorea Oppositae
Shan Zhu Yu	9 g	Fructus Corni Officinalis
Mu Dan Pi	9 g	Cortex Moutan Radicis
Fu Ling	15 g	Sclerotium Poriae Cocos
Bai Shao	9 g	Radix Paeoniae Lactiflorae
Dang Gui	9 g	Radix Angelicae Sinensis
Bai Jiang Cao	12 g	Herba cum Radice Patriniae
Chai Hu	6 g	Radix Bupleuri
Yan Hu Suo	6 g	Rhizoma Corydalis Yanhusuo
Xu Duan	9 g	Radix Dipsaci
Sang Ji Sheng	15 g	Ramulus Sangjisheng

Used in the treatment of pelvic inflammatory disease associated with Liver and Kidney deficiency.

GUI SHAO DI HUANG TANG (ANGELICA PEONIA REHMANNIA DECOCTION) MODIFIED

Dang Gui	9 g	Radix Angelicae Sinensis
Bai Shao	9 g	Radix Paeoniae Lactiflorae
Shu Di	9 g	Radix Rehmanniae Glutinosae Conquitae
Shan Zhu Yu	9 g	Fructus Corni Officinalis
Shan Yao	9 g	Radix Dioscorea Oppositae
Fu Ling	15 g	Sclerotium Poriae Cocos
Mu Dan Pi	9 g	Cortex Moutan Radicis
Ze Xie	15 g	Rhizoma Alismatis
Tu Si Zi	9 g	Semen Cuscatae
Du Zhong	6 g	Cortex Eucommiae Ulmoidis
Sha Ren	9 g	Fructus seu Semen Amomi

| Zhe Bei Mu | 6 g | *Fritillariae thunbergii Bulbus* |
| Zao Jiao Ci | 6 g | *Spina Gleditsiae Sinensis* |

Used in the treatment of PCOS Kidney-deficiency infertility, accompanied by irregular cycles and possibly some weight gain.

GUI SHAO DI HUANG TANG (ANGELICA PEONIA REHMANNIA DECOCTION) MODIFIED

Shu Di	12 g	*Radix Rehmanniae Glutinosae Conquitae*
Shan Yao	9 g	*Radix Dioscorea Oppositae*
Shan Zhu Yu	9 g	*Fructus Corni Officinalis*
Fu Ling	9 g	*Sclerotium Poriae Cocos*
Mu Dan Pi	9 g	*Cortex Moutan Radicis*
Ze Xie	6 g	*Rhizoma Alismatis*
Dang Gui	9 g	*Radix Angelicae Sinensis*
Bai Shao	9 g	*Radix Paeoniae Lactiflorae*
Dan Shen	9 g	*Radix Salviae Miltiorrhizae*
Sha Ren	6 g	*Fructus seu Semen Amomi*
Tu Si Zi	9 g	*Semen Cuscatae*
Bu Gu Zhi	9 g	*Fructus Psoraleae*
Xiang Fu	6 g	*Rhizoma Cyperi Rotundi*
He Huan Pi	9 g	*Cortex Albizziae Julibrissin*
Suo Yang	6 g	*Herba Cynomorii Songarici*
Lu Jiao Pian	6 g	*Cornu Cervi Parvum*
Zi Shi Ying	6 g	*Fluoritum*

For use by women with Kidney deficiency in preparation for doing IVF. This formula can be taken throughout the menstrual cycle.

GUI SHAO DI HUANG TANG (ANGELICA PEONIA REHMANNIA DECOCTION) MODIFIED

Shu Di	12 g	*Radix Rehmanniae Glutinosae Conquitae*
Shan Zhu Yu	9 g	*Fructus Corni Officinalis*
Shan Yao	9 g	*Radix Dioscorea Oppositae*
Dang Gui	9 g	*Radix Angelicae Sinensis*
Bai Shao	9 g	*Radix Paeoniae Lactiflorae*
Dan Shen	9 g	*Radix Salviae Miltiorrhizae*
Ji Xue Teng	9 g	*Radix et Caulis Jixueteng*
Mu Dan Pi	9 g	*Cortex Moutan Radicis*
Fu Ling	9 g	*Sclerotium Poriae Cocos*
Ze Xie	6 g	*Rhizoma Alismatis*
Sha Ren	6 g	*Fructus seu Semen Amomi*
Tu Si Zi	9 g	*Semen Cuscatae*
Bu Gu Zhi	6 g	*Fructus Psoraleae*
Xiang Fu	9 g	*Rhizoma Cyperi Rotundi*
Wu Yao	3 g	*Radix Linderae Strychnifoliae*
Yin Yang Huo	6 g	*Herba Epimedii*

Lu Jiao Pian	6g	Cornu Cervi Parvum
Zi Shi Ying	6g	Fluoritum
He Huan Pi	12g	Cortex Albizziae Julibrissin
Suan Zao Ren	9g	Semen Ziziphi Spinosae

For use during an IVF cycle in Phase 2 in certain restricted circumstances.

GUI SHAO DI HUANG TANG (ANGELICA PEONIA REHMANNIA DECOCTION) PLUS JIAN GU TANG
(STRENGTHEN AND CONSOLIDATE DECOCTION) MODIFIED

Nu Zhen Zi	9g	Fructus Ligustri Lucidi
Han Lian Cao	9g	Herba Ecliptae Prostratae
Shan Yao	9g	Dioscorea Oppositae
Shan Zhu Yu	9g	Fructus Corni Officinalis
Ji Xue Teng	9g	Radix et Caulis Jixueteng
Bai Shao	9g	Radix Paeoniae Lactiflorae
Dan Shen	9g	Radix Salviae Miltiorrhizae
Mu Dan Pi	9g	Cortex Moutan Radicis
Fu Ling	15g	Sclerotium Poriae Cocos
Ze Xie	9g	Rhizoma Alismatis
Sha Ren	6g	Fructus seu Semen Amomi
Yi Yi Ren	15g	Semen Coicis Lachryma-jobi
Dang Shen	9g	Radix Codonopsis Pilulosae
Bai Zhu	9g	Rhizoma Atractylodis Macrocephalae
Tu Si Zi	9g	Semen Cuscatae
Ba Ji Tian	9g	Radix Morindae Officinalis
Yin Yang Huo	9g	Herba Epimedii
Zao Jiao Ci	6g	Spina Gleditsiae Sinensis
Dan Nan Xing	6g	Rhizoma Arisaematis

Used to reinforce Kidneys and clear Damp in women (especially overweight women) preparing for IVF. This formula can be taken throughout the menstrual cycle.

GUI SHAO DI HUANG TANG (ANGELICA PEONIA REHMANNIA DECOCTION) PLUS TAO HONG SI WU TANG
(PERSICA CARTHAMUS FOUR SUBSTANCES DECOCTION) MODIFIED

Shu Di	9g	Rehmanniae Glutinosae Conquitae
Shan Yao	9g	Dioscorea Oppositae
Shan Zhu Yu	9g	Fructus Corni Officinalis
Dang Gui	9g	Radix Angelicae Sinensis
Bai Shao	9g	Radix Paeoniae Lactiflorae
Dan Shen	9g	Radix Salviae Miltiorrhizae
Mu Dan Pi	9g	Cortex Moutan Radicis
Fu Ling	9g	Sclerotium Poriae Cocos
Ze Xie	9g	Rhizoma Alismatis
Sha Ren	3g	Fructus seu Semen Amomi
Tu Si Zi	9g	Semen Cuscatae

Bu Gu Zhi	6g	*Fructus Psoraleae*
Xiang Fu	6g	*Rhizoma Cyperi Rotundi*
He Huan Pi	9g	*Cortex Albizziae Julibrissin*
Tao Ren	9g	*Semen Persicae*
Hong Hua	9g	*Flos Carthami Tinctorii*
Pu Huang	9g	*Pollen Typhae*
Wu Ling Zhi	9g	*Excrementum Trogopterori*

For use by women preparing for IVF to reinforce Kidneys and clear Blood stasis. It can be taken throughout the menstrual cycle.

GUI SHAO DI HUANG TANG (ANGELICA PEONIA REHMANNIA DECOCTION) WITH XIAO YAO SAN (BUPLEURUM AND TANGKUEI POWDER) AND GAN MAI DA ZAO TANG (LICORICE, WHEAT, AND JUJUBE DECOCTION) MODIFIED

Shu Di	9g	*Radix Rehmanniae Glutinosae Conquitae*
Shan Yao	9g	*Radix Dioscorea Oppositae*
Shan Zhu Yu	9g	*Fructus Corni Officinalis*
Dang Gui	9g	*Radix Angelicae Sinensis*
Bai Shao	9g	*Radix Paeoniae Lactiflorae*
Dan Shen	9g	*Radix Salviae Miltiorrhizae*
Fu Ling	9g	*Sclerotium Poriae Cocos*
Mu Dan Pi	9g	*Cortex Moutan Radicis*
Ze Xie	9g	*Rhizoma Alismatis*
Sha Ren	3g	*Fructus seu Semen Amomi*
Tu Si Zi	9g	*Semen Cuscatae*
Bu Gu Zhi	6g	*Fructus Psoraleae*
Xiang Fu	6g	*Rhizoma Cyperi Rotundi*
He Huan Pi	9g	*Cortex Albizziae Julibrissin*
Chai Hu	9g	*Radix Bupleuri*
Fu Xiao Mai	6g	*Semen Tritici Aestivi Levis*
Da Zao	6 pieces	*Fructus Zizyphi Jujuba*
Gan Cao	6g	*Radix Glycyrrhizae Uralensis*

Used to prepare for IVF by reinforcing Kidneys and regulating Liver and Heart Qi. This formula can be taken throughout the menstrual cycle.

GUI ZHI FU LING TANG (RAMULUS CINNAMOMI-PORIA DECOCTION)

Gui Zhi	9g	*Ramulus Cinnamomi Cassiae*
Fu Ling	9g	*Sclerotium Poriae Cocos*
Mu Dan Pi	9g	*Cortex Moutan Radicis*
Tao Ren	9g	*Semen Persicae*
Chi Shao	9g	*Radix Paeoniae Rubra*

Used in the treatment of fallopian tubes blocked by Cold-Damp. Also recommended in patent form as an addition to other formulas in the treatment of pelvic inflammatory disease if there are abdomen masses.

GUI ZHI FU LING TANG (RAMULUS CINNAMOMI-PORIA DECOCTION) MODIFIED

Gui Zhi	6g	Ramulus Cinnamomi Cassiae
Tao Ren	6g	Semen Persicae
Mu Dan Pi	9g	Cortex Moutan Radicis
Chi Shao	9g	Radix Paeoniae Rubra
Dan Shen	18g	Radix Salviae Miltiorrhizae
Wang Bu Liu Xing	6g	Semen Vaccariae
Che Qian Zi	9g	semen plantaginis
Fu Ling	9g	Sclerotium Poriae Cocos
Pu Gong Yin	12g	Herba Taraxaci Mongolici
Xiao Hui Xiang	3g	Fructus Foeniculi Vulgaris
Ju He	3g	Semen Citri Reticulatae
Chuan Lian Zi	9g	Fructus Meliae Toosendan
Xu Duan	9g	Radix Dipsaci
Huang Qi	18g	Radix Astragali

Used in the treatment of male infertility related to varicocele or antisperm antibodies.

GUI ZHI FU LING TANG (RAMULUS CINNAMOMI-PORIA DECOCTION) MODIFIED

Dang Gui	12g	Radix Angelicae Sinensis
Bai Shao	12g	Radix Paeoniae Lactiflorae
Chuan Xiong	6g	Radix Ligustici Wallichii
Yi Mu Cao	9g	Herba Leonuri Heterophylli
San Leng	12g	Rhizoma Sparganii
E Zhu	12g	Rhizoma Curcumae Zedoariae
Tao Ren	6g	Semen Persicae
Gui Zhi	6g	Ramulus Cinnamomi Cassiae
Fu Ling	15g	Sclerotium Poriae Cocos
San Qi	9g	Radix Pseudoginseng
Wu Ling Zhi	6g	Excrementum Trogopterori

Used in the treatment of large submucosal fibroids, with little or no complication by Kidney deficiency.

HUA YU LI SHI TANG (TRANSFORM BLOOD STASIS AND RESOLVE DAMP DECOCTION) MODIFIED

San Leng	12g	Rhizoma Sparganii
E Zhu	12g	Rhizoma Curcumae Zedoariae
Pu Huang	9g	Pollen Typhae
Wu Ling Zhi	9g	Excrementum Trogopterori
Shan Zha	9g	Fructus Crataegi
(Zhi) Da Huang	6g	Rhizoma Rhei
Tu Bie Chong	6g	Eupolyphagae seu Opisthoplatiae
Mo Yao	3g	Resina Commiphorae Myrrhae
Dang Gui	9g	Radix Angelicae Sinensis
Dan Shen	9g	Radix Salviae Miltiorrhizae

Bai Jiang Cao	9 g	Herba cun radice Patriniae
Lian Qiao	6 g	Fructus Forsythiae Suspensae
Hong Teng	9 g	Caulis Sargentodoxae
Xu Duan	9 g	Radix Dipsaci
Yin Yang Huo	9 g	Herba Epimedii
Gui Zhi	6 g	Ramulus Cinnamomi
Tai Zi Shen	12 g	Radix pseudostellariae

Used to treat endometriosis patients with a strong constitution, at times when not attempting to conceive.

HUO LUO XIAO LING DAN (REMOVE CHANNEL OBSTRUCTIONS FORMULA)

Mu Dan Pi	9 g	Cortex Moutan Radicis
Dan Shen	9 g	Radix Salviae Miltiorrhizae
Chi Shao	9 g	Radix Paeoniae Rubra
Wu Ling Zhi	9 g	Excrementum Trogopterori
Shan Zha	9 g	Fructus Crataegi
Chuan Niu Xi	9 g	Radix Cyathulae
Yu Jin	6 g	Tuber Curcumae
Ru Xiang	3 g	Gummi Olibanum
Chen Pi	6 g	Pericarpium Citri Reticulate
Gan Cao (Zhi)	6 g	Radix Glycyrrhizae Uralensis
Di Long	3 g	Lumbricus
Wu Gong	3 g	Scolopendra Subspinipes

Used in the management of ectopic pregnancy (early stage).

JIAN GU TANG (STRENGTHEN AND CONSOLIDATE DECOCTION) MODIFIED

Dang Shen	9 g	Radix Codonopsis Pilulosae
Bai Zhu	9 g	Rhizoma Atractylodis Macrocephalae
Shan Yao	9 g	Radix Dioscorea Oppositae
Yi Yi Ren	15 g	Semen Coicis Lachryma-jobi
Tu Si Zi	9 g	Semen Cuscatae
Ba Ji Tian	9 g	Radix Morindae Officinalis
Lu Jiao Pian	9 g	Cornu Cervi Parvum

Administered in the luteal phase to strengthen Kidney Yang by reinforcing Qi.

JIAN GU TANG (STRENGTHEN AND CONSOLIDATE DECOCTION) MODIFIED

Dang Shen	9 g	Radix Codonopsis Pilulosae
Bai Zhu	9 g	Rhizoma Atractylodis Macrocephalae
Shan Yao	9 g	Radix Dioscorea Oppositae
Yi Yi Ren	15 g	Semen Coicis Lachryma-jobi
Tu Si Zi	9 g	Semen Cuscatae
Ba Ji Tian	9 g	Radix Morindae Officinalis
Yin Yang Huo	9 g	Herba Epimedii

Shi Chang Pu	9 g	Rhizoma Acori Graminei
Dan Nan Xing	9 g	Rhizoma Arisaematis
Lu Lu Tong	9 g	Fructus Liquidambaris Taiwaniae
Di Long	9 g	Lumbricus
Wang Bu Liu Xing	9 g	Semen Vaccariae

Used in the luteal phase to clear Phlegm-Damp or Blood obstructions, while maintaining Kidney Yang.

JIAO AI SI WU TANG (GELATINUM ASINI ARTEMESIA FOUR SUBSTANCES DECOCTION) MODIFIED

E Jiao	9 g	Gelatinum Asini
Ai Ye	9 g	Folium Artemisiae
Dang Gui	9 g	Radix Angelicae Sinensis
Bai Shao	9 g	Radix Paeoniae Lactiflorae
Dan Shen	9 g	Radix Salviae Miltiorrhizae
Wu Ling Zhi	9 g	Excrementum Trogopterori
Pu Huang	9 g	Pollen Typhae
Gan Cao (Zhi)	6 g	Radix Glycyrrhizae Uralensis
Xu Duan	9 g	Radix Dipsaci

Used for threatened miscarriage due to Blood stagnation.

KANG MIAN YI HAO (IMMUNITY FORMULA FOR HELPING PREGNANCY #1)

Sheng Di	12 g	Radix Rehmanniae Glutinosae
Shan Zhu Yu	9 g	Fructus Corni Officinalis
Mai Dong	9 g	Tuber Ophiopogonis
Bai Shao	9 g	Radix Paeoniae Lactiflorae
Han Lian Cao	12 g	Herba Ecliptae Prostratae
Mu Dan Pi	9 g	Cortex Moutan Radicis
Dan Shen	30 g	Radix Salviae Miltiorrhizae
Huang Qi	30 g	Radix Astragali
Gui Ban	30 g	Plastrum Testudinis
Bie Jia	30 g	Carapax Amydae Sinensis
Huang Qin	9 g	Radix Scutellariae Baicalensis
Huang Bai	9 g	Cortex Phellodendri
Yu Zhu	15 g	Rhizoma Polygonati Odorati
Xu Chang Qing	9 g	Radix Cynanchi Paniculati
Zhi Gan Cao	9 g	Radix Glycyrrhizae Uralensis

This formula is used for women who have had recurrent miscarriage or who have been diagnosed with autoimmune disease that predisposes to miscarriage. It includes restricted products which require CITES certification.

KANG MIAN ER HAO (IMMUNITY FORMULA FOR HELPING PREGNANCY #2)

Dang Gui	9 g	Radix Angelicae Sinensis
Bai Shao	9 g	Radix Paeoniae Lactiflorae
Chuan Xiong	9 g	Radix Ligustici Wallichii

Tao Ren	9 g	Semen Persicae
Hong Hua	9 g	Flos Carthami Tinctorii
Yan Hu Suo	9 g	Rhizoma Corydalis Yanhusuo
Dan Shen	30 g	Radix Salviae Miltiorrhizae
Yi Mu Cao	18 g	Herba Leonuri Heterophylli
Gui Zhi	6 g	Ramulus Cinnamomi Cassiae
Xu Chang Qing	9 g	Radix Cynanchi Paniculati
Yin Yang Huo	15 g	Herba Epimedii
Tu Si Zi	9 g	Semen Cuscatae
Huang Qi	30 g	Radix Astragali
Gan Cao	9 g	Radix Glycyrrhizae Uralensis

This formula is prescribed for women with a history of recurrent miscarriage related to clotting factors or endometriosis or other forms of Blood stagnation.

LIU WEI DI HUANG TANG (SIX FLAVORS REHMANNIA DECOCTION)

Shu Di	9 g	Rehmanniae Glutinosae Conquitae
Shan Yao	9 g	Dioscorea Oppositae
Shan Zhu Yu	9 g	Fructus Corni Officinalis
Mu Dan Pi	9 g	Cortex Moutan Radicis
Fu Ling	9 g	Sclerotium Poriae Cocos
Ze Xie	9 g	Rhizoma Alismatis

While not used in its unmodified form in this text, this formula is the basis for all the prescriptions described here for infertility where Kidney deficiency is involved.

LONG DAN XIE GAN TANG (GENTIANA DRAINING THE LIVER DECOCTION)

Long Dan Cao	6 g	Radix Gentianae Scabrae
Huang Qin	9 g	Radix Scutellariae Baicalensis
Zhi Zi	9 g	Fructus Gardeniae Jasminoidis
Ze Xie	9 g	Rhizoma Alismatis
Mu Tong	9 g	Caulis Mutong
Che Qian Zi	9 g	Semen Plantaginis
Sheng Di	12 g	Radix Rehmanniae Glutinosae
Dang Gui	9 g	Radix Angelicae Sinensis
Chai Hu	9 g	Radix Bupleuri
Gan Cao (Zhi)	3 g	Radix Glycyrrhizae Uralensis

Used in the treatment of male infertility with Damp-Heat complications.

MAI WEI DI HUANG TANG (OPHIOPOGON AND REHMANNIA DECOCTION)

Mai Dong	12 g	Tuber Ophiopogonis
Wu Wei Zi	9 g	Fructus Schizandrae Chinensis
Shu Di	20 g	Radix Rehmanniae Glutinosae Conquitae
Shan Zhu Yu	15 g	Fructus Corni Officinalis
Shan Yao	12 g	Radix Dioscorea Oppositae

Fu Ling	12g	Sclerotium Poriae Cocos
Mu Dan Pi	9g	Cortex Moutan Radicis
Ze Xie	12g	Rhizoma Alismatis

Used to rescue and consolidate Yin after the use of Heat-clearing formulas treating Yin deficiency amenorrhea.

NEI YI ZHI TONG TANG (SIMPLIFIED ARREST PAIN DECOCTION)

Gou Teng	15g	Ramulus Uncariae Cum Uncis
Zi Bei Chi	9g	Mauritiae Concha
Dang Gui	9g	Radix Angelicae Sinensis
Chi Shao	9g	Radix Paeoniae Rubra
Wu Ling Zhi	9g	Excrementum Trogopterori
Yan Hu Suo	9g	Rhizoma Corydalis Yanhusuo
E Zhu	9g	Rhizoma Curcumae Zedoariae
Rou Gui	3g	Cortex Cinnamomi Cassiae
Quan Xie	1.6g	Buthus Martensi
Wu Gong	1.6g	Scolopendra Subspinipes
Mu Xiang	6g	Radix Saussureae seu Vladimiriae
Xu Duan	9g	Radix Dipsaci

Used before or during menstruation to treat period pain and Blood stasis associated with endometriosis.

SAN HE YIN (DISSIPATE AND HARMONIZE DECOCTION)

Da Huang	9g	Rhizoma Rhei
Mang Xiao	9g	Mirabilitum
Zhi Zi	6g	Fructus Gardeniae Jasminoidis
Huang Qin	6g	Radix Scutellariae Baicalensis
Lian Qiao	12g	Fructus Forsythiae Suspensae
Bo He	6g	Herba Menthae
Gan Cao (Zhi)	6g	Radix Glycyrrhizae Uralensis
Dang Gui	9g	Radix Angelicae Sinensis
Chuan Xiong	6g	Radix Ligustici Wallichii
Shu Di	12g	Radix Rehmanniae Glutinosae Conquitae
Chi Shao	9g	Radix Paeoniae Rubra

Used to clear Heat in the treatment of Yin deficiency amenorrhea.

SAN HUANG SI WU TANG (THREE YELLOWS FOUR SUBSTANCE DECOCTION)

Shu Di	15g	Radix Rehmanniae Glutinosae
Dang Gui	9g	Radix Angelicae Sinensis
Chuan Xiong	9g	Radix Ligustici Wallichii
Chi Shao	9g	Radix Paeoniae Rubra
Da Huang	6g	Rhizoma Rhei
Huang Lian	3g	Rhizoma Coptidis
Huang Qin	9g	Radix Scutellariae Baicalensis

Used to clear Heart- and Liver-Fire in the treatment of Yin deficiency amenorrhea.

472

SHAO FU ZHU YU TANG (LOWER ABDOMEN ELIMINATING STASIS DECOCTION)

Dang Gui	9 g	Radix Angelicae Sinensis
Chuan Xiong	6 g	Radix Ligustici Wallichii
Chi Shao	9 g	Radix Paeoniae Rubra
Xiao Hui Xiang	6 g	Fructus Foeniculi Vulgaris
Yan Hu Suo	6 g	Rhizoma Corydalis Yanhusuo
Wu Ling Zhi	6 g	Excrementum Trogopterori
Pu Huang	9 g	Pollen Typhae
Mo Yao	6 g	Myrrha
Rou Gui	6 g	Cortex Cinnamomi Cassiae
Gan Jiang	6 g	Rhizoma Zingiberis Officinalis

Used in the treatment of tubal blockage, amenorrhea or recurrent miscarriage due to Blood stagnation and Cold.

SHENG HUA TANG (GENERATING AND DISSOLVING DECOCTION)

Dang Gui	26 g	Radix Angelicae Sinensis
Chuan Xiong	9 g	Radix Ligustici Wallichii
Tao Ren	9 g	Semen Persicae
Pao Jiang	3 g	Rhizoma Zingiberis Officinalis
Gan Cao (Zhi)	3 g	Radix Glycyrrhizae Uralensis

Used in the management of inevitable miscarriage.

SHOU TAI WAN (FETUS LONGEVITY PILL)

Tu Si Zi	20 g	Semen Cuscatae
Du Zhong	9 g	Cortex Eucommiae Ulmoidis
Sang Ji Sheng	9 g	Ramulus Sangjisheng
E Jiao	9 g	Gelatinum Asini

Used for threatened miscarriage due to Kidney deficiency.

SI JUN ZI WAN (FOUR GENTLEMAN COMBINATION)

Ren Shen	9 g	Radix Ginseng
Bai Zhu	6 g	Rhizoma Atractylodis Macrocephalae
Fu Ling	6 g	Sclerotium Poriae Cocos
Gan Cao (Zhi)	3 g	Radix Glycyrrhizae Uralensis

This formula can be added to other formulas to help blood flow during menstruation if the Qi isn't leading the Blood sufficiently.

TAO HONG SI WU TANG (PERSICA CARTHAMUS FOUR SUBSTANCES DECOCTION)

Dang Gui	9 g	Radix Angelicae Sinensis
Shu Di	12 g	Radix Rehmanniae Glutinosae Conquitae
Chuan Xiong	6 g	Radix Ligustici Wallichii
Bai Shao	12 g	Radix Paeoniae Lactiflorae

Tao Ren	6g	Semen Persicae
Hong Hua	3g	Flos Carthami Tinctorii

Used during menstruation, to facilitate removal and restructuring of the endometrium.

TAO HONG SI WU TANG (PERSICA CARTHAMUS FOUR SUBSTANCES DECOCTION) PLUS SHI XIAO SAN (RETURN THE SMILE POWDER) MODIFIED

Dang Gui	9g	Radix Angelicae Sinensis
Chuan Xiong	6g	Radix Ligustici Wallichii
Shu Di	12g	Radix Rehmanniae Glutinosae Conquitae
Bai Shao	9g	Radix Paeoniae Lactiflorae
Tao Ren	6g	Semen Persicae
Hong Hua	3g	Flos Carthami Tinctorii
Pu Huang	9g	Pollen Typhae
Wu Ling Zhi	6g	Excrementum Trogopterori
Qian Cao Gen	6g	Radix Rubiae Cordifoliae
San Qi	6g	Radix Pseudoginseng

Used to control blood loss during a miscarriage.

TAO HONG SI WU TANG (PERSICA CARTHAMUS FOUR SUBSTANCES DECOCTION) MODIFIED

Dang Gui	9g	Radix Angelicae Sinensis
Chi Shao	9g	Radix Paeoniae Rubra
Chuan Xiong	6g	Radix Ligustici Wallichii
Tao Ren	9g	Semen Persicae
Hong Hua	9g	Flos Carthami Tinctorii
Gui Zhi	3g	Ramulus Cinnamomi Cassiae
Dan Shen	9g	Radix Salviae Miltiorrhizae
Shan Zha	6g	Fructus Crataegi
Pu Huang	9g	Pollen Typhae
Wu Ling Zhi	9g	Excrementum Trogopterori
Yan Hu Suo	12g	Rhizoma Corydalis Yanhusuo
Xiang Fu	9g	Rhizoma Cyperi Rotundi
Xu Duan	9g	Radix Dipsaci
Chuan Niu Xi	6g	Radix Cyathulae

Taken to prepare for IVF if there is marked Blood stasis. It can be taken throughout the menstrual cycle unless conception is attempted in which case it should be withdrawn a few days after ovulation.

TAO HONG SI WU TANG (PERSICA CARTHAMUS FOUR SUBSTANCES DECOCTION) MODIFIED

Dang Gui	12g	Radix Angelicae Sinensis
Bai Shao	9g	Radix Paeoniae Lactiflorae
Chuan Xiong	6g	Radix Ligustici Wallichii
Tao Ren	6g	Semen Persicae
Hong Hua	9g	Flos Carthami Tinctorii
Yi Mu Cao	9g	Herba Leonuri Heterophylli

Xiang Fu	12 g	*Rhizoma Cyperi Rotundi*
Ji Xue Teng	12 g	*Radix et Caulis Jixueteng*
Shan Zha	6 g	*Fructus Crataegi*
Dan Shen	12 g	*Radix Salviae Miltiorrhizae*
Chuan Niu Xi	6 g	*Radix Cyathulae*

For use during an IVF cycle Phase 1 in certain restricted circumstances.

WEN YANG HUA TAN FANG (WARM YANG AND TRANSFORM PHLEGM FORMULA)

(Zhi) Fu Zi	6 g	*Radix Aconiti Charmichaeli Praeparata*
Xu Duan	9 g	*Radix Dipsaci*
Yin Yang Huo	9 g	*Herba Epimedii*
Cang Zhu	9 g	*Rhizoma Atractylodes*
Chen Pi	6 g	*Pericarpium Citri Reticulate*
Fu Ling	9 g	*Sclerotium Poriae Cocos*
Zhi Ke	9 g	*Fructus Citri seu Ponciri*
Shan Zha	9 g	*Fructus Crataegi*
Hong Hua	6 g	*Flos Carthami Tinctorii*
Dan Nan Xing	9 g	*Rhizoma Arisaematis*

Used at midcycle (Phase 3) in a patient with a tendency to Damp accumulation.

WEN YANG HUA YU FANG (WARM YANG AND TRANSFORM STASIS FORMULA)

Gui Zhi	9 g	*Ramulus Cinnamomi Cassiae*
Hong Hua	6 g	*Flos Carthami Tinctorii*
Dang Gui	9 g	*Radix Angelicae Sinensis*
Chuan Xiong	6 g	*Radix Ligustici Wallichii*
Huai Niu Xi	9 g	*Radix Achyranthis Bidentatae*
Ji Xue Teng	15 g	*Radix et Caulis Jixueteng*
Yin Yang Huo	9 g	*Herba Epimedii*
Shu Di	9 g	*Radix Rehmanniae Glutinosae Conquitae*
(Zhi) Fu Zi	6 g	*Radix Aconiti Charmichaeli Praeparata*

Used at midcycle (Phase 3) by women with Cold or Yang-deficient symptoms.

XIANG SHA LUI JUN ZI WAN (SAUSSUREA AMOMUM SIX GENTLEMAN PILLS)

Dang Shen	*Radix Codonopsis Pilulosae*
Bai Zhu	*Rhizoma Atractylodis Macrocephalae*
Fu Ling	*Sclerotium Poriae Cocos*
Gan Cao (Zhi)	*Radix Glycyrrhizae Uralensis*
Chen Pi	*Pericarpium Citri Reticulate*
Ban Xia	*Rhizoma Pinelliae*
Mu Xiang	*Radix Saussureae seu Vladimiriae*
Sha Ren	*Fructus seu Semen Amomi*

Given in pill form to aid digestion of Yin tonic formulas given in the follicular phase.

XIANG SHA LIU JUN ZI TANG (SAUSSUREA AMOMUM SIX GENTLEMAN DECOCTION) MODIFIED

Dang Shen	12g	Radix Codonopsis Pilulosae
Bai Zhu	9g	Rhizoma Atractylodis Macrocephalae
Fu Ling	9g	Sclerotium Poriae Cocos
Gan Cao (Zhi)	9g	Radix Glycyrrhizae Uralensis
Chen Pi	6g	Pericarpium Citri Reticulate
Ban Xia	12g	Rhizoma Pinelliae
Mu Xiang	6g	Radix Saussureae seu Vladimiriae
Sha Ren	6g	Fructus seu Semen Amomi
Bai Jiang Cao	15g	Herba cum Radice Patriniae
Yi Yi Ren	20g	Semen Coicis Lachryma-jobi

Used in the treatment of pelvic inflammatory disease associated with Spleen Qi deficiency.

XIAO YAO SAN (FREE AND EASY POWDER)

Chai Hu	9g	Radix Bupleuri
Bai Shao	12g	Radix Paeoniae Lactiflorae
Dang Gui	9g	Radix Angelicae Sinensis
Bai Zhu	9g	Rhizoma Atractylodis Macrocephalae
Fu Ling	15g	Sclerotium Poriae Cocos
Sheng Jiang	3 slices	Rhizoma Zingiberis Officinalis Recens
Bo He	3g	Herba Menthae
Gan Cao (Zhi)	6g	Radix Glycyrrhizae Uralensis

Administered as part of the treatment of male infertility when there is a component of Qi stagnation.

XIAO YAO SAN (FREE AND EASY POWDER) WITH BU SHEN HUA TAN TANG (DECOCTION FOR RESTORING THE KIDNEY AND REMOVING PHLEGM) MODIFIED

Dang Gui	9g	Radix Angelicae Sinensis
Bai Shao	12g	Radix Paeoniae Lactiflorae
Chuan Xiong	6g	Radix Ligustici Wallichii
Chuan Niu Xi	9g	Radix Cyathulae
Gou Qi Zi	9g	Fructus Lycii Chinensis
Chai Hu	9g	Radix Bupleuri
Xiang Fu	12g	Rhizoma Cyperi Rotundi
Li Zhe He	9g	Semen Litchi
Xia Ku Cao	9g	Spica Prunellae Vulgaris
He Huan Pi	9g	Cortex Albizziae Julibrissin
Tu Si Zi	12g	Semen Cuscatae
Yin Yang Huo	9g	Herba Epimedii
Shu Di	9g	Radix Rehmanniae Glutinosae Conquitae
Shan Zhu Yu	9g	Fructus Corni Officinalis

Used for infertile PCOS patients where weight gain is not so marked.

XIAO YAO SAN (FREE AND EASY POWDER) PLUS JIN LING ZI SAN (GOLD BELL POWDER) MODIFIED

Chai Hu	9 g	Radix Bupleuri
Bai Zhu	12 g	Rhizoma Atractylodis Macrocephalae
Dang Gui	9 g	Radix Angelicae Sinensis
Bai Shao	15 g	Radix Paeoniae Lactiflorae
Fu Ling	15 g	Sclerotium Poriae Cocos
Gan Cao (Zhi)	3 g	Radix Glycyrrhizae Uralensis
Sheng Jiang	3 g	Rhizoma Zingiberis Officinalis Recens
Bo He	3 g	Herba Menthae
Chuan Lian Zi	9 g	Fructus Meliae Toosendan
Yan Hu Suo	9 g	Rhizoma Corydalis Yanhusuo
Ju He	9 g	Semen Citri Reticulatae

Used in the treatment of pelvic inflammatory disease related to Liver Qi stagnation.

XIANG SHA LIU JUN ZI TANG (SIX GENTLEMAN DECOCTION WITH AUCKLANDIA AND AMOMUM)

Bai Zhu Chao	12 g	Rhizoma Atractylodis Macrocephalae
Fu Ling	12 g	Sclerotium Poriae Cocos
Dang Shen	15 g	Radix Codonopsis Pilulosae
Ban Xia	9 g	Rhizoma Pinelliae
Sha Ren	6 g	Fructus seu Semen Amomi
Chen Pi	6 g	Pericarpium Citri Reticulate
Gan Cao (Zhi)	6 g	Radix Glycyrrhizae Uralensis
Mu Xiang	6 g	Radix Saussureae seu Vladimiriae

Used to reinforce Spleen function and support a weight loss program.

XIONG GUI PING WEI SAN (LIGUSTICUM ANGELICA BALANCING THE STOMACH POWDER)

Cang Zhu	Rhizoma Atractylodes
Chen Pi	Pericarpium Citri Reticulate
Hou Po	Cortex Magnoliae Officinalis
Gan Cao (Zhi)	Radix Glycyrrhizae Uralensis
Sheng Jiang	Rhizoma Zingiberis Officinalis Recens
Da Zao	Fructus Zizyphi Jujuba
Dang Gui	Radix Angelicae Sinensis
Chuan Xiong	Radix Ligustici Wallichii

Patent medicine used in conjunction with other formulas in the treatment of amenorrhea complicated with Phlegm-Damp.

XUE FU ZHU YU TANG (DECOCTION FOR REMOVING BLOOD STASIS IN THE CHEST)

Dang Gui	9 g	Radix Angelicae Sinensis
Sheng Di	9 g	Radix Rehmanniae Glutinosae

477

Chi Shao	6g	Radix Paeoniae Rubra
Chuan Xiong	6g	Radix Ligustici Wallichii
Tao Ren	12g	Semen Persicae
Hong Hua	9g	Flos Carthami Tinctorii
Chai Hu	3g	Radix Bupleuri
Zhi Ke	6g	Fructus Citri seu Poncili
Chuan Niu Xi	9g	Radix Cyathulae
Jie Geng	6g	Radix Platycodi Grandiflori
Gan Cao (Zhi)	3g	Radix Glycyrrhizae Uralensis

Used in the treatment of male infertility complicated by Blood stagnation.

XUE FU ZHU YU TANG (DECOCTION FOR REMOVING BLOOD STASIS IN THE CHEST) MODIFIED

Tao Ren	12g	Semen Persicae
Hong Hua	9g	Flos Carthami Tinctorii
Dang Gui	9g	Radix Angelicae Sinensis
Chuan Xiong	6g	Radix Ligustici Wallichii
Chi Shao	9g	Radix Paeoniae Rubra
Chuan Niu Xi	9g	Radix Cyathulae
Chai Hu	6g	Radix Bupleuri
Yi Mu Cao	9g	Herba Leonuri Heterophylli
Xiang Fu	9g	Rhizoma Cyperi Rotundi
Zhi Ke	9g	Fructus Citri seu Ponciri
Sheng Di	9g	Radix Rehmanniae Glutinosae
Gan Cao (Zhi)	3g	Radix Glycyrrhizae Uralensis

For treatment of amenorrhea caused by Blood stagnation.

YI GAN HE WEI YIN (RESTRAIN LIVER AND HARMONIZE THE STOMACH DECOCTION)

Su Ye	3g	Folium Perillae Frutescentis
Huang Lian	6g	Rhizoma Coptidis
Ban Xia	6g	Rhizoma Pinelliae
Zhu Ru	6g	Caulis Bambusae in Taeniis
Chen Pi	6g	Pericarpium Citri Reticulate
Gou Teng	15g	Ramulus Uncariae Cum Uncis
Huang Qin	9g	Radix Scutellariae Baicalensis
Sheng Jiang	3g	Rhizoma Zingiberis Officinalis Recens

Prescribed for morning sickness.

YI RU SAN (BENEFITING THE BREAST POWDER)

Chuan Bei Mu	6g	Bulbus Fritillariae Cirrhosae
Bai Shao	9g	Radix Paeoniae Lactiflorae
Qing Pi	6g	Pericarpium Citri Reticulatae Viride

Gou Teng	9 g	Ramulus Uncariae Cum Uncis
Chuan Niu Xi	9 g	Radix Cyathulae
(Sheng) Mu Li	15 g	Concha Ostreae
Mai Ya	30 g	Fructus Hordei
Chuan Lian Zi	9 g	Fructus Meliae Toosendan

Used for amenorrhea associated with hyperprolactinemia and Liver Qi stagnation.

YISHEN GUTAI TANG (NOURISH KIDNEY AND PROTECT FETUS) MODIFIED

Tu Si Zi	20 g	Semen Cuscatae
Du Zhong	15 g	Cortex Eucommiae Ulmoidis
Xu Duan	15 g	Radix Dipsaci
Sang Ji Sheng	15 g	Ramulus Sangjisheng
Bai Zhu	15 g	Rhizoma Atractylodis Macrocephalae
Huang Qin	9 g	Radix Scutellariae Baicalensis
Gou Qi Zi	12 g	Fructus Lycii Chinensis
Dang Shen	12 g	Radix Codonopsis Pilulosae
Bai Zhu	12 g	Rhizoma Atractylodis Macrocephalae
Da Zao	3 pieces	Fructus Zizyphi Jujuba
Sha Ren	3 g	Fructus seu Semen Amomi
He Shou Wu	12 g	Radix Polygoni Multiflori

This formula is prescribed to women who have become pregnant after experiencing a period of infertility.

YOU GUI WAN (RESTORING THE RIGHT PILL)

Shu Di	9 g	Radix Rehmanniae Glutinosae Conquitae
Shan Yao	9 g	Radix Dioscorea Oppositae
Shan Zhu Yu	9 g	Fructus Corni Officinalis
Tu Si Zi	9 g	Semen Cuscatae
Ba Ji Tian	9 g	Radix Morindae Officinalis
Lu Jiao Pian	9 g	Cornu Cervi Parvum

Used in the luteal phase to boost Kidney Yang by fostering Kidney Yin.

YOU GUI WAN (RESTORE THE RIGHT KIDNEY PILL) PLUS YU LIN ZHU (FERTILITY PEARLS) MODIFIED

Bai Zhu	12 g	Rhizoma Atractylodis Macrocephalae
Fu Ling	9 g	Sclerotium Poriae Cocos
Dang Gui	9 g	Radix Angelicae Sinensis
Bai Shao	9 g	Radix Paeoniae Lactiflorae
Shu Di	9 g	Radix Rehmanniae Glutinosae Conquitae
Shan Zhu Yu	9 g	Fructus Corni Officinalis
Shan Yao	9 g	Dioscorea Oppositae
Tu Si Zi	12 g	Semen Cuscatae
Xu Duan	12 g	Radix Dipsaci
Du Zhong	6 g	Cortex Eucommiae Ulmoidis

Ba Ji Tian	9 g	Radix Morindae Officinalis
Xiang Fu	9 g	Rhizoma Cyperi Rotundi
Gan Cao	3 g	Radix Glycyrrhizae Uralensis

For use during an IVF cycle in Phase 4b (restrictions on use of herbs during an IVF cycle are fewer in Phase 4).

YU LIN ZHU (FERTILITY PEARLS)

Dang Shen	12 g	Radix Codonopsis Pilulosae
Bai Zhu	9 g	Rhizoma Atractylodis Macrocephalae
Fu Ling	9 g	Sclerotium Poriae Cocos
Gan Cao (Zhi)	6 g	Radix Glycyrrhizae Uralensis
Dang Gui	9 g	Radix Angelicae Sinensis
Bai Shao	9 g	Radix Paeoniae Lactiflorae
Chuan Xiong	6 g	Radix Ligustici Wallichii
Shu Di	9 g	Radix Rehmanniae Glutinosae Conquitae
Tu Si Zi	9 g	Semen Cuscatae
Du Zhong	9 g	Cortex Eucommiae Ulmoidis
Lu Jiao Pian	9 g	Cornu Cervi Parvum

Used to strengthen Kidney Yang in the luteal phase by building Blood.

YU LIN ZHU (FERTILITY PEARLS) MODIFIED

Dang Shen	12 g	Radix Codonopsis Pilulosae
Bai Zhu	9 g	Rhizoma Atractylodis Macrocephalae
Fu Ling	9 g	Sclerotium Poriae Cocos
Gan Cao (Zhi)	6 g	Radix Glycyrrhizae Uralensis
Dang Gui	9 g	Radix Angelicae Sinensis
Bai Shao	9 g	Radix Paeoniae Lactiflorae
Chuan Xiong	6 g	Radix Ligustici Wallichii
Shu Di	9 g	Radix Rehmanniae Glutinosae Conquitae
Tu Si Zi	9 g	Semen Cuscatae
Du Zhong	9 g	Cortex Eucommiae Ulmoidis
Lu Jiao Pian	9 g	Cornu Cervi Parvum
San Leng	9 g	Rhizoma Sparganii
E Zhu	9 g	Rhizoma Curcumae Zedoariae
Pu Huang	9 g	Pollen Typhae
Chi Shao	9 g	Radix Paeoniae Rubra
Ru Xiang	6 g	Gummi Olibanum
Mo Yao	6 g	Myrrha

This version of Fertility Pearls is used to treat Blood stagnation with Kidney Yang deficiency in the luteal phase.

YU ZHU SAN (JADE CANDLE POWDER)

| Da Huang | 9 g | Rhizoma Rhei |
| Mang Xiao | 9 g | Mirabilitum |

Dang Gui	9 g	Radix Angelicae Sinensis
Chi Shao	9 g	Radix Paeoniae Rubra
Chuan Xiong	6 g	Radix Ligustici Wallichii
Sheng Di	15 g	Radix Rehmanniae Glutinosae
Gan Cao (Zhi)	3 g	Radix Glycyrrhizae Uralensis

Used to clear Liver-Fire in the treatment of Yin-deficiency amenorrhea.

YUAN ZHI CHANG PU YIN (POLYGALA ACORUS PILL)

Yuan Zhi	6 g	Radix Polygalae Tenuifoliae
Shi Chang Pu	9 g	Rhizoma Acori Graminei
Dang Gui	9 g	Radix Angelicae Sinensis
Chi Shao	9 g	Radix Paeoniae Rubra
Bai Shao	9 g	Radix Paeoniae Lactiflorae
Shan Zha	9 g	Fructus Crataegi
Fu Ling	9 g	Sclerotium Poriae Cocos
Chai Hu	6 g	Radix Bupleuri
Yu Jin	9 g	Tuber Curcumae
Dan Shen	9 g	Radix Salviae Miltiorrhizae
He Huan Pi	12 g	Cortex Albizziae Julibrissin

Used to safeguard ovulation if there is Liver Qi stagnation or Shen instability.

YUE JU ER CHEN WAN (GARDENIA LIGUSTICUM PILL)

Cang Zhu	Rhizoma Atractylodes
Shen Qu	Massa Fermenta
Chen Pi	Pericarpium Citri Reticulate
Fu Ling	Sclerotium Poriae Cocos
Ban Xia	Rhizoma Pinelliae
Xiang Fu	Rhizoma Cyperi Rotundi
Zhi Zi	Fructus Gardeniae Jasminoidis
Chuan Xiong	Radix Ligustici Wallichii

Patent medicine used in the treatment of Phlegm-Damp amenorrhea.

ZHEN WU TANG (TRUE WARRIOR DECOCTION)

(Zhi) Fu Zi	9 g	Radix Aconiti Charmichaeli Praeparata
Bai Zhu	6 g	Rhizoma Atractylodis Macrocephalae
Fu Ling	9 g	Sclerotium Poriae Cocos
Bai Shao	9 g	Radix Paeoniae Lactiflorae
Sheng Jiang	9 g	Rhizoma Zingiberis Officinalis Recens

Useful in treatment of both Kidney Yang and Spleen Qi deficiency; however, its use in the luteal phase has been superseded by Jian Gu Tang (see above).

Index

Page numbers followed by *f* indicate figures; *t*, tables; *b*, boxes.